SPRINGER PUBLISHING

T0075053

GET THE MOST FROM YOUR BOOK

Access your included eBook and educator resources today!

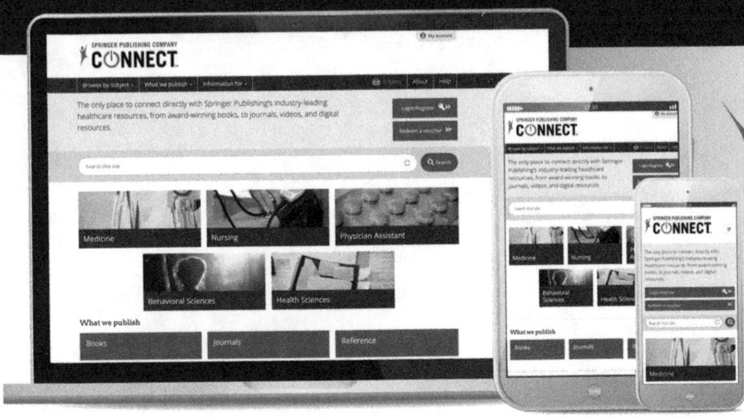

SPRINGER PUBLISHING CONNECT™

LCWBTHEH

eBook Access

Your print purchase of *Quality and Safety Education for Nurses, Third Edition,* includes **online access via Springer Publishing Connect™** to increase accessibility, portability, and searchability.

Insert the code at https://connect.springerpub.com/content/book/978-0-8261-6145-1 today!

Educator Resource Access

Let us do some of the heavy lifting to create an engaging classroom experience with a variety of educator resources included in your textbooks SUCH AS:

INSTRUCTOR'S MANUAL

POWERPOINTS

EBOOK

TEST BANK

Visit **https://connect.springerpub.com/** and look for the **"Show Supplementary"** button on your **book homepage** to see what is available to you! First time using Springer Publishing Connect? Email **textbook@springerpub.com** to create an account and start unlocking valuable resources.

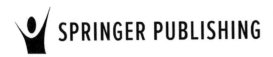

Quality and Safety Education for Nurses

Patricia Kelly Vana, MSN, RN, earned a diploma in nursing from St. Margaret Hospital School of Nursing, Hammond, Indiana; a baccalaureate in nursing from DePaul University in Chicago, Illinois; and a master's degree in nursing from Loyola University in Chicago, Illinois. She is professor emeritus, Purdue University Northwest, Hammond, Indiana. She has worked as a staff nurse, head nurse, travel nurse, school nurse, and nurse educator. Professor Kelly Vana has traveled extensively in the United States, Canada, and Puerto Rico, teaching hundreds of conferences for The Joint Commission, Resource Applications, Pediatric Concepts, and Kaplan, Inc. She currently teaches nationwide National Council Licensure Examination for Registered Nurses® (NCLEX-RN®) review courses for Evolve Testing & Remediation/Health Education Systems, Inc. (HESI), Houston, Texas. Professor Kelly Vana now volunteers part-time in a level one trauma center emergency department in Oak Lawn, Illinois, half the year. She volunteers part-time in an emergency department in Fort Myers, Florida, the other half of the year. She has been a nursing volunteer at the Old Irving Park Free Community Clinic in Chicago, Illinois, and a nursing volunteer at the Gladiolus Free Food Pantry in Fort Myers, Florida, for several years.

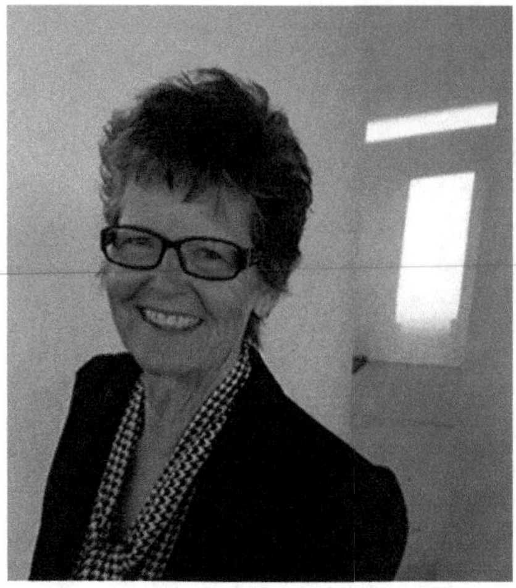

Professor Kelly Vana was director of quality improvement at the University of Chicago Hospitals and Clinics. She taught at Wesley-Passavant School of Nursing, Chicago State University, and was faculty and program director, Associate Degree Nursing at Purdue University Northwest, Hammond, Indiana. She has taught adult nursing, nursing leadership and management, nursing issues, nursing trends, quality improvement, legal aspects of nursing, and NCLEX-RN® reviews. Throughout her approximately 60-year nursing career, she has always maintained patient care contact, often working part-time as an agency staff RN in various emergency departments in Indiana, Illinois, Wisconsin, and Texas, often in addition to a full-time position in nursing education. Professor Kelly Vana has been a member of Sigma Theta Tau, the American Nurses Association, and the Emergency Nurses Association for many years. She has been listed in Who's Who in American Nursing, Notable American Women, and the International Who's Who of Professional and Business Women.

Professor Kelly Vana has served on the board of directors of Tri-City Mental Health Center, St. Anthony's Home, and the Mosby Quality Connection. She is co-editor/author of 11 nursing textbooks, including *Introduction to Quality and Safety Education for Nurses, Core Competencies*, First and Second Editions, with co-editors/authors Beth A. Vottero and Carolyn Christie-McAuliffe. Professor Kelly Vana is also co-editor/author of the Third Edition of *Introduction to Quality and Safety Education for Nurses, Core Competencies*, with co-editors/authors Beth A. Vottero and Gerry Altmiller. She is co-editor/author of *Kelly Vana's Nursing Leadership and Management,* with Janice Tazbir, co-editor/author, now in its Fourth Edition; Professor Kelly Vana is co-editor/author with Janice Tazbir of *Essentials of Nursing Leadership and Management*, now in its Third Edition; and *Nursing Delegation, Setting Priorities, and Making Patient Care Assignments* (with Maureen Marthaler, co-editor/author), now in its Second Edition. She contributed a chapter, "Preparing the Undergraduate Student and Faculty to Use Quality Improvement in Practice," to *Improving Quality*, Second Edition, by Claire Gavin Meisenheimer. Professor Kelly Vana also contributed a chapter on "Obstructive Lung Disease" to *Medical Surgical Nursing* by Rick Daniels. She has served as a national disaster volunteer for the American Red Cross and has also been a team member on healthcare relief trips to Nicaragua. Professor Kelly Vana currently lives with her husband, Ron, half the year in Oak Lawn, Illinois, and half the year in Fort Myers, Florida. Professor Kelly Vana can be reached at patkelly777@aol.com.

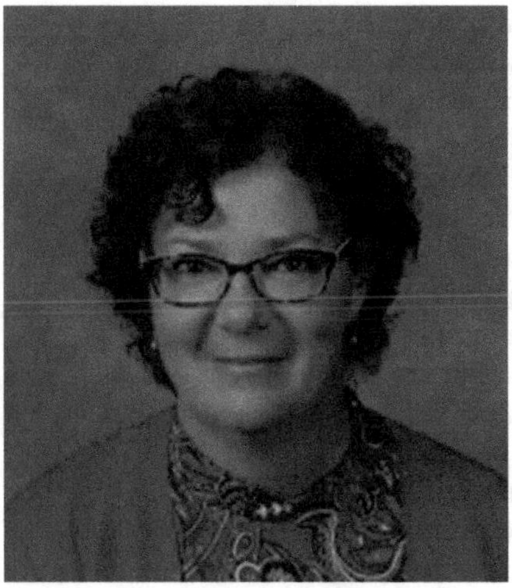

Beth A. Vottero, PhD, RN, CNE, earned a baccalaureate degree in liberal studies with a focus in business management from the University of Maine at Presque Isle; a baccalaureate degree in nursing from Valparaiso University; a master's degree in nursing from the University of Phoenix; and a PhD in nursing education from Capella University. Dr. Vottero currently is an associate professor of nursing at Purdue University Northwest, teaching courses including Evidence-Based Practice and Knowledge Translation at the doctoral level and Informatics as well as theory courses in the Graduate Nurse Educator program. At the undergraduate level, she teaches Quality and Safety for Professional Nursing Practice and Evidence-Based Quality Improvement in the Capstone course.

Dr. Vottero's background includes over 18 years as a staff and charge nurse. After completing her doctorate, Dr. Vottero coordinated and led a successful Magnet® redesignation for La Porte Hospital in La Porte, Indiana. She brought a desire to instill quality concepts to academia where she created an undergraduate quality course at Purdue Northwest focused on quality and safety in healthcare. Dr. Vottero is a deputy director of the Indiana Center for Evidence-Based Practice in Hammond, Indiana, a Joanna Briggs Institute (JBI) Collaborating Center. Through this association, she has completed systematic reviews on various topics. In collaboration with Dr. Lisa Hopp, she assisted in developing an Evidence Implementation Workshop to train nurses in translation science using an evidence-based quality improvement focus. Dr. Vottero is a certified comprehensive systematic review program trainer with JBI and conducts weeklong training for healthcare providers nationally.

Dr. Vottero has published chapters in Hopp and Rittenmeyer's *Introduction to Evidence-Based Practice: A Practical Guide for Nurses*; Bristol and Zerwekh's *Essentials of E-Learning for Nurse Educators*; and has developed case studies for Zerwekh and Zerwekh's *Nursing Today: Transitions and Trends*. She has published several articles on "Teaching Informatics" (*Nurse Educator QSEN Supplement)*, "Conducting a Root Cause Analysis" *(Nursing Education Perspectives*), and "3D Simulation of Complex Health Care Environments" (*Clinical Simulation in Nursing)*. Dr. Vottero is an active member of the QSEN Academic Task Force with multisite studies on Quality and Safety Education for Nurses (QSEN) teaching strategies. As a funded researcher through Purdue University, Dr. Vottero has studied factors affecting medication errors in the clinical setting. Dr. Vottero can be reached at bethvottero@pnw.edu.

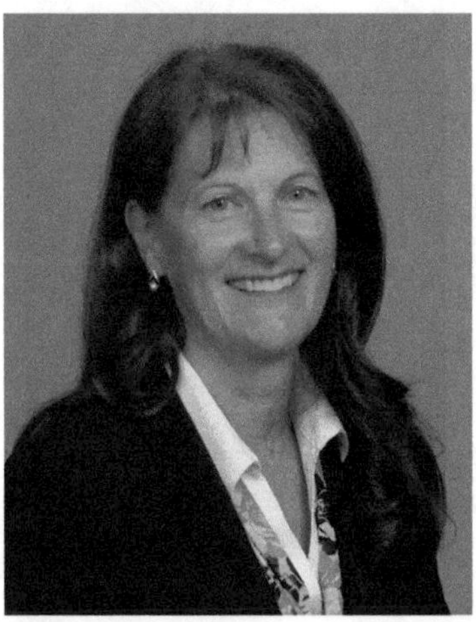

Gerry Altmiller, EdD, APRN, ACNS-BC, ANEF, FAAN, earned a diploma in nursing from Our Lady of Lourdes School of Nursing in Camden, New Jersey; a baccalaureate degree from La Salle University in Philadelphia; and an advanced practice degree as a clinical nurse specialist from Widener University in Chester, Pennsylvania. She later returned to Widener and earned her doctoral degree in higher education leadership. Dr. Altmiller is a professor of nursing at The College of New Jersey in Ewing, New Jersey. As a board-certified clinical nurse specialist, she has served in a consultant role for Einstein Healthcare Network in Philadelphia, Pennsylvania, for over a decade, supporting direct care nurses in their research, evidence-based practice, and quality improvement projects.

Dr. Altmiller has pioneered the integration of quality and safety competencies in nursing education since 2006 when she served as a faculty leader for one of the 15 pilot schools for the Quality and Safety Education for Nurses (QSEN) Collaboration. She is a national consultant for QSEN and director of the Quality and Safety Innovation Center at The College of New Jersey. She leads the QSEN Academic Task Force, creating opportunities for its 130 faculty members to network, share ideas, and conduct academic-focused research. Her work includes over 35 peer-reviewed publications, hundreds of presentations around the country, and the creation of many QSEN classroom and clinical teaching strategies available on the QSEN website. She has been awarded grants from the Agency for Healthcare Research and Quality and from the National League for Nursing. Dr. Altmiller was co-editor of a special QSEN issue of *Nurse Educator* and serves on the journal's editorial board.

Dr. Altmiller received a Lindback Award for distinguished teaching in 2014. Her work on constructive feedback led to the development, testing, and dissemination of support tools for nurse educators and learning tools for students to view feedback as an opportunity. She has developed and validated clinical evaluations framed in the QSEN competencies for all prelicensure clinical nursing courses and a nurse practitioner clinical evaluation framed in the graduate level QSEN competencies and aligned with The National Organization of Nurse Practitioner Faculties nurse practitioner core and practice doctorate competencies. Dr. Altmiller developed the beginning toolkit for the American Association of Colleges of Nursing (AACN) Essential Domain 5: Quality and Safety in 2021. Her research focuses on clinical evaluation, quality, and safety integration, creating a just culture in academia, and addressing communication challenges in both the education and practice environments. Dr. Altmiller can be reached at altmillg@tcnj.edu.

Quality and Safety Education for Nurses

Core Competencies for Nursing Leadership and Care Management

Third Edition

Patricia Kelly Vana, MSN, RN

Beth A. Vottero, PhD, RN, CNE

Gerry Altmiller, EdD, APRN, ACNS-BC, ANEF, FAAN

Editors

SPRINGER PUBLISHING

First Springer Publishing edition 2018

Springer Publishing Company, LLC
11 West 42nd Street, New York, NY 10036
www.springerpub.com
connect.springerpub.com/

Acquisitions Editor: Joseph Morita
Compositor: Exeter Premedia Services Private Ltd.

ISBN: 978-0-8261-6144-4
ebook ISBN: 978-0-8261-6145-1
DOI: 10.1891/9780826161451

SUPPLEMENTS:

SPRINGER PUBLISHING CONNECT™

A robust set of instructor resources designed to supplement this text is located at **http://connect.springerpub.com/content/book/978-0-8261-6145-1.** Qualifying instructors may request access by emailing **textbook@springerpub.com.**

Instructor's Manual: 978-0-8261-6146-8
PowerPoints: 978-0-8261-6147-5

22 23 24 / 5 4 3 2 1

Library of Congress Cataloging-in-Publication Data

Names: Vana, Patricia Kelly, 1941- editor. | Vottero, Beth A., editor. | Altmiller, Gerry, editor.
Title: Quality and safety education for nurses : core competencies for nursing leadership and care management / edited by Patricia Kelly Vana, MSN, RN, Beth A. Vottero, PhD, RN, CNE, Gerry Altmiller, EdD, APRN, ACNS-BC, ANEF, FAAN.
Other titles: Introduction to quality and safety education for nurses.
Description: Third edition. | New York, NY : Springer Publishing Company, [2022] | Revision of: Introduction to quality and safety education for nurses. 2018. Second edition. | Includes bibliographical references and index.
Identifiers: LCCN 2021052371 (print) | LCCN 2021052372 (ebook) | ISBN 9780826161444 (paperback) | ISBN 9780826161451 (ebook)
Subjects: LCSH: Nursing--Study and teaching.
Classification: LCC RT73 .I585 2022 (print) | LCC RT73 (ebook) | DDC 610.73071/1--dc23/eng/20211119
LC record available at https://lccn.loc.gov/2021052371
LC ebook record available at https://lccn.loc.gov/2021052372

Printed in the United States of America.

This book is dedicated by Patricia Kelly Vana to all the nurses and interprofessional health care team members working to save lives and support patients during the current Covid-19 crisis. It is also dedicated to her loving parents, Ed and Jean Kelly (her father was a safety engineer at Inland Steel Company, East Chicago, Indiana); to her charming, wonderful husband, Ron Vana; to her super sisters, Tessie Kelly Dybel and Kathy Kelly Milch; to her dear aunts and uncles, Aunt Pat and Uncle Bill Kelly and Aunt Verna and Uncle Archie Payne; her nephew, John Milch; her nieces, Natalie Dybel Bevil, Melissa Milch Arredondo, and Stacey Milch Monks; her nephews-in-law, Tracy Bevil, Peter Arredondo, and Derek Monks; her grandnephew, Brock Bevil; her grandniece, Reese Bevil; her nursing classmates and friends; and her fish, Homer. Know in your heart that Patricia loves you all!

Beth A. Vottero would like to thank her support, her rock, and her hero . . . her ever-patient husband, Dino. Thanks also go to her children Tom (Army Strong), Mitchell (ump extraordinaire), Micah (king of games), Michelle (ever-patient educator), and Trisha (the beautiful mother); to her amazing parents Tom and Judy, Ray and Dolly; and to her dog, Ben, who sat on a chair and stared at her for hours while she worked. To her super-human coworkers—you know who you are and how much you motivate her.

Gerry Altmiller dedicates this work to Cooper, Michelle, and Drew, the reason for everything she does, and to all the hard-working nurses in all sectors of practice and academia that see a better way to do it and take that work on, demonstrating fortitude, resilience, and ceaseless optimism about what is possible, earning the respect and admiration of many.

Contents

Contributors *xi*
Foreword Linda Cronenwett, PhD, RN (ret.), FAAN xiii
Preface *xv*
Acknowledgments *xix*

UNIT I: ROLE OF THE NURSE IN HEALTHCARE

1. **Patient Safety and Quality of Care as Measures of Nursing Competence** 3
   Gerry Altmiller

2. **Nurses as Leaders and Managers for Safe, High-Quality Patient Care** 41
   Sharon Wallace and Courtney Wallace

3. **Systems Thinking** 79
   Danielle Walker and Caitlin K. Dodd

4. **Legal and Ethical Aspects of Nursing Quality and Safety** 113
   Theodore M. McGinn and Patricia Kelly Vana

5. **Delegation and Setting Priorities for Safe, High-Quality Patient Care** 143
   Danette Ver Woert and Ruth I. Hansten

UNIT II: QUALITY AND SAFETY COMPETENCIES

6. **Person-Centered Care** 177
   Elizabeth Riley and Jamie L. Jones

7. **Interprofessional Teamwork and Collaboration** 225
   Gerry Altmiller

8. **Informatics** 257
   Beth A. Vottero

9. **Evidence-Based Nursing Practice** 287
   Beth A. Vottero

10. **Patient Safety** 317
    Christine Rovinski-Wagner and Peter D. Mills

11. **Quality Improvement Essentials** 361
    Anthony L. D'Eramo

12. **Quality Improvement Tools** 403
    Anthony L. D'Eramo

UNIT III: APPLICATION FOR PRACTICE

13. **Implementation Science** 443
Brant J. Oliver, Kolu Baysah Clark, and Christine Rovinski-Wagner

14. **Quality Improvement and Project Management** 473
Marianne K. Schallmo

15. **Population Health and the Role of Quality and Safety** 499
Rita M. Sfiligoj, Jesse Honsky, Shannon Wong, Rebecca L. Mitchell, and Mary A. Dolansky

16. **Professional Role Development in Patient Safety and Quality: Transitioning to Practice** 533
Loraine Hopkins Pepe

Appendix: Prelicensure Knowledge, Skills, and Attitudes 565
Glossary 575
Index 593

Contributors

Gerry Altmiller, EdD, APRN, ACNS-BC, ANEF, FAAN, Professor of Nursing, The College of New Jersey School of Nursing, Health, and Exercise Sciences; Director, The College of New Jersey Quality and Safety Innovation Center, Ewing, New Jersey

Kolu Baysah Clark, DNP, AGNP-BC, Fellow, Health Professions Education, Evaluation, and Research Fellowship, WRJ Veterans Administration Medical Center, White River Junction, Vermont

Anthony L. D'Eramo, MSN, RN, CPHQ, ISO Consultant, Region 1, VHA ISO Consultation Division, Office of Quality, Safety, and Value, Coventry, Rhode Island, Providence VA Medical Center, Providence, Rhode Island

Caitlin K. Dodd, DNP, RN, CNE, Assistant Professor of Professional Practice, Assessment and Evaluation Coordinator, TCU Nursing, Texas Christian University, Fort Worth, Texas

Mary A. Dolansky, PhD, RN, FAAN, Associate Professor of Nursing; and The Sarah C. Hirsh Professorship in Nursing, Frances Payne Bolton School of Nursing, Case Western Reserve University, Cleveland, Ohio

Ruth I. Hansten, PhD, MBA, BSN, RN, FACHE, Principal, Hansten Healthcare PLLC 3344 Parker Hill Road, Santa Rosa, California

Jesse Honsky, DNP, MPH, RN, PHNA-BC, Assistant Professor of Nursing, Frances Payne Bolton School of Nursing, Case Western Reserve University, Cleveland, Ohio

Jamie L. Jones, PhD, RN, CNE, Clinical Assistant Professor, College of Nursing, University of Arkansas for Medical Sciences, Little Rock, Arkansas

Patricia Kelly Vana, RN, MSN, Professor Emerita, Purdue University Northwest, College of Nursing, Hammond, Indiana, Faculty, Health Education Systems, Inc. (HESI), Houston, Texas

Theodore M. McGinn, JD, BBA, CPA, Managing Partner, Lavelle Law, Ltd., Schaumburg, IL

Peter D. Mills, PhD, MS, Director, VA National Center for Patient Safety Field Office, Veterans Affairs Medical Center, White River Junction, Vermont; Adjunct Associate Professor of Psychiatry, The Geisel School of Medicine at Dartmouth College, Hanover, New Hampshire

Rebecca L. Mitchell, DNP, MSN, APRN, Research Associate, Frances Payne Bolton School of Nursing, Case Western Reserve University, Cleveland, Ohio

Brant J. Oliver, PhD, MS, MPH, FNP-BC, PMHNP-BC, Associate Professor, Departments of Community & Family Medicine, Psychiatry, and the Dartmouth Institute, Geisel School of Medicine at Dartmouth and Dartmouth-Hitchcock Health, Lebanon, NH Senior Nurse Faculty Scholar, Health Professions Education, Evaluation, and Research Fellowship, WRJ Veterans Administration Medical Center, White River Junction, VT National Core Faculty (Improvement Methods and Analysis Curriculum Lead), Veterans Administration National Quality Scholars Fellowship, Houston, Texas

Loraine Hopkins Pepe, PhD, RN, NPD-BC, CCRN-K, Network Director of Nursing Education and Professional Development, Einstein Medical Center, Philadelphia, Pennsylvania

Elizabeth Riley, DNP, PED-BC, RNC-NIC, CNE, Clinical Assistant Professor, College of Nursing, University of Arkansas for Medical Sciences, Little Rock, Arkansas

Christine Rovinski-Wagner, MSN, ARNP, National Transformational Coach Captain, VHA Office of Veterans Access to Care, Faculty Scholar, VA Quality Scholars Fellowship Program, White River Junction, Vermont; Clinical Instructor in Community and Family Medicine, The Geisel School of Medicine at Dartmouth College, Hanover, New Hampshire

Marianne K. Schallmo, DNP, APRN, ANP-BC, Clinical Assistant Professor, Purdue University Northwest, College of Nursing, Hammond, Indiana

Rita M. Sfiligoj, DNP, MPA, MSN, RN, CCM, Assistant Professor of Nursing, Frances Payne Bolton School of Nursing, Case Western Reserve University, Cleveland, Ohio

Danette Ver Woert, PhD, MN, BSN, Assistant Professor of Nursing, Northwest University, College of Nursing, Kirkland, Washington

Beth A. Vottero, PhD, RN, CNE, Associate Professor of Nursing, Purdue University Northwest, College of Nursing, Deputy Director, Indiana Center for Evidence-Based Nursing Practice, Joanna Briggs Collaborating Center, Hammond, Indiana

Danielle Walker, RN, PhD, CNE, Assistant Professor, Texas Christian University, Harris College of Nursing and Health Sciences, Fort Worth, Texas

Courtney Wallace, MSN, RN, CPHQ, Clinical Manager, Progressive Care Unit, Confluence Health, East Wenatchee, Washington

Sharon Wallace, PhD, MSN, RN, CCRN-K, St. Martin's University, Instructor, Nursing, Lacey, Washington

Shannon Wong, MSN, RN, CPNP, Instructor, Frances Payne Bolton School of Nursing, Case Western Reserve University, Cleveland, Ohio

Foreword

With the publication of the 2003 Institute of Medicine Report, *Health Professions Education: A Bridge to Quality* (Greiner & Knebel, 2003), nursing and other health profession leaders were challenged to alter the process of professional development so that health professionals would graduate from their educational programs with the knowledge and competencies needed to both care for individual patients *and* continuously improve the quality, safety, and reliability of the healthcare systems in which they worked. The development of specific competencies related to patient-centered care, interprofessional teamwork and collaboration, evidence-based practice, safety sciences, quality improvement methods, and informatics were considered essential elements of future curricula. The *Quality and Safety Education for Nurses (QSEN)* initiative, funded by the Robert Wood Johnson Foundation from 2005 to 2012, supported faculty development to accomplish this paradigm shift in nursing education (Cronenwett et al., 2007).

The ensuing years brought many changes in the development, measurement, and execution of quality improvement and safety. Some changes improved patient care and the morale of health professionals. Others did not. For example, most healthcare institutions made great strides in developing quality and safety metrics, and many were transparent in sharing outcomes with staff and patient advisory groups as a basis for measuring efforts at quality improvement. On the other hand, many healthcare systems engaged staff in "chasing metrics" using superficial means, rather than supporting efforts to thoughtfully pursue theories of improvement that were relevant to local settings.

Today, healthcare is a complex enterprise. Multiple physicians and other health professionals are involved in a hospitalized patient's care. Patients and families often don't have the same nurse 2 days in a row, and much nursing care is delivered by various types of assistants and technicians. There are thousands of pieces of medical equipment, procedures and medications, and complex systems for documenting care. If you want to identify which professionals are responsible for the quality and safety of a particular patient's care, it can be hard to know who to hold accountable.

In fact, quality and safety outcomes are often more dependent on the way a healthcare microsystem (unit, clinic, or community-based setting) is designed to work than on the traits and skills of individual professionals. The reliability of the *system* is often what meets or fails to meet patient needs, in spite of the skills any one professional gives any one patient.

I congratulate the editors of the third edition of *Quality and Safety Education for Nurses: Core Competencies for Nursing Leadership and Care Management* on their commitment to continuously updating the resources needed by nursing leaders, faculty, and students who seek to develop or enhance their quality and safety competencies. The chapters and the contents of this edition align magnificently with new domains of the American Association of Colleges of Nursing (AACN) accreditation standards (2021). Whatever your level of education or role in nursing, this textbook is rich in resources to support your growth.

As you read (or guide others' learning using) this book, you are preparing yourself for your full obligation to your profession and the services nursing provides to patients and communities. To be a competent nurse means knowing what constitutes good care (as has always been true). But today, it also means knowing something about the actual care delivered in your unit or clinic and how it compares to expected or best practices. Furthermore, if you know there is a clinically significant gap between good care and the results of care in your local setting, being a competent health professional means using that knowledge and closing that gap. Thank you for reading this book, and for the commitment you thereby make to continuously improving your own quality and safety competencies. In doing so, you make healthcare better and safer for the communities we serve.

Linda Cronenwett, PhD, RN (ret.), FAAN
Professor and Dean Emeritus
University of North Carolina at Chapel Hill School of Nursing
Former Principal Investigator, *QSEN: Quality and Safety Education for Nurses*
(Funded by the Robert Wood Johnson Foundation, 2005–2012)

REFERENCES

American Association of Colleges of Nursing. (2021). *The Essentials: Core competencies for professional nursing education*. Author.

Cronenwett, L., Sherwood, G., Barnsteiner, J., Disch, J., Johnson, J., Mitchell, P., Sullivan, D. T., & Warren, J. (2007). Quality and Safety Education for Nurses. *Nursing Outlook, 55*(3), 122–131. https://doi.org/10.1016/j.outlook.2007.02.006

Greiner, A. C., & Knebel, E. (Eds.). (2003). *Health professions education: A bridge to quality*. National Academies Press. https://doi.org/10.17226/10681

Preface

The 1994 Institute of Medicine (IOM, now the National Academy of Medicine [NAM]) report, *America's Health in Transition: Protecting and Improving Quality*, highlighted the seriousness and pervasiveness of healthcare error rates and their effect on patient outcomes and morbidity and mortality rates. Then, in 2000, the IOM released the report, *To Err Is Human: Building a Safer Health System* (Kohn et al., 2000). This IOM report instantly received national attention from policy makers, healthcare providers, and consumers. The IOM report stated, "[A]t least 44,000 people and perhaps as many as 98,000 Americans, die in hospitals each year as a result of medical errors [that could have been prevented]" (p. 26). This IOM report caused major ripples throughout the healthcare system and highlighted the need to change how healthcare is delivered. Shockingly, recent research by Makary and Daniel (2016) has found that more than 250,000 deaths each year are the result of errors within healthcare. That means that after heart disease and cancer, patient safety errors are the third leading cause of death in the United States.

The 2001 release of the IOM report, *Crossing the Quality Chasm: A New Health System for the 21st Century*, spotlighted general problems in healthcare in an attempt to close the gap between what is known to provide quality healthcare and what is actually occurring in practice. This IOM report defined six principles for healthcare: Healthcare should be Safe, Timely, Effective, Efficient, Equitable, and Patient-centered (STEEEP).

The Quality and Safety Education for Nurses (QSEN) project began in 2005. Funded by the Robert Wood Johnson Foundation, QSEN addressed the challenge of preparing future nurses with the knowledge, skills, and attitudes (KSAs) necessary to continuously improve the quality and safety of the healthcare systems in which they work. QSEN stated that changes in healthcare needed to focus on the development of nursing competencies in patient-centered care, teamwork and collaboration, quality improvement, evidence-based practice, and informatics. Because of nurses' unique position at the front line of care, in direct contact with patients, often referred to as the "sharp end" of patient care, safety was added as a sixth QSEN competency. The QSEN initiative convened a national panel of experts to identify the core KSAs required for each of the six competencies. Information about the KSAs is available at qsen.org. QSEN also sponsors nursing conferences including an annual QSEN Forum to attract nursing leaders in academia and practice to share innovations and research in patient quality and safety.

The IOM report, *The Future of Nursing: Leading Change, Advancing Health* (2011), recommended that nurses practice to the full extent of their education; nursing education should be improved for seamless academic progression; nurses should be full partners with physicians and healthcare professionals in redesigning care in the United States; and there should be improved data collection for workplace planning and policy making. This IOM report further stated that strong leadership is critical if the vision of a transformed healthcare system is to be realized. The nursing profession must produce leaders throughout the healthcare system; from the bedside to the boardroom, nurses must engage with colleagues, subordinates, and executives so that together they can identify and achieve common goals (Bradford & Cohen, 1998). Nurses must be prepared for care management that incorporates their nursing skills with the ability to manage patient care in a complex healthcare system to optimize patient outcomes.

In 2021, the American Association of Colleges of Nursing (AACN) released *The Essentials: Core Competencies for Professional Nursing Education*. The new *Essentials* fully intertwines the QSEN competencies within 10 domains. The 10 domains reflect knowledge needed by nurses to effectively manage patient care within a complex healthcare setting. In addition, there are eight concepts that flow throughout each of the 10 domains. The new *Essentials* highlights the need to move past knowledge as evidence of competence and to move toward demonstrating competence within each domain throughout the nursing educational experience.

Every nurse is a nursing leader and manager, from the beginning frontline nurse who works directly with patients and takes action to ensure their safety and care quality, to the advanced practice nurse clinician, to the top federal nurse administrator in health services, scientific and academic organizations, and public health and community-based organizations. All of these nurses continuously work with the interprofessional team to ensure patient-centered, high-quality, safe, evidence-based care, utilizing informatics as appropriate.

WHY THIS BOOK?

The idea for this book was born when two of its editors, Patricia Kelly Vana and Dr. Beth A. Vottero, attended the 2011 QSEN Conference in Milwaukee, Wisconsin. This conference was designed to attract innovators and nurture faculty leaders for the improvement of quality and safety education through sharing of innovations in curricular design and teaching strategies that accomplish QSEN competency development. Patricia and Beth realized the need for this book to further the development of these objectives. For the first two editions, Patricia and Beth asked Carolyn Christie-McAuliffe from New York to be the third editor. When Carolyn was not available for the third edition, Patricia and Beth invited Dr. Gerry Altmiller, from New Jersey, to join them to continue to facilitate the development of a broad look at quality and safety. The co-editors have experienced the rapid evolution of quality and safety information in their clinical and academic practices and they identified the need for nursing students to understand foundational quality and safety principles as well as develop leadership and care management skills in their basic nursing preparation. The co-editors strongly believe in the need to organize existing information about quality, safety, leadership, and care management into one basic, easily understood textbook. The purpose of this book is to provide a comprehensive understanding of the essential QSEN competencies for nurses. As students graduate from nursing programs and transition into their practice role, they are expected to be able to use informatics, function within an interprofessional team, deliver patient-centered care, incorporate evidence-based nursing practice, focus on patient safety, and engage in quality improvement (QI) activities.

Many practical examples from real-life experiences are discussed in this text for students. The contributors to this text include nurse educators, nurse faculty, nurse researchers, library scientists, nurse administrators, nurse case managers, physicians, lawyers, nurse QI and patient safety practitioners, nurse practitioners, nurse entrepreneurs, psychologists, and others. The contributors are from all over the United States, emphasizing a broad view of quality and safety as well as leadership and care management. Each chapter includes interviews with experts in their respective healthcare field to provide an interprofessional team perspective.

ORGANIZATION

Quality and Safety Education for Nurses: Core Competencies for Nursing Leadership and Care Management, Third Edition, consists of 16 chapters. Each chapter provides nursing students and beginning nurses with a background and foundational knowledge of quality and safety to assist them in their role as nurses in today's healthcare environment.

CHAPTER FEATURES

Several chapter features are used throughout the text to provide the reader with a consistent format for learning. Chapter features include the following:

- Photos, tables, and figures to enhance student understanding
- Interviews with nurses from all sectors of healthcare to illustrate the chapter content
- Objectives that clearly state the chapter's learning goals and are mapped to the QSEN competencies as well as the *2021 AACN Essentials: Core Competencies for Professional Nursing Education*
- Opening Scenario, a brief entry-level clinical situation that relates to the chapter, with two or three critical thinking questions
- Key Concepts, a listing of the primary understandings the reader gains from the chapter
- Key Terms, a listing of important new terms defined in the chapter and identified within the chapter by bold type
- Critical Discussion Points for nurses, several questions to engage students in dialogue (guidelines for discussion are available to faculty online)
- Review Questions, with multiple-choice and alternative format National Council Licensure Examination for Registered Nurses® (NCLEX-RN®) style questions (answers to Review Questions are available to faculty online)
- Review Activities, to help students apply chapter content to patient care situations (guidelines for discussion are available to faculty online)
- Exploring Website Learning Activities
- References
- Suggested Readings
- QSEN Focused Learning Activities
- Leadership and Care Management Learning Activities

Special elements are sprinkled throughout several chapters to enhance student learning and encourage critical thinking and application of the knowledge presented. These include the following:

- Current Literature with a synopsis of key findings from nursing and healthcare literature
- Developing Clinical Judgment Boxes, formatted as a case study with questions that follow the NCSBN Clinical Judgment Measurement Model (NCJMM)
- Real World Interviews with healthcare leaders and managers, including nursing staff, clinicians, administrators, risk managers, faculty, nurses, physicians, patients, nursing assistive personnel, lawyers, pharmacists, hospital administrators, and others
- Case Studies to provide the nursing student with a patient care situation calling for clinical reasoning to solve an open-ended problem (answers to Case Study questions are available to faculty online)
- Answers to all questions, opening scenarios, and QSEN activities are available to faculty online.

HIGHLIGHTS OF THE TEXT

New to the third edition is a mapping of the 2021 AACN Essentials to each chapter. A robust online evolving clinical case study is available as an instructional supplement for faculty to guide teaching many chapter's content, with options for how students can use the case study for student learning. There are discussion questions for each section of the case study or there is guidance for a written paper assignment. The evolving case study pulls content from the text to guide the student into how to address an evidence-based quality improvement project as a new nurse.

Other highlights include:

- The six QSEN Competencies are covered in the text, each in a separate chapter.
- The six QSEN Competencies Knowledge, Skill, and Attitude (KSA) content placement in the book's chapters is identified in the Appendix.
- A strong foundation for evidence-based healthcare, with attention to high-quality, safe care, is emphasized throughout the text.
- Chapters include new information from national, federal, and state healthcare and nursing organizations.
- Leadership and management for frontline nurses are highlighted throughout the text and within each topic.
- Teamwork and interprofessional collaboration are emphasized throughout the text.
- There are many case studies and clinical discussion points for nurses throughout the chapters.

INSTRUCTOR RESOURCES

PowerPoint lecture slides for each chapter serve as guides for faculty presentations in the classroom. The instructor resources can be obtained by qualified instructors by emailing textbook@springerpub.com.

Patricia Kelly Vana
Beth A. Vottero
Gerry Altmiller

REFERENCES

Bradford, D. L., & Cohen, A. R. (1998). *Power up: Transforming organizations through shared leadership*. John Wiley & Sons.

Institute of Medicine. (1994). *America's health in transition: Protecting and improving quality*. National Academies Press. https://doi.org/10.17226/9147

Institute of Medicine. (2001). *Crossing the quality chasm: A new health system for the 21st century*. National Academies Press. https://doi.org/10.17226/10027

Institute of Medicine. (2011). *The future of nursing: Leading change, advancing health*. National Academies Press. https://doi.org/10.17226/12956

Kohn, L. T., Corrigan, J. M., Donaldson, M. S. (Eds.). (2000). *To err is human: Building a safer health system*. National Academies Press. https://doi.org/10.17226/9728

Makary, M., & Daniel, M. (2016). Medical error—The third leading cause of death in the U.S. *British Medical Journal*, *353*, i2139. https://doi.org/10.1136/bmj.i2139

Acknowledgments

A book such as this requires much effort and the coordination of many persons. Pat, Beth, and Gerry would like to thank all of the contributing authors for their time and effort in sharing their knowledge gained through years of experience in both clinical and academic settings. All of the contributing authors on all three editions worked within tight time frames to share their expertise. A special thanks to Jane A. Walker, PhD, RN, for her networking support.

We would like to acknowledge and sincerely thank the Springer Publishing Company team who worked to make this book a reality. Joseph Morita, senior acquisitions editor, and Hannah Hicks, assistant editor, are great people who worked hard to bring the third edition of this book to publication.

The three co-editors would like to thank the following nursing, medical, and librarian authors for their contributions to previous editions of this book:

Catherine C. Alexander, DNP, RN (Boston, Massachusetts)
Anne Anderson, DNP, MHSA, RN, CPHQ, NEA-BC (Winfield, Illinois)
Gail Armstrong, PhD, DNP, ACNS-BC, CNE (Aurora, Colorado)
Pauline Arnold, MSN, MSA, RN, HACP (LaPorte, Indiana)
Esther Bankert, PhD, RN (Utica, New York)
Amy J. Barton, PhD, RN, FAAN, ANEF (Aurora, Colorado)
Jodi L. Boling, MSN, RN, CNS (Indianapolis, Indiana)
Lindsay Bonaventura, MS, RN, FNP, BC (Chesterton, Indiana)
Kay Burke, MBA, BSN, RN, NE-BC (San Francisco, California)
Carolyn A. Christie-McAuliffe, PhD, FNP (Syracuse, New York)
Ashley Currier, MSN, RN, NE-BC (Chicago, Illinois)
Melinda Davis, RN, MSN, CCRN, CNL (Antioch, Tennessee)
Mary Gillaspy, MLS, MS (Woodland Park, Colorado)
Corinne Haviley, RN, MS, PhD (Winfield, Illinois)
Ronda G. Hughes, PhD, MHS, RN, CLNC, FAAN (Columbia, South Carolina)
Joanne M. Joseph, PhD (Utica, New York)
Andrea Lazarek-LaQuay, MS, RN (Syracuse, New York)
Patti Ludwig-Beymer, PhD, RN, CTN-A, NEA-BC, CPPS, FAAN (Hammond, Indiana)
Jerry A. Mansfield, PhD, RN, NEA-BC (Charleston, South Carolina)
Maureen T. Marthaler, RN, MS (Hammond, Indiana)
Karen L. McCrea, DNP, FNP-C (Washington, DC)
Joanne Belviso Puckett, EdM, RN (Lakenheath, United Kingdom)
Francia I. Reed, MS, RN, FNP-C (Utica, New York)
Kathleen Fischer Sellers, PhD, RN (Alfred, New York)
Danielle Scheurer, MD, MSCR, SFHM (Charleston, South Carolina)
Donna L. Silsbee, PhD, RHIA, CTR, CCS (Utica, New York)
J. Scott Thomson, MLIS, AHIP (North Chicago, Illinois)
Jamie L. Vargo-Warran, DM/IST, MSN, BSN, LSSGB (Rancho Cordova, California)
Cibele C. Webb, MSN Ed, RN (Mishawaka, Indiana)
Patrick M. Webb, MD (LaPorte, Indiana)
Kimberly J. Whalen, MLIS (Valparaiso, Indiana)

UNIT I

Role of the Nurse in Healthcare

CHAPTER 1

Patient Safety and Quality of Care as Measures of Nursing Competence

Gerry Altmiller

"There is no medicine like hope, no incentive so great, and no tonic so powerful as expectation of something tomorrow."

–Orison Swett Marden, 1894

Upon completion of this chapter, the reader should be able to:

1. Define elements of quality care and patient safety.
2. Identify drivers for quality and safety in care.
3. Discuss national organizations impacting healthcare improvement.
4. Analyze global perspectives of healthcare.
5. Explore the patient safety movement to improve quality and safety, reduce errors, and increase transparency.
6. Explore the role of Quality and Safety Education for Nurses (QSEN).
7. Discuss the integration of the six QSEN competencies and the knowledge, skills, and attitudes that underpin quality and safety in nursing education.
8. Apply the QSEN competencies to nursing practice.
9. Discuss nursing's role in quality and safety as direct care providers and healthcare leaders.
10. Analyze how quality of care and patient safety impact accreditation standards for nursing education programs and how it can be evaluated.

CROSSWALK

This chapter addresses the following:

QSEN Competency*:* Patient-Centered Care, Teamwork and Collaboration, Evidence-Based Practice, Quality Improvement, Safety, and Informatics

The American Association of Colleges of Nursing. (2021). *The essentials: Core competencies for professional nursing education.*

Domain 5 Quality and Safety

OPENING SCENARIO

A 64-year-old woman suffered a compound fracture of the femur in a motor vehicle accident. On admission to the emergency department, she was asked about medications she takes at home which she reported to be Fosamax (alendronate sodium) 70 mg by mouth once a week and Synthroid (levothyroxine) 75 mcg daily. She proceeded to the operating room quickly for an open reduction internal fixation of the right femur. During the surgery she had an unexpected complication of bleeding and required a transfusion of 2 units packed red blood cells. Postoperatively, she was transferred from the post anesthesia care unit to the ICU for a higher level of care than was anticipated for the recovery period due to concerns of further bleeding. It was identified in the ICU that the patient normally takes daily aspirin for arthritic pain which was not reported prior to the surgery because the patient didn't think of aspirin as a medication when asked.

1. *How was patient safety compromised in this situation?*
2. *What processes could have provided a higher level of safety for the patient?*
3. *What actions can be taken to improve the quality of care and prevent this type of error in the future?*

INTRODUCTION

For the past 20 years, the United States (U.S.) healthcare system has been focused on improving healthcare outcomes for patients and their families by improving the quality and safety of care. Rising healthcare costs, difficulty in accessing care, and research describing the state of the healthcare industry have signaled the need for improvement and driven accelerated change. Even with coordinated efforts and national initiatives, the complexity of healthcare has made change difficult and slow, with patients bearing the consequences. Despite being one of the wealthiest economies in the world and being among those countries that spend the most on healthcare, the United States continues to see poor coordination, ongoing variation in care and outcomes, disparities at all levels of acuity, and continuing injuries to patients.

Direct-care bedside nurses, as well as all nurses, have a significant leadership role to play in improving the quality and the safety of patient care. Nurses' work significantly influences the incidence of patient falls, pressure injuries, healthcare-acquired infections, appropriate pain management, overall quality improvement (QI), and patient safety. Nurses' work impacts mortality and morbidity rates, lengths of stay, development of complications, and patient satisfaction with care. The clinical reasoning skills of the nurse frequently serve to identify at-risk patients so that the interprofessional team can be alerted and begin the problem-solving process on behalf of patients.

This chapter provides an overview of the key concepts, drivers, and strategies for improving patient safety and quality care, setting the stage as the foundation of nursing work. Key terms will be defined. National and international initiatives to improve healthcare systems will be discussed. Nurses' role in quality and safety will be analyzed along with the origins and development of the Quality and Safety Education for Nurses (QSEN) competencies as a catalyst for improvement in nursing education. The transformation of nursing education from task-oriented instruction to the development of a new identity for nurses that demonstrates knowledge, skills, and attitudes that emphasize quality and safety in patient care will be fully explored. The role of nurses as healthcare leaders being champions for change will begin in this chapter and be examined throughout this text.

QUALITY OF CARE AND PATIENT SAFETY

Patients in hospitals and those who receive care from multiple healthcare providers at multiple sites of care are particularly vulnerable to safety and quality errors. Leaders in the United States have emphasized the need to redesign systems of care to better serve patients in the complex environment of the healthcare system. Much of this initiative began with the efforts of the Institute of Medicine (IOM), now the National Academy of Medicine (NAM), through their work to identify the requisite knowledge, skills, and attitudes necessary to provide safe, effective, high quality care. A series of reports from the IOM about the quality of America's healthcare (Greiner & Knebel, 2003, Kohn et al., 2000) disseminated healthcare research and evaluation and identified local as well as national policy changes that could be used to accelerate safety measures and QI. Following those reports, adoption of patient safety strategies and guidelines came quickly as the Centers for Medicare and Medicaid Services (CMS) stopped reimbursement for additional healthcare costs associated with events considered preventable that resulted in harm to patients (CMS, 2008). This forced hospital systems to either change or absorb those costs. Despite the efforts of the IOM and CMS, both government agencies, such as the Agency for Healthcare Research and Quality (AHRQ), and national healthcare quality organizations, such as The Leapfrog Group, report that while there have been some improvements, disparities and problems with quality and safety persist (AHRQ, 2011; The Leapfrog Group, 2020).

Healthcare quality refers to how well healthcare services for individuals and populations achieve desired health outcomes that are consistent with current professional knowledge and standards (IOM, 2001). **High-quality care** is defined as care that is safe, timely, effective, efficient, equitable, and patient centered, also referred to as STEEEP (Table 1.1), with no disparities between racial or ethnic groups (IOM, 2001). AHRQ expanded the definition of quality to include, "doing the right thing, at the right time, in the right way, to achieve the best possible results" (AHRQ, 2011). The IOM has recommended that quality can be improved on four levels:

- the patient level
- the health-delivery "microsystems" level, such as a surgical team or acute-care unit

TABLE 1.1 INSTITUTE OF MEDICINE'S DEFINITIONS OF STEEEP

	IOM TERM	DEFINITION
S	Safe	Avoiding injuries to patients from the care that is intended to help them
T	Timely	Reducing waits and sometimes harmful delays for both those who receive and those who give care
E	Efficient	Avoiding waste, including waste of equipment, supplies, ideas, and energy
E	Equitable	Providing care that does not vary in quality because of personal characteristics such as gender, ethnicity, geographic location, and socioeconomic status
E	Effective	Providing services based on scientific knowledge to all who could benefit, and refraining from providing services to those not likely to benefit
P	Patient-centered	Providing care that is respectful of and responsive to individual patient preferences, needs, and values, and ensuring that patient values guide all clinical decisions

Source: STEEEP Healthcare Goals. Compiled with information from the report, Institute of Medicine. (2001). *Crossing the quality chasm: A new health care system for the 21st century.* National Academies Press.

- the organizational level, such as hospitals and healthcare systems
- the regulatory and financial environment level in which those organizations operate (IOM, 2001)

The safety of the healthcare system is usually measured by its ability to prevent errors that cause harm to patients. An error may be an act of commission where someone does something wrong or an act of omission where someone fails to do what is required, with either type of events leading to an undesirable outcome or injury (AHRQ Patient Safety Network Glossary, n.d.). For many years healthcare had a shame and blame culture, punishing people for making mistakes, but in truth, rarely is an error the result of one person's actions. More often, it is the result of people working within a flawed system. Thinking about errors from this systems perspective has changed the culture in healthcare to support just culture principles. In a just culture, errors are addressed by looking at the system where the error occurred rather than the individual involved in the error so that mistakes can be addressed by error-proofing the system, making it very difficult for a mistake to reoccur. In doing so, patients are protected and the quality of care is improved.

An **adverse event** is any injury caused to a patient by the care received (AHRQ Patient Safety Network Glossary, n.d.). Adverse events, while not always errors, can cause serious injuries to patients, and many times can be prevented. Preventable adverse events such as falls and pressure injuries are considered to reflect care that falls below the accepted standard. Serious preventable adverse events can result in a patient death, loss of a body part, or permanent disability. Preventing adverse events is the work of all healthcare professionals through the development of policies that support quality and safety and through vigilant preoccupation with preventing errors and adverse events.

A **sentinel event** (sometimes referred to as a "never event") is any unanticipated event in a healthcare setting that reaches a patient and results in the patient's death, permanent harm, or such severe temporary harm it requires intervention to sustain life (The Joint Commission [TJC], 2017). When a sentinel event occurs that results in death or serious injury to a patient that is not related to the natural course of the patient's illness, it should be reported first within the organization according to policy. Reporting is essential because these are rare occurrences that should never happen. They require the full attention of the organization's leadership to investigate, identify causes, and develop processes to prevent any future reoccurrence. Nationally, 39 types of sentinel events are tracked by TJC including wrong-site surgery, medication errors, falls, perinatal events, and delays in treatment. Sentinel event data is compiled by TJC but organizations are not required to report sentinel events; reporting is voluntary and therefore it is estimated that the data represents only a small fraction of actual occurrences.

The term "**sharp end**" has been used to identify the point in a healthcare system where any healthcare provider works and gives care to patients. This point or sharp end of patient care is where errors may occur (Reason, 1990). Errors on the sharp end of patient care have often been considered to be the result of provider deficiencies such as careless behavior or lack of knowledge or skill. In fact, these sharp end errors have now been recognized to often be the result of flaws in the organization's system or due to extra-organizational issues such as healthcare regulators, payers, insurance administrators, economic policy makers, and technology suppliers, all of which are considered on the latent end of error. These latent end issues affect the behavior of care providers at the sharp end point of service and may lead to patient-care errors.

DRIVERS FOR QUALITY AND SAFETY

It is universally accepted that all people make mistakes, even the most competent of individuals. While errors can serve as the impetus for careful systematic review and process improvement, established national initiatives and core measures serve as a guide so that healthcare institutions can develop aims, identify shortfalls, and strive for excellence. Work by the AHRQ, CMS, and National Quality Forum (NQF) has led to the development of measures for improving the quality of care and patient safety. Many of these measures monitor the occurrence of adverse patient outcomes or injury (measures of patient safety) while others set the standard of care by ensuring that recommended care is available and used by all patients at the right time (measures of quality of care). When considered together, these measures can help healthcare organizations improve the value of care they provide to all patients.

Quality care and patient safety measures are primarily used in healthcare organizations, such as hospitals, nursing homes, and outpatient clinics. Most frequently used measures include the CMS Core Measures, AHRQ Quality Indicators, AHRQ Patient Safety Indicators, and NQF and the American Nurses Association (ANA) Nursing Sensitive Indicators (Table 1.2). Professional organizations and healthcare organizations also maintain quality of care and patient safety measures that can be found through websites of professional organizations and in peer-reviewed journal publications.

NATIONAL ORGANIZATIONS IMPACTING HEALTHCARE IMPROVEMENT

While the initial estimates in the IOM's *To Err Is Human* report proclaimed that each year there were about 98,000 preventable deaths in the United States (Kohn et al., 2000), a more recent study by Makary and Daniel (2016) found that more than 250,000 deaths each year are the result of healthcare error. That means that after heart disease and cancer, patient safety errors are the third-leading cause of death in the United States (Makary & Daniel, 2016). Recognizing the complex challenges of the healthcare system in working to address this, national organizations have provided resources and incentives to improve quality of care and patient safety.

There are three key agencies within the U.S. Department of Health and Human Services that are influential in shaping improvements in healthcare quality and patient safety: AHRQ, CMS, and the U.S. Food and Drug Administration (FDA). The AHRQ (www.ahrq.gov) is focused on producing evidence to make healthcare safer, higher quality, more accessible, and equitable, and working to make sure that evidence is understood and used. The CMS (www.cms.gov) has multiple roles that influence quality of care and patient safety. The CMS controls reimbursement for patients receiving federally supported healthcare through Medicare and Medicaid, so in that capacity, the CMS works with both public and private organizations to ensure quality care, promote efficient health outcomes, and make sure that CMS policies are used by healthcare organizations and clinicians as a prerequisite of receiving reimbursement payments for their services. The FDA (www.fda.gov) is responsible for protecting the public health by ensuring the safety, efficacy, and security of human and veterinary drugs, biological products, and medical devices; and by ensuring the safety of the nation's food supply, cosmetics, and products that emit radiation (FDA, 2018).

The organizations described in the text that follows have significant roles in influencing the quality of care and patient safety by working with government institutions, healthcare organizations, clinicians, and accreditation organizations. Many of them work together.

- The Institute for Safe Medication Practices (ISMP) is a private nonprofit organization that leads efforts to improve how medications are used, working to prevent medication errors and promote safe medication use. Through its national Medication Errors Reporting Program, healthcare professionals can report medication errors. Through

TABLE 1.2 EXAMPLES OF MEASURES OF PATIENT SAFETY AND MEASURES OF QUALITY OF CARE

MEASURE SET	EXAMPLES OF THE MEASURES	WHERE USED
Core Measures (CMS, 2017) Used to improve quality of care for common conditions www.cms.gov/Medicare/Quality-Initiatives-Patient-Assessment-Instruments/QualityMeasures/Core-Measures.html	Stroke: Received medication to prevent blood clots Immunization: Assessed for flu vaccine Heart failure: Received beta-blocker therapy for left ventricular systolic dysfunction Age-appropriate screening for colonoscopy Readmission: All-cause readmission rate following elective total hip or total knee replacement	Hospitals Health plan/ integrated delivery systems Individual clinician level
Patient Safety Indicators (AHRQ, 2017b) Used to improve the safety of inpatient care www.qualityindicators.ahrq.gov/Modules/psi_resources.aspx#techspecs	Rate of pressure ulcers Retained surgical item or unretrieved device fragment count Rate of central venous catheter-related bloodstream infections Rate of postoperative sepsis Transfusion reaction count Rate of accidental punctures or lacerations Rate of birth trauma–injury to neonate	Hospitals
Quality Indicators (AHRQ, 2017a) Used to improve quality of care https:// qualityindicators.ahrq.gov	**Prevention Quality Indicators** Perforated appendix admission rate Hypertension admission rate Urinary tract infection admission rate Uncontrolled diabetes admission rate Bacterial pneumonia admission rate	Hospitals
	Inpatient Quality Indicators Hip replacement mortality rate Heart failure mortality rate Acute stroke mortality rate Laparoscopic cholecystectomy rate Hysterectomy rate	Hospitals
	Pediatric Quality Indicators Neonatal mortality Pressure ulcers Transfusion reactions Postoperative hemorrhage or hematoma Postoperative respiratory failure	Hospitals
Nursing Sensitive Indicators (ANA, 2010; NQF, 2004) Used to improve the quality of nursing care www.qualityforum.org/improving_care_through_nursing.aspx	Falls with injury Nursing care hours per patient day Pressure injuries Rate of hospital-acquired infections Staffing mix (ratios of RNs, LPNs, and unlicensed staff)	Hospitals

AHRQ, Agency for Healthcare Research and Quality; ANA, American Nurses Association; CMS, Centers for Medicare and Medicaid Services; NQF, National Quality Forum.

its Medical Error Recognition and Revision Strategies program, the ISMP works directly and confidentially with pharmaceutical companies to prevent errors associated with confusing or misleading medication naming, labeling, packaging, and device design (www.ISMP.org).

- The NAM, formerly the IOM, is a private nonprofit organization that provides peer-reviewed evidence-based information and advice concerning health and health policy issues. The NAM released a series of 11 reports on quality and patient safety, starting with its seminal report, *To Err Is Human: Building a Safer Health System* (Kohn et al., 1999), followed by *Crossing the Quality Chasm* (IOM, 2001). The IOM also released the report, *The Future of Nursing: Leading Change, Advancing Health*, which was the original report that set forth a series of recommendations for nursing to have a greater role in the complex U.S. healthcare system (IOM, 2011).

- The NQF is a private nonprofit organization that conducts review processes and works with stakeholders to standardize healthcare performance measures aimed at reducing the occurrence of adverse events. A National Priorities Partnership, convened by the NQF, has issued sets of specific actions to reduce healthcare costs in three important areas: avoiding hospital readmissions, reducing emergency department overuse, and preventing medication errors (www.qualityforum.org).
- The Institute for Healthcare Improvement (IHI) is a private nonprofit organization that motivates and builds the will for change, partnering with patients and healthcare professionals to test new models of care to ensure the broadest adoption of best practices and effective innovations (www.ihi.org).
- TJC is a private nonprofit organization that operates accreditation programs for a fee to subscriber hospitals and other healthcare organizations. Hospitals seek reaccreditation every 3 years, a process through which TJC ensures that quality compliance requirements are met including core measures, safe practice measures, and process improvement efforts. TJC sets standards aimed at ensuring quality of care and patient safety and provides tools to meet those standards, such as the Sentinel Event Policy, Improving the Root Cause Analyses and Actions (RCA2) methodologies and techniques, and the National Patient Safety Goals (www.JointCommission.org). Accreditation is essential so that insurance companies are confident hospitals will provide the best care possible to their subscribers.
- The Leapfrog Group is a private nonprofit organization that collects and reports its Leapfrog Hospital Survey on hospital performance to improve the value of care and, through its Leapfrog Hospital Safety Grade, assigns letter grades to hospitals based on how they perform on patient safety measures (www.leapfroggroup.org).
- Healthcare Financial Management Association (HFMA) is a professional membership organization that represents leaders in healthcare finance with broad-based stakeholders in healthcare to provide education and coalition building to improve healthcare through best practices and standards. Through its Value Project, HFMA identified patient quality concerns (Table 1.3) and developed guides for value-driven care (HFMA, 2021).

For consumers, physicians, nurses, and other interested parties seeking information about quality of care and safety, CMS Hospital Compare is a government-sponsored website that provides performance measurement data. Selection of a zip code zone enables comparison between hospitals for core measurements that include scores for patient experience surveys (Hospital Consumer Assessment of Healthcare Providers and Systems [HCAHPS]) that are collected for all discharged patients, as well as infection rates, complication rates, timely and effective care, and many other aspects of the healthcare experience. Nurses can support patient choice by teaching consumers of healthcare how to use this resource by accessing the website at www.medicare.gov/care-compare/?providerType=Hospital&redirect=true.

TABLE 1.3 PATIENT QUALITY CONCERNS

Access	Make my care available and affordable
Safety	Do not hurt me
Outcomes	Make me better
Respect	Respect me as a person, not a case

Source: Data from Healthcare Financial Management Association. (2021). *The Value Project*. https://www.hfma.org/industry-initiatives/the-value-project.html

CASE STUDY

The risk manager at a community hospital reviewed occurrence report data trends over the last quarter and discovered an increasing trend of patients who arrived in the radiology department for an MRI who were not appropriate candidates due to having implanted metal devices. Speaking with the lead MRI technologist, concern was expressed that patients were not being correctly screened by the nurses on the units. The risk manager organized an interprofessional team from the nursing, medical, and MRI departments. After reviewing the MRI screening protocol, it was identified that a new scheduling system that had been put in place in the radiology department was so efficient at getting patients an MRI appointment, the unit nurses did not have time to complete an MRI patient screening between the time that the physician ordered the MRI and the time the patient went to the radiology department for the MRI. A new MRI screening protocol was immediately implemented in which the MRI order would now not be placed by the unit secretary until the RN communicated that the MRI patient screening was completed. This protected patients from a potential injury.

1. *Why is it important that patients with implants be identified on the unit by the nurse rather than later by the MRI technologist?*
2. *How did the risk manager's process of reviewing the MRI screening protocol contribute to solving this patient safety issue?*

Real World Interview

Courage does not always roar. … Sometimes courage is the quiet voice at the end of the day saying, "I will try again tomorrow."

–Mary Anne Radmacher

Earlier today following our daily safety huddle, I was out in our organization on "executive walking rounds." The ongoing COVID-19 pandemic is seeing a recurrent surge in cases within our medical center's service area. While we are prepared for the patients that will need our care, the prolonged work and home-life stress experienced by our workforce (with no end in sight!) has taken a significant toll.

In safety huddle today, our work teams reported high stress levels … and, as everyone knows, this is a known and insidious threat to patient safety. We consciously attempted to increase our pre-occupation with failure … talking about where and how we are vulnerable. We brainstormed some stress countermeasures. We also focused on the importance of sticking to our structured communication tools that we have been learning so as to decrease communication errors during team handoffs. All of this work we are doing in our safety huddle is now part of our organizational DNA.

As a leader, attending daily safety huddle and performing executive walking rounds are but a few of the ways that I try to keep my "sensitivity to operations" engaged—one of the five principles of an organization on the journey to high reliability. I am acutely aware of how integral to my daily work the focus of quality and safety have become.

For many of our newer staff, it is hard to remember a time when we didn't work this way ... but I actually do remember those times quite well. I remember being a Dean of a school of nursing when the QSEN work began. I remember my academic colleagues initially lamenting about our "packed curricula" and how there was simply no time in our baccalaureate and master's courses to have our students develop additional quality and safety-related competencies. Thank goodness at the time there was a simultaneous clear and compelling mandate driving the need for change in healthcare delivery systems and health professions education programs ... the responsibility to provide better and safer care for our patients.

Our students, as early as their first clinical experiences, quickly came to appreciate their developing knowledge and skills for safe practice, and for working and communicating effectively in teams. Being introduced to the necessity of improving care WHILE delivering care, and being given the tools to analyze and make these improvements, in fact, changed the way nursing students viewed their role. They were able to see themselves as agents for positive system change as well as advocates for their individual patients. These new competencies helped them to feel more confident as they were increasingly immersed in the complexities of contemporary care delivery. Making the required changes in our clinicians' educational curricula and within our healthcare organizations has taken years of painstaking work as well as sheer perseverance to keep at it. We have come a long way.

Admittedly, we have not yet achieved our goal of being 100% error free. Given the rising complexity of care, combined with the fact that the delivery of healthcare continues to largely be a human endeavor, this goal can, at times, feel elusive. When we have a mis-step that adversely affects a patient, it is hard not to become disheartened. All I know is that we need to have the will and the courage to keep at it.

Susan A. Reeves, EdD, RN, CENP
Executive Vice President
Dartmouth-Hitchcock Medical Center, Lebanon, New Hampshire

GLOBAL ADVANCES IN QUALITY AND SAFETY

Researchers and healthcare providers throughout the world have been actively involved in improving patient safety and quality of care with significant contributions from the United Kingdom, Canada, Australia, and the United States Even though some may consider the United States the leader in healthcare or in efforts to improve healthcare quality and patient safety, comparative studies by the Organisation for Economic Cooperation and Development (OECD), and The Commonwealth Fund, have consistently found that the United States does not have better healthcare outcomes than many industrialized nations, including countries in Europe, Australia, Canada, and Asia (OECD, 2021b; The Commonwealth Fund, 2020). This doesn't make sense when one considers that year after year, the United States continues to spend more on healthcare (per capita), than any other country in the world (OECD, 2021a). Despite spending more, Americans have poor health

TABLE 1.4 U.S. HEALTHCARE FROM A GLOBAL PERSPECTIVE

	TOTAL HEALTHCARE SPENDING PER CAPITA, 2019	INFANT MORTALITY PER 1,000 LIVE BIRTHS, 2019[a]	PERCENT OF POPULATION WITH OBESITY (BMI >30), 2019	SPENDING ON PHARMA-CEUTICALS PER CAPITA, 2019	LIFE EXPECTANCY AT BIRTH, 2019	PERCENT OF POPULATION WITH TWO OR MORE CHRONIC DISEASES, 2016
United Kingdom	$4,070	3.9	28.7	$469	81.3	14
Italy	$3,428	2.8	10.6	$590	83	-
Australia	$5,005	3.1	30.4	$673	82.6	15
France	$4,965	3.8	17	$653	82.6	18
Canada	$4,974	4.7	26.3	$806	82	22
Germany	$5,986	3.2	23.6	$823	81.1	17
Japan	$4,766	1.9	4.4	$838	84.2	-
United States	$10,586	5.8	40	$1,220	78.6	28

[a] Organisation for Economic Co-operation and Development. (2021b). *Infant mortality rates (2019).* https://data.oecd.org/healthstat/infant-mortality-rates.htm

Source: Data from The Commonwealth Fund. (2020). *International health care system profiles.* https://www.commonwealthfund.org/international-health-policy-center/countries

outcomes, including shorter life expectancy, greater prevalence of chronic conditions and obesity, and higher infant mortality rates (The Commonwealth Fund, 2020) (Table 1.4).

International organizations focused on improving the quality and safety of care work together bound by their common interests to improve the health of the world. The U.S.-based Joint Commission has an international component that has established the International Patient Safety Goals (Joint Commission International, n.d.) (Table 1.5). Each of these international goals can be related to the U.S.-based Joint Commission's patient safety goals. The World Health Organization (WHO) also continues to lead worldwide efforts to improve access to care and patient safety. Operating as the coordinating authority on international health within the United Nations, they have championed patient safety through their efforts to advocate for universal healthcare, to monitor public health risks, to coordinate responses to health emergencies, and to promote world-wide health and well-being. Around the world they intervene to improve the quality of the care provided for individuals regardless of country or circumstances.

TABLE 1.5 THE JOINT COMMISSION INTERNATIONAL PATIENT SAFETY GOALS

1.	Identify patients correctly
2.	Improve effective communication
3.	Improve safety of high-alert medications
4.	Ensure safe surgery
5.	Reduce the risk of healthcare-associated infections
6.	Reduce the risk of patient harm resulting from falls

Source: Data from Joint Commission International. (n.d.). *International patient safety goals.* http://www.jointcommissioninternational.org/improve/international-patient-safety-goals

CURRENT LITERATURE

CITATION

America is a health-care outlier in the developed world. (2018, April 16). *The Economist*. https://www.economist.com/news/special-report/21740871-only-large-rich-country-without-universal-health-care-america-health-care-outlier

DISCUSSION

America has some of the best hospitals in the world but it is also the only large rich country without universal healthcare coverage. About half of Americans have their health insurance provided by their employers. Healthcare costs can be financially ruinous for others. In 2016, America spent $10,348 per person on healthcare, roughly twice as much as the average for comparably rich countries. On average, both hospital cost and drug prices can be 60% higher in the United States than in Europe. The American Affordable Care Act expanded the health insurance system and cut the number of uninsured people from 44 million to 28 million but still left a gap among people not poor enough to qualify for Medicaid but not rich enough to buy private insurance.

The article claims that in the United States, prices for the same service can vary enormously. Having an appendix removed, for example, can cost anywhere from $1,500 to $183,000 depending on the insurer. Add to this the fact that nine of the 10 best-paid occupations in the United States involve medicine and doctors, who have little incentive to change the system.

IMPLICATIONS FOR PRACTICE

There is a tremendous amount of work to be done to improve quality and make healthcare more affordable, equitable, and accessible. Nurses must participate in the discussion about improving the healthcare system.

THE PATIENT SAFETY MOVEMENT TO IMPROVE QUALITY AND SAFETY

Errors in healthcare that harm patients cost approximately $20 billion each year (Rodziewicz et al., 2020). Medical errors, often referred to as never events because they are events that should never happen, continue to be a serious public health problem with many people experiencing adverse events that result in a longer hospital stay, permanent harm, the need for a life-sustaining intervention, or death. Errors happen because of a multitude of factors that include lack of education or experience, missed diagnoses, under- and over-treatment, and fatigue (Kohn et al., 2000). The financial constraints of hospitals can also impact patient safety. Often to decrease overhead, hospitals reduce nurse to patient ratios. For patients, being exposed to below targeted nurse staffing levels has been associated with increased mortality (Rodziewicz et al., 2020). By being in direct contact with patients, nurses are in a unique position to most likely be the last person able to stop a chain of events that may result in an error. Nurses are capable of preventing many errors from reaching the patient, but when error occurs, fear of punishment makes nurses and other healthcare professionals reluctant to report them. All errors need to be reported by members of the healthcare team, not just nurses, so that strategies can be implemented to error-proof the system, build a culture of safety, and prevent future errors. Organizations that have a culture of safety are nonjudgmental, acknowledge the risk and error-prone nature associated with healthcare, and focus on improving healthcare systems and processes. When an error does reach a patient, the team needs to work together to mitigate or decrease the seriousness of harm.

When something goes wrong and patients are harmed, it is difficult for clinicians, hospital leadership, and patients. When an adverse event occurs, it is important to respond in a timely manner. The Leapfrog Group recommends organizations take the following steps when an adverse event occurs:

1. Apologize to the patient and family.
2. Waive all costs related to the event and follow-up care.
3. Report the event to an external agency.
4. Conduct a root-cause analysis of how and why the event occurred.
5. Interview patients and families, who are willing and able, to gather evidence for the root cause analysis.
6. Inform the patient and family of the action(s) that the hospital will take to prevent future recurrences of similar events based on the findings from the root cause analysis.
7. Have a protocol in place to provide support for caregivers involved in never events, and make that protocol known to all caregivers and affiliated clinicians.
8. Perform an annual review to ensure compliance with each element of Leapfrog's Never Events Policy for each never event that occurred (www.leapfroggroup.org/influencing/never-events).
9. Make a copy of this policy available to patients upon request (The Leapfrog Group, n.d.).

Improvement of how care is delivered and improvement in patient outcomes from care received is a labor-intensive process that uses many staff and financial resources. Improvement processes include accurately looking at errors that occur from providing care; looking at areas where the quality of care can be improved through the early detection, prevention, and reporting of errors; and looking at improving performance on measures of quality care. Yet reporting errors or problems in quality of care is not straightforward. Federal and state governments, as well as private organizations, have used mandatory reporting systems for errors and instances of poor quality of care, yet they are often not effective in improving performance because of the fear that clinicians have of being punished with financial fines or punitive actions. As a result, errors continue to be underreported.

Patient safety and quality of care can improve in organizations where there is a culture of safety and a deep commitment to these priorities. Unfortunately, not all organizations demonstrate this. A survey by the AHRQ (2018) reported that there has been no increase in the performance measure of nonpunitive response to error and frequency of events reported, meaning healthcare workers did not believe reported errors would be addressed in a nonpunitive manner. This indicates that fear of punishment remains an obstacle to reporting errors. If nurses don't feel safe reporting errors, then risk and error-prone situations can't be corrected, which negatively affects the safety of care. The barriers for attaining a culture of safety include a lack of leadership, a culture where low expectations prevail, poor teamwork among colleagues, and poor communication within the organization. Achievement of a culture of safety requires that organizations acknowledge the high-risk nature of healthcare. Preoccupation with safety and the determination to achieve consistently safe operations serve as driving forces with an emphasis on systems improvement to support performance. Organizations that support a culture of safety encourage collaboration across ranks and disciplines to prevent errors and find solutions to patient safety problems. These organizations support just culture principles, meaning an employee can admit mistakes and trust that individual accountability will be balanced with investigation to determine whether the system is a safe and effective system or the system is set up to allow errors. Most importantly, proactive reporting of unsafe conditions and establishment of just culture principles in response to error allows candid discussion among employees in a blame-free environment so that patient safety concerns are dealt with quickly and effectively.

For many years efforts to improve patient safety and prevent errors were mostly managed by individual hospitals but as the national patient safety movement grew, CMS, which funds Medicare and Medicaid, and many private insurance companies instituted financial penalties to be applied to hospitals if and when sentinel events occurred. The penalty was that hospitals were not reimbursed from CMS for the cost of care associated with the aftermath of the sentinel event such as a longer hospital stay or a corrective surgical procedure because sentinel events are considered to be preventable and should not happen. These financial penalties, which have remained in place today, have motivated healthcare organizations to adopt prevention strategies to improve care and keep patients safe from harm. Over time, other harmful events that should never happen to a patient including pressure injuries, catheter-associated urinary tract infections, central line associated bloodstream infections, air embolisms, wrong type blood transfusions, and foreign objects left in surgical patients were also penalized with loss of reimbursement for services.

BOX 1.1 Developing Clinical Judgment

A staff nurse was assigned to care for five patients on a busy cardiac unit for weekend dayshift. Normally, each nurse is assigned four patients but one nurse called out sick and the nursing supervisor was unable to find a replacement. Midway through the Sunday morning shift while the nurse is administering medications to a patient, another of the nurse's five patients falls trying to get out of bed without assistance and sustains a wrist injury. The following Monday, the nurse manager, the weekend charge nurse, and the staff nurse meet to discuss the patient's fall. The nurse is worried about being blamed for the fall and being disciplined.

1. What cues might the nurse identify and consider in this situation?
2. What hypothesis will the nurse consider based on the available information?
3. What processes might the group apply in working to identify contributing factors for the patient's injury?
4. How can the three nurses work together to prevent future patient falls?

CURRENT LITERATURE

CITATION

Marsa, L. (2017, September). *Take charge of your health care: How to research a surgeon* (p. 20) https://www.aarp.org/health/conditions-treatments/info-2017/choose-a-surgeon-doctor-surgeries.html

DISCUSSION

Table 1.6 shows the most common surgeries for Americans over 50 years of age and the most common complications. In 2% to 4% of all cases, complications occur resulting in the patient needing to be readmitted to the hospital within 30 days.

IMPLICATIONS FOR PRACTICE

Nurses must be aware of the high incidence of complications in patients over age 50 undergoing these procedures. Increased awareness can support prevention. As direct caregivers, nurses are uniquely positioned to implement nursing care strategies to prevent complications.

TABLE 1.6 MOST COMMON SURGERIES AND COMPLICATIONS FOR AMERICANS OVER 50 YEARS OF AGE

SURGERY	COMPLICATION	OCCURRENCE
Cataract removal	Posterior capsule opacity	20%
Pacemaker implant	Hematoma	2.2% in patients over 70
Colectomy	Infection	12.4%
Coronary artery bypass	Atrial fibrillation	24%
Hip replacement	Dislocation	2%
Knee replacement	Blood clot	1%
Prostate removal	Bleeding	5.3%
Inguinal hernia	Infection	0.3% Open surgery 0.2% Laparoscopic surgery
Cholecystectomy	Infection	7.6% Open surgery 1% Laparoscopic surgery
Appendectomy	Infection	4.3% Open surgery 1.9% Laparoscopic surgery

The Cost of Achieving Quality and Safety

Across types of healthcare organizations, population needs coupled with available resources frequently determine service lines that can be provided. Reimbursement from insurance companies and CMS for Medicare and Medicaid patients, which represent a majority of healthcare users, support the day-to-day operations of most healthcare institutions. Healthcare salaries (Table 1.7) are a significant expense, with nurses making up the largest workforce segment in the hospital setting. Other costs include support services such as pharmacy, food service, and housekeeping, as well as technology-driven departments such as radiology, surgical services, and nuclear medicine. Quality and safety are impacted by the structure and processes an organization has in place as well as by the skill acquisition of caregivers and appropriate staffing available to meet the standards of care. A fundamental strategy to assure those baseline standards are met is through the accreditation process.

From a systems perspective, providing safe, high-quality care comes at a significant cost in terms of receiving and maintaining accreditation but the cost in human suffering and financial compensation of poor quality care far exceeds these amounts. TJC is the nation's oldest and largest standard setting and accrediting body for healthcare. This independent, not-for-profit organization is governed by physicians, administrators, nurses, quality experts, educators, and a consumer advocate, among others. The importance of accreditation cannot be overstated. CMS has made accreditation a requirement for reimbursement for care received by Medicare and Medicaid beneficiaries. Hospitals and free-standing healthcare centers in the United States must meet TJC accreditation standards every 3 years

TABLE 1.7 SELECTED HEALTHCARE SALARIES

ROLE	SALARY
CEO, Kenneth C. Frazier, Merck Pharmaceuticals	$22,570,328*
Physicians and surgeons	≥$208,000**
Nurse practitioner	$117,670**
Pharmacist	$128,710**
Registered nurse	$75,330**
Dietitian	$63,090**
Licensed practical nurse	$48,820**
Nursing assistant	$30,830**

*Salary.com 2019

**U.S. Bureau of Labor Statistics. (2021, September 8). Healthcare occupations: 2020 Median annual wage https://www.bls.gov/ooh/healthcare

or undergo review from a state survey agency in order to be reimbursed for care received by Medicare and Medicaid beneficiaries. A 2018 study (Lam et al., 2018) determined that there was little difference in patient outcomes between those institutions accredited by TJC and those reviewed by state agencies, seeming to indicate that regardless of which organization a healthcare institution chooses, it is the process of being reviewed by an outside agency that improves the quality and safety of the care provided.

Recognizing Healthcare Excellence

The most recognized award for excellence within a hospital is the Baldrige Award (American Society for Quality, 2021). The Baldrige Health Care Criteria for Performance Excellence provides guidance that many healthcare organizations have used to improve quality. Recipients of the Baldrige Award are selected based on the following Criteria for Performance Excellence:

1. **Leadership**: How upper management leads the organization and how the organization leads within the community.
2. **Strategy**: How the organization establishes and plans to implement strategic directions.
3. **Customers**: How the organization builds and maintains strong, lasting relationships with customers.
4. **Measurement, Analysis, and Knowledge Management**: How the organization uses data to support key processes and manage performance.
5. **Workforce**: How the organization empowers and involves its workforce.
6. **Operations**: How the organization designs, manages, and improves key processes.
7. **Results**: How the organization performs in terms of customer satisfaction, finances, human resources, supplier and partner performance, operations, governance, and social responsibility, and how the organization compares to its competitors.

The Criteria for Performance Excellence is based on a set of core values. Award recipient organizations are considered to have a role-model organizational management system that continuously makes improvements in delivering products and/or services, demonstrates efficient and effective operations, and provides a way of engaging and responding to customers and other stakeholders.

THE BEGINNING OF QUALITY AND SAFETY EDUCATION FOR NURSES

Nurses are key to ensuring and improving quality of care and patient safety for patients and families, as well as for the organizations in which they work. For many years, nursing education was focused on learning tasks. As the patient safety movement began to take hold after the landmark IOM publication *To Err Is Human: Building a Safer Health Care System* (Kohn et al. 2000), there was a new consciousness about quality and safety in U.S. healthcare systems. The IOM (Greiner & Knebel 2003) developed five competencies that all healthcare workers needed to have in order to be safe practitioners: patient-centered care (PCC), teamwork and collaboration, evidence-based practice (EBP), QI, and use of informatics. In 2005, a small group of thought leaders in nursing, funded by the Robert Wood Johnson Foundation, adopted those five competencies, added a sixth focused on safety, and developed the QSEN competencies (Cronenwett et al., 2007). What made the QSEN competencies significant is that they were focused on nursing work, translating the IOM competencies into language that aligned with nursing practice. Each competency was defined by knowledge, skill, and attitude statements (KSAs), resulting in a total of 162 KSAs to describe competent nursing.

The QSEN competencies challenged nursing education to move away from that task-oriented approach that had been used since the days of Florence Nightingale to a more global focus for developing competent nurses in the wider context of the complex healthcare system. This required a shift from the traditional approach of educating nurses to not only learn how to provide patients the care they need at the individual point of care, but to also focus on continuous improvement through systems thinking. **Systems thinking** is understanding and synthesizing the interactions and interdependencies within the healthcare system and how they influence care of the individual patient (Dolansky & Moore, 2013). This systems thinking created a significant shift for clinicians that tended to focus on the individual patient and their family, and not necessarily on how that patient and family affect and are affected by the larger population and system of care.

INTEGRATION OF THE QUALITY AND SAFETY EDUCATION COMPETENCIES INTO NURSING EDUCATION

The purpose of the QSEN competencies was to create a road map of sorts that could guide nurse educators, and nursing education as a whole, in redefining what nursing education should be. Generous funding from the Robert Wood Johnson Foundation provided the financial support for the work through four phases of development that spanned over 7 years. In Phase 1, a small group of nurse educators worked to define what the six competencies would be (Table 1.8) and identify the KSAs that aligned with each. KSAs are defined as **knowledge**: the fact or condition of having information and being learned; **skill**: the ability to use one's knowledge effectively and readily in execution or performance; and **attitude**: a mental position with regard to a fact or state (Merriam-Webster, 2021).

In Phase 2, schools of nursing from around the country were invited to apply for a grant to become a pilot school. Fifteen of the 53 schools that applied were funded for $25,000 each. The charge to the 15 pilot schools was to develop teaching strategies and faculty education tools that provided updated knowledge about safe systems and knowledge from safety science. **Safety science** is knowledge about safety-related issues, and the development of concepts, theories, principles and methods to understand, assess, communicate, and manage safety (Terge, 2014). Nurses and nurse educators have always thought about safety in nursing work but the new emphasis of the patient safety movement required new education strategies that used safety science to help to describe how errors and near misses

TABLE 1.8 THE QUALITY AND SAFETY EDUCATION FOR NURSES COMPETENCIES

Patient-centered care (PCC)	Recognize the patient or designee as the source of control and full partner in providing compassionate and coordinated care based on respect for the patient's preferences, values, and needs.
Teamwork and collaboration	Function effectively within nursing and interprofessional teams, fostering open communication, mutual respect, and shared decision-making to achieve quality patient care.
Evidence-based practice (EBP)	Integrate the best current evidence with clinical expertise and patient/family preferences and values for delivery of optimal healthcare.
Quality improvement (QI)	Use data to monitor the outcomes of care processes and use improvement methods to design and test changes to continuously improve the quality and safety of healthcare systems.
Safety	Minimize risk of harm to patients and providers through both system effectiveness and individual performance.
Informatics	Use information and technology to communicate, manage knowledge, mitigate error, and support decision-making.

Source: From Cronenwett, L., Sherwood, G., Barnsteiner, J., Disch, J., Johnson, J., Mitchell, P., Sullivan, D. T., & Warren, J. (2007). Quality and Safety Education for Nurses. *Nursing Outlook, 55*(3), 122–131. https://doi.org/10.1016/j.outlook.2007.02.006

are recognized and reported and provide ways to manage human factors that impact safe healthcare delivery. Safety science has its roots in high-performance industries such as aviation and nuclear power and is now being adapted for use in healthcare using processes such as checklists and web-based reporting systems to improve care. Educators needed teaching strategies to bring safety science to the classroom and clinical learning of nursing students. Many of the early teaching strategies developed were shared via the QSEN website (www.qsen.org).

Phase 3 focused on faculty development and sustainability. During this phase, faculty education was widespread with train the trainer programs provided across the United States. Work began to change the content of nursing textbooks, accreditation standards, the licensure examination, and the requirements to demonstrate competence. Lastly, Phase 4 expanded the competencies for application at the graduate level. The graduate level competencies mirrored the prelicensure QSEN competencies but had a greater focus on leadership. With each phase, the reach of QSEN became wider. Today, QSEN remains a national initiative for nurses, nurse educators, and nursing students that offers resources for integrating the IOM's recommendations into models of nursing education both in prelicensure and graduate nursing education.

Integration of the Knowledge, Skills, and Attitudes Into Nursing Curricula

The integration of the QSEN competencies and the KSAs that defined them into nursing education and practice was a gradual process. Early work included a Delphi Study (Barton et al., 2009) that identified the most appropriate place in the curriculum for specific KSAs to be introduced, where they should be reinforced, and where they should be demonstrated in practice Table 1.9 demonstrates how the authors of the Delphi Study suggest the QSEN competencies be integrated across prelicensure and undergraduate curricula to introduce and then emphasize concepts in the beginning, intermediate, and advanced phases of the student's education program.

TABLE 1.9 OVERVIEW OF DELPHI STUDY FINDINGS

QSEN COMPETENCY	BEGINNING INTRODUCTION	INTERMEDIATE INTRODUCTION	ADVANCED INTRODUCTION	BEGINNING EMPHASIS	INTERMEDIATE EMPHASIS	ADVANCED EMPHASIS
Patient-centered care	KSA competencies				KSA competencies	
Teamwork and collaboration	Skill and attitude competencies	Knowledge and skill competencies			Attitude competencies	Knowledge and skill competencies
Evidence-based practice	Knowledge and attitude competencies	Skill competencies			Knowledge and attitude competencies	Skill and attitude competencies
Safety	KSA competencies			Attitude competencies	KSA competencies	Knowledge competencies
Informatics	Skill and attitude competencies	Knowledge competencies			Skills competencies	Knowledge and attitude competencies
Quality improvement	Attitude competencies	Skill and attitude competencies	Knowledge competencies		Attitude competencies	KSA competencies

KSA, knowledge, skill, attitude; QSEN, Quality and Safety Education for Nurses.
Source: Data from Barton, A. J., Armstrong, G., Preheim, G., Gelmon, S. B., & Andrus, L. C. (2009). A national Delphi to determine developmental progression of quality and safety competencies in nursing education. *Nursing Outlook, 57*(6), 313–322. https://doi.org/10.1016/j.outlook.2009.08.003

Real World Interview

My initial exposure to QSEN was soon after I had joined the faculty at the University of Colorado, School of Nursing in 2000. I was working as a bedside RN on a busy 52-bed Med/Surg unit, and the University of Colorado hired me to teach Med/Surg to prelicensure nursing students. For many years as nursing faculty, I maintained my practice at 40%, and felt divided between two worlds (practice and academia). I became increasingly concerned that these two worlds felt distinct, unconnected, and separate from each other.

QSEN provided a vital common ground: patient safety and quality improvement. The QSEN competencies created the bridge I had been seeking between what I was seeing in practice and what I was teaching in the classroom. As I delved deeper into learning about preventable harm in healthcare, I developed a sense of urgency in how quality and safety needed to be foundational to all nursing care, and therefore foundational to nursing education. The University of Colorado became a pilot school for QSEN's early work, and I became deeply engaged in developing expertise about QSEN's competencies and exploring different ways to integrate these competencies into teaching early nursing students. Many colleagues doubted the value of introducing QSEN competencies to new nursing students. "We don't introduce systems thinking to nursing students until later in their education" was a common response. With early introduction of QSEN competencies to prelicensure students, I discovered the powerful impact the QSEN KSAs had on nursing students' developing clinical lens. New nursing students gravitated toward learning about preventing harm in healthcare and wanted to learn how to contribute to improving the healthcare system. I learned that QSEN provides a powerful catalyst, which infuses new nurses with an understanding of the impact that an individual nurse can have on patient outcomes and contributing to safer healthcare systems.

My work grew and developed to include teaching interprofessional teams of healthcare professionals in a 12-month program about leading and sustaining improvement in their healthcare microsystems. Individual nurses often have ideas about what needs to be improved, but do not know how to transition their ideas into actual improvements. This year-long team training was based on knowing that insights about how to improve patient outcomes often abound on healthcare teams, but few teams know how to actualize these insights. The QSEN KSAs provided the foundation and direction for much of this successful team-training program.

QSEN's relevance has never been more significant. The COVID-19 pandemic exposed a myriad of system gaps and chasms that require improvement work by nurses and healthcare teams. Leading nurses in this improvement work not only benefits patients and healthcare systems, but also connects nurses to the core joy of their work. Nurses are best able to provide optimal care when quality and safety are high priorities at every level. Helping nurses embrace improvement work as part of their nursing practice connects nurses to the joy of improvement and benefits all.

Gail Armstrong, PhD, DNP, RN, ACNS-BC, CNE
Professor, Assistant Dean of the DNP Program
Oregon Health & Science University School of Nursing

APPLYING THE QUALITY AND SAFETY EDUCATION COMPETENCIES IN PRACTICE

The QSEN competencies are each described by KSAs. Simply put, the knowledge is what needs to be understood by the practitioner to deliver competent care, skill pertains to the capabilities needed to achieve competency, and attitude describes the manner with which the work should be approached in order to be fully proficient in nursing practice. There are 162 total KSAs spread across the six competencies. While each of the QSEN competencies have specific KSAs, there is certainly overlap that occurs between them. For instance, to meet the competency of PCC, teamwork and collaboration as well as EBP are required. The next section will provide examples of some KSAs for each QSEN competency and some learning activities that support growth and development in the competencies at the beginning, intermediate, and advanced levels.

Patient-Centered Care

- K—Understand the multiple dimensions of PCC: Patient/family/community preferences and values; coordinate care; empower the patient; provide physical comfort and emotional support; involve family and friends.
- S—Elicit patient values, preferences, and expressed needs as part of clinical interview; implement the care plan; evaluate care; facilitate informed consent; build consensus.
- A—Value seeing healthcare situations through the patient's eyes; value patient's expertise with own health and symptoms.

The KSAs for PCC allow for not only the basic needs of the patient to be met (bathing, feeding, toileting) but for the patient needs to be met in a way that considers patient preferences and values in the delivery of care. For example, when would the patient like to be bathed? How does the patient like to be fed? What aspects of the care is the patient able to carry out independent of the nurse? Do family members want to be active participants in their loved one's care? Physical comfort and emotional support are one knowledge aspect of the larger PCC competency. Table 1.10 offers learning activities for PCC at the beginning, intermediate, and advanced levels of nursing education.

TABLE 1.10 PATIENT-CENTERED CARE LEARNING ACTIVITIES

LEVEL	LEARNING ACTIVITIES
Beginning level	Interview a patient about their diagnosis. What does the diagnosis mean to the patient? How does the patient's perspective of the diagnosis differ from that of the healthcare team? Write your understanding of the patient's perspective and share it with the patient. Ask the patient for feedback about accuracy and interpretation.
Intermediate level	Consider barriers to actively involving families in patients' healthcare processes. Examine system barriers like limited visiting hours in the ICU or inability of family to be present in the perioperative setting. Are there policies that interfere with family involvement? What is the history of these policies? Do they still make sense?
Advanced level	All patients hold different values. Consider how you would support patient-centered care for individuals or groups whose values differ from your own.

CASE STUDY

A new graduate nurse is caring for a complex patient who has been hospitalized for over 2 weeks. The patient and the family have expressed frustration and mistrust in the healthcare team because of poor communication among members of the team. An individualized care plan was developed based on the unique needs of the patient. After report, the charge nurse asks the new graduate nurse to read the plan of care for specific instructions related to the physical and psychosocial needs of the patient. The new graduate nurse states, "I don't have time to read the plan of care, I have so much to do. I will read it later." The charge nurse understands that reading the plan of care later in the shift does not allow the new graduate nurse to consider the patient's preferences, values, or needs and may compromise the delivery of PCC.

1. *Which QSEN competency should the charge nurse focus on expanding in the new nurse's practice?*
2. *Which resources for this QSEN competency might help the charge nurse in working with the new nurse?*
3. *Describe leadership attributes that would help this charge nurse support the new nurse in providing PCC.*

Teamwork and Collaboration

- K—Recognize scope of practice and roles of healthcare team members.
- S—Engage in standardized handoff communication during shift report, patient-care rounds, discharge, or interfacility transfer; assert own position/perspective in discussions about patient care.
- A—Value the personal contribution that team members make to achieve effective team functioning; contribute to resolution of conflict and disagreement.

The nurse is often at the center of communication for the healthcare team, frequently facilitates important patient-care transitions, and ensures all members of the team are aware of the patient's status. Teams act as a safety net for individual practice. Errors can easily occur when communication or roles are not clear. Standardizing communication works to prevent errors that occur from differences in communication styles and creates a framework that keeps all members informed. Table 1.11 offers learning activities for teamwork and collaboration at the beginning, intermediate, and advanced levels of nursing education.

TABLE 1.11 TEAMWORK AND COLLABORATION LEARNING ACTIVITIES

LEVEL	LEARNING ACTIVITIES
Beginning level	Explore the tools recommended for healthcare teams in the Team*STEPPS* program found at www.teamstepps.ahrq.gov. Consider which would be most helpful in preventing error and patient harm. See Chapter 7 for more information.
Intermediate level	Standardized report ensures all aspects of care are addressed. Provide report using the standardized report framework of your institution.
Advanced level	Assume a leadership role if reviewing a patient chart. Identify potential risks and opportunities for improvement.

CASE STUDY

John, a new graduate, just completed his 3-month orientation. He is given a complex patient assignment without the assistance of a preceptor. After receiving a quick bedside report from the night nurse, John notices that the patient is restless and has an elevated respiratory rate. He is concerned, but realizes the patient is not wearing his oxygen. He puts the nasal cannula on the patient and tells him he will be back to check on him. John gets behind in his work, but wants to make a good impression with his colleagues and decides not to ask for help. One hour later, the nursing assistant tells John that the patient is in respiratory distress. John checks the patient and decides to ask the charge nurse for help. After assessing the patient, the charge nurse calls the interprofessional rapid response team and tells John to bring the crash cart into the room. When the team arrives, they decide the patient is unstable and must be transferred to the ICU for close monitoring.

1. *What critical steps should John have taken to engage the interprofessional team sooner?*
2. *Describe the places where teamwork and communication could have been strengthened in this case.*
3. *Identify the quality and safety issues that emerged around teamwork and collaboration. What actions could have been taken to prevent the need for a patient transfer to the ICU.*

Evidence-Based Practice

- K—Describe EBP to include components of research evidence, clinical expertise, and patient/family values.
- S—Read original research and evidence reports related to area of practice; question rationale for routine approaches to care that result in less than desirable outcomes.
- A—Value the concept of EBP as integral to determining best clinical practice.

Research indicates that the implementation of EBP improves quality of care, improves patient outcomes, and decreases healthcare costs and empowers clinicians in their role as healthcare providers (Gallagher-Ford et al., 2020). Nurses play a key role in implementing the most current evidence into patient care processes. Table 1.12 offers learning activities for EBP at the beginning, intermediate, and advanced levels of nursing education.

TABLE 1.12 EVIDENCE-BASED PRACTICE LEARNING ACTIVITIES

LEVEL	LEARNING ACTIVITIES
Beginning level	Read a journal article that describes an evidence-based practice project. Consider if the content resonates with what you are seeing in practice.
Intermediate level	Review clinical guidelines used in the clinical setting. Consider the references for the guideline and how strong the evidence is that supports implementation of the guideline.
Advanced level	Become involved with an evidence-based practice project on the clinical unit. Conduct a search to find relevant articles that address the focus of the project.

Quality Improvement

- K—Explain the significance of variation and measurement in assessing quality of care; describe approaches for changing a process of care.
- S—Use tools (such as control charts and run charts) that are helpful for understanding variation; use measures to evaluate the effect of change.
- A—Appreciate that continuous QI is an essential part of the daily work of all healthcare professionals

QI is everyone's job. Nurses are well positioned to contribute to improvement by identifying where improvement is possible and participating to make system changes. As students progress through clinical courses, they will see many examples of nurses contributing to QI processes in the acute care setting. Table 1.13 offers learning activities for QI at the beginning, intermediate, and advanced levels of nursing education.

TABLE 1.13 QUALITY IMPROVEMENT LEARNING ACTIVITIES

LEVEL	LEARNING ACTIVITIES
Beginning level	Complete a QI project focused on improving something about yourself. Learn all the steps of the improvement process by using the teaching strategy: Quality Improvement Project for prelicensure nursing students. https://qsen.org/quality-improvement-project-for-prelicensure-nursing-students/
Intermediate level	Review the standardized checklist to prevent central line-associated bloodstream infection used by your institution. Identify how standardization protects patients.
Advanced level	Partner with someone who works in the QI department of your hospital. Shadow that person for 2 full days. Notice the focus of their work. Which patient outcomes is this department tracking? How are data gathered for these patient outcomes? Are any specific patient care processes tracked for these patient outcomes? What insight can nurses provide about the patient-care processes used to achieve these patient outcomes?

Safety

- K—Examine human factors and other basic safety design principles as well as commonly used unsafe practices, such as work-arounds and unapproved abbreviations.
- S—Demonstrate effective use of strategies to reduce the risk of harm to self or others; use organizational error reporting systems for near-miss and error reporting.
- A—Value the contributions of standardization/reliability to safety; value own role in preventing errors.

Safety competency emphasizes team strategies to promote safe care in a healthcare system rather than focusing on blaming individuals when errors occur. Accepting that humans make mistakes and that error occurs because the system allows it provides a focus for error-proofing the healthcare environment so that patient harm can be prevented. Table 1.14 offers learning activities for safety at the beginning, intermediate, and advanced levels of nursing education.

TABLE 1.14 SAFETY LEARNING ACTIVITIES

LEVEL	LEARNING ACTIVITIES
Beginning level	Identify and describe how to apply the National Patient Safety Goals. https://www.jointcommission.org/-/media/tjc/documents/standards/national-patient-safety-goals/2022/npsg_chapter_hap_jan2022.pdf
Intermediate level	Conduct a medication reconciliation on a patient in the clinical setting to create the most accurate list possible of all medications the patient is taking, including the drug name, dosage, frequency, and route and comparing that list against the prescriber's admission, transfer, and/or discharge orders with the goal of providing correct medications to the patient.
Advanced level	Visit the Institute for Safe Medication Report at www.ismp.org. View the error reporting page and discuss how reporting medication errors serves to help all healthcare providers.

Informatics

- K—Explain why information and technology skills are essential for safe patient care.
- S—Apply technology and information management tools to support safe processes of care.
- A—Value technologies supporting decision-making, error prevention, and care coordination

All members of a healthcare team contribute to an electronic health record that is used extensively to document shifting patient-care priorities but a broader view of informatics includes the use of informatics in computerized clinical alerts and decision management. For example, a clinical alert signals to the provider that the patient is eligible to receive the pneumonia or flu vaccine. Data used in decision management may come from patient records, diagnostic results, or providers' documentation. Table 1.15 offers learning activities for Informatics at the beginning, intermediate, and advanced levels of nursing education.

TABLE 1.15 INFORMATICS LEARNING ACTIVITIES

LEVEL	LEARNING ACTIVITIES
Beginning level	Many patients use internet resources to become educated about their diagnosis. Consider how nurses can direct patients to reputable sites for information.
Intermediate level	The QSEN website has an information and technology responsibilities teaching strategy with a posttest. Review and take the posttest to measure your knowledge. http://qsen.org/heath-informatics-and-technology-professional-responsibilities/
Advanced level	Discuss the qualities of an EHR system that makes it nurse friendly and useful. What qualities are most important to support nursing in the in-patient care setting?

EHR, electronic health records; QSEN, Quality and Safety Education for Nurses.

NURSES' ROLE IN QUALITY AND SAFETY AS DIRECT CARE PROVIDERS AND LEADERS

To effectively apply the six QSEN competencies within the wider context of complex healthcare systems, nurses need to think about how performance can be measured, how the strengths of each team member can be maximized to improve care delivery to patients and improve their outcomes, and what can be done in the healthcare system to assure quality and safety and prevent harm from unintended consequences of errors. Scoville et al. (2016) states all healthcare providers have two interdependent roles; one is to do the work and the other is to improve the work. Direct care nurses achieve this by not only providing safe high-quality care, but also by participating in QI initiatives, leading EBP projects to reduce unwanted variation, and working within the healthcare system to improve overall functioning and effectiveness of the day-to-day operations.

Direct care nurses demonstrate leadership when they use best practices and teach others about those practices. Working in organizations that support a culture of safety and promote open communication when an error does occur strengthens one's development as a professional nurse. Because nurses' work creates a connection between the patient and the entire healthcare system, nurses have been instrumental in developing checklists and other standardized tools to improve the quality of care and ensure patient safety. Standardized checklists have been proven successful particularly in operating rooms and other areas where multiple tasks need to be accomplished consistently to ensure quality and safety. Checklists protect against failure and establish a higher standard of baseline performance. Using standardized order sets, protocols, and other best practices support nurses and the entire healthcare team in preventing errors, ensuring quality care, and reducing variability and the potential for error.

Because nurses work at the sharp end of care in direct contact with patients, they are uniquely qualified to offer invaluable insights and perspectives about what is preventing effective and efficient care as well as how the quality and safety of care can be improved. Nurses tend to be resilient problem-solvers, meaning that if something does not work well while they are providing care to a patient, they may work around the "normal" way of doing things. These workarounds increase the opportunities for inconsistent care and inconsistent outcomes so nurses need to be diligent in addressing patient care processes that do not work well and seeking solutions to remedy them. Direct care nurses improve care when they address the flaws in the healthcare system instead of working around them.

BOX 1.2 Developing Clinical Judgment

In administering medication to a patient, the nurse sees that the medication administration record indicates the dose amount to be 5 mg. Because the dose seems high, the nurse decides to double check the order and confirms that the dose was transcribed incorrectly; that the dose was supposed to be 0.5 mg. Hospital policy is that when transcribing a dose, staff are required to always use a zero before a decimal when the dose is less than a whole unit. This is a national safety standard. This could have been a medication error that could have caused serious harm to the patient. The nurse wants the unit to be safe but doesn't want anyone to get in trouble for the mistake.

1. What cues might the nurse identify and consider in this situation?
2. What hypothesis will the nurse consider based on the available information?
3. How should this be addressed in a culture of safety?
4. What can the nurse do to protect patients from medication errors and promote safe medication practice on the unit?

Recognizing Nursing Excellence

The American Nurses Credentialing Center's (ANCC) Magnet Recognition Program® (2021) awards those healthcare organizations that achieve superior performance the designation of Magnet status, often referred to as the ultimate credential for high-quality nursing. The Magnet Recognition Program evaluates sources of evidence that create the foundational infrastructure for excellence, while the program's focus on results fosters a culture of quality and innovation. To achieve Magnet status, an organization participates in a rigorous review process where it must demonstrate support of professional clinical practice, promotion of excellence in the delivery of nursing services to patients, and implementation of healthcare processes that promote best nursing practices (ANCC, 2021).

Individual nursing excellence is also recognized through certification. Frequently hospitals compensate nurses for achieving certification in their specialty area. This individual credentialing requires licensed nurses to complete a specific number of education hours and/or hours of experience and take an examination to demonstrate mastery of a body of knowledge and acquired decision-making skills in a particular area of nursing practice, including nursing leadership roles. Certification is encouraged and supported by nursing leadership on all levels. The ANCC as well as other national nursing organizations offer certification opportunities for many nursing specialties (see www.nursecredentialing.org/Certification).

The Role of Nurse Leaders in Ensuring Quality and Safety

To support the role of nursing, the IOM released the report, *The Future of Nursing: Leading Change, Advancing Health* (IOM, 2011). This report significantly impacted nursing and nursing education as the key message of the report was that nurses need to take a greater leadership role across care settings in the increasingly complex U.S. healthcare system. The report emphasized that as the population ages and becomes increasingly diverse and complex, the roles, responsibilities, and education of nurses would need to change to effectively respond in order to improve healthcare for everyone. Because nurses represent the largest segment of the healthcare workforce, the IOM made these four overarching recommendations, that nursing should:

1. Be able to practice to the full extent of their education and training
2. Improve nursing education
3. Assume leadership positions and serve as full partners in healthcare redesign and improvement efforts
4. Improve data collection for workforce planning and policy making (IOM, 2011)

Five years later in 2015, the IOM released a report on the progress achieved on the IOM 2010 report recommendations (Altman et al., 2015 see Box 1.3), focusing on the areas of removing barriers to practice and care; transforming education; collaborating and leading; promoting diversity; and improving data collection. In this report, the IOM committee concluded that no single profession working alone would be able to meet the complex needs of patients and communities and therefore nurses should continue to develop skills and competencies in leadership and innovation and collaborate with other professionals to improve healthcare delivery and health system redesign. The report stressed that the nursing profession must continue to work with stakeholders both within and outside of nursing toward the achievement of the recommendations from the 2010 report in order to effect change in an evolving healthcare landscape (Altman et al., 2015). This vision is extended by the *Future of Nursing 2020–2030* report that charges nursing to take a significant role in the next decade to address the social determinants of health and continue to build a diverse and competent workforce to provide effective, efficient, equitable, and accessible care for all persons in all areas of the healthcare continuum (Wakefield et al., 2021).

BOX 1.3 Institute of Medicine Recommendations for *The Future of Nursing* Reports

IOM RECOMMENDATIONS—2010

- Remove scope of practice barriers.
- Implement nurse residency programs.
- Expand opportunities for nurses to lead and diffuse collaborative improvement efforts.
- Double the number of nurses with a doctorate by 2020.
- Build an infrastructure for collection and analysis of interprofessional healthcare workforce data.
- Increase the proportion of nurses with a baccalaureate degree to 80% by 2010.
- Ensure that nurses engage in lifelong learning.
- Prepare and enable nurses to lead change to advance health.

IOM RECOMMENDATIONS—2015

- Build common ground with other health professions groups around scope of practice and other issues in policy and practice.
- Create and fund transition-to-practice residency programs.
- Expand efforts and opportunities for interprofessional collaboration and leadership development for nurses.
- Make diversity in the nursing workforce a priority.
- Promote nurses' pursuit of doctoral degrees.
- Continue pathways toward increasing the percentage of nurses with a baccalaureate degree.
- Promote nurses' interprofessional and lifelong learning.
- Promote the involvement of nurses in the redesign of care delivery and payment systems.
- Improve workforce data collection.
- Communicate with a wider and more diverse audience to gain broad support for the Future of Nursing campaign objectives.

IOM RECOMMENDATIONS—2020–2030

- Develop a shared agenda to address social determinants of health (SDOH) and achieve health equity.
- Enable greater actions for the nurses to address SDOH in all practice settings.
- Implement structures, systems, and evidence-based interventions to promote nurses' health and well-being.
- Remove barriers that prevent nurses from practicing to the full extent of their education and training.
- Establish sustainable, flexible payment mechanisms to support nurses in both healthcare and public health.

(continued)

BOX 1.3 Institute of Medicine Recommendations for *The Future of Nursing* Reports (Continued)

- Incorporate nursing expertise for initiatives focused on SDOH and health equity.
- Ensure nursing education programs prepare nurses to address SDOH.
- Protect the nursing workforce during the response to public health emergencies such as the COVID-19 pandemic and natural disasters.
- Develop and support a research agenda and evidence base that describes the impact of nursing interventions on SDOH, environmental health, health equity, and nurses' health and well-being.

Sources: Data from Altman, S. H., Stith Butler, A., & Shern. (Eds.). (2015). *Assessing progress on the IOM report* The Future of Nursing. National Academies Press. https://doi.org/10.17226/21838; Institute of Medicine. (2011). *The future of nursing: Leading change, advancing health*. National Academies Press. https://doi.org/10.17226/12956; Wakefield, M. K., Williams, D. R., Le Menestrel, S., & Flaubert, J. L. (Eds.). (2021). *The future of nursing 2020–2030: Charting a path to achieve health equity*. National Academies Press. https://doi.org/10.17226/25982

ACCREDITATION AND EVALUATION OF QUALITY AND SAFETY EDUCATION FOR NURSES COMPETENCIES

Since the introduction of the QSEN competencies, nursing education has continued to evolve to meet the expectations of nursing practice. The AACN Essentials (2021) for nursing education identify 10 domains that reflect a competency-based guide for curriculum development and design that emphasizes quality and safety, person-centered care, systems thinking, interprofessional collaboration, evidence-based practice, informatics, and many of the other concepts that underscored the QSEN competencies (Table 1.16). The

TABLE 1.16 AMERICAN ASSOCIATION OF COLLEGES OF NURSING ESSENTIALS DOMAINS

Domain 1	Knowledge for Nursing Practice
Domain 2	Person-Centered Care
Domain 3	Population Health
Domain 4	Scholarship for the Nursing Discipline
Domain 5	Quality and Safety
Domain 6	Interprofessional Partnerships
Domain 7	Systems-Based Practice
Domain 8	Informatics and Healthcare Technologies
Domain 9	Professionalism
Domain 10	Personal, Professional, and Leadership Development

Source: Data from American Association of Colleges of Nursing. (2021). *The essentials: Core competencies for professional nursing education.* https://www.aacnnursing.org/Education-Resources/AACN-Essentials

AACN Essentials will set the standard for nursing program accreditation and serve as the overarching principles that signal competency if nurses are to be practitioners that positively impact their local healthcare setting as well as the larger scope of the profession. Future work will focus on developing valid and reliable methods for measuring competency achievement and methods to support transfer of these competencies into the practice setting.

The 162 KSAs of the QSEN competencies remain relevant today and provide a scaffold that all nurses can use across the span of their nursing career. The QSEN competencies provide the foundation for clinical learning and practice expectations. Validated clinical evaluations framed in the QSEN competencies that define level-appropriate expectations are available for every prelicensure clinical nursing course (Nursing Fundamentals, Psychiatric, Pediatric, Maternal-Baby, Medical-Surgical Acute and Chronic Care, and Community Health Nursing) (Altmiller, 2019) as well as graduate level nurse practitioner clinical practicum courses (Altmiller & Dugan, 2021); these are available for free download at: https://qsicenter.tcnj.edu. As new graduates enter the workforce, many will enroll in nurse residency programs where the QSEN competencies will frame their professional development and transition into practice (see Chapter 16). As nurses grow in their roles and assume the leadership position of charge nurse in their units and participate in the acculturation of other nurses into the profession, the QSEN competencies will remain a constant framework that describes the work of nurses and the expectations for safe, high-quality patient care. The QSEN competencies create a vision for nursing that is meaningful at all levels of practice and can serve as the inspiration, motivation, and purpose for continuing professional development throughout one's career.

END-OF-CHAPTER RESOURCES

KEY CONCEPTS

1. Healthcare quality refers to how well healthcare services for individuals and populations achieve desired health outcomes that are consistent with current professional knowledge and standards (IOM, 2001).
2. Several organizations have significant roles in influencing the quality of care and patient safety; these include the ISMP, NAM, NQF, IHI, TJC, The Leapfrog Group, and HFMA.
3. Data from CMS Hospital Compare provides information on the quality of care provided to patients in hospitals and includes information about patients' experiences (HCAHPS), timely and effective care, complications, readmissions and deaths, use of medical imaging, payment, and value of care.
4. Even though some may consider the United States as the leader in healthcare or in efforts to improve healthcare quality and patient safety, comparative studies by the OECD, the United Kingdom, and The Commonwealth Fund, among others, have consistently found that the United States does not have better healthcare outcomes than other industrialized nations, including countries in Europe, Australia, Canada, and New Zealand (The Commonwealth Fund, 2020; OECD, 2021b).
5. Despite spending more on healthcare, Americans have poor health outcomes, including shorter life expectancy, greater prevalence of chronic conditions, and higher infant mortality rates (The Commonwealth Fund, 2020).
6. Poor U.S. healthcare outcomes do not make sense when you consider the fact that year after year, the United States continues to spend more on healthcare (per capita) than any other country in the world (OECD, 2021a).
7. The majority of hospitals in the United States are required by the CMS to meet TJC accreditation requirements to be reimbursed for care received by Medicare and Medicaid beneficiaries, who represent the majority of hospitalized patients.
8. Nurses are key to ensuring and improving quality of care and safety for patients and families, as well as for the organizations in which they work.
9. The QSEN competencies were a nursing initiative funded by Robert Wood Johnson following the 2003 IOM report, *Health Professions Education: A Bridge to Quality*, where competencies in quality and safety were recommended for all health professions students.
10. All six of the QSEN competencies, that is, PCC, QI, safety, teamwork and collaboration, EBP, and informatics, are integral aspects of nursing clinical practice.
11. Each of the six QSEN competencies has KSA elements that help operationalize each competency for practice.
12. There are quality care and patient safety measures that are used primarily in healthcare organizations, such as hospitals, nursing homes, and outpatient clinics; these include the CMS Core Measures, AHRQ Quality Indicators, AHRQ Patient Safety Indicators, and the NQF and the ANA Nursing Sensitive Indicators.
13. Strategies to reduce unwarranted variation and ensure predictable and favorable patient-care outcomes have proven successful in improving healthcare quality and patient safety; these include developing checklists and other standardized tools, using best practices, working in an organization with a culture of safety, and clear communication when an error does occur.

14. Workarounds may occur when something doesn't work well while nurses are providing care to a patient and they work around the "normal" way of doing things. These workarounds increase the opportunities for inconsistent care and inconsistent outcomes.

15. The U.S.-based Joint Commission has an international component that has established the International Patient Safety Goals that are used worldwide.

16. The Baldrige Health Care Criteria for Performance Excellence has been used by many healthcare organizations to improve quality.

17. The ANCC Magnet Recognition Program awards healthcare organizations that have achieved superior nursing performance and is often referred to as the ultimate credential for high-quality nursing.

18. The QSEN competencies are fundamental components of accreditation standards for nursing programs and are integrated into beginning, intermediate, and advanced level nursing courses.

CRITICAL DISCUSSION POINTS

1. Is all healthcare error preventable? Explain.
2. Are there similarities in the measures of patient safety and the measures of quality of care (Table 1.2)?
3. How do nursing-sensitive indicators help maintain high-quality care?
4. Describe how the safety practices of the individual nurse affect the larger healthcare system.

KEY TERMS

> Adverse event
> Attitude
> Errors
> Healthcare quality
> High-quality care
> Knowledge
> Safety science
> Sentinel events
> Sharp end
> Skill
> Systems Thinking

REVIEW QUESTIONS

Answers to Review Questions appear in the Instructor's Manual. Qualified instructors should request the Instructor's Manual from textbook@springerpub.com.

1. A group of emergency department nurses are asked to develop an action plan to improve the time between when a patient presents with chest pain and when the electrocardiogram is completed. Which of the following would be helpful when working on a QI effort like this? *Select all that apply.*

   A. Identify an interprofessional group of individuals to help review current performance.

B. Compare current hospital emergency department data results to benchmark comparison information reported on a national website.

C. Post current hospital performance data results openly for staff in the nursing lounge.

D. Identify whose fault it is when the electrocardiogram is not being done quickly for patients with chest pain.

E. Create a system to report colleagues that create a delay in electrocardiogram completion.

2. A staff nurse is interested in making QI in the overall care of patients with heart failure. Where would be most helpful to look for data and information to begin work for these improvements?

   A. Explore the IHI website (www.IHI.org), which includes white papers, evidence-based protocols, blogs, and improvement stories that can be applied to patients with heart failure.

   B. Review the National Cancer Institute's website, which includes facts and statistics related to cancer care, resources, and latest research developments.

   C. Review drug companies' websites to see if there are any new medications available to treat heart failure.

   D. Google "heart failure" to see if you can get access to the latest treatment options for this patient population.

3. An 87-year-old patient was admitted to an acute care hospital with an advanced directive that stipulates that the patient not be resuscitated in the event of a cardiac or respiratory arrest. On Day 3 of the patient's hospitalization, the patient experiences a cardiac arrest and a code blue is called. The code blue lasts for an hour. The patient's heart rhythm is restored. When notified of the event, the family is very upset. When the family arrives at the hospital, what should the nurse caring for the patient do?

   A. Apologize, but state that the patient was a full code, which means he must be resuscitated.

   B. Apologize, and assure the family that the attending physician and the nurse manager will be notified they have arrived and will be coming to speak with them.

   C. Notify the family that the advance directive is not legal or binding and that the family needed to tell the nurse specifically that the patient did not want to be resuscitated.

   D. Tell the family to try to focus on the positive, that their family member is still alive.

4. A new graduate nurse is learning what it means to have the hospital accredited by TJC. Which of the following are Joint Commission quality compliance requirements? *Select all that apply.*

   A. Billing models

   B. Core measures

   C. Safe practice measures

   D. Process improvement efforts

   E. Disciplinary standards to address errors

5. Errors in healthcare happen for a multitude of reasons. Which of the following are possible reasons patients might experience a healthcare error? *Select all that apply.*
   A. A patient is misdiagnosed at the time of admission.
   B. Nurses are working with an infusion pump they are unfamiliar with.
   C. The nursing unit is short-staffed for the day.
   D. Staff are fatigued nearing the end of a shift.
   E. Staff adhere to processes as outlined in the policy and procedure manual.

6. What is a common cause of errors within healthcare settings?
   A. Uncaring professionals
   B. Incompetent caregivers
   C. Communication between caregivers
   D. Disorganized processes within the system

7. The nurse is participating in a team meeting with the patient, dietitian, physician, and social worker. The nurse recalls that the patient had expressed that spirituality was important to her. A pastoral care representative is not present and the nurse contacts pastoral care to be included in the meeting. This inclusion is an example of implementing which QSEN competency?
   A. Teamwork and collaboration
   B. Safety
   C. Patient-centered care
   D. Informatics

8. The nurse is caring for a patient with heart failure that is relocating to a different state. The patient has a primary care provider in his new state and intends to follow up as instructed upon discharge. He states he would like to identify an acute care hospital in his new state that is adept in caring for heart failure patients, in the event that he needs to be admitted and asks for a recommendation. Which would be the *best* suggestion to the patient so that he may make a well-informed, objective decision?
   A. Explain that hospitals publicly report their quality data associated with caring for heart failure patients on the Hospital Compare website and instruct him where he can retrieve this information.
   B. Tell him to ask members in the community or family and friends where they have had good experiences and feel safe.
   C. Instruct the patient that he should ask his primary care provider for a recommendation.
   D. Recommend the patient visit the websites of hospitals in the community where he is moving.

9. A medical resident enters a patient's room to complete a physical assessment. The nurse notices that the resident did not wash her hands before entering the room. The nurse gently reminds the resident to use the hand sanitizer before touching the patient. This reminder is an example of meeting which of the following QSEN competencies? *Select all that apply.*
   A. Safety
   B. Quality improvement
   C. Patient-centered care
   D. Teamwork and collaboration
   E. Informatics

10. The primary nurse is caring for a patient admitted to the unit from a nursing home with a Stage III pressure injury. In reviewing the electronic health record, the nurse notes a discrepancy in the patient's wound care procedures and calls the wound care nurse to consult and ensure a consistent plan of care. The wound care nurse assesses the patient and provides the necessary information reflecting the standard of care. The primary nurse is practicing which of the QSEN competencies? *Select all that apply.*

A. Quality improvement
B. Safety
C. Teamwork and collaboration
D. Patient-centered care
E. Informatics
F. Evidence-based practice

REVIEW ACTIVITIES

1. What patient safety challenges do you see in hospitals or in outpatient care sites?
2. Consider how nurses impact patients. Identify the resources available to nurses that help them determine if the work they are doing is effective and if the care they are providing in their unit meets national standards.
3. A patient's family complains to the nurse about the care being rendered to the patient. What strategies framed in the QSEN competencies might a nurse use to address the family's concerns and ensure that the patient is receiving high-quality care?

EXPLORING THE WEB

1. Read through the summary of recommendations for two reports in the Quality Chasm series (go to www.nap.edu/catalog/21895/quality-chasm-series-health-care-quality-reports) and look at the list of recommendations. What is surprising about these recommendations?
2. Access the QSEN website at www.qsen.org. Choose the link to the QSEN competencies and review the KSAs for each competency. Consider how knowledge, skill, and attitude are all required to achieve each competency.
3. Access the Lewis Blackman Story at www.youtube.com/watch?v=Rp3fGp2fv88. Consider how a nurse could have intervened at any point to save Lewis's life. Identify the multiple opportunities throughout Lewis's hospital stay in which a nurse could have spoken up to get Lewis the care he needed.

REFERENCES

Agency for Healthcare Research and Quality. (n.d.). *TeamSTEPPS™ fundamentals course: Module 1. Introduction: Instructor's slides.* https://www.ahrq.gov/teamstepps/instructor/fundamentals/module1/igintro.html

Agency for Healthcare Research and Quality. (2011). *Health care quality still improving slowly, but disparities and gaps in access to care persist, according to new AHRQ reports.* https://archive.ahrq.gov/news/newsletters/patient-safety/66.html

Agency for Healthcare Research and Quality. (2017a). *Inpatient quality indicators.* https://www.qualityindicators.ahrq.gov/modules/iqi_resources.aspx

Agency for Healthcare Research and Quality. (2017b). *Patient safety indicators overview.* https://www.qualityindicators.ahrq.gov/modules/psi_resources.aspx

Agency for Healthcare Research and Quality. (2018). *SOPS hospital database.* https://www.ahrq.gov/professionals/quality-patient-safety/patientsafetyculture/hospital/hosp-reports.html

Agency for Healthcare Research and Quality. (2021). *Patient safety network glossary.* https://psnet.ahrq.gov/glossary

Altman, S. H., Stith Butler, A., & Shern, L. (Eds.). (2015). *Assessing progress on the IOM report* The Future of Nursing. National Academies Press. http://www.nationalacademies.org/hmd/Reports/2015/Assessing-Progress-on-the-IOM-Report-The-Future-of-Nursing.aspx

Altmiller, G. (2019). Content validation of Quality and Safety Education for Nurses (QSEN) pre-licensure clinical evaluation instruments. *Nurse Educator, 44*(3), 118–121. https://doi.org/10.1097/NNE.0000000000000656

Altmiller, G., & Dugan, M. (2021). Content validation of the quality and safety framed clinical evaluation for nurse practitioner students. *Nurse Educator, 46*(3), 159–163. https://doi.org/10.1097/NNE.0000000000000936

American Association of Colleges of Nursing. (2021). *The essentials: Core competencies for professional nursing education.* https://www.aacnnursing.org/Education-Resources/AACN-Essentials

American Nurses Association. (2010). *Nursing-sensitive indicators.* https://nursingandndnqi.weebly.com/ndnqi-indicators.html

American Nurses Credentialing Center. (2021). *Practice standards.* https://www.nursingworld.org/organizational-programs/pathway

American Society for Quality. (2021). *Malcolm Baldrige National Quality Award (MBNQA).* http://asq.org/learn-about-quality/malcolm-baldrige-award/overview/overview.html

Barton, A. J., Armstrong, G., Preheim, G., Gelmon, S. B., & Andrus, L. C. (2009). A national Delphi to determine developmental progression of quality and safety competencies in nursing education. *Nursing Outlook, 57*(6), 313–322. https://doi.org/10.1016/j.outlook.2009.08.003

Centers for Medicare and Medicaid Services. (2008). *Medicare takes new steps to help make your hospital stay safer.* https://www.cms.gov/Newsroom/MediaReleaseDatabase/Fact-sheets/2008-Fact-sheets-items/2008-08-045.html

Centers for Medicare and Medicaid Services. (2017). *Hospital Compare.* https://www.cms.gov/medicare/quality-initiatives-patient-assessment-instruments/hospitalqualityinits/hospitalcompare.html

The Commonwealth Fund. (2020). *International health care system profiles.* https://www.commonwealthfund.org/international-health-policy-center/countries

Cronenwett, L., Sherwood, G., Barnsteiner, J., Disch, J., Johnson, J., Mitchell, P., Sullivan, D. T., & Warren, J. (2007). Quality and Safety Education for Nurses. *Nursing Outlook, 55*(3), 122–131. https://doi.org/10.1016/j.outlook.2007.02.006

Dolansky, M. A., & Moore, S. M. (2013). Quality and Safety Education for Nurses (QSEN): The key is systems thinking. *The Online Journal of Issues in Nursing, 18*(3). http://ojin.nursingworld.org/quality-and-safety-education-for-nurses.html

Gallagher-Ford, L., Thomas, B. K., Connor, L., Sinnott, L., & Melnyk, B. M. (2020). The effects of an intensive evidence-based practice educational and skills building program on EBP competency and attributes. *Worldviews on Evidence-Based Nursing, 17*(1), 71–81. https://doi.org/10.1111/wvn.12397

Greiner, A. C., & Knebel, E. (Eds.). (2003). *Health professions education: A bridge to quality.* National Academies Press. https://www.nap.edu/catalog/10681/health-professions-education-a-bridge-to-quality

Healthcare Financial Management Association. (2021). *The Value Project*. https://www.hfma.org/industry-initiatives/the-value-project.html

Institute of Medicine. (2001). *Crossing the quality chasm: A new health system for the 21st century*. National Academies Press. https://www.ncbi.nlm.nih.gov/books/NBK222274

Institute of Medicine. (2011). *The future of nursing: Leading change, advancing health*. National Academies Press. http://nationalacademies.org/HMD/Reports/2010/The-Future-of-Nursing-Leading-Change-Advancing-Health.aspx

Joint Commission International. (n.d.). *International patient safety goals*. http://www.jointcommissioninternational.org/improve/international-patient-safety-goals

The Joint Commission. (2017). *Initiatives. Transforming care at the bedside*. http://www.ihi.org/Engage/Initiatives/Completed/TCAB/Pages/default.aspx

The Joint Commission. (2021). *International patient safety goals*. https://www.jointcommissioninternational.org/standards/international-patient-safety-goals

Kohn, L. T., Corrigan, J. M., & Donaldson, M. S. (Eds.). (2000). *To err is human: Building a safer health system*. National Academies Press. https://www.nap.edu/read/9728/chapter/1

The Leapfrog Group. (n.d.). *Never events*. http://www.leapfroggroup.org/influencing/never-events

The Leapfrog Group. (2020). *Reports on hospital performance*. https://www.leapfroggroup.org/ratings-reports

Lam, M., Figueroa, J., Feyman, Y., Reimold, K. E., Orav, E. J., & Jha, A. (2018). Association between patient outcomes and accreditation in US hospitals: Observational study. *British Medical Journal, 363*, k4011. https://doi.org/10.1136/bmj.k4011

Makary, M. A., & Daniel, M. (2016). Medical error—the third leading cause of death in the US. *British Medical Journal*, *353*, i2139. https://doi.org/10.1136/bmj.i2139

Merriam-Webster. (2021). merriam-webster.com.

National Quality Forum. (2004). *National voluntary consensus standards for nursing-sensitive care: An initial performance measure set*. Author. https://www.qualityforum.org/Publications/2004/10/National_Voluntary_Consensus_Standards_for_Nursing-Sensitive_Care__An_Initial_Performance_Measure_Set.aspx

Organisation for Economic Co-operation and Development. (2021a). *Health spending 2019*. https://data.oecd.org/healthres/health-spending.htm

Organisation for Economic Co-operation and Development. (2021b). *Infant mortality rates 2019*. https://data.oecd.org/healthstat/infant-mortality-rates.htm

Reason, J. (1990). *Human error*. Cambridge University Press.

Rodziewicz, T., Houseman, B., & Hipskind, J. (2020). Medical error prevention. *StatPearls*. https://www.ncbi.nlm.nih.gov/books/NBK499956

Scoville, R., Little, K., Rakover, J., Luther, K., & Mate, K. (2016). *Sustaining improvement*. IHI White Paper. Institute for Healthcare Improvement. http://www.ihi.org/resources/Pages/IHIWhitePapers/Sustaining-Improvement.aspx

Terge, A. (2014). What is safety science? *Safety Science, 67*, 15–20. https://doi.org/10.1016/j.ssci.2013.07.026

U.S. Food and Drug Administration. (2018). *What we do*. https://www.fda.gov/about-fda/what-we-do

Wakefield, M. K., Williams, D. R., Le Menestrel, S., & Flaubert, J. L. (Eds.). (2021). *The future of nursing 2020–2030: Charting a path to achieve health equity*. National Academies Press. https://doi.org/10.17226/25982

SUGGESTED READINGS

Dekker, S. (2011). *Patient safety: A human factors approach*. CRC Press.

Gawande, A. (2011). *The checklist manifesto: How to get things right*. Picador.

The Joint Commission. (n.d.). *Initiatives. The IHI Triple Aim initiative*. http://www.ihi.org/Engage/Initiatives/TripleAim/Pages/default.aspx

The Joint Commission. (n.d.). *Sentinel event policy and procedures*. https://www.jointcommission.org/sentinel_event_policy_and_procedures

Institute of Medicine. (2001). *Crossing the quality chasm: A new health system for the 21st century*. https://www.nap.edu/catalog/10027/crossing-the-quality-chasm-a-new-health-system-for-the

Kohn, L. T., Corrigan, J. M., & Donaldson, M. S. (Eds.). (2000). *To err Is Human: Building a safer health system*. National Academy Press. https://www.nap.edu/read/9728/chapter/1

Mossialos, E., Wenzl, M., Osborn, R. & Sarnak, D. (Eds.). (2016). *2015 international profiles of health care systems: Australia, Canada, China, Denmark, England, France, Germany, India, Israel, Italy, Japan, The Netherlands, New Zealand, Norway, Singapore, Sweden, Switzerland, and the United States*. The Commonwealth Fund.

Wakefield, M. K., Williams, D. R., Le Menestrel, S., & Flaubert, J. L. (Eds.). (2021). *The future of nursing 2020–2030: Charting a path to achieve health equity*. National Academies Press.

CHAPTER 2

Nurses as Leaders and Managers for Safe, High-Quality Patient Care

Sharon Wallace and Courtney Wallace

"A leader is anyone who takes responsibility for finding the potential in people and processes, and who has the courage to develop that potential."

–Brené Brown, 2018

Upon completion of this chapter, the reader should be able to:

1. Discuss the value of enhancing the leadership skills of nurses at the bedside, who are on the frontline of patient care.
2. Apply leadership and management theories to transform nursing practice to improve care.
3. Compare the roles and education of nurses leading and managing safe, quality care in hospital healthcare settings.
4. Explore what motivates nurses on the frontline of patient care to lead and manage quality improvement.
5. Describe the organizational structure typically found in hospital healthcare settings.
6. Use examples to illustrate how leadership and management influence an organization's culture.
7. Identify major events that mark the advancement of nursing as a profession.
8. Examine why professional nurses take part in a life-long endeavor of professional development and continuing education.
9. Explore local, national, and global nursing organizations to discover the benefits of membership.
10. Identify resources to support innovation for nurses leading change for safe, high-quality patient care.
11. Discuss nursing leadership and management skills for crisis management.

CROSSWALK

This chapter addresses the following:

QSEN Competency: *Patient-Centered Care, Teamwork and Collaboration, Quality Improvement*

The American Association of Colleges of Nursing. (2021). *The essentials: Core competencies for professional nursing education.*

Domain 5: Quality and Safety
Domain 9: Professionalism
Domain 10: Personal, Professional, and Leadership Development

OPENING SCENARIO

Jordan is receiving bedside shift report from Vincent, a new nurse. Vincent is nervous about giving the report in front of the patient. Vincent starts to give report but does not include important information. Jordan notices Vincent is not using the unit bedside shift report tool. Jordan reviews the chart with Vincent and identifies several missed orders and a critical lab value that Vincent did not report to the healthcare provider. Jordan is concerned that other things may have been missed but does not want to give feedback to Vincent in front of the patient. The nurses finish bedside shift report and step out into the hall.

1. What feedback can Jordan give Vincent, the new nurse?
2. What will happen if Jordan does not give Vincent feedback?
3. What can Jordan do to improve bedside shift report for Vincent and the team?

INTRODUCTION

Florence Nightingale is credited with being the founder of modern nursing, but her legacy is much more. Nightingale transformed healthcare by leading in a time of crisis and working to measure and understand how environmental conditions influenced patient outcomes. In the 1800s, Nightingale's work was seen by many as disruptive and innovative. Today the nursing profession considers her work foundational to quality and process improvement. In the words of Nightingale, "for us who nurse, our nursing is a thing, which, unless in it we are making progress every year, every month, every week, take my word for it, we are going back. The more experience we gain, the more progress we can make" (Ulrich, 2020, p. 110).

Progress and change cannot be made without excellent nursing leadership and management. To answer the *Future of Nursing*'s (Institute of Medicine, 2011) clarion call to lead change and to continue in the footsteps of Nightingale to improve quality to influence patient outcomes, more nurses are needed to expand their leadership skills and gain experience leading change. Taking up this leadership challenge may require some nurses to transform their thinking about leading and managing care at the bedside. The first step is to acknowledge that anyone who is responsible for caring for others is a leader (Rigolosi, 2013). The next step is to develop leadership and management skills that demonstrate a powerful shift in mindset, followed by bold actions (Yantis, 2017). Leadership is a core competency of professional nursing practice (American Association of Colleges of Nursing [AACN], 2021). All nurses, no matter the role, have an indispensable role to lead in providing safe, quality patient care.

This chapter will discuss the value of enhancing the leadership skills of nurses at the bedside, on the frontline of patient care. Leadership and management theories to transform nursing practice will be applied to demonstrate how they can improve care. The roles and education of nurses leading and managing in hospital healthcare settings will be described, as will motivations for bedside nurses on the frontline of patient care to lead and manage quality improvement (QI). This chapter introduces readers to the organizational structure of a hospital healthcare setting and explains how nursing leadership and management influence the culture of an organization. Major events that have marked the advancement of nursing as a profession will be explored. Professional nurses need to engage in a life-long endeavor of professional development and continuing education. Membership in professional nursing organizations and reading current literature about changing standards and expectations within the profession of nursing support that need. This chapter will provide direction for foundational nursing leadership and management skills that enhance safe, high-quality patient care in all areas of nursing from bedside care to crisis management.

VALUE OF ENHANCING LEADERSHIP SKILLS OF NURSES AT THE BEDSIDE

Leadership is the ability to motivate a person or persons to achieve common goals. **Management**, in businesses such as healthcare, refers to the structure that maintains an environment so that members of the organization can work to achieve the mission and vision of the organization. Nurses are knowledgeable about barriers to positive patient outcomes; with enhanced clinical leadership skills and strong management skills, nurses can drive QI from the bedside. This calls for nurses to develop a skill set that includes QI processes, data management, and strategies and tactics to lead change (Lacey et al., 2017). Nurses can also enhance their ability to drive QI by learning skills to lead interprofessional teams and facilitate interprofessional training and collaborative QI projects (Baernholdt et al., 2019). Communication is a core competency of nursing practice and leadership and management. The Agency for Healthcare Research and Quality (AHRQ) has developed tools and strategies to enable nurses and other healthcare professionals to create safer, higher quality processes for communication using Team*STEPPS* (2015). These tools are explored in Chapter 7. Learning effective communication strategies is an important leadership skill that all nurses need.

APPLY LEADERSHIP AND MANAGEMENT THEORY TO TRANSFORM NURSING PRACTICE TO IMPROVE CARE

Healthcare is rapidly changing, and the role nursing leadership plays in healthcare is increasingly complex. The term **frontline nurse** is the designation used to describe nurses that provide direct patient care, leading from the bedside. In a hospital healthcare setting, direct responsibility and accountability to patients and families begins with bedside nurses. **Bedside nurses** provide direct patient care; the designation is often used interchangeably with staff nurse or frontline nurse. Direct care positions implement evidence-based practice and create safe transitions across healthcare settings to provide high-quality patient care. Some examples of how these nurses advance the plan of care safely include that they observe policy to identify patients accurately by using two patient identifiers and that they conduct medication reconciliation for every patient, verifying the patient's medication list is complete and accurate without duplication whenever a patient is admitted, transferred, or discharged.

Nurses at the bedside adhere to and promote principles of safety and safe practices to administer medications. They review and clarify healthcare provider orders and use **nursing surveillance,** which is the process to identify threats to safety and quality care such as physiological deterioration and adverse events, including unintended injury, complications, or harm in the hospital healthcare setting (Boamah, 2018). Nurses at the bedside apply universal health literacy precautions to minimize the use of healthcare jargon and facilitate **shared decision-making,** which is a collaborative interprofessional approach to patient- and family-centered care. An example of a health literacy precaution that is frequently used by nurses at the bedside is teach-back. Using teach-back, a nurse can provide important patient teaching and then confirm that the patient and family understand the medical information that has been explained and understand how to implement self-care management to prevent readmission, by having the patient and family teach it back to the nurse. Resources for universal health literacy precautions and teach-back are available from the AHRQ (2014).

To augment leadership and management skills, bedside nurses can develop a systems mindset and make use of systems thinking, discussed in Chapter 3, as well as work to transform care through continuous improvement, both of which are features of management theory (Table 2.1). Bedside nurses must become adept at interpreting cues in the environment and building relationships in the healthcare setting to effectively delegate, collaborate, participate as interprofessional team members, and lead unit-based committees and interprofessional teams in the evolving healthcare environment. They can develop skills in building relationships, which is a key feature of authentic leadership and leadership theory (Table 2.2). A supportive environment for bedside nurses to enhance skills and learn techniques for team-based communication and conflict negotiation can help to build a team-based culture (Meliniotis, 2020).

Nursing leaders, managers, and bedside nurses use leadership and management theory to provide a better understanding of how to implement their roles as leaders and managers and fulfill their responsibilities to themselves, patients, other nurses, other interprofessional

TABLE 2.1 MANAGEMENT THEORY

THEORY	DESCRIPTION	MAJOR THEMES AND DISCUSSION	APPLICATION TO NURSING
Theory X and Theory Y	Contrasting theories based on manager's beliefs about what motivates people; some people are self-motivated to do work, and some are not.	Managers who believe that people have little motivation, dislike their work, and therefore need to be controlled follow the authoritarian, or Theory X, model. These managers are described as "micromanagers." Managers who believe that people have pride in their work, are self-motivated, and enjoy the challenge of the work follow the participative, or Theory Y, model. These managers delegate to their team and provide little oversight.	Nurse managers can use both Theory X and Theory Y depending on the situation but tend to favor one over the other. Theory X may be more useful when quick decisions need to be made, for instance, in a crisis. Theory Y may be used when overseeing a team of experienced nurses who would need little oversight.

(continued)

TABLE 2.1 MANAGEMENT THEORY (*continued*)

THEORY	DESCRIPTION	MAJOR THEMES AND DISCUSSION	APPLICATION TO NURSING
Systems Theory	Describes how different subsystems such as a hospital unit, relate to other subsystems within the larger system in the hospital, such as the radiology or medical records departments.	A complex healthcare system is made up of multiple smaller subsystems, such as departments, service lines, or units. A complex healthcare system has its own culture and climate within and among the different subsystems or units. Feedback allows units to adapt and grow in response to the feedback within and among the different subsystems such as another unit. Harmony within and among the subsystems is not always possible.	Nurse managers utilize systems theory to understand how their patient care unit functions within and among the larger hospital system.
Chaos Theory	Describes how even in chaos, patterns and predictions can be made.	Healthcare environments are prone to chaos. The use of protocols and procedures helps to create order and understanding in a chaotic environment. Small changes can result in significant differences; also known as the butterfly effect.	Nurse managers can use this theory to understand and prepare for the unexpected (chaos) in healthcare, for instance, not knowing what kind of patient will present to the emergency department for care.
Deming's Theory of Management	Organizations can achieve quality through continuous process improvement and transformation.	Healthcare can be transformed by engaging care providers in continual improvement of healthcare processes. Process improvement is achieved by using the PDCA cycle.	Nurse managers can engage staff by using the PDCA cycle to make incremental changes to improve processes and outcomes.

PDCA, plan do check act.

Sources: From Northouse, P. G. (2018). *Introduction to leadership: Concepts and practice* (4th ed.). SAGE Publication; Rigolosi, E. L. M. (2013). *Management and leadership in nursing and health care: An experiential approach* (3rd ed.). Springer Publishing Company; W. Edwards Deming Institute. (n.d.). *Dr. Deming's 14 points for management*. https://deming.org/explore/fourteen-points

TABLE 2.2 LEADERSHIP THEORY

THEORY	DESCRIPTION	MAJOR THEMES AND DISCUSSION	APPLICATION TO NURSING
Trait Leadership	Leaders have certain personal traits or characteristics that influence their ability to lead.	Leaders are born with certain personal traits or characteristics that cannot be taught or developed. Good leaders are often described as having traits such as integrity, empathy, assertiveness, good decision-making skills, and likability. Note that no specific trait nor any combination of traits will guarantee success as a leader.	Nursing leaders have traits or characteristics that are helpful when leading others. These traits may include intelligence, self-confidence, determination, integrity, or sociability. Nurses demonstrate trait leadership when deciding how the team will best accommodate the day's admissions and discharges.
Transactional Leadership	Transactional leaders influence and motivate others by what they offer in exchange (i.e., the transaction).	Transactional leaders use incentives or consequences in transactions to motivate others to change behavior or performance. If incentives are attractive and consequences are undesirable, changes in behaviors or performance can be achieved.	Transactional nursing leaders can motivate others to meet goals by offering incentives such as a more desirable weekend day off for covering a short shift during the week. Transactional nursing leaders can utilize consequences such as disciplinary action for tardiness to motivate people to be on time.
Transformational Leadership	Transformational leaders lead by example and encourage, inspire, and motivate followers to go above and beyond, raising both motivation and morality.	Transformational leaders inspire followers through establishing and sharing clear goals. Transformational leaders gain followers by building relationships, supporting their growth, and allowing for transformation, creativity and innovation. Transformational leaders sustain followers with enthusiasm and passion.	Transformational nursing leaders behave and act in ways they want the team to behave and act. A unit charge nurse demonstrates this by offering assistance with patient care to busy colleagues.

(continued)

TABLE 2.2 LEADERSHIP THEORY (*continued*)

THEORY	DESCRIPTION	MAJOR THEMES AND DISCUSSION	APPLICATION TO NURSING
Lewin's Leadership Styles: Autocratic, Democratic, and Laissez-Faire	Leaders can utilize three different leadership styles with emphasis on the decision-making process of each style (i.e., autocratic, democratic, and laissez-faire).	Autocratic leaders are "hands on" leaders. They make decisions without consulting the team even if the team's input would be helpful. An autocratic style of leadership can lead to low morale and high staff turnover.	Autocratic nursing leadership works well in emergencies when decisions must be made quickly. Nurses may use this style when deciding to call a rapid response.
		Democratic leaders actively seek out and request opinions from the team before making decisions. A democratic style can be ineffective if decisions need to be made quickly.	Democratic nursing leadership works well when there is time to get feedback and team input is important. Nurses may use this style in determining change of shift assignments.
		Laissez-faire leaders are "hands off" leaders; they give the team freedom to manage their work and deadlines. A laissez-faire style is associated with high job satisfaction but may not be the most efficient or effective leadership style.	Laissez-faire nursing leadership works well when the team is highly qualified and motivated. Nurses may use this style in determining a QI project for the unit.
Hersey and Blanchard Situational Leadership	Leaders utilize strategies based on the abilities and motivation of the people they lead in various situations.	People who lack skill and lack motivation need to have clear direction to complete tasks. People who lack skill but are enthusiastic can be encouraged and supported to complete tasks. People who have skill but lack motivation must be encouraged to take a more active role as part of the team to problem-solve or make decisions. People who have skill and are enthusiastic can be delegated tasks.	People's skill level and motivation is different based on each task performed. Nursing leaders can use different approaches in different situations to support people to meet goals and complete tasks.

(*continued*)

TABLE 2.2 LEADERSHIP THEORY (*continued*)

THEORY	DESCRIPTION	MAJOR THEMES AND DISCUSSION	APPLICATION TO NURSING
Authentic Leadership	Authentic leaders motivate people, developing high levels of trust by practicing their values and developing strong relationships.	Authentic leaders are self-aware of their behaviors and how that behavior influences their decision-making. Authentic leaders are described as having high levels of integrity, transparency, reliability, credibility, and compassion.	Nursing leaders are perceived as being authentic and genuinely caring, motivating people and environments to flourish. Authentic leadership is when the charge nurse helps a colleague complete patient care when the colleague is overwhelmed.
Servant Leadership	Servant leaders serve the needs of others and the team before their own needs or the organization's needs.	Servant leaders build trust by focusing on the individual to promote growth both personally and professionally. The individual is committed to the organization because they feel valued by the leader.	Nursing servant leaders do not ask their team to do something they would not do themselves.

QI, quality improvement

Sources: From Northouse, P. G. (2018). *Introduction to leadership: Concepts and practice* (4th ed.). SAGE Publication; Rigolosi, E. L. M. (2013). *Management and leadership in nursing and health care: An experiential approach* (3rd ed.). Springer Publishing Company; Sfantou, D. F., Laliotis, A., Patelarou, A. E., Sifaki-Pistolla, D., Matalliotakis, M., & Patelarou, E. (2017). Importance of leadership style towards quality of care measures in healthcare settings: A systematic review. *Healthcare*, *5*(4), 73. https://doi.org/10.3390/healthcare5040073

team members, and to the profession of nursing. While leadership style significantly effects quality measures in health settings (Sfantou et al., 2017), it is useful to understand that no one leadership or management theory is regarded as the best approach to leadership or management, but transformational leadership has been associated with higher nurse satisfaction and better patient care outcomes (Boamah, 2018; Press Ganey, 2020). **Nurse managers** are nurses who are responsible for controlling part of a healthcare organization, such as one or more patient care units. Transformational leadership by unit-based nurse managers has been found to influence an ethic of care and a culture that enables staff to preserve human dignity in vulnerable patients (Gustafsson & Stenberg, 2017). Healthcare organizations that apply transformational leadership theory create the ideal environment to promote safe patient care, which is attained with high-quality nursing leadership and management across the continuum of nursing and at all levels of the healthcare system.

Theories that approach leadership based on traits (intelligence, self-confidence, determination, integrity, sociability) or style (authoritarian, democratic, laissez-faire) focus on the leader and are described as leader centric (Northouse, 2018). Servant leadership, a contemporary style of leadership, focuses on followers and followership (Northouse, 2018). Followers follow the leader because they believe in the goals of the leader. Leaders may use engagement as a metric to assess followership. Nursing engagement directly correlates with measures of quality, safety, and surveillance capacity by nurses (Press Ganey, 2020).

A positive work culture has been identified as a key component of nurse engagement (Meliniotis, 2020). Leaders need to know if followers are actively engaged or not because without followership, organizational goals cannot be met.

ROLES AND EDUCATION OF NURSES LEADING AND MANAGING QUALITY CARE

Nurses at the bedside as well as nurse managers and administrators are responsible and accountable to lead in providing safe, quality care. Differences in those responsibilities distinguish the professional designation and characterize the roles of each. Education and certification options are associated with each nursing role. Professional designations for nursing roles in the hospital setting include bedside nurse, nurse preceptor, nurse champion, nurse educator, unit charge nurse, clinical nurse leader (CNL), unit-based nurse manager, director of nursing (DON), and **chief nursing officer (CNO)**. Table 2.3 describes the professional designation for nursing roles and education of nurses who are leading and managing safe, quality care. The highest-ranking nurse in the organization is the CNO, who oversees the entire department of nursing and is charged with maintaining standards of care. The CNO operates on the executive level, interacting with other executives that make up the organization's C-suite. The **C-suite** refers to the executive managers of the team. Most common C-suite members include the chief executive officer (CEO), chief operating officer (COO), chief financial officer (CFO), and CNO.

Nurses have several educational avenues to obtain registered nurse (RN) licensure, including diploma education, associate degree, bachelor's degree, and accelerated pathways to a bachelor's or a master's degree. As a professional RN, many nurses can become certified in a specialty. Certification validates that nurses have the knowledge, skills, and attitudes to lead change and manage patient care at the bedside. Many bedside nurses who

TABLE 2.3 ROLES AND EDUCATION OF NURSES LEADING AND MANAGING SAFE QUALITY CARE

NURSES LEADING AND MANAGING SAFE QUALITY CARE	ROLES OF NURSES	EDUCATION AND OPTIONS FOR CERTIFICATION
Bedside Nurse	The bedside nurse is a member of the interprofessional team and uses the nursing process and leadership and management skills to collaborate with the team and all staff to assure the delivery of evidence-based safe, high quality patient- and family-centered care The bedside nurse monitors patient care delivery and cultivates innovative ideas to problem-solve and improve care outcomes. The bedside nurse uses the chain of command and speaks up, as needed, to assure safe, high-quality patient care.	The bedside nurse is eligible for registered nurse licensure by way of diploma education, associate or bachelor's degree, or an accelerated pathway to a bachelor's or master's degree. The bedside nurse has the option to seek specialty certification.

(continued)

TABLE 2.3 ROLES AND EDUCATION OF NURSES LEADING AND MANAGING SAFE QUALITY CARE (*continued*)

NURSES LEADING AND MANAGING SAFE QUALITY CARE	ROLES OF NURSES	EDUCATION AND OPTIONS FOR CERTIFICATION
Nurse Preceptor	The nurse preceptor supports growth and development of new staff and students. The nurse preceptor aids in the transition from nursing education to nursing practice through utilization of the nursing process to determine learning needs, establish goals, and evaluate outcomes; gives timely feedback to new nursing staff; and coaches new nursing staff in critical thinking and leadership to ensure safety and quality.	The nurse preceptor is a licensed registered nurse by way of diploma education, associate or bachelor's degree, or an accelerated pathway to a bachelor's or master's degree. The nurse preceptor usually participates in additional education to precept others and has the option to seek specialty certification.
Nurse Champion	The nurse champion is committed to implementing organizational or unit-based change. The nurse champion is an implementation-related role, held by a nurse internal to the organization, who is knowledgeable of the organization's unique values and culture and works to drive change; this nurse is enthusiastic, personable, and persistent.	The nurse champion is a licensed registered nurse by way of diploma education, associate or bachelor's degree, or an accelerated pathway to a bachelor's or master's degree. The nurse champion assumes a leadership role in QI initiatives and has the option to seek specialty certification.
Nurse Educator	The nurse educator develops, implements, and evaluates staff education. Education can be initial and ongoing and meets annual regulatory training requirements. The nurse educator role may be a unit-based, department based, or system-wide role.	The nurse educator is a licensed registered nurse by way of diploma education, associate or bachelor's degree, or an accelerated pathway to a bachelor's or master's degree. The nurse educator role may require a master's degree in the hospital healthcare setting and other healthcare settings. The nurse educator has the option to seek specialty certification.
Unit Charge Nurse	The unit charge nurse organizes and supports nursing care for the shift within a nursing unit. The unit charge nurse is an experienced unit-based leader with a clear understanding of the organization and serves as a resource to provide real time feedback for nurses and to ensure standards of practice and unit goals are met.	The unit charge nurse is a licensed registered nurse by way of diploma education, associate or bachelor's degree, or an accelerated pathway to a bachelor's or master's degree. The unit charge nurse has the option to seek specialty certification.

(*continued*)

TABLE 2.3 ROLES AND EDUCATION OF NURSES LEADING AND MANAGING SAFE QUALITY CARE (*continued*)

NURSES LEADING AND MANAGING SAFE QUALITY CARE	ROLES OF NURSES	EDUCATION AND OPTIONS FOR CERTIFICATION
Clinical Nurse Leader	The clinical nurse leader focuses on best practices, evidence-based QI, evaluation, and outcomes management at the bedside or point of patient care. The clinical nurse leader may choose to become certified as a CNL.	The clinical nurse leader is a formal leadership role that requires a master's degree. The clinical nurse leader has the option to seek specialty certification. The AACN offers clinical nurse leader (MSN-CNL) certification.
Unit-Based Nurse Manager	The **unit-based nurse manager** usually manages several units in a hospital healthcare setting. The unit-based nurse manager collaborates with hospital leadership and frontline nursing staff to identity priorities and interventions to meet unit, nursing department, and hospital goals. Additional duties include developing unit-specific goals, hiring and managing staff, and planning the unit budget. The unit-based nurse manager uses strategies to support the implementation of interventions for professional development and to provide timely feedback on staff goals.	The unit-based nurse manager is a licensed registered nurse by way of diploma education, associate or bachelor's degree, or an accelerated pathway to a bachelor's or master's degree. The unit-based nurse manager is a formal leadership and management role that usually requires a master's degree. The unit-based nurse manager has the option to seek specialty certification. The AONL offers the CNML certification.
Director of Nursing	The director of nursing oversees all nursing managers and the operations of all nursing units, and uses benchmarks such as the NDNQI* or the HCAHPS† patient satisfaction scores to evaluate patient outcomes and establish hospital-wide nursing goals.	The director of nursing is a licensed registered nurse by way of diploma education, associate or bachelor's degree, or an accelerated pathway to a bachelor's or master's degree. The director of nursing is a formal leadership and management role that usually requires at least a master's degree. The NE-BC certification can be obtained through the ANCC.
Chief Nursing Officer	The chief nursing officer provides vision for nursing across the institution and takes action to join the hospital board of directors and C-suite‡ leadership team to support the development and implementation of an organization-wide patient safety program. This role is ultimately responsible for all facets of nursing care, planning, and budgeting.	The chief nursing officer is a licensed registered nurse by way of diploma education, associate or bachelor's degree, or an accelerated pathway to a bachelor's or master's degree. The chief nursing officer is a formal leadership and management role that usually requires a master's or doctorate degree. The NE-BC and NEA-BC certifications can be obtained through the ANCC.

(*continued*)

TABLE 2.3 ROLES AND EDUCATION OF NURSES LEADING AND MANAGING SAFE QUALITY CARE (*continued*)

NURSES LEADING AND MANAGING SAFE QUALITY CARE	ROLES OF NURSES	EDUCATION AND OPTIONS FOR CERTIFICATION
Assistive Personnel	The assistive personnel assist the bedside nurse to deliver patient- and family-centered care.	The assistive personnel complete training or certification but are not licensed.
Nursing Student	The nursing student delivers patient- and family-centered care using the nursing process. The nursing student is paired with a bedside nurse or nurse preceptor, to provide safe, high-quality care to patients.	The **nursing student** is enrolled in an accredited nursing program and is in good standing at a school of nursing. The nursing student typically enters the hospital healthcare setting during the first clinical nursing course in the program.

AACN, American Association of Colleges of Nursing; ANCC, American Nurses Credentialing Center; AONL, American Organization of Nursing Leadership; CNL, clinical nurse leader; CNML, Certified Nurse Manager and Leader; CNO, Chief Nursing Officer; DON, Director of Nursing; NEBC, Nurse Executive Board Certified; NEA-BC, Nurse Executive Advanced Board Certified; QI, quality improvement.

*National Database of Nursing Quality Indicators (NDNQI): This database was originally developed by the ANA and managed by the University of Kansas School of Nursing. NDNQI was acquired by Press Ganey in 2014.

†Hospital Consumer Assessment of Healthcare Providers and Systems (HCAHPS): A national standardized survey of patients' perspective of hospital care (https://www.cms.gov/Medicare/Quality-Initiatives-Patient-Assessment-Instruments/HospitalQualityInits/HospitalHCAHPS).

‡C-suite refers to the C-suite executives. This term usually refers to high-ranking administrators with a C for chief in the title of the position.

want to demonstrate leadership and management of care in a specialty choose to become certified. Certification is available for 183 specialty areas including medical–surgical, progressive care, critical care, emergency, trauma, pediatric, and geriatric nursing. For a complete list of common nursing certifications and the awarding agency, visit https://nurse.org/articles/nursing-certifications-credentials-list.

To demonstrate leadership and management in a formal role at the bedside, nurses can choose the CNL role. This role was developed by the AACN to improve the quality of patient care outcomes in hospitals and other healthcare settings. AACN offers clinical nurse leader (MSN-CNL) certification. Nurses who want to achieve roles such as nursing professional development (NPD) specialist or nursing informatics specialist, can do so by obtaining a graduate degree specific to the specialty role. These roles are also eligible for specialty certification. The American Nurse Credentialing Center (ANCC) offers these and many other nursing specialty certifications.

Professional designations for nurse leader and manager roles include unit-based nurse manager, DON, and CNO. Education for formal leadership and management nursing roles minimally requires a bachelor's degree in nursing or a master's degree in nursing with a bachelor's in another area. A master's degree is preferred in many formal leadership and management roles. Typical advanced degrees nurse leaders and managers may obtain include master's degrees in nursing administration, nursing management, executive leadership, or health systems management. Certification for this group of leaders and managers can include certified nurse manager and leader (CNML) and certified executive nursing practice (CENP) obtained through the American Organization for Nursing

Leadership (AONL). More information for these certifications is available at www.aonl.org/initiatives/certification. Designations of nurse executive board certified (NE-BC) and nurse executive advanced board certified (NEA-BC) can be obtained through the ANCC with more information available at www.nursingworld.org/our-certifications.

Understanding the relationship between roles, decision-making responsibility, and accountability initially can involve a steep learning curve for new bedside nurses. The same is true for nurses who are new to the charge nurse role, for nurses that change to a new position or nursing specialty, and even for students who are adjusting to new experiences and roles throughout their nursing education. It can be challenging for nurses in new experiences to determine which member(s) of the healthcare team to consult with to make patient care decisions and understand who needs to be informed in different situations. The **RACI Matrix** is a helpful tool that can facilitate understanding the relationships between roles and decision-making (Harned, 2019). RACI is an acronym for Responsible, Accountable, Consulted, and Informed (American Society for Quality, 2016). Table 2.4 illustrates the RACI Matrix for roles and decision-making.

Bedside nurses have direct responsibility and accountability to patients. This responsibility and accountability includes the nurse's role to transform the culture of care so that patient- and family-centered care becomes the norm in the hospital healthcare setting. The goal of patient- and family-centered care is to improve individual health outcomes and provide care that is meaningful and valuable to patients and families. Nurses at the bedside can do this by developing and advancing the plan of care with the patient and family, instead of for the patient and family. Shared decision-making based on a collaborative interprofessional approach is a building block of patient- and family-centered care. Furthering patient- and family-centered care in the hospital healthcare setting requires bedside nurses to improve this process of care. Integrating shared decision-making that includes the patient, family, and interprofessional team into the process of care is necessary for the development of patient- and family-centered care outcomes.

The AHRQ (2014) has developed the SHARE approach to support bedside nurses and interprofessional team members to integrate shared decision-making into the process of care. SHARE is an acronym for Seeking the patient's participation, Helping the patient to explore and compare treatment options, Assessing the patient's values and preferences, Reaching a decision with the patient, and Evaluating the patient's decision (AHRQ, 2014). This five-step process was developed to guide the dialogue between the patient, family, bedside nurse, and interprofessional team. Nurses at the bedside can lead discussion about care using the SHARE approach to engage patients and families and interprofessional team members in shared decision-making. Box 2.1 lists the five steps of the SHARE approach to shared-decision making.

TABLE 2.4 RACI MATRIX FOR ROLES AND DECISION-MAKING

RACI	MATRIX FOR ROLES AND DECISION-MAKING
Responsibility	When responsible, the nurse owns the work, decision, or objective. It is the nurse's responsibility to do what needs to be done. Several people can be jointly responsible for the work.
Accountability	When accountable, the nurse owns the work and must sign off or approve when the work, decision, or objective is completed. The nurse can delegate work according to scope of practice. The nurse who is accountable can also be the nurse who is responsible.
Consulted	When consulted, the nurse or other members of the healthcare team must give input before the work can be started, completed, or accepted.
Informed	Members of the healthcare team who are informed must be kept notified of progress, but they do not need to be consulted.

BOX 2.1 The SHARE Approach to Shared Decision-Making

The SHARE Approach
Five Steps to Shared Decision-Making

1. Seek your patient's participation.
2. Help your patient to explore and compare treatment options.
3. Assess your patient's values and preferences.
4. Reach a decision with your patient.
5. Evaluate your patient's decision.

Sources: From Agency for Healthcare Research and Quality. (2014). *The SHARE approach—essential steps of shared decision making: Quick reference guide.* https://www.ahrq.gov/health-literacy/professional-training/shared-decision/tools/resource-1.html

CASE STUDY

Mr. Ritchie has been hospitalized five times over the last 6 months for heart failure. He tells his nurse he doesn't want to continue to come to the hospital; he is tired of tests and new medications, and he misses his dog. Mr. Ritchie is frustrated and does not know what to do and asks the nurse to help. The nurse recently learned about the SHARE model and wants to develop a patient-centered care plan with Mr. Ritchie.

1. *What healthcare team members should the nurse collaborate with to support the patient?*
2. *What options would the nurse expect to discuss with the team and Mr. Ritchie?*
3. *What evaluation would indicate Mr. Ritchie is satisfied with the care plan?*

When the bedside nurse implements a patient- and family-centered approach to care, the patient's decisions form the plan of care and the quality measures used to assess the patient-centered care outcomes. The bedside nurse assumes accountability that a patient-centered plan of care developed using shared decision-making embodies the values and cultural preferences of the individual person. This approach to care has consistently been part of nursing science and practice (Clarke & Fawcett, 2016). However, the healthcare system is not always aligned with the bedside nurse's responsibility and accountability to the patient even though the bedside nurse is central to the negotiation of care. To be accountable to the patient, the bedside nurse may make an exception to a unit policy or work to change it to support the patient's care decisions and improve the patient's experience. For example, if the patient has identified who is allowed to visit and when the patient would like to have visitors, the nurse at the bedside may honor the patient-centered care plan by working with the unit-based manager and unit leaders to modify unit visiting policy to advocate for the goals of the patient. This decision is an example of clinical leadership from the bedside nurse to create a healing environment for the patient and family. Quality of care is linked to bedside nurses' clinical leadership and the trust developed in the relational style of leadership. Boamah (2018) describes the components of this leadership style as demonstrating idealized influence, supported by inspirational motivation to provide individualized consideration. This mutually beneficial relationship results in the nurse trusting that clinical leadership decisions will be supported by the unit-based nurse manager.

The unit-based nurse manager role is to oversee and coordinate daily operations of one or more units within the hospital healthcare setting to implement the hospital's mission. To accomplish this, the unit-based nurse manager establishes goals for the unit(s) that align with and fulfill the hospital's mission, and measure and evaluate goal attainment. The oversight and coordination elements of the unit-based nurse manager's role include hiring and coaching of personnel, planning the budget and finances, and assuring appropriate resources such as supplies and equipment.

Unit-based nurse managers are charged with developing a yearly expense, revenue, and capital budget for each unit they operate (Johnson & Smith, 2017). The **budget** is an estimate of revenues and expenses for a set amount of time, often annualized. It is balanced by resources and expenditures. Resources are allocated to hospital units to support the unit's goals. Managers strategically align resources to achieve targeted outcomes, aware that clinical outcomes impact unit budgets and unit budgets impact clinical outcomes. The principal resources included in a hospital unit's budget are people, training, equipment, and supplies. It is easy to become familiar with the language used in budgets by comparing it to a personal budget. For example, the unit budget refers to revenue and expenses. In a personal budget, revenue would be a person's income, and expenses would be the debits made by the person to pay for needs such as food and rent. Spending for day-to-day activities is comparable to the unit operating budget, which outlines the funds needed for daily operations. Biweekly and monthly financial reports show the status of the budget. If there is a difference between the estimated and actual cost of the operations, the unit-based nurse manager will develop a variance report which details how to adjust personnel and supplies to attain budget targets across the fiscal year (Johnson & Smith, 2017).

The unit-based nurse manager recognizes the relationships between budgeting, staffing, and promoting patient safety to support quality care outcomes. This may include adjusting the staff and skill mix of assistive personnel and licensed personnel for safety. If the need arises, the unit-based nurse manager may adjust the ratio of novice to expert nurses on a shift to facilitate new nurse orientation to the unit and to ensure support needed to deliver safe patient care. The unit-based nurse manager may allocate resources to support relief for staff to take breaks and have uninterrupted mealtime. Unit-based nurse managers contribute to safety and quality by establishing and upholding policies and procedures based on evidence that create work process standards. Coordinating new staff onboarding and orientation with ongoing staff training and educational requirements can also be part of the role.

The unit-based nurse manager's proximity to the frontline of patient care makes assessing the well-being of staff and taking the pulse of the unit a significant component of this leadership role. They demonstrate skill in the role by listening to what nurses say, as well as what nurses do not say. That active listening allows the unit-based nurse manager to recognize when staff are experiencing change fatigue or burnout or when the work is overwhelming the staff. It is important that the unit-based leadership team, which includes nurse preceptors, nurse champions, nurse educators, unit charge nurses, and the unit-based nurse manager, role model the Quality and Safety Education for Nurses (QSEN) competency of Teamwork and Collaboration, demonstrating respect for the unique attributes that all members bring to the nursing team of each hospital unit.

The role of the CNO is to lead an organization at the highest nursing level. The CNO is responsible for an organization's long-term strategic planning for nursing and its sustainability into the future. The strategic plan developed by the CNO supports the mission, vision, values, and long-term goals of the organization. This nursing leader's role is to inspire a shared vision that motivates nursing managers and leaders as well as the bedside staff members of the entire nursing department to implement the action steps of the strategic plan. The CNO role is responsible to plan hospital-wide budgeting for personnel, supplies, and equipment, and to ensure that nursing units meet the policy, regulatory, and accreditation requirements for nursing patient care services, provide evaluation of staff performance, and participate in continuous QI. CNOs forge collaboration with other services and departments within the organization, as well as outside of the organization.

The CNO's role includes understanding future-oriented trends in healthcare and leadership. Several trends nursing leaders must proactively respond to include the call for nurses to earn advanced degrees and certifications, the need to improve quality of care and the patient experience, the importance of addressing cybersecurity, and the need to create environments that support staff retention. An important future-oriented focus includes developing millennial nurses, generally those born between 1981 and 1994, which is the largest cohort generation of the nursing workforce, and supporting intergenerational team approaches to nursing care (McCarthy, 2020). The leadership of the CNO sometimes is reactive. Leading during uncertain times such as during the COVID-19 pandemic required CNOs to frame that incredibly difficult period for nurses as an unprecedented healthcare event and, during the period that followed, work to promote well-being in nursing leaders, managers, bedside nurses, and assistive personnel. The CNO can support techniques for resilience and strategies to take back control ceded to such unprecedented events. Often this involves supporting staff to access mental health help when needed as a way to develop resilience and manage the anxiety, stress, and depression that can result from feeling powerless.

No one wants to be powerless, yet many people, including nurses, have difficulty with the concept that power is an integral component of a leadership role. Brown (2020) describes how leaders work from different positions of power and identifies four types of power: (a) power over, (b) power with, (c) power to, and (d) power within. Leaders who believe power is finite and protect their power work from a position of power over others. Leaders who work from the positions of power with, power to, and power within believe that power is infinite and therefore they share power with others. Transformational leaders and servant leaders are examples of leadership styles that work from an infinite view of power. Table 2.5 describes the positions of power with bedside nursing examples.

In practice, bedside nurses commonly make use of power with and power to when engaging patients and families in patient-centered care. Nurses use power within when working in healthy work environments to express ideas, suggestions, and concerns. Many nursing units have unit-based nursing councils, led by a bedside nurse. These unit-based

TABLE 2.5 POSITIONS OF POWER AND EXAMPLES OF BEDSIDE NURSING

POWER	EXAMPLE OF NURSES AT THE BEDSIDE USE
Leaders who use power over believe power is finite and use fear to protect and hoard power.	Telling a patient to take medications without explaining them Telling a patient that they must have blood drawn without providing clear and understandable information for why the blood tests are necessary
Leaders who use power with, power to, and power within believe power is infinite and grows when shared with others.	Teaching a patient about their medication when administering them Teaching a patient and family strategies to prevent fall injuries Asking a patient their preference regarding aspects of care

Source: Data from Brown, B. (Host). (2020, October 21). Brené with Joe Biden on empathy, unity, and courage [Audio podcast episode]. In *Unlocking Us With Brené Brown*. Cadence 13. https://brenebrown.com/podcast/brene-with-joe-biden-on-empathy-unity-and-courage

nursing councils provide opportunities for bedside nurses to identify concerns and work toward resolution to improve care. They provide a collective voice for bedside nurses. Nurses at the bedside have the power to lead change and improve quality and safety by voicing concerns, particularly when the concerns are about unsafe practices (Cole et al., 2019). It is vital for nursing leaders and managers to facilitate a culture of safety that supports nurses using their voice and power to improve safety and quality outcomes (Nembhard et al., 2015; Zeng & Xu, 2020). Leaders across the continuum of nursing need to take responsibility to co-create a culture and mindset for patient safety because silence can lead to harm. Transformational and authentic leadership promote trusting relationships between the leader and the follower (Zeng & Xu, 2020), which influence nurses' voice and willingness to report concerns (Nembhard et al., 2015). For example, inadequate staffing is a safety threat and remaining silent could result in a patient receiving improper or incomplete care. Bedside nurses are the closest to the issue of inadequate staffing and need to be proactive in addressing concerns. Issues impacting safe, quality care can be improved by evidence-based nurse-to-patient ratios, increased levels of education for nurses, ensuring unit staff has the proper skill mix, and standardizing transition to practice and nurse residency programs discussed in Chapter 16.

Real World Interview

When I first learned that the hospital administration was working to support the formation of unit-based nursing councils in the hospital, I just knew it was something I wanted to be a part of. Every member of our nursing unit has a voice and something to contribute. A unit-based nursing council provides the opportunity and venue for every member of the nursing unit to share their voice and impact not only our patients' care, but the environment for staff, and the organization's well-being as a whole. I have been researching the literature and attending unit-based council meetings on other units in preparation for our first meeting. We are going to review the unit-based council draft charter which outlines expectations, and then develop some shared goals for our unit-based council. We plan to start small and show the nursing team some successes and then tackle larger issues and processes.

Just as I am preparing to lead the unit-based council, new nurses can prepare to lead at the bedside. I encourage new nurses to come to work prepared with an understanding of your unit's standards of care. Know where to find your resources, policies, protocols, reference documents – and use them! Do not be afraid to ask for help. Have courage and confidence in knowing that you are part of a team and can speak up for safety. And lastly, join your unit-based council to share your ideas for quality improvement. We are all learning together on our journey.

Leah Soto, RN
Unit-Based Council Chair
Progressive Care Unit at Confluence Health, Wenatchee, Washington

MOTIVATING NURSES ON THE FRONTLINE OF PATIENT CARE TO LEAD AND MANAGE QUALITY IMPROVEMENT

Nurses value safety and quality and act to enhance these core values for individual patients, hospital processes, and healthcare systems when they lead and manage QI projects. Bedside nurses may initiate a project for a number of reasons that may include improving some aspect of care to address unmet patient and family needs, addressing an environment determined to be unsafe, or just increasing the efficiency and effectiveness

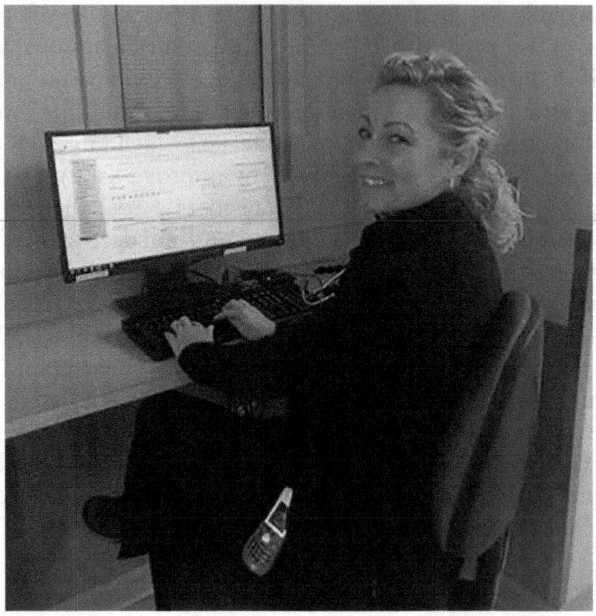

FIGURE 2.1 Leah Soto, RN, Researching Unit-Based Councils.

of nursing practice. The development of the Behavioral Emergency Support Team (BEST) code response (Tommasini et al., 2020) is an example of nurses being motivated by an unsafe environment to initiate a QI project. Frontline nurses in a 400-bed academic medical center collaborated with members of an interprofessional team to manage patient aggression and violent behavior in the workplace. The BEST code response brought resources to the bedside and coordinated an interprofessional response to behavioral emergencies. In its first year, BEST responded to 64 codes and no patient or staff sustained injury (Tommasini et al., 2020). Evaluation of effectiveness indicated the support offered by BEST also decreased staff burnout (Tommasini et al., 2020).

An example of an individual nurse leading change and managing QI is Robin Cogan, a school nurse and an advocate for children and families from an urban school district located in Camden, New Jersey, who implemented a QI project to improve the lives and welfare of school children. So impactful on the social determinants of health was Nurse Cogan's work that she was invited to give testimony about providing quality care to school children at the Summer 2019 *Future of Nursing 2020–2030* meeting (Cogan, 2020). The influence of nurses to affect change is an outcome of leadership. The implementation of focused projects that serve others illustrate nurses' resolve to manage QI, improve patient care outcomes, and lead change in diverse healthcare settings.

ORGANIZATIONAL STRUCTURES IN HOSPITAL HEALTHCARE SETTINGS

The structure of organizations in hospital healthcare settings vary by type, size, and service lines offered. Service lines integrate clinically related conditions and procedures across a system of care such as surgical services or maternal care. The American Hospital Association ([AHA], n.d.) reports that in the United States, 85% (5,198) of hospitals are community hospitals and 10% (616) are non-federal psychiatric hospitals. In addition, 56% (2,937) of community hospitals are not-for-profit, with 25% (1,296) being investor-owned for-profit community hospitals. About two-thirds of community hospitals are

BOX 2.2 Developing Clinical Judgment

Joe, a staff nurse, is having lunch with some other nurses from the cardiac care unit. During the conversation, one of the nurses asks the group if they have noticed an increase in readmissions for heart failure. The nurse reports seeing a few of the same patients' names on the unit bed board coming back in month after month. Two of the patients Joe is assigned have heart failure and were in the hospital earlier this year.

1. What cues might Joe identify in this situation?
2. What hypothesis will Joe consider based on the available information?
3. What other information should Joe gather to determine if readmissions are increasing?
4. Which members of the interprofessional team would have the expertise to address the situation?

system-affiliated or part of a large healthcare system; 65% are located in urban areas and 35% are in rural areas (AHA, n.d.).

Every hospital has a system of governance and all nurses should understand that structure. A hospital organization is typically governed by a board of directors. Members of the hospital board generally have a fiduciary (financial) duty and legal and ethical responsibility to the hospital and the hospital mission. Many hospitals use an organizational chart as a graphic representation of reporting structures within the healthcare organization. Figure 2.2 depicts a hospital organizational chart and reporting structure. In this representation, the reporting structure has five management levels. Staff are not considered management level. The organizational chart includes the board of directors, CEO, CNO, chief information officer, chief financial officer, chief quality officer, chief medical officer, chief operating officer, and chief human resources officer, which are typical high-level management roles within most hospitals. This level is followed by directors, managers, and staff.

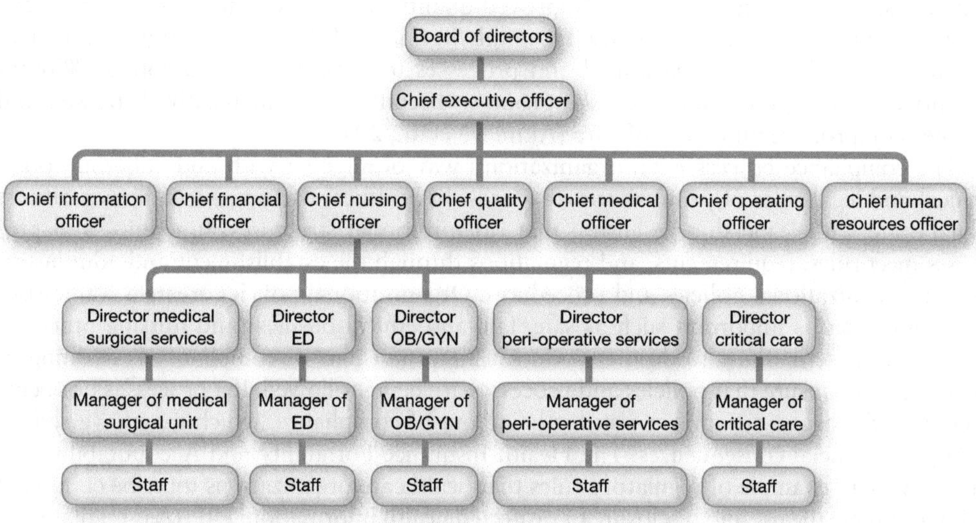

FIGURE 2.2 Example of Organizational Chart.

Hierarchical organizational structures are common and work well for the purposes of clear lines of reporting, responsibility, and accountability. Conversely, hierarchal organizational structures can be slow to make decisions due to the multilevel chain of command. Administrative leaders and managers in organizations with a multilevel chain of command can be perceived as disconnected from the frontline staff. This type of organizational structure often results in work group silos that make it difficult to communicate outside of the hierarchical organizational structure. In nursing, a common reporting structure is for the staff, which can include unit-based clerks, nursing assistant personnel, bedside nurses, nurse preceptors, charge nurses, nurse champion, nurse educator, and CNL, to report to the unit-based nurse manager. The unit-based nurse manager reports to the DON, the DON reports to the CNO, and the CNO reports to the CEO.

The leaders and managers of a hospital healthcare setting engage in strategic planning and goal setting that aligns with the mission and vision of the organization. Strategic planning creates a direction for practice and is proactive in identifying the steps toward goals. The actionable steps needed to reach goals are developed with goal statements, interventions, and timelines for monitoring and evaluation. Actionable steps identify and describe what must be done to achieve the goals. Some common goals that many hospitals have include transitioning to a value-based payment model, compliance, risk management, integration of technology, resource alignment, and investing in QI. Each of these topics will be introduced with a brief description and purpose.

Healthcare is transitioning from a fee-for service model to a value-based payment model. **Fee-for service** provides payment for each service that is rendered. Examples are diagnostic tests such as laboratory samples, x-rays, or office visits. **Value-based purchasing (VBP)** is an incentive program that rewards quality of services provided based on patient outcomes. The incentive of VBP is designed to improve the quality of care and the patient experience. The measures selected to evaluate outcomes of care include mortality and complications, healthcare-associated infections (HAIs), patient safety, patient experience, process, efficiency, and cost reduction (Centers for Medicare and Medicaid Services, 2020). The hospital value-based payment model does not reimburse for poor outcomes, thus linking payment to value and financial incentives to improve outcomes of care (AHA, n.d.).

Akinleye et al. (2019) identified an association between the financial status of hospitals, quality outcomes, and patient safety. Study findings show that financially stable hospitals have better quality and safety outcomes. One reason is that financial stability permits hospitals to allocate resources to develop systems that reliably result in quality outcomes. The VBP model rewards improved quality and safety outcomes with financial incentives which sustain the quality. Hospitals in financial decline typically do not steer resources into developing personnel and processes to improve care outcomes. Without incentive bonuses, these hospitals are prone to become more financially distressed and further compromise outcomes of care (Akinleye et al., 2019).

The compliance process is an organization's way of aligning with and adhering to the ethical and legal rules of professional standards. In healthcare settings, compliance officers collaborate with leadership to ensure that organizational structures, functions, and processes meet rules, requirements, and regulations through the establishment and administration of organizational policies and procedures. Organizational policies create a framework to outline what is important such as safe, fair, and ethical business and nursing practices. Procedures describe how to do the work. An important part of compliance is auditing or monitoring to ensure that policies and processes are being followed. If a process is not being followed, the organization is at risk for being out of compliance, which may have serious safety or financial consequences. The Health Insurance Portability and Accountability Act (HIPAA) is an example of regulatory rules that healthcare organizations must be compliant with to protect the use and disclosure of protected health information. HIPAA is regulated by the Department of Health and Human Services and enforced by the Office for Civil Rights.

Proactive assessment of risk is a complementary process to compliance. Risk management is the process of identifying, assessing, and mitigating risks. Often risk centers around patient and staff safety but can also include financial and business processes. Opportunities for actual or potential risk frequently result in development or review of policy or procedure to define and outline ways to prevent or reduce risk. Bedside nurses need to recognize the financial health of the institution is affected by their work.

Technological advances have significant impacts on compliance and risk management. The use of barcode medication administration has reduced the risk of medication error. Hard stops that prevent a user from proceeding without noting an alert in electronic health records (EHRs) support clinical decision-making while also ensuring compliance and reducing risk. On-screen computer reminders can be used to alert the bedside nurse to unfinished or undocumented care. For example, if a fall risk assessment has not been completed, a practice alert or pop-up will inform the bedside nurse while the nurse is working in the EHR. This simple alert prompts the bedside nurse to complete the screening tool and implement fall prevention protocols to increase safety and prevent a patient fall. Integrating practice alerts into the EHR requires thoughtful planning to minimize the effect of repeated alerts on staff developing alert fatigue (Ancker et al., 2017). Workarounds or informal practices that may develop in response to using EHRs also have the potential to significantly impact compliance and risk management.

CURRENT LITERATURE

CITATION

Driscoll, A., Grant, M. J., Carroll, D., Dalton, S., Deaton, C., Jones, I., Lehwaldt, D., McKee, G., Munyombwe, T., & Asten, F. (2018). The effect of nurse-to-patient ratios on nurse-sensitive patient outcomes in acute specialist units: A systematic review and meta-analysis. *European Journal of Cardiovascular Nursing, 17*(1), 6–22. https://doi.org/10.1177/1474515117721561

DISCUSSION

Driscoll et al. (2018) found that higher levels of bedside nurse staffing have been shown to influence outcomes by decreasing in-hospital mortality. Medication errors, pressure injuries, restraint use, HAIs, and pneumonia decreased as well. The researchers found that outcomes for aspirin use and the number of patients receiving percutaneous coronary intervention (PCI) within 90 minutes of arrival at the hospital, which is the gold standard for PCI, increased with appropriate nurse staffing (Driscoll et al., 2018).

IMPLICATIONS FOR PRACTICE

Findings of this study demonstrate bedside nurse staffing reductions have a negative effect on outcomes and consequently will reduce the hospital's financial stability.

Resources in alignment with the mission contribute to quality outcomes while supporting the financial health of the institution. Resources are misaligned when bedside nurse staffing reductions result in unfinished or missed nursing care. Every level of the organizational chart must have a mindset that equates investing resources in appropriate nurse staffing levels and QI to reduced mortality and improved quality outcomes. Sepsis, a systemic infection, is associated with high mortality and requires prompt intervention. Lasater et al. (2020) found the patient–nurse staffing ratio was associated with improved sepsis outcomes. Findings of the study indicate that it is not enough to implement the sepsis bundle. Implementation of the sepsis bundle must be delivered without delay to impact sepsis care outcomes and save lives, and that relies on bedside nurses. Nursing resources must be aligned to facilitate prompt implementation of the sepsis bundle to reduce mortality and readmission among patients with sepsis (Lasater et al., 2020). Steps needed to improve sepsis care outcomes include standard bedside nurse staffing levels. Administrators must recognize that generating a return on investment and standard bedside nurse staffing levels are not mutually exclusive (Akinleye et al., 2019). Financial performance and QI goals are not likely to increase without accounting for the relationship between bedside nurse staffing levels and quality outcomes.

BOX 2.3 Developing Clinical Judgment

The unit-based nursing council identifies that the personal protective equipment (PPE) worn by staff has been tearing and asks their manager to support a proposal to change a safety protocol related to the equipment. The manager reviews the proposal, agrees the change is needed, and submits the proposal to the safety committee. The safety committee reviews the proposal and decides not to make the change because of budgetary constraints.

1. What cues might the unit-based nursing council members identify?
2. What hypothesis will the members consider based on the available information?
3. What options does the nursing council have in response to this decision?
4. How can the council members and the manager be effective leaders in response to this situation?

LEADERSHIP AND MANAGEMENT INFLUENCE AN ORGANIZATION'S CULTURE

The culture of an organization has a profound influence on safety and quality for nurses and patients. A **culture of safety** is one that generates trust related to transparency of processes, including reporting and learning from unsafe conditions, to pursue safety. Organizations that support a culture are preoccupied with preventing errors and welcome suggestions for improvement from all members. Tenure, data, work environment, and culture have been found to influence nurses' perception of a culture of safety (Nembhard et al., 2015).

Adopting a culture of safety is an underpinning of being a **high-reliability organization,** which is one that experiences fewer than anticipated harmful events despite working in highly complex environments such as healthcare. Comparable to air traffic control towers, high-reliability organizations consistently accomplish complex, high stakes work without causing harm. High-reliability organizations are transparent and focus on processes and systems, have situational awareness, and create a workplace environment that gives deference to frontline expertise (AHRQ, 2019). Leadership is inclusive, collaborative, and responsive. Leaders encourage people to speak out and act when needed to ensure safety.

As discussed earlier, bedside nurses perform complex, high stakes work through their interactions with patients and play an integral role in maintaining a high reliability organization through their vigilant surveillance at the point of care. Nurses' work includes purposeful and ongoing intervention to acquire, interpret, and synthesize data to make clinical decisions that prevent harm. The close proximity of their work at the bedside allows them to identify near miss events, which are errors caught before reaching the patient. Because they are aware of the potential for failure in the complex and dynamic workplace of healthcare, through surveillance, nurses are able to interrupt adverse events when technical and organizational systems fail (Henneman, 2017). By engaging in the practice of surveillance, bedside nurses influence a culture of safety and contribute to the high reliability of the organization.

EVENTS TO MARK THE ADVANCEMENT OF NURSING AS A PROFESSION

The World Health Organization (WHO) designated both 2020 and 2021 the International Year of the Nurse and Midwife. This honor celebrated the 200th anniversary of the birth of Florence Nightingale (1820–1910) but further celebrated the significant role that nurses played during the COVID-19 pandemic that killed over 3.7 million people worldwide at the time of this writing (Our World in Data, 2021). This distinction is a significant acknowledgement of the value of nurses around the globe. The legacy of Nightingale still inspires the development of nursing as a profession. QSEN has reframed the nursing role from being task-oriented to a being a role driven by the knowledge, skills, and attitudes to lead safety and QI from the bedside (Altmiller & Hopkins-Pepe, 2019). The integration of QSEN competencies into nursing education marks another significant step in the development of nursing as a profession. The QSEN competencies are now heavily represented as domains in the AACN *Essentials* (2021), which are the core competencies for nursing education.

In the practice environment, the ANCC Magnet Recognition Program® speaks to the value of the nursing profession. **Magnet status** is granted by the ANCC to hospitals that have exemplary nursing care based on criteria to ensure excellent patient outcomes and high job satisfaction.

The Magnet Recognition Program influences an organizations' leadership and culture to commit to nursing excellence and align nursing goals to improve patient outcomes. More on the Magnet Recognition Program is described in Chapter 1.

An essential component of Magnet status is that hospitals have an effective shared governance structure. **Shared governance** is a practice model designed to integrate core values of nursing as a means to achieve quality care (Anthony, 2004). Through this model, bedside nurses are empowered to be involved in decision-making over their practice. In a shared governance structure, every nursing discipline across the hospital is represented by bedside nurses from that discipline in organized councils that have a role in the organization's power structure. This representation gives voice to nursing in regards to all facets of nursing work.

Nurses serving on boards is another significant marker in the advancement of nursing as a profession. The American Association of Retired Persons (AARP), the Nurses on Boards Coalition (NOBC), and the Robert Wood Johnson Foundation collaborated to advance nurse leadership on boards to raise the leadership voices of nurses. The goal to have nurses fill 10,000 board seats was reached in 2020, giving voice to the unique perspective of nurses in the work to achieve more effective and efficient healthcare systems. This is a significant accomplishment toward quality and safety because nurses are well suited to serve on boards and advocate for the needs of patients (Harper & Benson, 2019) and evidence indicates quality and safety measures decline when clinicians do not serve on boards (Satiani & Prakash, 2016).

Real World Interview

Nursing has come a long way from the original iteration of the bedside nurse. Nursing has evolved to differentiate itself from medicine, to stand on its own as both an art and a science. Looking forward, nursing has come full circle back to Florence Nightingale to influence the healthcare industry and examine environmental factors that affect quality and safety. One thing that has not changed, however, is the nursing process of assessment, diagnosis, outcomes/planning, implementation, and evaluation. The nursing process has guided me as a bedside nurse, as a nurse manager, and now as a board member of a public district community hospital. I never pictured myself as a politician, yet I saw an oppor-

tunity. The board did not have one healthcare member guiding decisions of the hospital. I felt like I had a responsibility to the community and had to offer my knowledge and skills. While there certainly has been a lot of learning along the way about governance, my background as a nurse has helped me to ask the right questions and to assess the needs of the hospital and the district. We have spent the last several years as a board educating ourselves about new ways of thinking of quality and safety. We have taken the conversation from reviewing data to systems evaluations. We are connecting what our job is with what everyone else is doing in the organization. We look to them for feedback. Nurses specifically have a collective voice that can draw attention to improvements needed for safe patient care and quality outcomes. I would encourage any, and all, nurses to find and use their voice. Leaders are listening.

Mary Murphy, EdD, BSN, RN
Vice Chair, Commissioner
Lake Chelan Health, Chelan, Washington

PROFESSIONAL DEVELOPMENT AND EDUCATION IS A LIFE-LONG ENDEAVOR

The clinical environment is constantly changing and so is our understanding of it. Data from the 2018 National Sample Survey of Registered Nurses (NSSRN) shows those involved in nursing are more diverse and better educated than 10 years ago (Brassard, 2020). Nurses are seeking a higher level of competence and want to make progress, becoming more aware of others' cultures to develop cultural sensitivity (Carr & Knutson, 2015). Bedside nurses who want to have a career that is varied or who want to travel prepare for change and stay current with new software, technology, hardware, and medications (Ausmed, 2020). Specialty certification is another way to stay current and improve knowledge, skills, and patient outcomes (Halm, 2021). Halm suggests that future research in this area focus on the "dose" or the percent of certified bedside nurses needed on a given nursing unit to identify the link between specialty certification and outcomes, as well as specialty certification and reduction of harm. Improved self-rated health later in life is another reason to pursue life-long learning. Yamashita et al. (2019) suggest that life-long learning should be included as a health-promoting factor. This was supported by study findings that indicate that although formal education is a strong social determinant of health, participation in life-long learning can reduce the effect of this relationship (Yamashita et al., 2019).

BENEFITS OF MEMBERSHIP IN NURSING ORGANIZATIONS

Professional nursing organizations are dedicated to the development of members and advancing the nursing profession as a whole. Through membership, nurses are provided ongoing opportunities for continuing education, certification, research, scholarships, collaboration, and a platform for representation. Local, national, and international and global professional nursing organizations host annual meetings and conferences with opportunities for networking. Many publish their own peer-reviewed journal to provide specialty-specific research, evidence-based practice, and professional information for members, providing access to experts and mentors in specialty areas and offering career advice and assistance.

The largest professional nursing organization in the United States, the American Nurses Association (ANA), is the principal professional nursing organization that represents the nation's 4 million registered nurses. The ANA advocates for nurses and the public and focuses primarily on the career development of nurses. Two professional organizations shaping the future of nursing education are the AACN and the National League for Nursing (NLN). These organizations provide standards and support accreditation for nursing education programs across the nation. The National Student Nurse Association (NSNA) is the first professional nursing organization many student nurses join and is supported by students and nursing faculty alike. Sigma Theta Tau International is the honor society of the nursing profession. It is active in more than 90 countries and supports the scholarship of nurses around the globe. The American Association of Critical-Care Nurses works to facilitate the work of nurses working in critical care roles. The organization is a champion in promoting healthy work environments for patients, nurses, and the healthcare team through evidence-based standards for a healthy work environment. These standards include skilled communication, true collaboration, effective decision-making, appropriate staffing, meaningful recognition, and authentic leadership (AACN, 2020). The American Organization for Nursing Leadership is a national professional organization with a mission and vision to shape healthcare through innovative and expert nursing leadership. Many of their members participate in conferences and development workshops to enhance leadership skills and share ideas and strategies with other leaders working to advance health in their own institutions.

LEARNING SYSTEMS AND INNOVATION FOR SAFE, HIGH-QUALITY PATIENT CARE

In healthcare, the best nursing leadership is needed at every level to bring together the top-down approach and bottom-up approach to lead QI. This distributed approach to leadership presents an opportunity to bring together vision and action from both bedside caregivers and nurse administrators to transform the outcomes of care (Harvey, 2020). Bringing the top and bottom together will enable bedside nurses to create a better system to achieve better outcomes (Godin, 2018).

Becoming a **learning system** that learns from adverse event reporting as a way to optimize performance and deliver greater value through focusing on continual improvement, innovation, quality, and safety improves the patient experience. Learning systems do not measure safety and quality with the goal of compliance to hinder innovation, nor does measurement and compliance change practice (McCormack, 2017). Instead, learning systems aggregate, measure, and share information to learn from clinical practice and identify clinical risk to improve systems (Cross, 2018).

The Center for Care Innovation and Transformation, established by the AONL, offers resources for nurses who want to transform care at the bedside or transform the culture of care (AONL, n.d.). Today's complex healthcare challenges need innovative solutions. Rebecca Love (TEDx Talks, 2018) points out that nurses are natural innovators who, on average, develop 27 workarounds each shift. The ANA and Johnson & Johnson founded *See You Now*, an innovation podcast to highlight the work of nurses who are changing the future of healthcare with innovative ideas, processes, and protocols to improve quality.

Nightingale was innovative in her quest to improve quality and save lives. So was the 1950 nurse inventor of neonatal phototherapy, Sister Jean Ward (Cosier, 2017). Elise Sorenson was the nurse inventor of the ostomy bag in 1954. Anita Dorr, another nurse innovator, developed the crash cart in 1968 (Cosier, 2017). Fast forward to the year 2021. Brian Mohika, another innovator, has invented CathWear, underwear for patients with catheters and leg bags (Wofford, 2021).

Innovation centers are emerging in hospitals and health systems to find solutions to challenges in healthcare and support the innovative ideas of clinicians, scientists, and employees. Although research findings show that innovation centers have different structures and purposes, they share certain characteristics that include collaborative spaces, flattened hierarchies, a diverse pool of expertise and experience, interprofessional partnerships, and boundary spanning (Cresswell et al., 2020). Boundary spanning describes the roles of individuals who cross boundaries within and across organizations. Nurse innovators Andrea Jordan and Andrew Bell crossed boundaries to collaborate with engineers and developed novel devices to meet unmet patient needs by designing an assistive handset device to fit with a patient-controlled analgesia pump and user friendly pediatric anal dilators for young children who had anoplasty surgery for Hirschsprung's disease (Andrews et al., 2020). These bedside nurses saw a need and met it with innovative thinking that changed nursing care to improve the experience for patients, proving that disruptive innovation comes from the ground up (Chowdhury, 2012).

LEADERSHIP AND MANAGEMENT SKILLS TRANSFER TO CRISIS MANAGEMENT

Leaders at every level of an organization are tested during crisis. The COVID-19 pandemic exposed significant gaps in the pandemic preparedness of the United States. The U.S. response to the COVID-19 pandemic was characterized by chaos and uncertainty. This response exacerbated healthcare's challenges to contain transmission of a novel virus, determine best practices for treatment, and protect essential workers–all without a roadmap. The U.S. federal government was unable to deliver an adequate supply of PPE to safeguard its workforce. More unexpected events occurred when healthcare workers confronted the first pandemic surge in the United States. The usual strategies for infectious disease containment–hygienic practices, social distancing (Figure 2.3), travel restrictions, and quarantine—were implemented by states in patchwork fashion or were resisted by segments of the public (Gostin et al., 2020). Disinformation and distrust of experts became an obstacle to controlling the transmission of COVID-19. The effectiveness of the disinformation campaign to persuade people against wearing face masks was staggering. In July 2020, Gallup revealed only 44% of Americans indicated they always wore a mask outside their home (Brenan, 2020). Gallup completed this survey at the same time COVID-19 cases were surging in several states.

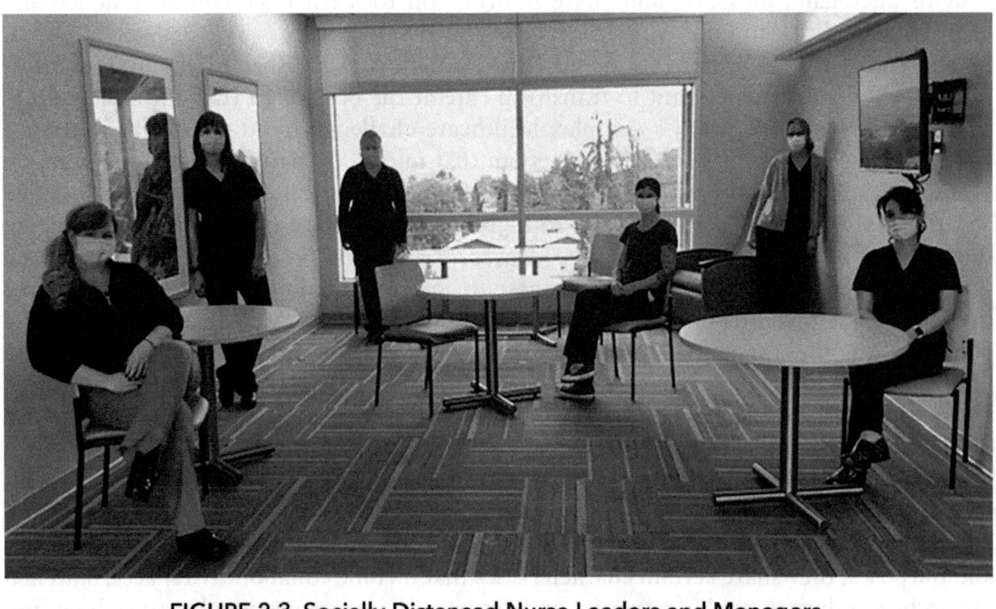

FIGURE 2.3 Socially Distanced Nurse Leaders and Managers.

Forster et al. (2020) describe the COVID-19 pandemic as an administrative code blue. Navigating this type of turbulent environment requires the adaptive thinking of nursing leaders and managers to engender trust during organizational crisis and chaotic times. Transparency and prioritizing the safety and well-being of staff are essential behaviors and skills when leading and managing during disaster. Transparent communication precedes trust and supports open dialogue between leaders, managers, and nurses at the bedside. It is crucial for nurse managers to be visible on nursing units and for them to listen to staff. Throughout the pandemic, volumes of information and rapidly changing conditions had to be interpreted in short spans of time, creating the need for more frequent communication (Scherer, 2020). Listening to staff concerns and conveying empathy about the effect of policy and protocol frequently changing, and the unexpected circumstances staff experienced due to the pandemic, helped nurse managers know what support nurses needed to accomplish the work and be able to care for patients and self. Staff shortages coexisted with staff furloughs when elective procedures and chronic illness care was shut down, absent of a strategy to reassign or cross-train staff. Chronic hospital understaffing and inability to meet surge capacity exacted a toll on staff well-being and hindered the pandemic response efforts (Lasater et al., 2021).

At most hospitals, a dedicated unit was established to convert a shared space between the ICU and the progressive care unit (PCU) to cohort patients with COVID-19. The ICU and PCU nurse managers would co-manage the COVID-19 unit and implement a team-based surge staffing model. Rapid cycle orientation to the team model introduced the ICU and PCU staff to nursing skills for non-ICU nurses in a team nursing model, meaning an ICU nurse might be paired with two PCU nurses to care for a group of COVID-19 patients. Several PCU staff also cross-trained to the ICU. To facilitate communication and teamwork, each shift needed to start with a COVID-19 huddle. Nurses at the bedside would assume the role of huddle leaders and developed a huddle checklist to standardize the process. COVID-19 huddle leaders would introduce team members by name and devise teams to align patient needs with nurse competencies.

Within a short time after the first pandemic surge, bedside nurses started to innovate care delivery with rapid-cycle QI. Hospitals across the country shared ideas and strategies for managing the crisis and supporting frontline staff. Improvements were initiated for team nursing orientation, cross-training, communication, resources, and equipment. Safety and workflow solutions developed organically as nurses were able to draw upon the benefit of experience, gained at the bedside in the shared COVID-19 unit. Redesign included building a medication room in the hallway of the COVID-19 units. Nurses at the bedside used continuous process improvement to optimize function and eliminate waste. The hallway medication room redesign facilitated easy access to equipment and reduced the number of steps bedside nurses had to take to obtain a patient's medications, respiratory care supplies, and a select supply of patient care items (T. Holder, personal communication, September 12, 2020).

When new challenges emerged on the COVID-19 unit, bedside nurses took the lead to problem-solve. For instance, after the bedside nurse would don PPE and entered a patient's room, it was difficult to communicate with the healthcare team outside the patient's room. The power to fix this challenge came from within for bedside nurses. The nurses who set out to resolve this issue discovered a way to preserve PPE and communicate a patient's vital signs and proning schedules (turning patients in prone position to improve breathing) by using a dry erase marker to write on the window glass in the wall of the patient's room. Extension tubing sets for intravenous infusions were used to position infusion pumps outside of patient rooms in the COVID-19 unit. This innovation reduced the frequency of the nurse's exposure, preserved PPE, and facilitated administration and surveillance of intravenous medication infusions. Bedside nurses continued to track changes and implement updates to the plan, process, policy, and procedures with each COVID-19 surge.

Early lessons from the pandemic reveal that to respond more effectively, administrative leaders and CNLs must increase their knowledge of emergency preparedness and disaster response (Veenema et al., 2020). Nurses must be informed of the legal and ethical elements of decision-making in disaster, including crisis standards of care (ANA, n.d.). **Crisis standards of care** are the significant changes in operations or ability to provide the established level of care because of a catastrophic or emergency event such as a pandemic or earthquake. These were established to provide a framework in the event healthcare systems experience a substantial change to usual operations during disaster. Demand is defined by surge capacity, which includes conventional, contingent, or crisis situations, and need for a corresponding level of space, staff, and supplies (Watkins, 2020). The conventional capacity is consistent with daily operations. Contingent capacity indicates space, staff, and supplies are not consistent with daily operations, but can be adapted short term to provide care equivalent to the usual level. Crisis capacity occurs when space, staff, and supplies that have been adapted are not consistent with the usual level of care and circumstances of the disaster require a significant adjustment to the usual level of care consistent with crisis standards. Decision-making in crisis is guided by ethical principles to appropriate use and distribution of available resources. Duty to care, transparency, consistency, and accountability are examples of these principles (Watkins, 2020).

The COVID-19 pandemic has served to highlight the leadership of women. Data supported that women leading countries performed better than men leading countries in this crisis (Cuthbertson, 2020). Anecdotal support reported in the popular press suggests that better outcomes have been associated with proactive policies and clear communication. Another explanation offered is that women have a trust advantage; research shows that women take a relational approach to leadership (Post et al., 2019). The relational behaviors women use to anticipate and manage emotion elicit trust.

Recognizing how a pandemic unfolds helps leaders and managers to anticipate points in time when staff are most vulnerable to physical and psychological distress (Medical Association of Georgia, 2020). It is when the demands of the pandemic are dwindling that the psychological and physical impact of grief, mourning, exhaustion, and posttraumatic stress disorder are likely to come about for healthcare workers (Medical Association of Georgia, 2020).

Nurses must reliably care for themselves during a crisis. Nurses must realize that self-care is not a separate task from their everyday work; it is how they must do their work (MobLab Team, 2018). Nurse leaders are positioned to support and sustain the healthcare workforce by establishing a multidisciplinary pandemic resilience task force to identify and implement new practices for COVID-19 and for future disasters (Medical Association of Georgia, 2020). Unit-based nurse managers can accelerate development of resilience by identifying nurse champions to connect with bedside nurses at the frontline and share resilience strategies. Creating a culture of care and modeling it allows people to be mindful of collective wellbeing, and their own well-being (MobLab Team, 2018). Nurses in the video, *Philadelphia Nurses Go Viral Dancing to Ciara's 'Level Up'* (www.youtube.com/watch?v=SKdCfWYSj4I) model self-care and resilience strategies. The video of nurses from a Philadelphia hospital reveals a culture of caring and collective well-being. In a presentation delivered in 2021, Dr. Tachibana, senior vice president of quality and safety, and CNO of a leading healthcare system in the Pacific Northwest, shared 15 lessons learned while leading the COVID-19 pandemic response. In lesson #12, Dr. Tachibana affirmed self-care is not self-indulgence, it is vital (Tachibana, 2021). Moreover, self-care is how nurses level up to care for a nation in crisis. The COVID-19 pandemic demonstrated to the world the ability of bedside nurses to transfer their everyday leadership skills to meet the challenges of, and turn the tide on, a devastating world-wide disaster.

CASE STUDY

Identify a leadership or management theory that can be used during a crisis.

1. *Describe how leadership and management theory apply to crisis management.*
2. *How might a bedside nurse use leadership and management theory during a crisis?*
3. *How might a nurse manager use leadership and management theory during a crisis?*

END-OF-CHAPTER RESOURCES

KEY CONCEPTS

1. Bedside nurses are vital to safe quality care. Enhancing the skill set of bedside nurses will drive QI and increase safety.
2. Frontline nurses can apply leadership and management theory to improve the safety and quality of care.
3. Bedside nurses use surveillance to identify threats to safety and quality care such as physiological deterioration and adverse events, unintended injury, complications, or harm in the hospital healthcare setting.
4. The educational backgrounds of nurses and their roles vary, but all nurses have an important role to lead and manage quality care.
5. Nursing leaders, managers, and bedside nurses use leadership and management theory to provide a better understanding of how to implement their roles as leaders and managers and fulfill their responsibilities to themselves, patients, other nurses, other interprofessional team members, and to the profession of nursing.
6. Leaders and managers take part in strategic planning and goal setting to align these with the mission and the vision of the organization.
7. The culture of an organization impacts safety and quality. Inclusive, collaborative leadership is associated with healthy workplace environments.
8. Unit-based nursing councils provide an opportunity for bedside nurses to identify concerns and work toward resolution to improve care by providing a collective voice for bedside nurses.
9. Nursing continues to develop as a profession, with a notable shift to a role driven by knowledge, skills, and attitudes, that lead to improving patient outcomes at the bedside.
10. Improvement in care has been driven by value-based purchasing which rewards quality by providing hospitals reimbursement based on outcomes.
11. All nurses should understand the system of governance at their hospital.
12. Nurses become life-long learners as a natural consequence of a highly complex healthcare environment that is constantly changing.
13. Nursing organizations offer a myriad of opportunities to network, enhance professional development, and connect with a mentor.
14. Current thinking suggests innovative thinking and learning systems are required to build a better healthcare system. Disruptive innovation is likely to come from nurses at the bedside.
15. Transparent communication, open dialogue, presence on the unit, listening to learn from frontline staff, and having empathy are transferable skills for nurses who are leading and managing during crisis.

CRITICAL DISCUSSION POINTS

1. How does the culture of an organization or unit influence quality and safety outcomes?
2. Consider the position of a unit-based nurse educator. Write three SMART goals for a workshop the unit-based nurse educator is teaching for preceptors focusing on mentoring new staff and students about quality and safety.
3. VBP strategies improve quality and safety?

4. Managers are accountable to the budgets of their departments. Is there a time when it is acceptable to sacrifice quality and safety for budgetary reasons?
5. Compare and contrast how the charge nurse and bedside nurse would utilize resources, policies, protocols, and reference documents.
6. How is the health of a community impacted when a nurse serves on an advisory board in the community?

KEY TERMS

- Bedside nurses
- Budget
- C-suite
- Chief nursing officer
- Crisis standards of care
- Culture of safety
- Fee-for-service model
- Frontline nurse
- High-reliability organization
- Leadership
- Learning systems
- Magnet status
- Management
- Nurse managers
- Nursing surveillance
- RACI matrix
- Shared decision-making
- Shared governance
- Value-based purchasing

REVIEW QUESTIONS

Answers to Review Questions appear in the Instructor's Manual. Qualified instructors should request the Instructor's Manual from textbook@springerpub.com.

1. The unit-based nurse manager motivates the team by exchanging rewards for performance outcomes. This is a characteristic of which type of leader?
   A. Transformational leader
   B. Transactional leader
   C. Servant leader
   D. Trait leader
2. Juan is a new nurse manager of a pediatric unit. He wants to learn more about leadership and management by attending a strategic planning workshop. Which of the following are part of the strategic planning process? *Select all that apply*.
   A. Developing long-term goals
   B. Reviewing the mission and vision
   C. Reviewing the budget
   D. Researching ways to achieve the goals
   E. Identifying organizational values

3. Heather is a nurse on the medical unit. She notices that staff used to quickly respond to bed alarms to prevent patient falls but now they just casually walk to the alarm. Heather recognizes this could impact patient safety. Identify actions Heather can take to help prevent falls in this scenario. *Select all that apply.*

   A. Model the behaviors she desires to see in her peers.

   B. Report staff behavior to the unit-based nurse manager.

   C. Join the fall prevention committee to learn more about fall prevention.

   D. Speak to staff individually to identify and understand drivers for the behavior.

   E. Try to answer all the bed alarms herself.

4. Mary is a nurse manager on a busy unit. She notices that the patient satisfaction scores have been decreasing over the last several months. She decides to make a plan to improve the scores. Which of the following actions should Mary take as a first step?

   A. Seek help from her nursing director.

   B. Ignore the issue; it will resolve on its own.

   C. Develop a plan to improve the scores.

   D. Discuss the concerns at a staff meeting.

5. Some managers are leaders but not all leaders are managers. Which of the following qualities are associated with leaders? *Select all that apply.*

   A. Help develop solutions to problems.

   B. Inspire the team.

   C. Provide discipline.

   D. Provide feedback.

   E. Approve timecards.

6. In response to staffing shortages, a manager has been hiring outside agency nurses to prevent the unit from not having enough nurses to care for the patients. Staff nurses on the unit council are concerned that the increased number of outside agency staff that are not familiar with unit policies is putting patient safety at risk. Which of the following actions should members of the unit council take as a first step?

   A. Develop educational programs to assist the outside agency nurses.

   B. Supply the outside agency nurses with the unit safety policy.

   C. Seek help from the unit-based nurse manager.

   D. Conduct chart reviews of the patients of outside agency nurses to assess safety behaviors.

7. Bedside nurses are working on a project to improve bedside report with a checklist. Which of the following is a simple but effective way for them to gain the support of team members?

   A. Threaten that they will be disciplined by the manager if they don't participate.

   B. Ask for support for the project because it will improve patient safety.

   C. Mandate that bedside report is the way report will be given.

   D. Ignore the team and go directly to the unit-based nurse manager to have it approved as policy.

8. Nursing surveillance refers to the bedside nurse's ability to do which of the following?
   A. Observe colleagues as they work to ensure they are doing things correctly.
   B. Identify threats to the patient's safety and quality care such as deteriorating status.
   C. Maintain a healthy work environment by identifying threatening patient visitors.
   D. Review policies to ensure they are being followed by staff and achieving positive outcomes.
9. A group of bedside nurses in a cardiac unit are self-motivated and active participants in the governance of the unit. More than half serve on the unit council. They work as a unit to cover staffing shortages and a third of them are certified in their specialty. Which of the following management theories would be the best fit with this group?
   A. Theory X
   B. Systems theory
   C. Theory Y
   D. Deming's theory of management
10. A bedside nurse is seeking to learn more about the nursing unit and understand the policies that guide the falls prevention effort on the unit. The nurse attends hospital-sponsored continuing education and completes the requirements for leading the efforts. On the unit, the nurse serves as a mentor regarding falls prevention and provides guidance to peers. Which role best describes the role of this staff nurse?
   A. Clinical nurse leader
   B. Nurse champion
   C. Unit charge nurse
   D. Nurse preceptor

REVIEW ACTIVITIES

1. How does innovation improve quality and safety?
2. Consider how staffing shortages impact patient and staff safety. Identify risks to patients and staff when staffing shortages occur.
3. A bedside nurse wants to assume a greater role in the leadership of the unit. What strategies might the nurse use?

EXPLORING THE WEB

1. View this short video clip: www.youtube.com/watch?v=VJAwy3krWzQ (2.09 minutes) to hear why nurses become certified. Investigate how many nurses hold one or more certifications from the AACN. What would it take to achieve this goal? What leadership and management skills are needed for specialty certification?
2. Explore the Florence Nightingale Museum website at www.florence-nightingale.co.uk. Identify several quality and safety strategies that are still used today.
3. View the video: *Shirtless Dancing Guy* at www.ted.com/talks/derek_sivers_how_to_start_a_movement?language=en. In 3 minutes, Sivers narrates the video to describe the relationship between the dance leader and the first follower of this impromptu dance. How do the roles of leader and first follower apply in nursing?

A robust set of instructor resources designed to supplement this text is located at **http://connect.springerpub.com/content/book/978-0-8261-6145-1.** Qualifying instructors may request access by emailing **textbook@springerpub.com.**

REFERENCES

Agency for Healthcare Research and Quality. (2014). *The SHARE approach—essential steps of shared decision making: Quick reference guide*. https://www.ahrq.gov/health-literacy/professional-training/shared-decision/tools/resource-1.html

Agency for Healthcare Research and Quality. (2015). *About TeamSTEPPS®*. https://www.ahrq.gov/teamstepps/about-teamstepps/index.html

Agency for Healthcare Research and Quality. (2019b). *Patient safety primer. High reliability*. Patient Safety Network. https://psnet.ahrq.gov/primer/high-reliability

Akinleye, D. D., McNutt, L., Lazariu, V., & McLaughlin, C. C. (2019). Correlation between hospital finances and quality and safety of patient care. *PloS One, 14*(8), Article e0219124. https://doi.org/10.1371/journal.pone.0219124

Altmiller, G., & Hopkins-Pepe, L. (2019). Why quality and safety education for nurses matters in practice. *The Journal of Continuing Education in Nursing, 50*(5), 199–200. https://doi.org/10.3928/00220124-20190416-04

American Association of Colleges of Nursing. (2021). *The essentials: Core competencies for professional nursing education*. https://www.aacnnursing.org/Education-Resources/AACN-Essentials

American Association of Critical-Care Nurses. (n.d.). *Healthy work environments*. https://www.aacn.org/nursing-excellence/healthy-work-environments

American Hospital Association. (n.d.). *Current and emerging payment models*. https://www.aha.org/advocacy/current-and-emerging-payment-models

American Nurses Association. (n.d.). *Crisis standards of care: COVID-19 pandemic*. https://www.nursingworld.org/~496044/globalassets/practiceandpolicy/work-environment/health--safety/coronavirus/crisis-standards-of-care.pdf

American Organization for Nurse Leaders. (n.d.). *Care innovation & transformation*. https://www.aonl.org/education/cit

American Society for Quality. (2016). *RACI matrix*. https://asqservicequality.org/glossary/rasic-or-raci-matrix

Ancker, J. S., Edwards, A., Nosal, S., Hauser, D., Mauer, E., & Kaushal, R. (2017). Effects of workload, work complexity, and repeated alerts on alert fatigue in a clinical decision support system. *BMC Medical Informatics and Decision Making, 17*(1), Article 36. https://doi.org/10.1186/s12911-017-0430-8

Andrews, R., Greasley, S., Knight, S., Sireau, S., Jordan, A., Bell, A., & White, P. (2020). Collaboration for clinical innovation: A nursing and engineering alliance for better patient care. *Journal of Research in Nursing, 25*(3), 291–304. https://doi.org/10.1177/1744987120918263

Anthony, M. K. (2004). Shared governance models: The theory, practice, and evidence. *Online Journal of Issues in Nursing, 9*(1), Manuscript 4. https://ojin.nursingworld.org/MainMenuCategories/ANAMarketplace/ANAPeriodicals/OJIN/TableofContents/Volume92004/No1Jan04/SharedGovernanceModels.aspx

Baernholdt, M., Feldman, M., Davis-Ajami, M. L., Harvey, L. D., Mazmanian, P. E., Mobley, D., Murphy, J. K., Watts, C., & Dow, A. (2019). An interprofessional quality improvement training program that improves educational and quality outcomes. *American College of Medical Quality, 34*(6), 577–584. https://doi.org/10.1177/1062860618825306.

Boamah, S. (2018). Linking nurses' clinical leadership to patient care quality: The role of transformational leadership and workplace empowerment. *Canadian Journal of Nursing Research, 50*(1), 9–19. https://doi.org/10.1177/0844562117732490

Brassard, A. (2020). *Newly released survey data show nurses more diverse, better educated*. The Future of Nursing: Campaign for Action. https://campaignforaction.org/newly-released-survey-data-show-nurses-more-diverse-better-educated

Brenan, M. (2020, July 13). *Americans' face mask usage varies greatly by demographics*. Gallup. https://news.gallup.com/poll/315590/americans-face-mask-usage-varies-greatly-demographics.aspx

Brown, B. (2018). *Dare to lead: Brave work, tough conversations, whole hearts*. Random House.

Brown, B. (Host). (2020, October 21). Brené with Joe Biden on empathy, unity, and courage [Audio podcast episode]. In *Unlocking Us With Brené Brown*. Cadence 13. https://brenebrown.com/podcast/brene-with-joe-biden-on-empathy-unity-and-courage

Carlson, K. (2020). *Preparing for nursing career transitions*. https://www.ausmed.com/cpd/articles/preparing-for-nursing-career-transitions

Carr, B., & Knutson, S. (2015). Culturally competent school nurse practice. *NASN School Nurse, 30*(6), 336–342. https://doi.org/10.1177/1942602X15605169.

Centers for Medicare and Medicaid Services. (2020). *The hospital value-based purchasing (VBP) program*. https://www.cms.gov/Medicare/Quality-Initiatives-Patient-Assessment-Instruments/Value-Based-Programs/HVBP/Hospital-Value-Based-Purchasing

Clarke, P. N., & Fawcett, J. (2016). Nursing knowledge driving person-centered care. *Nursing Science Quarterly, 29*(4), 285–287. https://doi.org/10.1177/0894318416661110

Chowdhury, J. (2012). Hacking health: Bottom-up innovation for healthcare. *Technology Innovation Management Review*, 31–35. https://timreview.ca/sites/default/files/article_PDF/Chowdhury_TIMReview_July2012_1.pdf

Cogan, R. (2020). Future of Nursing 2020–2030 Philadelphia town hall: Lessons shared from a relentless school nurse. *NASH School Nurse, 35*(2), 74–78. https://doi.org/10.1177/1942602X19896836

Cole, D. A., Bersick, E., Skarbek, A., Cummins, K., Dugan, K., & Grantoza, R. (2019). The courage to speak out: A study describing nurses' attitudes to report unsafe practices in patient care. *Journal of Nursing Management, 27*(6), 1176–1181. https://doi.org/10.1111/jonm.12789

Cosier, S. (2017). *8 medical inventions created by nurses*. mentalfloss.com/article/500467/8-medical-inventions-created-nurses.

Cresswell, K., Williams, R., Carlile, N., & Sheikh, A. (2020). Accelerating innovation in health care: Insights from a qualitative inquiry into United Kingdom and United States innovation centers. *Journal of Medical Internet Research, 29*(2), e19644. https://doi.org/10.2196/19644

Cross, S. R. H. (2018). The systems approach at the sharp end. *Future Healthcare Journal, 5*(3), 176–180. https://doi.org/10.7861/futurehosp.5-3-176

Cuthbertson, A. (2020, July 25). *Coronavirus tracked: How women leaders outperform men during pandemic*. INDEPENDENT. https://www.independent.co.uk/news/world/coronavirus-cases-women-men-leaders-countries-data-a9635396.html

Driscoll, A., Grant, M. J., Carroll, D., Dalton, S., Deaton, C., Jones, I., Lehwaldt, D., McKee, G., Munyombwe, T., & Astin, F. (2018). The effect of nurse-to-patient ratios on nurse-sensitive patient outcomes in acute specialist units: A systematic review and meta-analysis. *European Journal of Cardiovascular Nursing, 17*(1), 6–22. https://doi.org/10.1177/1474515117721561

Forster, B. B., Patlas, M. N., & Lexa, F. J. (2020). Crisis leadership during and following COVID-19. *Canadian Association of Radiologists Journal*, *71*(4), 421–422. https://doi.org/10.1177/0846537120926752

Godin, S. (2018, December 6). Perfect processes. *Seth's Blog*. https://seths.blog/2018/12/perfect-processes

Gostin, L. O., Cohen, I. G., & Koplan, J. P. (2020). Universal masking in the United States: The role of mandates, health education, and the CDC. *The Journal of the American Medical Association, 324*(9), 837–838. https://doi.org/10.1001/jama.2020.15271

Gustafsson, L., & Stenberg, M. (2017). Crucial contextual attributes of nursing leadership towards a care ethics. *Nursing Ethics*, *24*(4), 419–429. https://doi.org/10.1177/0969733015614879

Halm M. A. (2021). Specialty certification: A path to improving outcomes. *American Journal of Critical Care 30*(2), 156–160. https://doi.org/10.4037/ajcc2021569

Harned, B. (2019). *How to clear project confusion with a RACI chart*. TeamGantt. https://www.teamgantt.com/blog/raci-chart-definition-tips-and-example

Harper, K. J., & Benson, L. S. (2019). The importance and impact of nurses serving on boards. *Nursing Economic$*, 37(4), 209–212. https://www.nursesonboardscoalition.org/wp-content/uploads/The-Importance-and-Impact-of-Nurses-Serving-on-Boards.pdf

Harvey, G. (2020). Perspectives: Leadership for quality improvement. *Journal of Research in Nursing*, *25*(5), 494–497. https://doi.org/10.1177/1744987120938924

Henneman, E. A. (2017). Recognizing the ordinary as extraordinary: Insight into the "Way We Work" to improve patient safety outcomes. *American Journal of Critical Care, 26*(4), 272–277. https://doi.org/10.4037/ajcc2017812

Institute of Medicine. (2011). *The future of nursing: Leading change, advancing health*. National Academies Press. http://nationalacademies.org/HMD/Reports/2010/The-Future-of-Nursing-Leading-Change-Advancing-Health.aspx

Institute for Safe Medication Practices. (2020, April 3). *Clinical experiences keeping infusion pumps outside the room for COVID-19 patients*. https://www.ismp.org/resources/clinical-experiences-keeping-infusion-pumps-outside-room-covid-19-patients

Johnson, C. S., & Smith, C. M. (2017). Preparing nursing professional development practitioners in their pivotal leadership role. *Journal for Nurses in Professional Development*, *33*(6), 316–317. https://doi.org/10.1097/NND.0000000000000392.

Lacey, S. R., Goodyear-Bruch, C., Olney, A., Hanson, D., Altman, M. S., Varn-Davis, N. S., Brinker, D., Lavandero, R., & Cox, K. S. (2017). Driving organizational change from the bedside: The AACN Clinical Scene Investigator Academy. *Critical Care Nurse*, *37*(4), e12–e25. https://doi.org/10.4037/ccn2017749.

Lasater, K. B., Sloane, D. M., McHugh, M. D., Cimiotti, J. P., Riman, K. A., Martin, B., Alexander, M., & Aiken, L. H. (2020). Evaluation of hospital nurse-to-patient staffing ratios and sepsis bundles on patient outcomes. *American Journal of Infection Control, 49*(7), 868–873. https://doi.org/10.1016/j.ajic.2020.12.002

Lasater, K. B., Aiken, L. H., Sloane, D. M., French, R., Martin, B., Reneau, K., Alexander, M., & McHugh, M. D. (2021). Chronic hospital nurse understaffing meets COVID-19: An observational study. *BMJ Quality & Safety, 30, 639–647*. https://doi.org/10.1136/bmjqs-2020-011512

McCarthy, A. (2020). Develop millennial leaders with generation collaboration. *American Nurse, 15*(12), 5–7, 49. https://www.myamericannurse.com/wp-content/uploads/2020/12/an12-Millennial-1123.pdf

McCormack, B. (2017). Compliance versus innovation in evidence-based nursing. *Worldviews on Evidence-Based Nursing*, *14*(3), 173–174. https://doi.org/10.1111/wvn.12240

Medical Association of Georgia. (2020). *Health care workforce resilience*. https://www.mag.org/wp-content/uploads/2020/08/COVID19FAQFactSheet.pdf

Meliniotis, C. (2020, October 23). The rewards of teamwork and productive leadership in healthcare today. *American Nurse*. https://www.myamericannurse.com/the-rewards-of-teamwork-and-productive-leadership-in-healthcare-today

MobLab Team. (2018, June 5). *Why self-care and collective wellbeing are critical to winning change*. https://mobilisationlab.org/stories/moblab-live-self-care-collective-wellbeing

Nembhard, I. M., Labao, I., & Savage, S. (2015). Breaking the silence: Determinants of voice for quality improvement in hospitals. *Health Care Management Review, 40*(3), 225–236. https://doi.org/10.1097/HMR.0000000000000028

Northouse, P. G. (2018). *Introduction to leadership: Concepts and practice* (4th ed.). SAGE Publication.

Our World in Data. (2021). *Coronavirus pandemic (COVID-19)*. https://ourworldindata.org/coronavirus

Post, C., Latu, I. M., & Belkin, L. Y. (2019). A female leadership trust advantage in times of crisis: Under what conditions? *Psychology of Women Quarterly, 43*(2), 215–231. https://doi.org/10.1177/0361684319828292

Press Ganey. (2020). *Press Ganey nursing special report: The far-reaching impact of nursing excellence*. https://www.pressganey.com/resources/white-papers/2020-nursing-special-report

Rigolosi, E. L. M. (2013). *Management and leadership in nursing and health care: An experiential approach* (3rd ed.). Springer Publishing Company.

Satiani, B., & Prakash, S. (2016). It is time for more physician and nursing representation on hospital boards in the US. *Journal of Hospital & Medical Management, 1*, 2. https://hospital-medical-management.imedpub.com/it-is-time-for-more-physician-and-nursing-representation-on-hospital-boards-in-the-us.php?aid=9753

Scherer, L. (2020). 4 changes every healthcare team must make to prepare for the next pandemic. *Florence Health*. https://www.florence-health.com/professions/np-view-professional/4-changes-every-healthcare-team-must-make-to-prepare-for-the-next-pandemic

Sfantou, D. F., Laliotis, A., Patelarou, A. E., Sifaki-Pistolla, D., Matalliotakis, M., & Patelarou, E. (2017). Importance of leadership style towards quality of care measures in healthcare settings: A systematic review. *Healthcare, 5*(4), 73. https://doi.org/10.3390/healthcare5040073

Tachibana, C. (2021, May 6). *COVID-19 pandemic: Lessons learned*. Keynote Speaker, School of Nursing Research Day, Pacific Lutheran University.

TEDx Talks. (2018). *Nurse innovation: Saving the future of healthcare | Rebecca Love | TEDxBeaconStreet* [Video]. YouTube. https://www.youtube.com/watch?v=IPBcRW8NQPY-MAG Fact Sheet

Tommasini, N., Laird, K., Cunningham, P., Ogbejesi, V. C., & Jansen, L. (2020). Building a successful behavioral emergency support team. *American Nurse Journal, 15*(1), 42–45. https://www.myamericannurse.com/building-a-successful-behavioral-emergency-support-team

Ulrich, B. (2020). Year of the nurse: Celebrating the 200th anniversary of the birth of Florence Nightingale. *Nephrology Nursing Journal, 47*(2), 109–111.

Veenema, T. G., Meyer, D., Bell, S. A., Couig, M. P., Friese, C. R., Lavin, R., Stanley, J., Martin, E., Montague, M., Toner, E. Schosh-Spana, M., & Cicero, A. (2020, June 10). *Recommendations for improving national nurse preparedness for pandemic response: Early lessons from COVID-19*. The Johns Hopkins Center for Health Security. https://www.centerforhealthsecurity.org/our-work/publications/recommendations-for-improving-national-nurse-preparedness-for-pandemic-response--early-lessons-from-covid-19

Watkins, S. (2020). *What are crisis standards of care?* Washington State Nurses Association. https://www.wsna.org/news/2020/what-are-crisis-standards-of-care

Wofford, P. (2021). Nurse invents underwear for patients with catheters and leg bags. *Nurse.org*. https://nurse.org/articles/nurse-foley-catheter-underwear-clothing

Yamashita, T., Bardo, A. R., Liu, D., & Yoo, J. W. (2019). Education, lifelong learning and self-rated health in later life in the USA. *Health Education Journal, 78*(3), 328–339. https://doi.org/10.1177/0017896918809500

Yantis, C. (2017). Here's what it means to level up. *Thought Changer*. https://www.thoughtchangerblog.com/2017/06/heres-what-it-means-to-level-up.html

Zeng, J., & Xu, G. (2020). Linking ethical leadership to employee voice. *Social Behavior and Personality, 48*(8), Article e9200. https://doi.org/10.2224/sbp.9200

SUGGESTED READINGS

American Association of Critical-Care Nurses. (n.d.). *AACN synergy model for patient care*. https://www.aacn.org/nursing-excellence/aacn-standards/synergy-model

Andrews, R., Greasley, S., Knight, S., Sireau, S., Jordan, A., Bell, A., & White, P. (2020). Collaboration for clinical innovation: A nursing and engineering alliance for better patient care. *Journal of Research in Nursing, 25*(3), 291–304. https://doi.org/10.1177/1744987120918263

Duquesne University School of Nursing. (2020, April 14). *Top concerns for nurse leaders*. https://onlinenursing.duq.edu/blog/top-concerns-for-nurse-leaders

Scott, P. A., Harvey, C., Felzmann, H., Suhonen, R., Habermann, M., Halvorsen, K., Christiansen, K., Toffoli, L., & Papastavrou, E. (2019). Resource allocation and rationing in nursing care: A discussion paper. *Nursing Ethics, 26*(5), 1528–1539. https://doi.org/10.1177/0969733018759831

Zenger, J., & Folkman, J. (2020). Research: Women are better leaders during a crisis. *Harvard Business Review*. https://hbr.org/2020/12/research-women-are-better-leaders-during-a-crisis

CHAPTER 3

Systems Thinking

Danielle Walker and Caitlin K. Dodd

"Systems thinking is a mixed bag of holistic, balanced, and often abstract thinking to understand things profoundly and solve problems systematically."

–Pearl Zhu, 2018

Upon completion of this chapter, the reader should be able to:

1. Identify the theoretical principles of a system and apply it to nursing practice.
2. Define systems thinking.
3. Apply systems thinking to nursing practice.
4. Identify the origins of systems thinking in healthcare.
5. Analyze the impact of systems thinking on quality and safety processes within complex healthcare.
6. Examine ways to foster systems thinking in professional practice.
7. Explore the role of leadership as a component for systems thinking.

CROSSWALK

This chapter addresses the following:

QSEN Competency: Patient-Centered Care, Teamwork, Evidence-Based Practice, Quality Improvement, Safety

The American Association of College of Nursing. (2021). The essentials: Core competencies for professional nursing education.

Domain 1: Knowledge for Nursing Practice
Domain 2: Person-Centered Care
Domain 5: Quality and Safety
Domain 7: Systems-Based Practice

OPENING SCENARIO

Mrs. J, a patient in the emergency department (ED), has called the patient advocate hotline to complain about spending the night in the ED. She states, "It's loud, I can't sleep and I can't have visitors. My son always helps me remember what everyone is telling me. When am I going to get a room?" The patient advocate contacts the nurse to determine if they can help Mrs. J. The nurse tells the advocate that Mrs. J has been assigned a room on the second floor since 10 p.m. yesterday but the room is not available. The nurse has noticed this has become a more common problem and notifies the nurse manager. The manager runs a report and realizes patients are waiting in the ED to be moved to a room over 4 hours longer this month than last month. The manager brings the concerns to other managers at the monthly managers' meeting. The group decides to form a committee to look into the problem further.

1. What is the initial problem? For what reasons might a patient wait in the ED for a room?
2. How does waiting for a room in the ED impact patient outcomes, quality care, or safety concerns?
3. Make a list of the factors that may contribute to patients in the ED waiting for rooms.

INTRODUCTION

The world is made up of seemingly disconnected pieces, but upon closer inspection every action is connected, and many small, interconnected parts create the whole. Connections are everywhere, in every action taken, in everything. For example, a tree is just a tree, but it is also part of a larger forest and an entire ecosystem. The tree serves a purpose within the forest ecosystem; it is a home for animals, it provides shade for plants beneath it, and it produces the oxygen people breathe. If one tree fails to thrive, the entire system is impacted. As humans who breathe air, it can be easy to overlook that a single tree is an important functional part of a larger system like the forest and is just one of many parts that make up a more complex whole. Systems thinking allows people to observe and understand each part and how all components together interact and create a whole. In healthcare, systems thinking offers a common language and process with which to organize thinking to minimize error and work to create consistent outcomes every time.

Because systems provide order that can improve outcomes and safety, many fields, such as aviation and automobile manufacturing, retail, and technology companies, have embraced the concept of systems thinking. In healthcare, systems thinking is considered a key component to providing safe, high-quality care (Dolansky & Moore, 2013; Dolansky et al., 2020). The application of systems thinking is identified as a core competency for practice in *The Future of Nursing* report (Institute of Medicine [IOM], 2011) and is included as a component for licensing and accreditation by governing agencies such as The Joint Commission (TJC). This chapter will define the principles of systems thinking and apply it to nursing practice. It will explore the impact of systems thinking on quality and safety in healthcare and examine ways to foster systems thinking in professional practice and leadership roles.

DEFINE THE THEORETICAL PRINCIPLES OF A SYSTEM

What makes a **system**? Merriam-Webster's (n.d.) dictionary defines a system as a group of interconnected parts that, when combined, form a whole that works or moves as a unit. Other definitions describe a system as parts or groups of parts that work together toward a specific purpose (Kim, 1999). For example, riders on a bus or tools in a tool box are just a collection of parts—not a system. But a football team or an automobile is a system because each is composed of many interrelated parts that have a specific purpose. In a system, each of the parts contributes to the overall functioning of the whole. For a football team, each player has a specific purpose such as blocking, throwing, and catching. For an automobile, each part allows it to operate safely. If one part is missing, the whole of the system is impacted; a pass might be missed or the brakes may malfunction. This same concept applies to the significance of the parts within any system. An important function of the system is to provide feedback. **Feedback** is information produced that can be used to evaluate a system. When a system provides feedback, it indicates how the system is working. For an automobile, if the check engine light comes on, it is providing feedback that something is wrong with a component of the automobile's engine.

One way to determine if something is a system is to ask four simple questions: (a) Do these parts have a common purpose?(b) Do all the parts contribute to the system working effectively? (c) Does the order of the parts contribute to system performance? and (d) Does the system provide feedback? If it is a system, the answer will be yes to all four questions (Kim, 1999).

Ludwig von Bertalanffy in 1968 originally developed general systems theory (GST) to create a set of universal principles for general systems by looking at a system as one unit (Von Bertalanffy, 1968). In GST, systems are composed of four major elements. **Input** is the material or energy that goes into the systems. **Process** is the actions that happen within the system to create an output. **Output** is what results from the process. Lastly, feedback, as previously stated, is the information produced that can be used to evaluate the system. Applying the example of the football team as a system, the input is when they meet in the huddle before executing a play. The play is the process and the outcome is movement up or down the field. Feedback would be provided in the form of data such as the score or watching tape of previously played games. Additionally, von Bertalanffy identified two types of systems: open and closed. A **closed system** is one that does not interact with the environment, whereas an **open system** does interact with the environment (Von Bertalanffy, 1968). An example of a closed system is a computer not connected to the internet. The computer can work perfectly within its programs without an internet connection. But once the computer is connected to the internet it becomes part of an open system, now able to interact with thousands of other computers.

Systems can also be simple or complex. A **simple system** has a single path to only one answer. A **complex system** consists of many parts or smaller systems that interact with each other or the environment. A complex system has many paths that can be followed to create many answers. It is difficult to predict the behavior of complex systems because of the relationships within the system as well as interactions with the environment that impact the behavior of the system (Cordon, 2013). A computer is an example of a complex system. Systems can be open or closed and complex or simple all at once. Using the previously noted terminology, the human body would be described as an open, complex system (Cordon, 2013).

An example of an open system is a healthcare team because it interacts with the environment through material, people, energy, and information. A healthcare team includes multiple people working together to improve the health outcomes of patients. The team must exchange information about the patient among itself, and interact with the environment by working with the patient and family members to properly care for a patient. Exchanging information among itself would include inputs such as the information put into the electronic charting system for the pharmacy to dispense medication and processes such as double checking for utilization of best practices. The obvious members of the open system are physicians and nurses, but for the team to truly be effective, it must include all who are involved in the system, from the chef in the kitchen preparing meals to the technology support person ensuring the electronic health record is working correctly. Each of these members of the team is connected in the open system, directly or indirectly, to ensure the patient receives safe, high-quality care.

Thinking about the whole of the system is guided by processes. Complex systems consist of groupings of processes (Johnson et al., 2008). Processes are vital to the healthcare system to ensure safety, standardize practice, and improve health outcomes. Examples of standardized processes include those used for medication administration, patient registration, report given between providers, and documentation of patient care. Often multiple processes are combined during patient transfers between care units. There is a process for giving report to the receiving nurse, a process for transporting the patient, and a process for accepting the new patient on the new unit. Each of these individual processes interact to make one complex system for transferring patients. As nurses, it is important to evaluate processes within the healthcare environment as individual components of the larger system in order to improve care.

Since Von Bertenaffly's initial work, many scholars have studied systems theory and made extensive contributions to the science of systems. **Systems science** is an interdisciplinary field that studies the nature of systems and applies systems concepts to improve outcomes (Mobus & Kalton, 2015). Many nursing theories that guide current practice are based on systems theory. Two common nursing theories that utilize a systems approach are Neuman's System Model and Roy's Adaptation Model. Neuman's System Model was created in 1970 and is based on the idea that the human body is an open system that works to achieve balance and adaptation through the internal and external environment (Başoğul & Buldukoğlu, 2020; Neuman & Fawcett, 2011). The body has lines of defense and resistance changed by each individual's psychological, sociocultural, developmental, and spiritual growth that allow or prevent environmental factors from affecting the body system (Neuman & Fawcett, 2011). Roy's Adaptation Model is a conceptual framework for nursing that combines the principles of systems theory and adaptation theory into a single set of assumptions (Roy, 2009). Roy's Adaptation Model views the person in continuous interaction with the environment. It is the nurse's role to manage the environment, or factors impacting the patient's current situation (Ursavaş et al., 2014).

SYSTEMS THEORY IN OTHER FIELDS

Healthcare has adapted many of the systems processes used from other fields. Toyota's production systems, often called lean manufacturing systems or just-in-time systems, are systems based on making vehicles quickly and efficiently (Toyota, n.d.). In manufacturing, this process makes it possible for the production system to stop quickly when a problem occurs and ensure volume meets demand (Toyota, n.d.). The overall goal in this process is to eliminate waste and use the most efficient options possible (Toyota, n.d.). The Toyota manufacturing process is then able to reduce cost and improve safety in their manufacturing plants by immediately stopping the system when problems occur. The system in this case is the production line and it involves the machines, orders, and people that work on the line. The aim of Lean Management in healthcare is to provide cost-effective, innovative quality care to patients through utilization of essential resources. Lean healthcare uses principles focused on continuous improvement by using analytical tools to identify waste and areas for improvements with patient flow, supplies, and processes (Udod et al., 2020). Lean is discussed in Chapter 11.

The aviation industry uses the Safety Management System to provide a systematic approach for reaching safety goals and includes four components: safety policy, safety risk management, safety assurance, and safety promotion/culture (Federal Aviation Administration [FAA], 2019). Safety policy (the establishment of safe processes and procedures), safety risk management (the risk assessment process), and safety assurance (review of the effectiveness and notification of new hazards) work together in a cyclical loop for continual improvement (FAA, 2019). The safety promotion/culture includes training and the creation of a safety mindset for those working within the industry and encompasses the other three components (FAA, 2019). The Safety Management System meets the definition of a system because all system components are interrelated, all parts contribute in a certain order to the effective functioning of the system, and feedback is readily provided from continual improvement. TJC applies the Safety Management System from the aviation industry to the adoption of patient safety systems within healthcare organizations. TJC (2021) describes a patient safety system as standardized safety policies and reporting process, methods to evaluate and improve safety processes and systems, and a safety culture.

These previously described systems were successful in improving the quality and safety of their products while decreasing costs and improving efficiency. Because of these successes, healthcare has begun to model systems from these industries to promote safety leading to improved patient outcomes and decreased costs within organizations.

DEFINE SYSTEMS THINKING

In its simplest form, **systems thinking** is a mental model to solving problems within a complex system that considers structures, patterns, and cycles (Cordon, 2013). For a nurse, using systems thinking allows the caregiver to recognize patterns and interactions in order to understand how actions impact each other (Dolansky & Moore, 2013). With systems thinking, the nurse can assess not only the problem at hand but begin to determine how all of the providers and interventions work in concert to correct or improve the patient's problem.

Systems thinking has four key principles: (a) looking at the big picture, (b) recognizing patterns, (c) reflective practice, and (d) willingness to adapt or change perceptions (Plack et al., 2019; Stalter et al., 2017). The next sections will explore each of these concepts.

LOOKING AT THE BIG PICTURE

As a systems thinker, it is important to identify all aspects of the system, not just the one aspect with which one interacts. Like the example at the beginning of the chapter, nurses need to be able to see beyond the tree and consider all the components of the forest. When working to solve a problem, a nurse must evaluate more than just what initially caused the problem (Stalter et al., 2017). This is often called having a global perspective. A global perspective, or looking at the big picture, requires comprehensive evaluation of any part that impacts an event or circumstance. Healthcare consists of many separate yet connected processes. Looking at the big picture requires identifying interdependency of different processes. Problems in healthcare are rarely isolated issues (Trbovich, 2014). Take for example the concept of homelessness. Homelessness is often seen as a problem that can be easily addressed by simply providing an individual a place to live, but that does not fix the problems associated with homelessness. Individuals experiencing homelessness are more likely to have physical and mental health problems, which leads to increased needs and costs in healthcare (Fowler et al., 2019). To help improve the problems associated with homelessness, whether for the individual or the society at large, complex systems must be navigated and reviewed. Help for homelessness starts with short-term systems solutions; however, for long-term success, evaluations must occur regarding education, employment, housing, healthcare, and many other aspects (Fowler et al., 2019). So, while the problem of homelessness might first appear to be an individual issue of not having a home, it is really a complex problem which requires the ability to navigate multiple complex systems if it is to be solved.

RECOGNIZING PATTERNS

Recognizing patterns seems like a simple task and one that is easily mastered. But in a complex system, recognizing patterns in data or trends across time can be challenging. To be able to recognize patterns, a nurse must be able to identify connections between systems or processes, visualize how one interaction is interdependent on another interaction, understand cause-and-effect relationships, and continually request and assess feedback (Plack et al., 2019; Stalter et al., 2017).

For example, most organizations communicate specific isolation measures or requirements through signs on the patients' door. Of course, having a sign does not ensure that everyone follows the recommended procedures to prevent the spread of infection from room to room. The work of Hoang et al. (2017) describes how, at one facility, a nurse recognized that signage was consistently not followed. An interprofessional group was created to gather input from frontline staff about why the protocols were not being followed. The team evaluated current signage and created a new product with fewer words and larger icons, which improved employee compliance. Noticing the relationship between behavior and a process allowed the interprofessional group to improve adherence to isolation precautions and impact infection control rates.

REFLECTION

Questions are the key to reflection and are at the heart of systems thinking. Asking oneself the right questions to elicit new thoughts, connections, and opportunities is an important skill to develop as a nurse (Plack et al., 2019). Schon (1983) identified three types of self-reflection: reflection in action, reflection on action, and reflection for action (Table 3.1).

WILLINGNESS TO CHANGE

Consistent reflective practice will lead to a transformation. Transformation is simply dramatic change (Stalter et al., 2017). A systems thinker must be willing to reflect on one's behavior or assumptions and make changes to one's actions or beliefs. It may require modifying one's thoughts about the way something functions. Willingness to change is a commitment to continuous improvement which nurtures a culture of proactive responses rather than reactions (Stalter et al., 2017). Being willing to change may mean being an

TABLE 3.1 THREE TYPES OF REFLECTION

TYPE OF REFLECTION	DEFINITION	QUESTIONS TO ENCOURAGE REFLECTION
Reflection in action	Using knowledge as one works to solve the problem (commonly referred to as thinking on your feet).	Is this going as expected? Can something be changed to make the outcome better?
Reflection on action	Happens after a person has completed the problem-solving. It is thinking through what one knows about the problem or the situation. This type of reflection can help review performance and evaluate outcomes.	Was that the expected outcome? How did my actions impact the outcome?
Reflection for action	Is thinking about the outcome and anticipating the possible outcomes of the problem. This type of reflection helps improve future actions.	What was learned from this experience? How could something be done different next time? How can the system be changed to prevent this from happening again?

advocate for system change. As a systems thinker, the nurse is equipped to identify necessary process changes, make other members of the healthcare team understand the rationale for changes, and then implement appropriate system adjustments (Trbovich, 2014).

CASE STUDY

Patient satisfaction surveys have come back with concerns regarding the extensive amount of time it takes for call lights to be answered. The unit manager wants to identify ways to decrease the amount of time it takes for call bells to be answered to increase patient satisfaction and prevent any resulting concerns regarding falls or pain control. Consider how the nurse manager might use the mental model for systems thinking to answer the questions that follow.

1. *What is the problem the unit needs to address?*
2. *What patterns should the nurse manager consider regarding this issue?*
3. *What systemic structures should the nurse manager review?*
4. *What shared vision should be created for the unit to improve this issue?*

Real World Interview

On a typical COVID vaccine hub day, we provide 3,000 vaccinations to our community in 8 hours. We did not start out providing this many in one day; it was a process. My role changed many times in the last year, but I adapted already developed systems and processes to each new project I undertook. When the COVID pandemic surged, I began managing COVID testing and, eventually, vaccine distribution. Getting shots in arms quickly and efficiently for employees and the community was the goal. I started working 100-hour weeks with a team of three people (a manager and two nurse supervisors), with about 30 staff to work for each vaccine session) to vaccinate 300 people a day. As the vaccine's availability increased, we knew we had to scale up our services (we now have about 200 staff working at the hub). We relied on our medical center's best practices to create a large-scale vaccination drive-thru site.

One of the biggest challenges was moving from a situation where I could see every part of the system functioning to a system so widely spread that I could no longer physically see all of its components. I had to rely on our leaders (that I assigned in each work area) and ensure that we had processes to allow everyone to do their jobs effectively. The biggest challenge was drawing up vaccines, knowing how many people would not show-up for appointments, and ensuring no vaccines were wasted. The first week I struggled. I didn't have any information from past large-scale hubs to rely on, and I wasn't confident in my decisions. By the following week, I assessed data trends in the morning related to how many people were coming for their appointments and used that information to determine the number of vaccines to prepare for the afternoon. As we got more experienced at the hub process, I analyzed data trends more clearly. I learned to look at other factors that influenced people's actions such as the news and the environment. When eligibility criteria changed, our numbers of no-shows for appointments also changed. If it was rainy or cold weather, I knew I could expect more people not to come. We created a backup system to use if our estimations were off, and we implemented a process for a cue of people waiting so that all extra doses were used. Every week, as we run the COVID vaccination clinic, we learn something and apply what we learn to the next clinic.

Kim-Dung Mai, BSN, RN, CMSRN
Nurse Manager II, COVID Vaccination Clinic
Baylor Scott and White All Saints Medical Center, Fort Worth, Texas

APPLYING SYSTEMS THINKING TO NURSING PRACTICE

Upon graduation, nurses are expected to work in a variety of settings and be able to coordinate care across settings and with diverse teams, make decisions and solve problems at the bedside, and participate in error detection and prevention (Dolansky & Moore, 2013; Johnson et al., 2008; Stalter & Mota, 2018). To be successful in these endeavors, the nurse must employ systems thinking. For new-to-practice nurses, it is easy to focus solely on assessment data or inputs and the processes needed to care for the individual patients the nurse is assigned to, but the larger healthcare system inputs and processes greatly impact the care the nurse can deliver. Understanding and respecting how the nurse and patient interact with the healthcare system creates better outcomes for patients. Figure 3.1 demonstrates growth from an individual care mindset to a system's care mindset.

Kim (2000) devised a four-step model or process for applying systems thinking as demonstrated in Table 3.2. The first step in applying systems thinking is identifying the problem. When a patient falls, nurses respond immediately by providing care for the patient. This dangerous event can repeat over and over if that is where the response stops. But after the immediate concern is resolved, a systems thinker begins to wonder how many falls happen daily, weekly, or monthly and what were the circumstances or context for falls? Is there a pattern? Moving from focusing on the problem or event and thinking about patterns is the next step in the systems thinking process. Thinking at this level identifies patterns that can be adjusted so that smoother processes or systems are in place to allow for more effective care, but this step still does not help prevent reoccurrence. In the third step, a systems thinker evaluates all the factors that contribute to the system or its processes; this step is the systematic structure step of applying systems thinking (Kim, 2000). In this step, the systems thinker is trying to understand the whole picture through patterns and relationships. Thinking like this involves evaluating system structures and includes a review of the physical environment, organizational structures, and individual actions, which may uncover inconsistencies identified in the patterns and relationships so that future problems can be prevented (Kim, 2020). The final step in applying systems thinking is developing a shared vision for all involved. Transformation occurs within that shared vision (Kim, 2000). It is important to note that reflection, although an important attribute of systems thinking, was not identified specifically within any of the individual steps of systems thinking application because systems thinking requires reflection throughout the entire process.

The context for systems thinking, although presented linearly, is a dynamic process. Each layer can be used to inform the layer preceding or following it. This method for systems thinking can be utilized within current practice frameworks such as the nursing

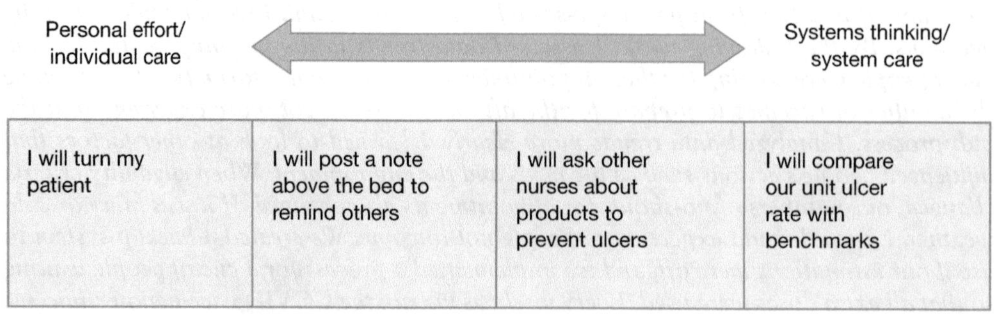

FIGURE 3.1 Continuum of Systems Thinking.

Source: Reprinted with permission from Dolansky, M. A., & Moore, S. M. (2013). Quality and Safety Education for Nurses (QSEN): The key is systems thinking. *Online Journal of Issues in Nursing, 18*(3), 1–12. https://doi.org/10.3912/OJIN.Vol18No03Man01. Figure 2 Knowing the attributes of systems thinking allows the nurse to apply them in practice.

TABLE 3.2 APPLICATION OF THE FOUR STEP SYSTEMS THINKING PROCESS TO PATIENT CARE

STEPS OF THE SYSTEM THINKING PROCESS	APPLICATION OF THE SYSTEMS THINKING PROCESS
Identify the problem	A patient falls on the unit. This is not the first patient fall this week and the nurse begins to contemplate why falls are happening.
Recognize patterns	Unit data is evaluated and determines falls happen most often when a patient reports needing to use the restroom.
Evaluate systemic structures	The nurse evaluates the: **Physical environment** - Are beds lowered? Is the path to the bathroom clear? Are nonslip socks available? Are side rails up? **Organizational structures** - Has staffing been sufficient to meet unit needs? Has the unit been educated about how to prevent falls? Does the unit and hospital value and emphasize the importance of minimizing falls? **Individual actions** - Are nurses or unlicensed personnel completing hourly rounding? Are call lights being answered within 5 minutes? Does the nurse think helping patients up from bed is a valuable use of time?
Develop a shared vision	After recognizing patterns and evaluating systemic structures, the nurse begins to work with the unit to create a plan for decreasing falls. Together the nursing staff and unlicensed personnel agree to answer the call bell system and respond to requests for help and share rounding responsibilities by rotating each hour. On odd hours nurses will round on patients and include checking if patients need assistance to the bathroom. On even hours unlicensed assistive personnel will round.

clinical judgment model or nursing process. Later in this chapter, different tools and practices will be presented to create a clear understanding of the process of systems thinking so that the concepts can be applied to problems that arise in the clinical practice setting.

Real World Interview

As a leader my mantra is "Seek first to understand." I have to be acutely cognizant of my blind spots, assumptions, and perspectives because these factors inform how I interact with others and the decisions I make daily in my job. I try and ask myself often, "How is XY decision going to impact each person involved, whether directly or indirectly?" Thinking holistically about everyone's roles, what is important to them, what are their values, and what are their needs are important components of systems thinking.

Often, we work alone in our silos or pockets. We find out belatedly that there are duplicates of work, or worse, we are actively working in ways that are in direct conflict with each other. It is so easy to just do your work and not think about the entire system and how everything connects together. In my role I oversee simulation education. One day, nurses were running a simulation on the unit but somehow the physicians were unaware. When the simulated code situation was called overhead, physicians came running to help, leaving actual patients for what they thought was a higher priority. As we reviewed that situation we thought: How could we have missed that? Why weren't the physicians notified in advance? And most importantly, why isn't the entire interprofessional team needed in that scenario part of the simulation? None of us ever work alone. In the end, the simulation helped us realize something we never even intended and helped us evaluate an overarching systems issue.

Diana Singer, MSN, RN, CCRN-K, CNE, C-TAGME
Executive Director
Academic Affairs, JPS Health Network, Fort Worth, Texas

IDENTIFY THE ORIGINS OF SYSTEMS THINKING IN HEALTHCARE

The healthcare system is an open, complex, adaptive system where many smaller systems are interacting together. Health systems are considered adaptive because they are composed of individuals, patients, and families who have the capacity to learn and change based on experiences. These interactions and behaviors cause variation within the system (Cordon, 2013). The healthcare system has been called the most complex system ever created (Plack et al., 2019) and a branch of systems-related theory has been developed to describe it. **Healthcare systems science** is the application of systems thinking to the healthcare setting to improve quality, outcomes, and costs for patients and populations (Dolansky et al., 2020; Hwang & Park, 2017).

To determine uses of systems thinking in healthcare, it is important to understand the purpose of healthcare systems. The primary purpose is to promote, restore, or maintain health (World Health Organization, 2000). The systems incorporated into healthcare ultimately seek to improve the quality of care provided to effectively achieve that purpose through multiple pathways. The IOM identified six key areas to guide improvements to the healthcare system (2001). Healthcare should be safe, effective, patient centered, timely, efficient, and equitable. The current systems in place are designed to enhance or improve care in all of these key areas.

Often healthcare is described in silos, with each occupation or field working within its specialty area with little to no interaction with people outside of that field. For safe, quality patient care, healthcare professionals need to interact with each other and utilize a systems thinking framework to provide care. A simple systems framework applied often in healthcare is the nested healthcare delivery system (Figure 3.2). The patient is always at the center of care provided. The interprofessional team works together with the patient to manage the patient's healthcare needs. The interprofessional team is employed by the

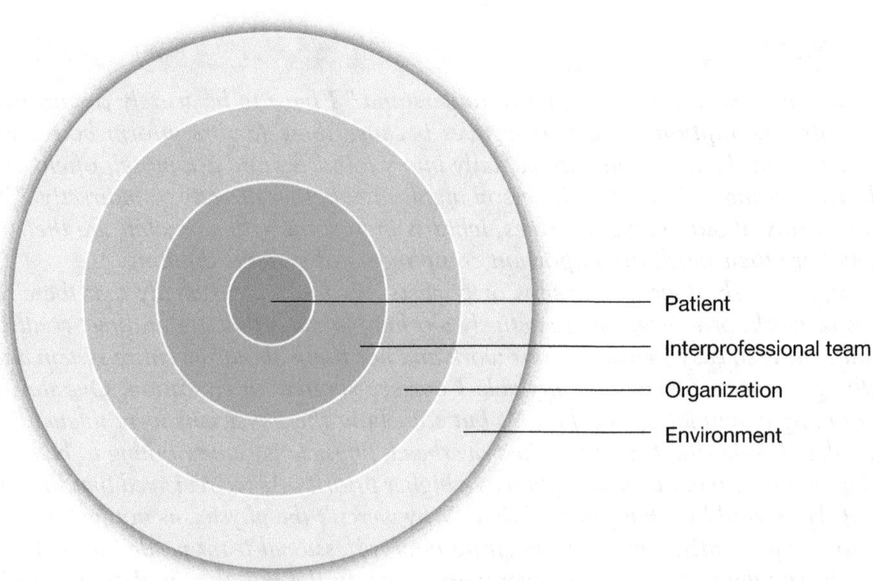

FIGURE 3.2 Four-Level Nested System of Healthcare Delivery.

Source: Adapted from Reid, P. P., Compton, W. D., Grossman, J. H., & Fanjiang, G. (Eds.). (2005). *Building a better delivery system: A new engineering/health care partnership.* National Academies Press. https://doi.org/10.17226/11378

TABLE 3.3 NESTED LEVEL OF HEALTHCARE DELIVERY AND SAMPLE QUESTIONS

Patient	What was the patient doing before the problem occurred? How can we solve this problem with the patient?
Interprofessional Team	Does the patient have multiple providers? Are the providers working together to optimize care and outcomes? Did the treatment plan work? Were the interventions evidence-based practice and following the established policy and procedures? Are all providers following the same procedures for treating breathing problems?
Organization	Are the needed supplies available? Are the appropriate personnel available? Are there policies that improve access or decrease access to care? Is the organization supportive of the solution?
Environments	Was the patient being treated for the problem before entering the hospital? Can the patient afford to pay for medication or care? Does insurance cover the care provided? Does the patient have transportation access to future treatment or medications? Are future treatment options geographically attainable? Can the patient work and seek treatment? Is the family supportive of treatment?

organization such as a hospital or nursing home. The organization supports the interprofessional team and provides resources, structures, policies, and procedures. The environment impacts all the levels: the patient, interprofessional teams, and organizations. The environment influences how the healthcare delivery system can function. Licensing and regulations such as those dictated by TJC illustrate the role of the environment within the nested healthcare delivery system.

The four-level nested system of healthcare delivery uses the terms, "microsystems," "mesosystems," and "macrosystems" to describe the different levels within the framework. Examples of microsystems are the patient, the interprofessional team, the organization, and the environment. The collection of microsystems that make up clinics or divisions of care form mesosystems. Mesosystems are accountable to the macrosystem, which is the overarching hospital system formed from all the microsystems working within it. The macrosystem of the healthcare network is impacted by other micro, meso, and macro systems such as government regulations, the ability to pay for healthcare, or resources within the community that contribute to the health and well-being of the patients. Problems or changes in the microsystems within any macro system can change the quality of care the patient receives or the outcome (Reid et al., 2005). The visual model of circles or systems nested within each other communicates the interconnectedness of all aspects of healthcare, demonstrating how the interprofessional team cannot work alone or in a silo; it is always connected to the patient, organization, and environment (Table 3.3).

HISTORICAL DEVELOPMENT OF SYSTEMS THINKING IN HEALHCARE

In 2000, the IOM report *To Err Is Human* (Kohn et al., 2000) placed a national spotlight on patient safety and outcomes within the healthcare system by informing Americans about the volume of patient deaths from preventable medical errors. Although this landmark report was published over 20 years ago, hospital executives still cite safety and quality as a priority issue confronting hospitals (Federico, 2018). Today it is estimated that preventable harm is the third-leading cause of death in the United States (Frankel et al.,

2017). Since the initial IOM report, healthcare organizations have sought to advance safety and quality through the application of a systems perspective.

To initially improve patient safety and therefore outcomes, healthcare organizations adopted standardized systems or processes to reduce variation in care provided. But these systems can still be ineffective when they are not holistic (Federico, 2018), do not consider how one process impacts another, and do not involve all stakeholders (Frankel et al., 2017). A total systems approach is essential in effective patient safety and quality (Johnson et al., 2008). Initially industries such as aviation and the auto industry adopted a total systems approach. Seeing that success, healthcare modeled its systems after them, applying many of the key concepts.

To create a total systems approach, healthcare organizations applied organization-wide systems thinking methods to improving safety and quality, ending the siloed processes that had been in place for many years (National Steering Committee for Patient Safety, 2020). The Agency of Healthcare Research and Quality (AHRQ) developed the concept of a learning health system to explain this approach. A **learning health system** is one in which all members of the healthcare team are acting as change agents, engaging in consistent, holistic evaluation of the organization. All feedback gained is applied to the healthcare system to improve care (AHRQ, 2019). If it sounds similar to systems thinking, it is. A learning health system is simply one where systems thinking is applied across the entire organization at all levels and it is an approach that is redefining quality and safety and is fundamental to quality improvement (QI; Bates & Singh, 2018; Dolansky & Moore, 2013). The Institute for Healthcare Improvement (IHI) *Safer Together: A National Action Plan to Advance Patient Safety* (National Steering Committee for Patient Safety, 2020) embraced this concept and is working to impact patient safety through system-wide safety processes that reach across the entire care continuum and involve all stakeholders. Additionally, TJC emphasizes the importance of a learning system to improve patient safety and quality (TJC, 2021).

A high-reliability organization in healthcare is a learning health system dedicated to the goal of zero error or, in the context of healthcare, zero harm. Imagine an aircraft carrier with planes constantly coming and going with ever-changing conditions; however, everyone on board, no matter their status, prioritize safety and can make adjustments as needed to ensure safe operations continue (AHRQ, 2019). A high-reliability organization in healthcare would have this same focus on safety with all members of the healthcare team, despite their role, being able to use their clinical judgment to identify and make adjustments as needed in response to concerns. The healthcare industry is adopting models similar to those of high-reliability organizations in other industries, such as Toyota in the auto industry, which is well known for its effective cost saving measures, safe practices, and ability to sustain these practices across long time periods (Polonsky, 2019).

In healthcare, high-reliability organizations have a commitment to patient safety and goal of no harm supported by a constant awareness of failures, a commitment to continual observations, and through motivation for continual improvement (Polonsky, 2019). These organizations recognize that errors do not occur because of one-time mistakes or the actions of one person. These organizations as a whole are continually providing feedback and making changes to improve the system of patient care. A major difference between high-reliability organizations and other healthcare organizations is that high-reliability organizations make drastic changes instead of focusing on small incremental steps (Polonsky, 2019). Systems thinkers within these organizations take time to reflect on the patterns and processes used and identify changes that will drastically change the way care is delivered. High-reliability organizations continually evaluate the systems within, recognize when something is not working, and make the needed changes to ensure their commitment to zero harm is maintained.

An example of an organization that has achieved the status of high reliability is the Cleveland Clinic. The Cleveland Clinic has sustained a high level of safety and quality over a prolonged period of time, adopting a culture with a zero-harm policy and a team-oriented approach. Through these changes, the healthcare organization has been able to improve patient outcomes, increase healthcare provider satisfaction, and decrease healthcare provider burnout (Cheney, 2019). To reach the goals of a high-reliability organization, the Cleveland Clinic standardized policies and created a culture that values each member of the healthcare team for their concerns and perspectives on safety (Cheney, 2019). All members of the healthcare team know that their concerns are valued and their ideas are validated through continual feedback from staff, healthcare providers, and leadership. Because of this culture and their established processes, the Cleveland Clinic is able to make consistent, real time changes to the way care is being delivered, continually supporting the work to achieve the goal of zero harm. Through these high-reliability ideals, the Cleveland Clinic has been able to make significant improvements in patient care that include reducing the readmission rates, improving hypertension control, and reducing severe safety events (Cheney, 2019), demonstrating how systems thinking can lead to positive improvements in patient outcomes.

CURRENT LITERATURE

CITATION

Owings, A., Graves, J., Johnson, S., Gilliam, C., Gipson, M., & Hakim, H. (2018). Leadership line care rounds: Application of the engage, educate, execute, and evaluate improvement model for the prevention of central line–associated bloodstream infections in children with cancer. *American Journal of Infection Control, 46*(2), 229–231. https://doi.org/10.1016/j.ajic.2017.08.032

DISCUSSION

Central lines are a common source of hospital-acquired infections. One hospital organization initiated multidisciplinary bedside leadership line care rounds (LLCRs) to improve the implementation of central line associated bloodstream infections (CLABSI) care bundles. The CLABSI care bundles identified actions that must occur for every patient, every time, in order to prevent infection. The LLCRs were utilized to engage the nursing staff in completing the requirements for the CLABSI bundles and to engage the patients themselves and family members in the prevention of infections (Owings et al., 2018). This healthcare organization realized that it was not enough to simply provide nursing staff with the elements of the evidence-based care bundle. There needed to be a change to the overall system where everyone involved was engaged in preventing infections. The LLCRs in this study worked to identify barriers to implementation, whether that was a knowledge deficit or non-adherence to the bundle interventions, which in turn allowed for continual training and created a feeling of empowerment for those involved.

IMPLICATIONS FOR PRACTICE

A systems thinking lens was applied to the nested levels of the healthcare system in this example. The four principles of applying systems thinking to clinical practice—(a) identifying the problem, (b) recognizing patterns, (c) evaluating systemic structure, and (d) developing a shared vision—are highlighted in this case study. Most importantly, the nurses evaluated system structures to improve adherence to the new process. Because the nurses took time to evaluate system structures, the healthcare organization developed a shared vision.

ORGANIZATIONS THAT FOSTER SYSTEMS THINKING IN HEALTHCARE

There are many government-funded and private organizations dedicated to the improvement of health outcomes through a systems-based approach. The organizations in Table 3.4 are examples of organizations whose mission is to encourage, educate, and advise healthcare professionals on ways to improve and incorporate systems-based thinking to provide safe, quality care. These organizations offer free training, education courses, and resources to anyone who signs up for an account.

DISCUSS THE IMPACT OF SYSTEMS THINKING ON QUALITY AND SAFETY PROCESSES

Nurses are often leading the way in QI and patient safety measures using the concepts of systems thinking. Nurses use clinical judgment to continually analyze systems, recognize patterns, and develop changes to improve care being delivered. The application of effective systems thinking to nursing practice is a strong predictor of safe nursing care (Moazez et al., 2020). Nurses' systems thinking skills have been shown to decrease medication errors, enhance QI efforts, and improve interprofessional interactions (Dolansky & Moore, 2013).

TABLE 3.4 ORGANIZATIONS FOSTERING SYSTEMS THINKING IN HEALTHCARE

ORGANIZATION	KEY INITIATIVES RELATED TO SYSTEMS THINKING	WEB ADDRESS
AHRQ	Delivery System Research Initiative	www.ahrq.gov/practiceimprovement/delivery-initiative/index.html
IHI	High-Reliability Organizations Safer Together: A National Action Plan to Address Patient Safety	www.ihi.org/resources/Pages/Publications/Is-Your-Organization-Highly-Reliable.aspx www.ihi.org/Engage/Initiatives/National-Steering-Committee-Patient-Safety/Pages/National-Action-Plan-to-Advance-Patient-Safety.aspx
QSEN	The Six Competencies for Nursing Education	https://qsen.org/competencies/pre-licensure-ksas
NAHQ	NAHQ Healthcare Quality Competency Framework	https://nahq.org/education/nahq-healthcare-quality-competency-framework
NQF	NQF Quality Positing System, a database of NQF endorsed measures	www.qualityforum.org/Measures_Reports_Tools.aspx
TJC	National Patient Safety Goals	www.jointcommission.org/standards/national-patient-safety-goals

AHRQ, Agency for Healthcare Research and Quality; IHI, Institute for Healthcare Improvement; QSEN, Quality and Safety Education for Nurses; NAHQ, National Association for Healthcare Quality; NQF, National Quality Forum; TJC, The Joint Commission.

Incorporation of systems thinking competencies into guiding frameworks of nursing education highlight the importance of systems thinking in providing safe and effective care. While systems thinking is not one of the identified six QSEN competencies, it is woven throughout the knowledge, skills, and attitudes within each of the six competencies. This next section will explore examples of how nurses are solving problems within the healthcare organizations through the lens of systems thinking.

EXAMPLE 1: MEDICATION ADMINSTRATION

One of the most common healthcare errors involves medication administration. While the act of administering a medication seems simple, it actually involves a complex systems approach, with many different systems interacting before the point of care. To safely administer medications, nurses learn different safety strategies, such as the five rights of medication administration or the 5+5 steps or the eight steps. Whichever strategy the nurse employs, it is important to recognize that these steps focus on the nurses' role in medication administration, but as a systems thinker, the roles of other healthcare providers need to be considered as well.

Technological advances have been made in medication administration systems including bar coding medication, computerized order entry, and electronic health recorders; however, medication errors still occur. Often medication errors occur because of distractions or interruptions at some point in the system (Bucknall et al., 2019). Consider how often nurses gather medications for administration only to be stopped by a call light, family member, patient, or ringing phone before they even reach the patient's room to administer the medication. Systems thinking has allowed organizations to have some success in reducing the amount of medication errors by limiting distractions during medication administration, increasing awareness for potential errors during the medication administration process, involving patients in their medication administration, and double checking high-risk medications between providers (Bucknall et al., 2019).

The ability of the individual nurse to practice and utilize systems thinking can reduce medication errors (Hwang & Park, 2017). Flynn et al. (2016) describe how one organization initiated a systems change to reduce the number of interruptions during medication administration. By looking at interruptions holistically, they recognized that interruptions may not be intentional and that others may not understand or "see" the nurse as busy. This led to a simple visual representation strategy designed to signify when a nurse is engaged in medication administration. Nurses clearly identified they were in the process of medication administration by wearing a sash, noting on the communication board when they were completing the medication administration process, and forwarding phone calls to the main desk. The evidence-based changes made during this QI project modified the complex process of medication administration. The simple process of nurse-led medication administration did not change, but the visual adaptations impacted how others interacted with the nurses during medication administration. This example demonstrates how a systems thinking approach significantly decreased the number of interruptions nurses experienced during medication administration, resulting in decreased medication errors (Flynn et al., 2016). The nurses in this example demonstrated the QSEN competency of safety by examining human factors and the limits of safety enhancing technologies, designing system improvements, and valuing their role in preventing medication errors.

CASE STUDY

A hospital system is working to decrease door to balloon times for patients who present to the ED with ST elevation myocardial infarctions (STEMI). Door to balloon is the amount of time that occurs between when a patient enters the ED with STEMI to the time the patient's blocked coronary artery is opened via a percutaneous coronary intervention. The hospital goal for door to balloon times is 90 minutes but that goal was only being met 80% of the time. Hospital administration determined that a task force should be created to determine changes needed to the process in order to meet this goal 100% of the time.

1. ***Who should be members of the task force?***
2. ***Utilizing a systems thinking approach, what processes should be analyzed for changes?***
3. ***What evidence should the task force gather related to changing the policy and procedures?***

EXAMPLE 2: HOSPITAL-ACQUIRED INFECTIONS

Common hospital-acquired infections include catheter associated urinary tract infections (CAUTI), CLABSI, ventilator associated pneumonia (VAP), and *Clostridium difficile* (*C-diff*). At one hospital CAUTI rates were high despite well researched, evidence-based solutions for prevention and sterile insertions. A systems thinking approach was utilized to address the problem.

At one hospital, a bedside nurse and an identified CAUTI champion initially recognized their unit had higher CAUTI rates than other units in the hospital. Some units had zero infections while their unit's infection rate was 18.7%. An interprofessional team was formed to review the current processes related to urinary catheters, study all possible contributors to CAUTI rates, and discuss the problem with a diverse group of stakeholders. Following data collection about the current system, a nurse-driven protocol was created to facilitate a shared vision regarding the need for an indwelling catheter. The protocol outlined the process for the nurse to analyze the amount of time the patient had the indwelling catheter, review the patients' diagnosis, and consult with the interprofessional team as needed to facilitate earlier removal of unnecessary catheters (Schiessler et al., 2019). A year after implementation, the hospital unit only had one CAUTI infection compared to five the previous year (Schiessler et al., 2019).

This example of systems thinking demonstrates how interprofessional teams can work together to develop policies that support safer care. The nurse champion and team looked at the problem holistically, recognized patterns over time across settings, evaluated contributing factors, reflected on the opinions and perceptions of all stakeholders, and facilitated change through the creation of a revised protocol. As the new protocol is utilized, systems thinking is also employed by the individual nurse to demonstrate understanding of cause and effect and utilizes reflection to make practice changes. In solving patient care problems, systems thinking is necessary to consider all aspects of the problem and find an effective solution.

The nurses in this example demonstrated the QSEN competency of QI by recognizing that nurses are part of the systems of care process that impacts outcomes, seeking information about outcomes of care in their patient population, developing a protocol to make process of care explicit, and appreciating the value of continuous QI.

BOX 3.1 Developing Clinical Judgment

It has been well established that good hand hygiene is essential for the prevention of infection. Nurses wash their hands with the provided alcohol hand gel as they enter and exit patients' rooms. Recently a nurse has begun to notice the hand sanitizer systems are empty in many patients' rooms. Staff often become distracted before finding hand sanitizer and, because the sanitizer systems are empty, are failing to clean their hands after patient contact. The nurse begins to wonder about how the holders get filled, how often, and by whom.

1. What **CUES (Assessment)** should the nurse consider?
2. What **HYPOTHESIS (Diagnosis)** should the nurse consider?
3. What **ACTION (Plan and Implement)** will be most effective for the nurse to take to improve adherence to hand washing?
4. What **OUTCOME (Evaluation)** metric will determine successful QI?

EXAMPLE 3: LENGTH OF STAY

Many healthcare organizations struggle with variations in patient length of stay (LOS) and patients being in the ED for extended periods because beds are not available to move them to. This leads to an increased cost for the organization and patient dissatisfaction. Molla et al. (2018) describes how an interprofessional QI team identified the problem, recognized the holistic process involved in movement of patients, and made system-wide changes to improve patient outcomes. Because the process of discharging a patient involves multiple systems and team members, the QI department within this organization started by identifying patterns related to discharge, such as a lack of medication reconciliation or the need for patient transport, and created targeted interventions within the discharge process to improve the timeliness of discharge (Molla et al., 2018). They sought input from everyone involved in the discharge process before initiating a large process change.

Traditionally, patients were assigned a healthcare provider and then a bed anywhere in the hospital. The assigned healthcare provider traveled across the hospital to see and care for patients. With the new process, patients were not assigned a provider until they were placed in a room. This allowed the healthcare providers to be centralized geographically and reduced the amount of time needed to travel from place to place (Molla et al., 2018). The healthcare providers, along with members of the interprofessional team, could now more easily participate in daily rounding. Daily rounding was also modified to include a specific bundle of items related to discharge and patients' needs (Molla et al., 2018). The bundle worked to create a systematic process that reduced variations in care. Limiting geographic spread of care providers and incorporating discharge bundles improved the time of discharge orders and physical discharges of the patients.

Nursing leadership within the organization monitored the interprofessional rounds and provided feedback on the outcomes of the QI project (Molla et al., 2018). The feedback, a necessary component of the process, allowed the team to identify successes and areas for improvement, ultimately leading to the system functioning more effectively. The nurses in this example demonstrated the QSEN competency of teamwork and collaboration by understanding the role and scopes of practices of all team members, soliciting input from all members of the team, and valuing system solutions for effective team functioning.

BOX 3.2 Developing Clinical Judgment

The hospital has well-established evidence-based procedures in place to prevent post-op surgical infections. A nurse who works on a surgical unit has noticed an increase in the number of post-op surgical infections in patients. The unit has recently been short staffed leading to the use of float pool nurses and a large amount of new hires. The nurse begins to wonder how well the procedures are being followed.

1. What **CUES (Assessment)** should the nurse consider?
2. What **HYPOTHESIS (Diagnosis)** should the nurse consider?
3. What **ACTION (Plan and Implement)** will be most effective for the nurse to take to improve the rate of surgical site infections?
4. What **OUTCOME (Evaluation)** metric will determine successful QI?

EXAMINE WAYS TO FOSTER SYSTEMS THINKING IN PRACTICE

Systems thinking is a learned skill that requires dedicated preparation through instruction, reflective practices, and personal experience (Dolansky & Moore, 2013; Plack et al., 2019). This section will provide strategies to include in a personal systems thinking toolkit. Included are strategies for identifying, describing, analyzing, and evaluating a system and its performance. All the strategies provided will require holistic thinking, recognition of patterns, reflective practice, and willingness to change perceptions.

SELF-ASSESSMENT

Assessing personal systems thinking skill level is an important component of becoming an effective systems thinker. The Systems Thinking Scale (STS) is a 20-question test designed to assess systems thinking abilities in new graduates (Dolansky et al., 2020). The test takes less than 10 minutes to complete. The more items marked "most of the time" the better the ability to employ systems thinking in professional nursing practice. As experience and personal mastery of nursing practice improves, so will the ability to use systems thinking. It may be helpful to come back to the STS on a routine basis to assess growth across time and identify areas that need concentrated improvement (Table 3.5).

The Waters Center for Systems Thinkers offers 14 habits of the mind for systems thinkers (Box 3.3). Routinely going through this checklist and reflecting on these habits is another way to assess systems thinking growth across time and identify areas for improvement.

CASE STUDY

Mr. J has pain described as 5 on a scale of 0 to 10. The healthcare provider has ordered morphine for pain management. The new graduate nurse is working with the assigned senior staff nurse to provide care for the patient. During medication administration the nurse reviews the medication administration record (MAR) and obtains the necessary vial of morphine. The staff nurse hands the vial to the new nurse and states, "This is to be given IV." The medication is administered without incident. As the new nurse provides report to the oncoming staff nurse, they review the MAR for medications needed that shift. The oncoming nurse asks, "Why did you give the morphine IV, it is ordered IM?" The nurse recognizes a medication error occurred.

1. *What is the new graduate nurse and staff nurse's immediate next steps to address the problem?*
2. *Identify the relationships that impact the medication administration process in this case study.*
3. *Identify systems factors that could have impacted the medication administration process.*
4. *Reflect on some beliefs, values, or assumptions within the new graduate nurse/senior nurse relationship that may have impacted the medication administration process.*

STRATEGIES TO LEARN HOW TO BECOME A SYSTEMS THINKER

Root cause analysis was initially developed to analyze industrial accidents but is now widely deployed as an error analysis tool in healthcare to identify underlying problems that increase the likelihood of error while avoiding the trap of focusing on mistakes by individuals. The fishbone technique for root cause analysis is used to determine cause-and-effect relationships related to patient safety or QI (Connelly, 2018). It is commonly utilized to review an error or near miss to determine systems changes that can prevent repeated error in the future. The fishbone technique helps the learner to visually consider multiple pre-identified system factors that may have impacted the problem (Dolansky & Moore, 2013; Plack et al., 2019). Identified system factors to include in a standard root cause analysis are people, equipment, process, materials, environment, and management. More can be found about constructing a fishbone diagram in Chapter 11.

Causal loop diagrams are visual stories about a problem or issue created through the connecting of loops that represent variables within the system and show the links between them (Lannon, n.d.). By visualizing the causes of the issues, it is easier to analyze what factors may be contributing to the problems or potential causes of behavior. There are four main parts of a causal loop diagram: the variables, links between variables, interconnection of variables, and the expected outcome of the interconnections and links (Lannon, n.d.). A step-by-step procedure for creating causal loop diagrams is provided in Box 3.4.

An example casual loop diagram about customized meal ordering in the hospital cafeteria is provided in Figure 3.3. The hospital initiates customized meal ordering services for patients from a diverse set of options in order to increase patient satisfaction with food services. The customizable menus initially caused an increase in patient satisfaction. However, as patients' requests for different food options increase, the delivery time for meals becomes extended and the kitchen staff complain of being overworked.

Concept Mapping

A concept map is a visual representation of information often used in nursing to help students organize and represent knowledge of a subject. Concept mapping requires reflective practices, critical thinking, understanding of clinical situations, and viewing situations holistically. Concept mapping starts with the main idea in the center and then flows out from that point to demonstrate connections as a way to break down large concepts to specific aspects. Figure 3.4 is an example of a concept map for a patient who is having trouble breathing. The concept map considers the patients, current presentation,

TABLE 3.5 SYSTEMS THINKING SCALE

20-Item Systems Thinking Scale					
Instructions: Please read each of the statements and place an "X" in the answer box that indicates frequency of agreement with the statement:					
WHEN I WANT TO MAKE AN IMPROVEMENT...	**NEVER**	**SELDOM**	**SOME OF THE TIME**	**OFTEN**	**MOST OF THE TIME**
1. I seek everyone's view of the situation.					
2. I look beyond a specific event to determine the cause of the problem.					
3. I think understanding how the chain of events occurs is crucial.					
4. I include people in my work unit to find a solution.					
5. I think recurring patterns are more important than any one specific event.					
6. I think of the problem at hand as a series of connected issues.					
7. I consider the cause and effect that is occurring in a situation.					
8. I consider the relationships among coworkers in the work unit.					
9. I think that systems are constantly changing.					
10. I propose solutions that affect the work environment, not specific individuals.					
11. I keep in mind that proposed changes can affect the whole system.					
12. I think more than one or two people are needed to have success.					
13. I keep the mission and purpose of the organization in mind.					
14. I think small changes can produce important results.					
15. I consider how multiple changes affect each other.					
16. I think about how different employees might be affected by the improvement.					
17. I try strategies that do not rely on people's memory.					
18. I recognize system problems are influenced by past events.					
19. I consider the past history and culture of the work unit.					
20. I consider that the same action can have different effects over time, depending on the state of the system.					

Source: Reprinted with permission from Dolansky, M. A., Moore, S. M., Palmieri, P. A., & Singh, M. K. (2020). Development and validation of the Systems Thinking Scale. *Journal of General Internal Medicine, 35*(8), 2318, Figure 3. https://doi.org/10.1007/s11606-020-05830-1

BOX 3.3 Habits of Mind for Systems Thinkers

A systems thinker:

- Seeks to understand the big picture.
- Observes how elements within a system change over time, generating patterns and trends.
- Recognizes that a system's structure generates behavior.
- Identifies the circular nature of complex cause-and-effect relationships.
- Makes meaningful connections within and between systems.
- Changes perspectives to increase understanding.
- Tests assumptions.
- Considers the issue fully and resists coming to a quick conclusion.
- Considers how mental models affect current reality and the future.
- Uses understanding of system structure to identify possible leverage actions.
- Considers short-term, long-term, and unintended consequences of actions.
- Pays attention to accumulations and their rates of change.
- Recognizes the impact of time delays when exploring cause-and-effect relationships.
- Checks results and change actions if needed, a process known as "successive approximation."

Note: Adapted from Habits of a System Thinker. Thinking Tools Studio: https://thinkingtoolsstudio.org/cards. WatersCenterST.org and www.ThinkingToolsStudio.org

BOX 3.4 How to Create Causal Loop Diagrams

1. Select variable names using nouns that can be represented or changed over time.
2. Identify verbs that link the variables together and how they change each other. These links between variables can be positive or negative depending on what occurs after.
3. Determine if the loop is reinforcing, meaning one change leads to another in the same direction, or balancing, meaning keeping the variable at the current state.
4. Talk through the loops to explain the causes and solutions to the problem.

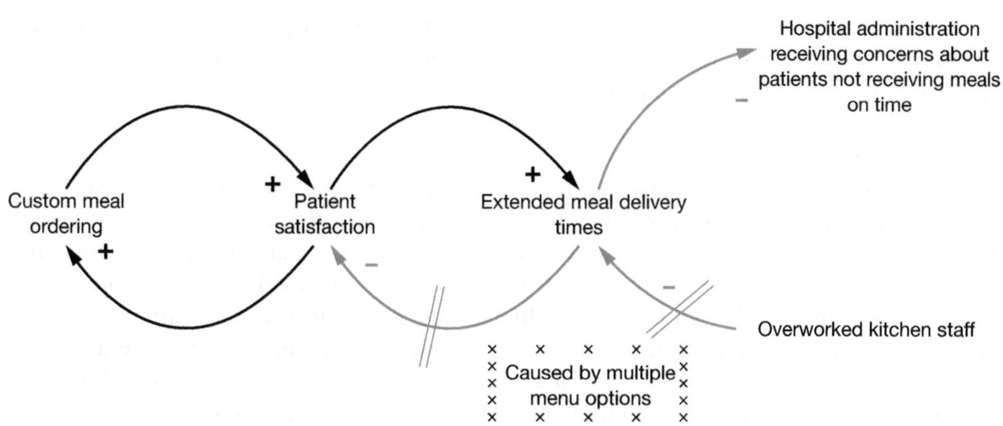

FIGURE 3.3 Example of a Causal Loop Diagram.

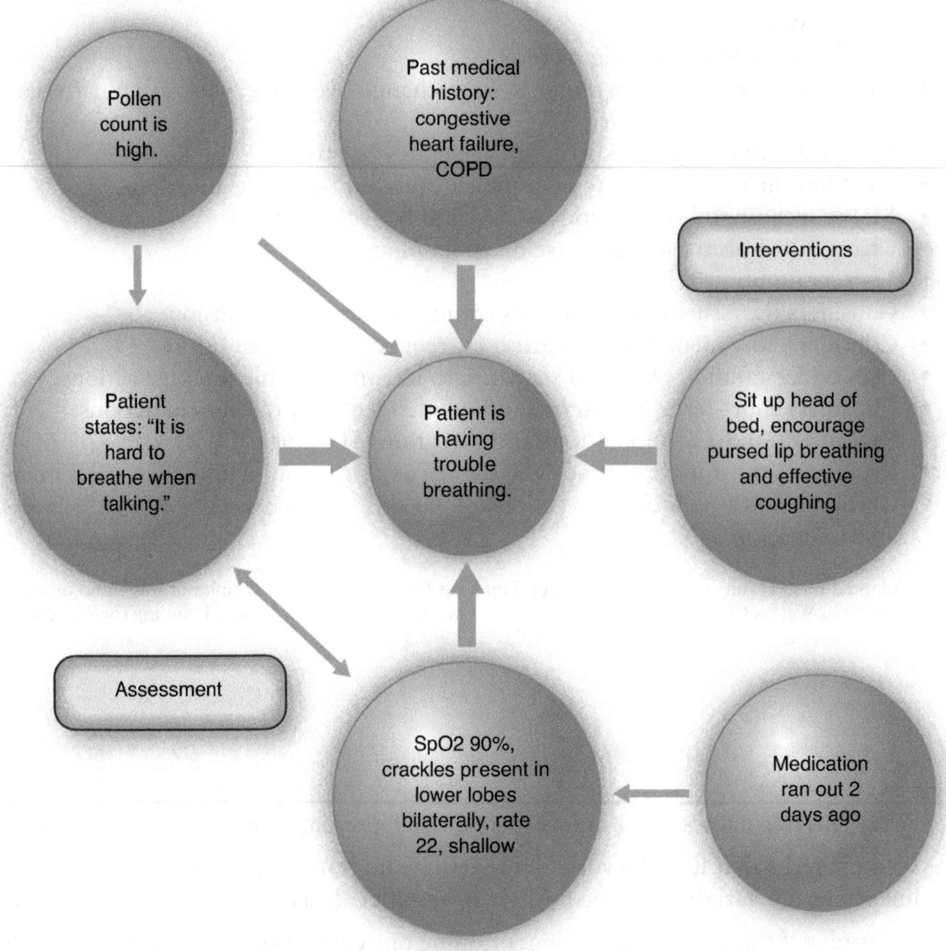

FIGURE 3.4 Example of a Concept Map.

COPD, chronic obstructive pulmonary disease.

as well as factors that may have led to the breathing problems and ways to improve the patient's, breathing. More about concept mapping is available at www.unthsc.edu/center-for-innovative-learning/concept-mapping.

Left-hand column technique:

The **left-hand column technique** is a way to analyze difficult conversations by visualizing spoken words in relation to personal perceptions, opinions, or thoughts that were occurring at the same time. This technique allows examination of how perceptions, opinions, and thoughts influence interactions in different situations. The left-hand column technique can be especially helpful with communication. In difficult conversations, there can be unspoken messages or interpretations that are incorrect. To use this technique to analyze a specific conversation, first make two columns on a page and recreate what was said in a list in the right-hand column. As demonstrated in Table 3.6, the left-hand side column allows a space to document what was being thought or felt when that comment was made (Senge, 2006). After completion, self-reflect is written between the two columns. Use these questions to

TABLE 3.6 EXAMPLE OF A LEFT-HAND COLUMN REFLECTION

WHAT THE STUDENT WAS THINKING OR FEELING	WHAT WAS SAID
I did it wrong! Did I harm the patient? How am I supposed to do it?	Nurse Preceptor: "Why did you do it that way?" Student: "I don't know"
Why is the nurse asking this? She is wrong. I did it correctly.	Nurse Preceptor: "Our policy and procedure handbook states you should always clean IV ports with alcohol before and between medication administration to prevent infection." Student: "I did do that, didn't you see"?
I am embarrassed that I missed the in between step. I know to do that. I demonstrated it in my check off last week. I wonder why I didn't do it in the patient's room?	Nurse Preceptor: "You did clean with alcohol before injecting the saline flush but you didn't clean with alcohol in between the saline flush and the medication. Students: "Oh, well that seems like a silly rule. I didn't touch it anyways."

guide reflection. What was the purpose of the conversation? Did the conversation accomplish the intended goals? How did personal assumptions contribute to this interaction? Why weren't the thoughts and feelings written in the left-hand column articulated during the conversation? What other communication techniques can be used to achieve the purpose of the conversation? By asking ourselves these reflective questions while reviewing the spoken and unspoken aspects of communication, nurses can better identify how one's individual words and actions affect others and the overall system (Plack et al., 2019; Senge, 2006).

The Iceberg Model Challenge

The **iceberg model challenge** is a method for viewing a problem holistically rather than focusing on a single individual problem by considering what lies beneath the actual problem that is visible. Just like an iceberg, frequently only 10% of the problem is readily apparent while 90% of the supporting structure is hidden underwater. The hidden structure of a problem generates the perceived concerns and determines the visible (above water) outcomes. The iceberg model applies different lenses to view the system and explore patterns or events that may cause a problem to occur. The four levels of the iceberg model are the events (what is easily visible), patterns of behavior, system structure, and mental models (all unseen; Waters Center for Systems Thinking, 2021). In each level there are guiding questions to help process through the problem and encourage deeper understanding (Table 3.7). The Waters Center for Systems Thinking provides free courses on the iceberg strategy and many other systems thinking strategies on their website at https://thinkingtoolsstudio.org/courses/04-iceberg.

DISCUSS THE ROLE OF LEADERSHIP AS A COMPONENT FOR SYSTEMS THINKING

Nurses in management or at the bedside are the leaders in the application of systems thinking to improve patient quality and care. Safe nursing care and systems thinking are directly correlated (Moazez et al., 2020). Nurses who have higher systems thinking scores are more likely to report positive safety culture contributions such as using the established reporting system to report a medication error. Additionally, these same nurses are less likely to be involved in an adverse patient event (Hwang & Park, 2017). Systems thinking allows a nurse at the bedside or a nurse leader to transform patient care for a unit or an entire hospital by identifying problems, recognizing new possibilities for change, evaluating current processes, and developing an action plan or shared vision. Nurse leaders must model systems thinking through their actions and actively work to encourage and develop systems thinking in those they lead.

Systems thinking is a fundamental competency in effective leadership (American Organization for Nursing Leadership, 2021). As nurses apply systems thinking at the bedside they are developing leadership skills. The components of systems thinking and the steps required to apply it to practice emphasize qualities of effective leadership such as communication, working with others in a holistic and comprehensive manner, strategic problem-solving though pattern and relationship identification, self-reflection, and a shared vision. Solving a problem is rarely simple. Solutions are often multifaceted, interdependent, and complex. The tools provided in this chapter can help nurses solve problems and communicate effectively at all levels. Nurses and nurse leaders should routinely complete the Systems Thinking Scale and review the Habits of Mind for Systems Thinkers to identify strengths in their systems thinking and areas where they can improve.

Nurses leading to improve patient care through systems thinking is illustrated throughout this chapter. Schiessler et al. (2019) began their CAUTI prevention protocol because a bedside nurse, CAUTI champion, and a charge nurse recognized inconsistencies in the

TABLE 3.7 ICEBERG MODEL CHALLENGE

LEVEL	QUESTIONS FOR EVALUATING THE SYSTEM	EXAMPLE
Event	What happened?	A medication error
Patterns over time	What has been happening? What are trends over time? Have changes occurred?	The medication was ordered IV and was administered IM. This is the third instance of this medication being given by the wrong route on this unit in the last year. A new group of physicians recently started performing surgeries at the facility. The number of daily procedures is increasing.
System structure	What factors influence the identified patterns (policies, behavior, physical environment, etc.)? Are their relationships between influencing factors?	An increased number of orders are for IV injections. Previous orders for that medication were IM. Daily procedures are increasing. Nurses are taking care of more patients at a time. Metrics are hung on the wall for length of stay and satisfaction with care. Nurses are busier with more patients to care for since the new doctors arrived. A new group of doctors has changed the routine. Nurses feel like they are being judged by how quickly they can provide care.
Mental model	What assumptions, beliefs, and values do I and others have about the event, structures, or system?	Nurses value providing safe and efficient care. On this unit patients are consistently admitted and discharged. Efficiency and speed is valued. Nurses made assumptions about medication order based on how it was always done and did not stop to perform necessary safety double checks.

IM, intramuscularly; IV, intravenously.

Source: Adapted from Iceberg Model. https://thinkingtoolsstudio.org/resources/iceberg-with-graphics/downloads Copyright 2020 Waters Center for Systems Thinking. www.WatersCenterST.org and www.ThinkingToolsStudio.org

discussion of indwelling catheter use in their unit. The program Flynn et al. (2016) implemented to limit interruptions during medication administration was inspired by a keynote speaker heard by nurses who were attending a national conference. All nurses are leaders, and each has the ability to effect change through the use of systems thinking whether for an individual patient or an entire healthcare system. At the bedside or in upper management, nurses are leaders. As healthcare becomes more complex, the roles within the system are increasingly interdependent and nurses will be required to continue to apply systems thinking in an increasingly robust manner to affect change, improve care, and improve the healthcare delivery system (Institute of Medicine (US) Committee on the Robert Wood Johnson Foundation Initiative on the Future of Nursing, at the Institute of Medicine, 2011).

BOX 3.5 Developing Clinical Judgment

Bedside reporting can improve patient satisfaction and is a way to provide family-centered care. A nurse has been asked by the manager to create a policy regarding the use of bedside reporting on the unit. Currently, nurses complete shift reports at the nurses' station and many use that time to have a cup of coffee and lean on the counter to write while listening. The nurse begins to wonder what might be preventing bedside reporting from happening on the unit regarding the staff attitude, the space, and the equipment.

1. What **CUES (Assessment)** should the nurse consider?
2. What **HYPOTHESIS (Diagnosis)** should the nurse consider?
3. What **ACTION (Plan and Implement)** will be most effective for the nurse to take when creating a policy about bedside reporting?
4. What **OUTCOME (Evaluation)** method will be completed to measure the success of the plan?

END-OF-CHAPTER RESOURCES

KEY CONCEPTS

1. Systems are everywhere and can be simple or complex, open or closed.
2. There are four components of a system: input, output, outcome, and feedback.
3. Open systems are impacted by their environment.
4. Healthcare is made up of complex adaptive systems.
5. Effective systems reduce variation or error.
6. Systems thinking focuses on four key principles: looking at the big picture, recognizing patterns, reflective practice, and willingness to adapt or change perceptions.
7. A four-step process can help apply systems thinking to practice. The four steps are identifying the event, determining patterns, evaluating systemic structures, and finally creating a shared vision.
8. Nurses are systems thinkers and drivers of QI efforts.
9. Using a systems thinking approach can improve patient safety and quality of care.
10. Systems thinking is embedded in current QI methodologies.
11. Learning health systems are organizations that are engaged in continuous QI empowering all to be change agents.
12. High-reliability organizations consistently perform at high levels of safety over prolonged periods of time.
13. Systems thinking requires practice and experience in order to effectively integrate it into practice.

CRITICAL DISCUSSION POINTS

1. Think about how systems thinking can be applied during change of shift report. How are the four phases of systems thinking utilized during shift report?
2. Think about a patient who is diagnosed with congestive heart failure and end-stage renal disease. Considering the fourlevels of the nested healthcare system, who should be included on the interprofessional team?
3. A nurse made a medication error. The nurse gave the wrong dose of a medication because the nurse did not realize that two tablets were needed. Think about how the iceberg challenge can be utilized to look at this problem holistically.
4. Take the systems self-evaluation quiz. Write a 60-second reflection on the findings and identify an area of improvement for a systems thinker.
5. A patient has a fall. Review Figure 3.1 Continuum of Systems Thinking and consider how the patient's fall can be analyzed from a personal effort to a systems thinking effort.

KEY TERMS

> Causal loop diagram
> Closed system
> Complex system
> Concept map

- > Feedback
- > Healthcare systems science
- > High-reliability organization
- > Iceberg model challenge
- > Input
- > Learning health system
- > Left-hand column technique
- > Open system
- > Output
- > Process
- > Root cause analysis
- > Simple system
- > System
- > Systems science
- > Systems thinking

REVIEW QUESTIONS

Answers to Review Questions appear in the Instructor's Manual. Qualified instructors should request the Instructor's Manual from textbook@springerpub.com.

1. Determine which of the following options are systems. *Select all that apply.*
   A. Medication administration
   B. Catheter insertion kit
   C. Hospital bed
   D. PYXIS
   E. Supply room
2. When nurses are working to minimize interruptions during medication administration by evaluating the physical environment, they are applying which step of the systems thinking process?
   A. Identifying the problem
   B. Looking for patterns
   C. Identifying systemic structures
   D. Embracing a shared vision
   E. Reflecting
3. Which is an example of a nurse providing patient care from a systems thinking approach?
   A. The nurse turns a patient every 2 hours.
   B. The nurse helps a team member to turn the patient.
   C. The nurse advocates for adequate nutrition for the patient and turns the patient every 2 hours.
   D. The nurse reviews current research studies on pressure ulcer prevention.
4. Examine the systems approaches that follow and determine which ones will improve patient care. *Select all that apply.*
   A. Systems are designed to minimize error by creating the same outcome every time.
   B. Systems are designed to minimize error by allowing practitioners to use clinical judgment.
   C. Systems are designed to minimize error by creating a shared purpose.
   D. Systems are designed to minimize error by decreasing waste.

5. Compared to traditional healthcare organizations, what do high-reliability organizations strive to achieve? *Select all that apply.*
   A. Makes changes one unit at a time to evaluate the effect
   B. Makes changes system wide to create a dynamic change in the process
   C. Has a goal of zero harm
   D. Continually evaluates systems and processes for areas of change
6. A nurse is trying to identify patterns and causes for the increased falls on the unit this month. What strategies would be most effective to help the nurse identify relationships and patterns? *Select all that apply.*
   A. Concept mapping
   B. Casual loop diagram
   C. Left-hand column technique
   D. Root cause analysis
7. A nurse is working on discharge planning with an interprofessional team. The conversation has ended abruptly and left the nurse confused and frustrated. What strategy would be most helpful for the nurse to use to evaluate the conversation from a systems perspective?
   A. Iceberg challenge
   B. Concept mapping
   C. Left-hand column technique
   D. Root cause analysis
8. A nursing student witnessed healthcare providers not following the proper personal protective equipment (PPE) guidance related to infection control procedures. To evaluate the concern, the nursing student is surveying staff knowledge, skills, and attitudes related to infection prevention protocols. What question asked by the student is within the patterns of events level using a systems thinking mental model?
   A. What is the current policy for infection prevention protocols?
   B. What are the hospital-acquired infection rates on this unit within the last 6 months?
   C. How do isolation signs get put into place?
   D. Who is responsible for infection prevention?
9. Which items that follow identify change from a systems viewpoint? *Select all that apply.*
   A. Fall rates have improved since initiating hourly rounding.
   B. Staff has scanned all required inventory this month for billing.
   C. Wait times have increased in the ED following a new triage policy.
   D. Training on new patient lifts has increased the use of patient lifts on the unit.
10. Determine which of the statements that follow by the nurse represent the four principles of systems thinking. *Select all that apply.*
   A. The nurse recognizes their patient has a pressure ulcer.
   B. The nurse realizes that patients who are intubated are more likely to have a pressure ulcer.
   C. The nurse talks to a patient who has experienced a pressure ulcer.
   D. The nurse creates a new policy related to patient movement to prevent pressure ulcers.

REVIEW ACTIVITIES

1. What type of a system is a classroom? Identify and classify all the elements of a classroom. What are the structures, patterns, inputs, outcomes, environment, and feedback?
2. At a clinical facility, find the policy and procedure related to handwashing. After reviewing the protocol, observe the practices of the healthcare providers around you. Interview a nurse about their hand washing knowledge, skills, and attitudes. After investigating, identify all possible factors that can impact handwashing compliance (people, equipment, materials, environment, and management). Identify relationships between factors or patterns that can emerge from compliance of handwashing. Draw a concept map representing the relationships and factors involved in handwashing compliance.
   A. Examples that can be applied to different factors
   B. People: role, training, personal views/beliefs related to handwashing, how busy they are
   C. Materials: water, soap, sinks, hand sanitizer, effects of soap or hand sanitizer on skin
   D. Management: feedback provided, handwashing audits
   E. Environmental (culture): organizational culture, accountability, value of evidence-based practice
   F. Environmental (physical): placement of sinks, hand sanitizer
3. What makes an effective systems thinker? Review the 14 habits of mind for a systems thinker. Identify three to five statements as personal areas for improvement. List ways to improve abilities in these areas or questions that can be asked to remind a nurse of this habit.

EXPLORING THE WEB

1. On the qsen.org website under the education tab, navigate to strategies and find the teaching strategy: A Virtual Clinical Learning Experience/Reflection Using Transformational Leadership and Systems Thinking. Complete the activity: https://qsen.org/leadership-to-use-systems-thinking-a-virtual-clinical-learning-experience
2. On the qsen.org website under the education tab, navigate to strategies and find the teaching strategy: Systems Thinking for Quality Improvement: Innovative Teaching Strategy for Advanced Practice. Complete the activity: https://qsen.org/systems-thinking-for-quality-improvement-innovative-teaching-strategy-for-advanced-practice
3. Access the Thinking Tools Studio created by the Waters Center for Systems Thinking: https://thinkingtoolsstudio.org/login. Sign up to take the free courses offered. Under the courses tab explore the "habits" or "tools" courses. All the courses offered are designed for applying systems thinking.
4. Access the IHI website at www.ihi.org. Select IHI Open School. Select Courses and Certificates. Select course number QI 202: Addressing Small Problems to Build Safer, More Reliable Systems and complete the course.
5. Explore the Institute for Healthcare Improvement. Under topics, explore the systems and reliability topic. This tab contains videos, personal stories, activities, and more about highly reliable organizations and using systems to improve outcomes: www.ihi.org/Topics/Reliability/Pages/default.aspx

6. Investigate the Cleveland Clinics ConsultQD page: https://consultqd.clevelandclinic.org/. Under specialties choose Nursing. Read about real world applications of systems thinking to improve care and interviews from nurse experts at the Cleveland Clinic.

REFERENCES

Agency for Healthcare Research and Quality. (2019). *About learning health systems*. https://www.ahrq.gov/learning-health-systems/about.html

American Organization for Nursing Leadership. (2021). *AONL nurse leader competencies*. https://www.aonl.org/resources/nurse-leader-competencies

Başoğul, C., & Buldukoğlu, K. (2020). Neuman systems model with depressed patients: A randomized controlled trial. *Nursing Science Quarterly, 33*(2), 148–158. https://doi.org/10.1177/0894318419898172

Bates, D. W., & Singh, H. (2018). Two decades since *To Err Is Human*: An assessment of progress and emerging priorities in patient safety. *Health Affairs, 37*(11), 1736–1743. https://doi.org/10.1377/hlthaff.2018.0738

Bucknall, T., Fossum, M., Hutchinson, A. M., Botti, M., Considine, J., Dunning, T., Hughes, L., Weir-Phyland, J., Digby, R., & Manias, E. (2019). Nurses' decision-making, practices and perceptions of patient involvement in medication administration in an acute hospital setting. *Journal of Advanced Nursing, 75*(6), 1316–1327. https://doi.org/10.1111/jan.13963

Cheney, C. (2019). *Health systems and hospitals in pursuit of high reliability*. HealthLeaders. https://www.healthleadersmedia.com/clinical-care/health-systems-and-hospitals-pursuit-high-reliability

Connelly, L. (2018). Voice of the process. *MedSurg Nursing 27*(4), 262–263. http://www.medsurgnursing.net/archives/18jul/262.pdf

Cordon, C. (2013). System theories: An overview of various system theories and its application in healthcare. *American Journal of Systems Science, 2*(1), 13–22. http://article.sapub.org/10.5923.j.ajss.20130201.03.html

Dolansky, M. A., & Moore, S. M. (2013). Quality and Safety Education for Nurses (QSEN): The key is systems thinking. *Online Journal of Issues in Nursing, 18*(3), 1–12. https://doi.org/10.3912/OJIN.Vol18No03Man01

Dolansky, M. A., Moore, S. M., Palmieri, P. A., & Singh, M. K. (2020). Development and validation of the Systems Thinking Scale. *Journal of General Internal Medicine, 35*(8), 2314–2320. https://doi.org/10.1007/s11606-020-05830-1

Federal Aviation Administration. (2019). *Safety Management System (SMS)*. https://www.faa.gov/about/initiatives/sms

Federico, F. (2018). Is your organization highly reliable? *Healthcare Executive, 33*(1), 76–79. http://www.ihi.org/resources/Pages/Publications/Is-Your-Organization-Highly-Reliable.aspx

Flynn, F., Evanish, J. Q., Fernald, J. M., Hutchinson, D. E., & Lefaiver, C. (2016). Progressive care nurses improving patient safety by limiting interruptions during medication administration. *Critical Care Nurse, 36*(4), 19–35. https://doi.org/10.4037/ccn2016498

Fowler, P. J., Hovmand, P. S., Marcal, K. E., & Das, S. (2019). Solving homelessness from a complex systems perspective: Insights for prevention responses. *Annual Review of Public Health, 40*(1), 465–486. https://doi.org/10.1146/annurev-publhealth-040617-013553

Frankel, A., Haraden, C., Federico, F., & Lenoci-Edwards, J. (2017). *A framework for safe, reliable, and effective care* [White Paper]. Institute for Healthcare Improvement and Safe & Reliable Healthcare. http://www.ihi.org/resources/Pages/IHIWhitePapers/Framework-Safe-Reliable-Effective-Care.aspx

Hoang, T., Harris, J., Givan, M., Sisk, M., Brinkman, M., Eustace, A., Gibson, V., Jewell, R., & Abo, R. (2017). Using design thinking to re-design isolation signs. *American Journal of Infection Control, 45*(6, Suppl.), S116–S117. https://doi.org/10.1016/j.ajic.2017.04.202

Hwang, J.-I., & Park, H.-A. (2017). Nurses' systems thinking competency, medical error reporting, and the occurrence of adverse events: A cross-sectional study. *Contemporary Nurse, 53*(6), 622–632. https://doi.org/10.1080/10376178.2017.1409081

Institute of Medicine. (2001). *Crossing the quality chasm: A new health system for the 21st century.* National Academies Press. https://doi.org/10.17226/10027

Institute of Medicine Committee on the Robert Wood Johnson Foundation Initiative on the Future of Nursing, at the Institute of Medicine. (2011). *The future of nursing: Leading change, advancing health*. National Academies Press. https://doi.org/10.17226/12956

Johnson, J., Miller, S., & Horowitz, S. (2008). Systems-based practice: Improving the safety and quality of patient care by recognizing and improving the systems in which we work. In K. Henriksen, J. B. Battles & M. A. Keyes (Eds.), *Advances in patient safety: New directions and alternative approaches* (Vol. 2) (AHRQ Publication No. 08-0034-2). Agency for Healthcare Research and Quality. https://www.ncbi.nlm.nih.gov/books/NBK43731

The Joint Commission. (2021). *Comprehensive accreditation manual for hospitals* (pp. PS-1–PS-48). https://www.jointcommission.org/-/media/tjc/documents/standards/ps-chapters/camh_04a_ps_all_current.pdf

Kim, D. (1999). *Introduction to systems thinking*. https://thesystemsthinker.com/introduction-to-systems-thinking

Kim, D. (2000). *Systems thinking tools: A user's reference guide.* Pegasus Communications. https://thesystemsthinker.com/systems-thinking-tools-a-users-reference-guide

Kohn, L. T., Corrigan, J. M., & Donaldson, M. S. (Eds.). (2000). *To err is human: Building a safer health system.* National Academies Press. https://doi.org/10.17226/9728

Lannon, C. (n.d.). *Causal loop construction: The basics.* https://thesystemsthinker.com/causal-loop-construction-the-basics

Merriam-Webster. (n.d.). *System.* In Merriam-Webster.com dictionary. https://www.merriam-webster.com/dictionary/system

Moazez, M., Miri, S., Foroughameri, G., & Farokhzadian, J. (2020). Nurses' perceptions of systems thinking and safe nursing care: A cross-sectional study. *Journal of Nursing Management, 28*(4), 822–830. https://doi.org/10.1111/jonm.13000

Mobus, G. E., & Kalton, M. C. (2015). *Principles of systems science*. Springer.

Molla, M., Warren, D. S., Stewart, S. L., Stocking, J., Johl, H., & Sinigayan, V. (2018). A lean Six Sigma quality improvement project improves timeliness of discharge from the hospital. *Joint Commission Journal on Quality & Patient Safety, 44*(7), 401–412. https://doi.org/10.1016/j.jcjq.2018.02.006

National Steering Committee for Patient Safety. (2020) *Safer together: A national action plan to advance patient safety.* Institute for Healthcare Improvement. http://www.ihi.org/SafetyActionPlan

Neuman, B., & Fawcett, J. (Eds.). (2011). *The Neuman systems model* (5th ed.). Pearson.

Plack, M. M., Goldman, E. F., Scott, A. R., & Brundage, S. B. (2019). *Systems thinking in the healthcare professions: A guide for educators and clinicians*. The George Washington University. https://hsrc.himmelfarb.gwu.edu/cgi/viewcontent.cgi?article=1000&context=educational_resources_teaching

Polonsky, M. S. (2019). High-reliability organizations: The next frontier in healthcare quality and safety. *Journal of Healthcare Management, 64*(4), 213–221. https://doi.org/10.1097/jhm-d-19-00098

Reid, P. P., Compton, W. D., Grossman, J. H., & Fanjiang, G. (Eds.). (2005). *Building a better delivery system: A new engineering/health care partnership*. National Academies Press. https://doi.org/10.17226/11378

Roy, C. (2009). *The Roy Idaptation Model*. Prentice Hall.

Schiessler, M. M., Darwin, L. M., Phipps, A. R., Hegemann, L. R., Heybrock, B. S., & Macfadyen, A. J. (2019). Don't have a doubt, get the catheter out: A nurse-driven CAUTI prevention protocol. *Pediatric Quality & Safety, 4*(4), e183. https://doi.org/10.1097/pq9.0000000000000183

Schön, D. A. (1983). *The reflective practitioner: How professionals think in action.* Ashgate.

Senge, P. (2006). *The fifth discipline.* Doubleday.

Stalter, A. M., & Mota, A. (2018). Using systems thinking to envision quality and safety in healthcare. *Nursing Management, 49*(2), 32–39. https://doi.org/10.1097/01.NUMA.0000529925.66375.d0

Stalter, A. M., Phillips, J. M., Ruggiero, J. S., Scardaville, D. L., Merriam, D., Dolansky, M. A., Goldschmidt, K., Wiggs, C., & Winegardner, S. (2017). A concept analysis of systems thinking. *Nursing Forum, 52*(4), 323–330. https://doi.org/10.1111/nuf.12196

Toyota (n.d). *Toyota production system.* https://global.toyota/en/company/vision-and-philosophy/production-system

Trbovich, P. (2014). Five ways to incorporate systems thinking into healthcare organizations. *Biomedical Instrumentation & Technology, 48*(s2), 31–36. https://doi.org/10.2345/0899-8205-48.s2.31

Udod, S. A., Duchscher, J. B., Goodridge, D., Rotter, T., McGrath, P., & Hewitt, A. D. (2020). Nurse managers implementing the lean management system: A qualitative study in Western Canada. *Journal of Nursing Management, 28*, 221–228. https://doi.org/10.1111/jonm.12898

Ursavaş, F. E., Karayurt, Ö., & İşeri, Ö. (2014). Nursing approach based on Roy Adaptation Model in a patient undergoing breast conserving surgery for breast cancer. *The Journal of Breast Health, 10*(3), 134–140. https://www.ncbi.nlm.nih.gov/pmc/articles/PMC5351537

Von Bertalanffy, L. (1968). *General system theory.* George Braziller.

Waters Center for System Thinking. (2020). *Habits of a system thinker.* Thinking Tools Studio. https://thinkingtoolsstudio.org/cards

Waters Center for System Thinking. (2021). *Tools course #4: The iceberg* [MOOC]. Thinking Tools Studio. https://thinkingtoolsstudio.waterscenterst.org/courses/tools

World Health Organization. (2000). *The world health report 2000: Health systems: Improving performance.* Author. https://www.who.int/whr/2000/en/whr00_en.pdf?ua=1

Zhu, P. (2018). *Problem solving master: Frame problems systematically and solve problem creatively*. Lulu Press.

SUGGESTED READINGS

Dolansky, M. A., & Moore, S. M. (2013). Quality and Safety Education for Nurses (QSEN): The key is systems thinking. *Online Journal of Issues in Nursing, 18*(3), 1–12. https://doi.org/10.3912/OJIN.Vol18No03Man01

Gandhi, T. K., Feeley, D., & Schummers, D. (2020). Zero harm in health care: How a comprehensive systems-focused approach can help to prevent all types of harm in health care. *NEJM Catalyst Innovations in Care Delivery, 1*(2). https://doi.org/10.1056/CAT.19.1137

Hwang, J.-I., & Park, H.-A. (2017). Nurses' systems thinking competency, medical error reporting, and the occurrence of adverse events: A cross-sectional study. *Contemporary Nurse: A Journal for the Australian Nursing Profession, 53*(6), 622–632. https://doi.org/10.1080/10376178.2017.1409081

Institute for Healthcare Improvement. (2019). *Patient safety essentials toolkit.* Institute for Healthcare Improvement. http://www.ihi.org/resources/Pages/Tools/Patient-Safety-Essentials-Toolkit.aspx

Moazez, M., Miri, S., Foroughameri, G., & Farokhzadian, J. (2020). Nurses' perceptions of systems thinking and safe nursing care: A cross-sectional study. *Journal of Nursing Management, 28*(4), 822–830. https://doi.org/10.1111/jonm.13000

National Steering Committee for Patient Safety. (2020). *Safer together: A national action plan to advance patient safety.* Institute for Healthcare Improvement. https://www.ihi.org/SafetyActionPlan

Plack, M. M., Goldman, E. F., Scott, A. R., & Brundage, S. B. (2019). *Systems thinking in the health-care professions: A guide for educators and clinicians*. The George Washington University. https://hsrc.himmelfarb.gwu.edu/cgi/viewcontent.cgi?article=1000&context=educational_resources_teaching

Senge, P. (2006). *The fifth discipline*. Doubleday.

Stalter, A. M., & Mota, A. (2018). Using systems thinking to envision quality and safety in healthcare. *Nursing Management, 49*(2), 32–39. https://doi.org/10.1097/01.NUMA.0000529925.66375.d0

Stalter, A. M., Phillips, J. M., Ruggiero, J. S., Scardaville, D. L., Merriam, D., Dolansky, M. A., Goldschmidt, K., Wiggs, C., & Winegardner, S. (2017). A concept analysis of systems thinking. *Nursing Forum, 52*(4), 323–330. https://doi.org/10.1111/nuf.12196

CHAPTER **4**

Legal and Ethical Aspects of Nursing Quality and Safety

Theodore M. McGinn and Patricia Kelly Vana

"As a nurse, we have the opportunity to heal the heart, mind, soul and body of our patients, their families and ourselves. They may not remember your name, but they will never forget the way you made them feel."

–Maya Angelou

Upon completion of this chapter, the reader should be able to:

1. Identify the three branches of the United States (U.S.) Federal Government.
2. Explore the role of administrative agencies.
3. Describe how law shapes the practice of nursing.
4. Discuss the four elements of negligence or malpractice.
5. Discuss the nurse's independent responsibility to deliver quality care to patients.
6. Review responsibility of the nurse to follow hospital guidelines and physician's orders.
7. Analyze obligations under the Health Insurance Portability and Accountability Act of 1996 (HIPAA).
8. Identify Medicare Home Health Certification requirements.
9. Describe the Federal Anti-Kickback Statute, the Stark Law, and the Civil Monetary Penalties Law
10. Discuss whistleblower claims.
11. Review the International Council of Nurses Code of Ethics, the American Nursing Association Code of Ethics, and the underlying ethical principles that guide nursing practice.
12. Identify steps of the ethical decision-making process.

CROSSWALK

This chapter addresses the following:

QSEN Competency: Safety

The American Association of Colleges of Nursing (AACN). (2021). *The Essentials: Core competencies for professional nursing education.*

Domain 5: Quality and Safety
Domain 9: Professionalism
Domain 10: Personal, Professional, and Leadership Development

OPENING SCENARIO

A medical-surgical nurse with 15 years of experience has an excellent reputation for providing safe patient care and building rapport with patients and their families. Late one evening, an emergency department (ED) nurse calls with handoff report for an admission to the medical-surgical unit. During report, the nurse learns that while in the ED for the past 14 hours, the patient has been uncooperative, difficult to manage, and lashing out at staff and other patients. The patient was in a motor vehicle accident and tested positive for both alcohol and drugs. Upon arrival to the ED, the examination of the patient revealed two broken ribs, bruising on his chest, and multiple facial lacerations. The ED nurse states that the patient is currently stable and must be moved immediately because they are expecting multiple patients with critical injuries to arrive in the ED shortly. Currently, the medical-surgical unit is short-staffed because a nurse called out sick and could not be replaced. The patient arrives on the medical-surgical unit and is quiet and withdrawn. His initial vital signs include a pulse rate of 110 and blood pressure of 90/50. These assessment findings concern the nurse, who makes a note to recheck the patient's vitals after assessing the nurse's other patients. Within an hour of admission and before the nurse has an opportunity to reassess the patient, the patient experiences a cardiac arrest and dies. Three weeks after the incident, the medical-surgical nurse is informed that a lawsuit has been filed and the nurse has been named as a defendant.

1. Will the nurse be arrested and have to go to jail?
2. Should the nurse call the patient's family and apologize?
3. Is the nurse's license to practice in jeopardy of being lost?
4. Should the nurse hire a lawyer?

INTRODUCTION

The law provides guidance for the way people live and, in many instances, for the manner in which people conduct their work. The healthcare system is highly regulated with laws and regulations that guide the way nurses interact with patients and identify the rights that patients can legally expect during healthcare delivery. These laws and regulations derive from federal statutes, state statutes, state common law, and administrative rules and codes. The result is that nurses may feel bombarded with laws and regulations.

The role of the nurse in direct patient care and in the expanding roles that nurses now occupy in the healthcare system make it imperative that nurses understand the current legal system and their role in complying with the laws and regulations governing the practice of nursing. Advances in technology and healthcare are constantly changing the care that is reasonably expected to be provided to the patient. As an integral part of the healthcare system that has significant interaction with patients and families, nurses must not only stay current with emerging healthcare trends and risks, but they must also assume leadership in designing healthcare systems and processes to support those trends and minimize the risks.

This chapter will describe the three branches of the United States (U.S.) federal government and the role of administrative agencies. This chapter will also consider how law shapes the practice of nursing. It will discuss the four elements of negligence and malpractice and review the nurse's independent responsibility to deliver quality care to patients. The nurse's obligations under the Health Insurance Portability and Accountability Act of 1996 (HIPAA) as well as Medicare home health certification requirements will be explored. The chapter discusses the Anti-Kickback Law, the Stark Law, and the Civil

Monetary Penalties Law. The common ethical principles and theories that influence nursing practice such as whistleblower claims, the International Council of Nurses Code of Ethics, and the American Nursing Association Code of Ethics will be described along with the steps of the ethical decision-making process.

THREE BRANCHES OF THE U.S. FEDERAL GOVERNMENT

The U.S. Constitution established three branches of the federal government: (a) the executive branch, (b) the legislative branch, and (c) the judicial branch. Each branch has specific and occasionally overlapping roles and duties. This structure puts in place a **separation of powers**, which are strategic checks and balances designed to prevent one branch from overpowering the others. For example, the U.S. Supreme Court may declare a law passed by Congress and signed into law by the president as unconstitutional.

The **executive branch** of the federal government consists of the office of the president of the United States. The executive branch of the government carries out laws and shapes the agenda for the country. This agenda is based on the platform of the president's respective political party and is also often based on how the president seeks to advance their personal agenda. The president has a significant role in making law. Although the president does not write legislation, the president must approve any bill passed by Congress in order for it to become law. The president may also veto a bill, preventing it from becoming a law, but Congress may overturn the veto.

The president is responsible for the execution and implementation of federal laws, often through the delegation of authority to members of the Cabinet and through numerous governmental agencies. The president is also the Commander in Chief, responsible for defending the country and leading the United States Armed Forces. The president can sign treaties, issue executive orders, declare states of emergency, make appointments to the judiciary, and grant pardons.

The **legislative branch** of the federal government has the responsibility under the U.S. Constitution to make laws. This legislative branch of government is also known as Congress. It is comprised of the House of Representatives and the Senate. The Founding Fathers were very intentional when they defined the duties of the legislative branch and when they set the terms for holding office. The members of the House of Representatives are elected to 2-year terms. Currently, there are 435 members of the House of Representatives. The number of representatives each state has in the House of Representatives is directly proportional to the respective state's population. In contrast, members of the Senate are elected to 6-year terms. Each state has two senators, for a total of 100 senators. The structure in the Senate was designed to prevent the more populous states from overpowering the less populous states.

Federal laws always begin in one of the bodies of Congress. Either the Senate or the House of Representatives will draft a bill, and members of that body of Congress will vote on the bill. If the vote on the bill passes, the bill is then considered in the other body of Congress for passage. If the bill passes in both bodies of Congress, the president has the power to sign the bill into law, or veto the bill and prevent it from becoming law. After the president signs a bill, it becomes official law, otherwise known as a "statute" or "code."

The legislative branch also has the power to tax and spend. It may regulate interstate commerce, borrow money, and ratify treaties signed by the president. The legislative branch has the sole power to approve members appointed by the president to the judicial branch. Finally, the legislative branch has the sole power of impeachment of the president, judges, and members of Congress.

The **judicial branch** of the federal government has the responsibility of interpreting federal laws and assuring that the laws are in compliance with the U.S. Constitution. The

Supreme Court justices who comprise the judicial branch are appointed by the president and approved by Congress. Justices of the federal courts are appointed for lifetime terms. This is intended to assure that federal justices are not subject to the whims of the electorate who may seek to have a federal or Supreme Court Justice removed from their position because of rendering a decision in a manner that might have been contrary to others, political beliefs. Justices are expected to base their decisions only on the facts of the case at hand and their interpretation of the law relevant to the case (and not base their decisions on politics).

ADMINISTRATIVE AGENCIES

The legislative branch and the executive branch of the government often delegate authority to governmental administrative agencies. These federal governmental administrative agencies may be created under the Cabinet of the president. Other federal governmental administrative agencies are created by Congress through statute. In addition, the 50 states have a web of state governmental administrative agencies in existence. Regardless of the source, federal and state governmental administrative agencies permeate the landscape of America.

One of the most influential federal administrative agencies in the healthcare industry is the U.S. Department of Health and Human Services (HHS). This federal agency consists of 11 operating units that influence laws surrounding many aspects of the healthcare delivery system, including payment of healthcare services, regulation of medication and healthcare devices, vaccine programs, healthcare research, and patient safety. These federal administrative agencies can also develop regulations, but they often run into difficulties with some of the other branches of government, such as when Congress refuses to allocate dollars to fund the programs created under the regulations. Table 4.1 lists the federal agencies under the HSS and briefly describes their most important functions. Many of these HHS agencies are familiar to nurses working both in direct patient care and in administration.

CASE STUDY

President Jones was elected in 2020 on a campaign promoting tax code reform. Unfortunately for President Jones, the other political party has control of Congress. After several months of inaction, President Jones becomes impatient and orders the Internal Revenue Service to reduce the effective tax rates across the board.

1. *Is the president's order constitutional?*
2. *Is the president part of the legislative branch?*
3. *Will the Supreme Court uphold President Jones' orders?*

THE ROLE OF THE LAW IN SHAPING NURSING PRACTICE

The federal government is responsible for carrying out those powers specifically delegated to it in the U.S. Constitution. All other powers are reserved to the states. The U.S. Constitution does not directly address the regulation of nursing. Therefore, the states are the bodies that have created most of the nursing regulations. Moreover, the law that governs individual nursing practice is dependent upon the particular state where the individual nursing practice takes place. There are also many state and federal laws which govern

TABLE 4.1 U.S. DEPARTMENT OF HEALTH AND HUMAN SERVICES (HHS) AGENCIES AND FUNCTIONS

U.S. DEPARTMENT OF HEALTH AND HUMAN SERVICES (HHS) AGENCY	MOST IMPORTANT FUNCTIONS
The Administration for Children and Families	Promotes the economic and social well-being of families, children, individuals, and communities through a range of educational and supportive programs in partnership with states, tribes, and community organizations.
The Administration for Community Living	Increases access to community support and resources for the unique needs of older Americans and people with disabilities.
AHRQ	Produces evidence to make healthcare safer, higher quality, more accessible, equitable, and affordable, and works within HHS and with other partners to make sure that the evidence is understood and used.
The Agency for Toxic Substances and Disease Registry	Prevents exposure to toxic substances and the adverse health effects and diminished quality of life associated with exposure to hazardous substances from waste sites, unplanned releases of toxic substances, and other sources of environmental pollution.
CDC	Protects the public health of the nation by providing leadership and direction in the prevention and control of diseases and other preventable conditions and responds to public health emergencies.
CMS	Combines the oversight of the Medicare program, the federal portion of the Medicaid program, the State Children's Health Insurance Program (CHIP), the Health Insurance Marketplace, and related quality assurance activities.
FDA	Ensures that food is safe, pure, and wholesome; human and animal drugs, biological products, and medical devices are safe and effective; and that electronic products that emit radiation are safe.
HRSA	Provides healthcare to people who are geographically isolated and economically or medically vulnerable.
The Indian Health Service	Provides American Indians and Alaska Natives with comprehensive health services by developing and managing programs to meet their health needs.
NIH	Supports biomedical and behavioral research within the United States and abroad, conducts research in its own laboratories and clinics, trains promising young researchers, and promotes the collecting and sharing of healthcare knowledge.

AHRQ, Agency for Healthcare Research and Quality; CDC, Centers for Disease Control and Prevention; CMS, Centers for Medicare & Medicaid Services; FDA, Food and Drug Administration; HRSA, Health Resources and Services Administration; NIH, National Institutes of Health.

the healthcare industry and influence the practice of nursing. Nurses are regulated by both criminal law and civil law as well as by both statutory law and common law.

Criminal Law Versus Civil Law

Law is divided into two separate categories: criminal law and civil law. The primary distinction between the two categories relates to the particular goal of the law in question: Is the law designed to punish the wrongdoer for crimes against society? If so, then it is criminal law. Examples of criminal law include traffic violations, assault or battery, burglary, and murder. On the other hand, civil law aims to address a wrong against an individual or group of individuals by providing for compensation to the victim or victims. Examples of civil law include negligence, breach of contract, and/or infringement of trade secrets. There are many differences in procedure, purposes, and objectives for these two categories of law.

One of the most significant differences between criminal law and civil law is the burden of proof required in any legal proceeding. In a criminal law proceeding, the prosecution must prove their case beyond a reasonable doubt. For a civil law proceeding, the plaintiff (the person who brings a case against another in a court of law) must prove its case by a "preponderance of the evidence," meaning that the plaintiff must prove the defendant more likely than not committed the actions in question. Another important distinction is that in a criminal law proceeding, the case is initiated by the prosecution, who is working on behalf of the government. Criminal law proceedings are referred to as criminal prosecutions. In a civil law proceeding, the legal case is initiated by private individuals or entities.

Another difference between criminal law and civil law relates to the resolution of the case. In a criminal law proceeding, if the prosecution is successful, the defendant is required to spend time incarcerated in jail or is assessed a fine. In a civil law proceeding, if the plaintiff is successful, the defendant has to reimburse the plaintiff for the amount of damages determined by the court.

Statutory Law Versus Common Law

The category of civil law is further divided into two additional categories: statutory law and common law. **Statutory laws** are written laws that derive from a legislative body, such as those written statutes from the U.S. Congress, a state legislative body, or a municipal board of trustees of a city or town. Members of these legislative bodies are elected by the citizens of their respective communities. An example of statutory law would be the state **nurse practice act (NPA)** that is enacted by the various states to govern the licensure process for nurses.

Common law is the body of law that has been created through the application of prior court decisions, such as precedents to a unique set of facts; it has been developed by judges, courts, and other special courts or tribunals appointed to deal with a particular problem. If a similar matter has been heard by a court in the past, a court will generally follow the prior court's decision and apply the reasoning given in the earlier case to the matter that is pending before the court at that time. This is referred to as "precedent." Examples of the common law in action would be judicial opinions created through the application of prior court decisions, such as precedents to negligence, malpractice, or breach of contract lawsuits that have been rendered in prior negligence, malpractice, or breach of contract lawsuits.

Nurse Practice Acts

The nursing profession is regulated by NPAs, which are laws that have been enacted by state governments to protect the public's health, safety and welfare by overseeing and ensuring the safe practice of nursing. NPAs vary by state but generally include a definition of the scope of nursing practice allowed in the state, the types of nursing licenses allowed, and the requirements for each license. Types of nursing licenses may include licensed practical nurse/licensed vocational nurse (LPN/LVN), registered nurse (RN), and advanced practice registered nurse (APRN). NPAs also dictate grounds for disciplinary action and remediation, standards for nursing education programs, and the authority and power of the State Board of Nursing.

The purpose of NPAs is to protect the public's health, safety and welfare. They are designed to shield the public from nurses who lack the minimum qualifications to perform competent nursing services. In addition, NPAs contain protections to punish and/or suspend any nurse who fails to follow proper protocol or otherwise engages in unsafe practices. NPAs define the minimum requirements in order to obtain a nursing license within a particular state. All nurses can view their state's NPA at the National Council of State Boards of Nursing website: www.ncsbn.org/npa.htm.

In addition to NPAs, state legislatures and agencies also enact certain administrative codes and rules that regulate the nursing profession. Such administrative codes and rules contain additional minimum requirements for nurses in practice and define different disciplinary structures for misconduct. The administrative codes and rules typically will allow a state governing body the right to suspend or revoke a license for the following acts:

- engaging in conduct likely to defraud or harm the public or demonstrating a willful disregard for the health, welfare, or safety of a patient
- departing from or failing to conform to standards of practice
- engaging in behavior that crosses professional boundaries (such as signing wills or other legal documents of patients) not related to healthcare
- engaging in sexual conduct with a patient
- demonstrating actual or potential inability to practice nursing with reasonable skill, safety, or judgment by reason of illness; use of alcohol, drugs, chemicals, or any other material; or as a result of any mental or physical condition (Illinois Administrative Code, Title 68, Section 1300.90)

NPAs also set forth the number of hours of continuing education required in order to maintain the current status of state licensure. For example, in the state of Illinois, licensed nurses are required to complete 20 hours of approved continuing education per 2-year license cycle (Illinois Administrative Code, Title 68, Section 1300.130). Many states have similar requirements designed to ensure continuing education and competency.

All individuals entering into nursing practice must become familiar with their particular state's NPA. Failure to understand and comply with one's NPA can jeopardize one's nursing license and the ability to legally practice nursing within a state. Moreover, such failure may also subject an individual nurse to charges of negligence and malpractice, including fines and license revocation.

Healthcare organizations define the manner in which nurses are to practice in specific work settings through policies and procedures. It is important that these policies and procedures are not only descriptive of the work nurses are performing in the organization but that they also are compliant with the state's NPA. Because these policies and procedures may be used in court to both determine the standard of care for nurses in a negligence or malpractice case and to assess whether a nurse was in compliance with the standard of care, clarity and specificity of these policies and procedures is essential. Periodic review and revision of an organization's policies and procedures is essential to assure that they are aligned with the NPA, and consistent with current nursing technological and clinical standards.

THE FOUR ELEMENTS OF NEGLIGENCE OR MALPRACTICE

Negligence is a failure to exercise the care that a reasonably prudent person would exercise in like circumstances. **Malpractice** is one form of negligence and is defined as improper, illegal, or negligent professional activity or treatment by a healthcare practitioner, lawyer, or other professional. A suit for negligence or malpractice is a civil suit brought by a person to recover damages from the individual or entity that caused such damages. A party bringing a negligence or malpractice suit must prove, by a preponderance of the evidence, the four elements in a healthcare negligence or malpractice suit (Box 4.1).

BOX 4.1 The Four Elements in a Healthcare Negligence or Malpractice Suit

1. A duty of care was owed to the patient.
2. A breach occurred in that duty.
3. Any injury was proximately caused by the breach in duty of care.
4. There were damages.

Duty of Care Owed to Patient

Duty of care is the legal obligation of professionals to deliver a certain standard of care when performing acts which could directly or indirectly harm others. The element of duty of care is generally the easiest of the four elements to prove in a healthcare negligence or malpractice case. A duty of care is often viewed as a social contract that requires members of a society to behave responsibly toward one another.

Because negligence or malpractice is part of states' common law, the applicable law depends on the state where the conduct took place. Each state may have a slightly different legal interpretation of the law. In many states, the test for duty of care is whether the harm to the patient due to the nurse's actions was foreseeable. Many states weigh the following factors to determine if a duty of care exists:

- foreseeability of harm (was the injury likely to occur as a result of the conduct?)
- degree of likelihood of harm (was the injury certain to occur or merely a possibility?)
- relationship of the parties (did the nurse have a relationship with the patient?)
- policy of preventing harm (is it important to society to prevent this sort of harm?) and
- available alternative conduct (how could the nurse have handled the situation differently?).

Once a duty of care has been established, a nurse is expected to use the degree of skill, knowledge, and care that would be offered by a similarly trained nurse in a similar situation. It is important to note that a nurse is not expected to guarantee a perfect result or outcome, but a nurse is expected to conform to specific standards of care.

Duty of care may vary in some unique situations. For example, a nurse while exercising at a local health club may encounter someone having a heart attack. In such a situation, public policy eliminates the duty of care; the nurse is not obligated to assist the person having a heart attack. Contrast that situation with a Good Samaritan case, where a nurse or other well-meaning citizen comes to the aid of a person who, outside of a hospital or doctor's office, has sustained a physical injury or is in physical peril or harm. Courts want to encourage people to render aid to those in need. If the law of negligence were not modified in the case of the Good Samaritan, people would be discouraged from getting involved in rendering aid to those in need.

Although Good Samaritan laws vary by state, there are a few principles which are universally accepted. Good Samaritan laws generally apply when someone renders aid to an individual in an emergency on a voluntary basis without the expectation of remuneration or compensation. In most states, it is acknowledged that a person, even a person with medical or nursing training, is not required to come to the aid of someone who has been injured, but if they elect to do so, they must act in a manner that is reasonable. For example, they cannot come to the scene, offer assistance, and then decide they need to leave and abandon the patient. In many states, the reasonable person standard is used to judge the conduct of the nurse in these situations rather than the standard of the reasonable nurse professional; in other words, a nurse in this situation would only be expected to do what a non-nurse would normally be able to do. This is due to the fact that when rendering care or assistance as a Good Samaritan, a nurse would not have access to the tools and support they might have when practicing in a formal healthcare setting.

A Breach in the Duty of Care

A **breach in duty** of care occurs when a nurse or other healthcare professional has a duty of care toward another person but fails to live up to the accepted standard of care. A breach in duty of care can be either an act of commission (doing something but doing it incorrectly) or an act of omission (not doing what was expected or ordered). The expectation of duty is dictated by practice standards. Healthcare institutions adhere to standards of care that emerge from research and evidence-based literature, which continuously evolves as researchers discover new treatment modalities for providing safe and effective care.

Expert testimony and scholarly evidence-based articles and practice guidelines can be used in a trial to establish whether or not the nurse acted in accordance with best and acceptable standards of care. A failure to conform to hospital policies and procedures is evidence of a breach in duty of care. The policies, procedures, and the nurse's adherence to them are supported or refuted and disproved by a nurse expert, who is credible in light of their experience and background. Determining the applicable standard of care is the crux of the legal debate on whether a duty of care was breached. Generally, the standard of care is how a reasonable nurse would treat a patient under the same circumstances. Note that the standard of care in one community may be different in another community and, as previously mentioned, the standard of care is always evolving based on healthcare research and the development of best practices.

CASE STUDY

Mary, an RN, is busy with four patients. She receives a new order for an intravenous piggyback (IVPB) medication from the healthcare provider, and orders it from the pharmacy for her patient. When the unit clerk tells Mary that her patient's IVPB medication has arrived from the pharmacy, Mary quickly picks up the medication bag and begins the infusion. A few minutes later, the patient becomes short of breath. As Mary assesses the patient, she notes to her horror that she mistakenly hung another patient's IVPB medication for this patient.

1. *Is this an error of omission or commission? Explain.*
2. *Is a problem like this the fault of the provider, the hospital, the nurse, the pharmacy department, or the patient care unit, or all of them?*
3. *Was this medication error and patient harm a foreseeable breach in the duty of care?*

Injury Proximately Caused by the Breach in Duty of Care

The third element of negligence or malpractice is injury proximately caused by a breach in the duty of care. Proximate cause of injury consists of successfully proving that a patient was indeed injured, and that a breach in the duty of care was the cause of the injury sustained. Proximate cause is very difficult to prove or to get a jury to understand. Nurses often care for patients who are already vulnerable and might be subject to exacerbations of their condition or further injury by the very nature of their condition. Thus, it can be difficult to prove that an injury was not part of the natural progression of the patient's illness or that the injury would not have occurred except for the breach in the duty of care.

In addition, many times a patient may have contributed towards their own injury (for example, a patient may have intentionally pulled out an intravenous line providing medication). This is known as contributory negligence. If a lawyer for the defendant can prove contributory negligence, the amount of a patient's monetary award for damages is reduced. Lawyers who seek to prove this element of negligence or malpractice rely upon experts to establish proximate cause.

Note there may be multiple parties responsible for a patient injury. For instance, imagine a physician makes the wrong diagnosis, and then a nurse, who knows that what the physician diagnosed was incorrect, continues to follow the physician's orders and the patient receives the wrong treatment. In this situation, both the physician and nurse are at varying levels of fault. This is known as comparative negligence. In this situation, a court will allocate responsibility among the parties based on their respective level of fault.

Damages

The fourth element of negligence or malpractice is that the attorney for the plaintiff (the patient) must present evidence that, as a result of the conduct of the nurse, the plaintiff suffered some type of economic or physical damages. The goal of civil litigation, like negligence or malpractice, is to award compensation (damages) and/or make the injured patient whole. Courts may award the patient damages for a variety of reasons, including:

- actual cost of reversing or caring for the injury
- future anticipated economic losses because of the injury
- pain and suffering
- emotional distress that those close to the injured person might have sustained while witnessing the harm to a loved one
- punitive damages, where the plaintiff (patient) seeks an amount to punish the nurse or the organization for particularly egregious bad conduct

The maximum amount of money that can be awarded as damages varies from state to state and, in rare cases, there may be a partial or limited immunity from liability (if the claim is against a governmental entity). The damages awarded may be covered under the malpractice insurance policy that has been purchased by the healthcare organization employing the nurse. If a nurse is sued, then the insurance policy will require the insurance company to pay for an attorney to defend the nurse, but the insurance policy does not necessarily cover the plaintiff's (the patient) attorney fees. Rather, the plaintiff's attorney receives a contingency fee, usually a third of what is awarded to the plaintiff. The malpractice insurance policy generally covers attorney's fees incurred by the nurse as a defendant and any money paid to the plaintiff to compensate for injuries.

Some states have set a cap on the amount of punitive damages that can be awarded, whereas other states have set a ratio between the amount of actual damages in the case and the amount of punitive damages that can be awarded. A table that lists the limits to punitive damages in each of the 50 states and the District of Columbia is available at www.mondaq.com/unitedstates/insurance-laws-and-products/762574/sky39s-the-limit-a-50-state-survey-of-damages-caps-and-the-collateral-source-rule. Some states focus on the ability of the defendant to pay based on their income or net worth.

Sometimes, a patient can receive both compensatory damages (to pay the patient back for the injury suffered) and punitive damages (to discipline the defendant for the wrongdoing). For example, a court could award a patient $100,000 for their injuries, and also award punitive damages of $50,000 against the hospital for allowing such an injury to occur. The patient would then recover $150,000 total. The United States Supreme Court has set a limit on punitive damages. Punitive damages cannot exceed a 10:1 ratio and cannot be more than 10 times the compensatory award given. For example, if the trial court or jury awards $200,000 in compensatory award given, then the court must give less than $2,000,000 in punitive damages, with the only exception being that the case was extremely egregious or shocking to the court. In many states, no punitive damages may be awarded if there are no compensatory damages in the case.

In today's litigious environment, all professionals must take care to ensure that they perform their duties compliant with reasonable care. Malpractice claims against nurses are increasing, with more than $90 million paid in nurses' malpractice claims over a 5-year period (Relias Media, 2016). Table 4.2 identifies common causes of nursing malpractice (McGuire & Mroczek, 2017). All nurses must understand their responsibilities in order to avoid common causes of nursing malpractice.

CURRENT LITERATURE

CITATION

Brous, E. (2020). The elements of a nursing malpractice case, Part 4: Harm. *American Journal of Nursing, 120*(3), 61–64. https://doi.org/10.1097/01.NAJ.0000656360.21284.50

DISCUSSION

This last article in a four-part series discusses harm, the last of the four elements required to prevail in a malpractice lawsuit. In order to succeed, a plaintiff must demonstrate duty (discussed in Part 1, July 2019), breach (discussed in Part 2, September 2019), causation (discussed in Parts 3A and 3B, November 2019 and January 2020), and harm, Part 4 (discussed here in the final installment of the series). The author states that nurses can reduce their liability exposure by understanding the four elements of a malpractice lawsuit and practicing in accordance with acceptable standards of practice.

IMPLICATIONS FOR PRACTICE

The author states that nurses should:

- Maintain professional liability insurance to provide coverage for off-duty events and licensure defense.
- Be aware of what creates a nurse–patient relationship and triggers the duty of reasonable care.
- Avoid work-arounds or deviations from organizational policies and procedures.
- Maintain clinical competency including awareness of standard-of-practice changes.
- Engage the chain of command with patient concerns and pursue concerns to resolution.
- Document in a manner that permits accurate reconstruction of patient assessment, notification of others, and the sequence of events.

INDEPENDENT RESPONSIBILITY OF NURSES TO DELIVER QUALITY PATIENT CARE

One of the nurse's responsibilities is to follow hospital guidelines and physician orders to deliver quality patient care. However, the fact that a nurse may have followed hospital

TABLE 4.2 COMMON CAUSES OF NURSING MALPRACTICE[†]

NURSING MALPRACTICE	EXAMPLE
Negligent Infliction of Emotional Stress	In *Spangler v. Bechtel* (958 N.E.2d 458 [2011]), the Supreme Court found that the defendants, which included a nurse-midwife, could be liable for negligent infliction of emotional distress following the death of the plaintiff's stillborn child.
Burns	In *Pillers v. Finley Hospital* (2003 Iowa App. LEXIS 792), the Court concluded that a nurse was liable, along with the physician, when the nurse applied a tourniquet to the plaintiff, as ordered, prior to surgery. Prep solution leaked around the tourniquet, resulting in chemical burns to the plaintiff's thigh.
Falls	The California Third Circuit Court in *Massey v. Mercy Medical Center Redding* (180 Cal. App. 4th 690 [2009]) concluded that expert testimony was not necessary to prove a nurse's negligence in preventing a 65-year-old patient, who had recently had surgery, from falling.
Failure to Properly Diagnose	The Supreme Court of Kansas held that the defendant's advance practice nurse and physician failed to diagnose the decedent's urinary tract infection, which later caused the decedent's death (*Puckett v. Mt. Carmel Reg'l Med. Ctr.*, 290 Kan. 406, 2010).
Assault and Battery	The Illinois Fifth Circuit Court of Appeals found a nurse and hospital guilty of battery, alleging that the nurse attending the plaintiff-patient observed and touched her without her permission, citing religious standards and beliefs (*Cohen v. Smith*, 269 Ill. App 3d 1087 5th Cir. 1995).
HIPAA* Violations	In *Guardo v. Univ. Hosps., Geneva Medical Center* (2015-Ohio-1492), the Eleventh District Court of Appeals in Ohio upheld the defendant-hospital's decision to terminate the plaintiff-nurse due to an unwarranted disclosure of HIPAA*-protected information by the nurse.
Breach of Privilege	The Fourth District Ohio Court of Appeals found that the defendant-nurse and physician breached the physician-patient privilege by revealing the plaintiff's pregnancy to the plaintiff's parents. The liability extended to the nurse as well as to the physician because the nurse contacted the plaintiff's parents at the supervising physician's direction (*Hobbs v. Lopez*, 96 Ohio App. 3d 670 [4th Dist. 1994]).
Failure to Observe/ Report	Reviewing a decision of the Nevada State Board of Nursing, the Supreme Court of Nevada upheld the Board's determination that the plaintiff-nurse had, among other things, failed to "observe the conditions, signs and symptoms of a patient, to record the information or to report significant changes to the appropriate persons" in treating one of the nurse's patients. The nurse did not deliver medication to a patient in a timely manner, and the patient subsequently passed away. Additionally, the nurse back-timed the order for the medication in his report (*Nevada State Bd. of Nursing v. Merkley*, 113 Nev. 659 [1997]).
False Imprisonment	The Supreme Court of Mississippi held in *Lee v. Alexander* (607 So. 2d 30 [1992]) that "all who united in the illegal commitment are equally liable" in a false imprisonment case. This finding would extend to nurses who take part in a patient's involuntary confinement.
Medication Errors	The Fourth Circuit Court of Appeals in Louisiana agreed that the district courts should not instruct the jury to consider an "intervening cause." Intervening causes are separate and distinct actions that may have caused or contributed to the injury in question. In that case, the patient suffered an adverse reaction to a drug administered, and the patient's reaction was not monitored by the attending nurse (*Cagnolatti v. Hightower*, 692 So. 2d 1104 [La.App. 4 Cir. 1996]. However, the defendants raised an "intervening cause" argument by claiming that the patient suffered both an adverse reaction to the drug *and* a stroke, which would be the cause-of-death. The court determined the drug was the "cause-in-fact" of the death.

*Health Insurance Portability and Accountability Act of 1996 (HIPAA).

[†]Note that malpractice claims against nurses are increasing, with more than $90 million paid in nurses' malpractice claims over a 5-year period (Relias Media, 2016).

guidelines or a physician or nurse practitioner's prescribed order does not relieve the nurse of the duty to use reasonable care to deliver safe patient care. If a nurse receives conflicting orders from multiple prescribers, the nurse may legally delay execution of the order until satisfying which order is correct. In addition, some states may hold that the nurse not only has the legal ability but a legal obligation to follow through on which order is correct.

While nurses are expected to follow prescribed orders from physicians and nurse practitioners, many courts have determined there is an exception to this general rule: when the nurse or other hospital employee knows the prescriber's orders are "not in accordance with normal medical practice." In this situation, nurses have an affirmative duty to take action. If a nurse or other hospital employee fails to report changes in a patient's condition and/or question a prescriber's orders when they are not in accord with standard medical practice, and the omission results in injury to the patient, the hospital, the prescriber, and the nurse will be liable for negligence. Moreover, a nurse has a duty not to obey instructions of a prescriber which are obviously negligent or dangerous. The independent responsibility of the nurse to deliver quality care to patients is clear.

So, what should a nurse do if they receive prescriber instructions which are obviously negligent or dangerous? The first step should be to discuss the concern with the prescriber. It is possible that the prescriber made an error and the nurse is catching it before it gets to the patient. The nurse may also consult as appropriate with the pharmacist, nurse colleagues, or the charge nurse, and, if the concern remains unresolved, the nurse can use the hospital chain of command to consult with the nursing supervisor and other administrators to address the issue. The nurse should never modify the course set by the prescriber just because the nurse holds a different view. The duty of diagnosis and treatment belongs with the physician or nurse practitioner. However, in a negligent or dangerous patient care situation, the nurse has a duty to use appropriate channels to protect the patient and maintain safety.

Real World Interview

One day, early in my nursing career, I made rounds with a surgeon and helped him change a surgical dressing on his new post-op patient. As he changed the dressing, we saw that stool was leaking from the incision. We finished the dressing, left the room, and I asked the surgeon what was going to happen with the leaking stool. He said, I am concerned about it but I'll just watch it for a while. I was a new nurse and thought that must be okay.

Then I was off duty for 2 days. When I returned to work, the patient was spiking a temperature and his stool drainage had increased. As I thought about it then, I thought the surgeon had probably nicked the bowel during surgery and that more action might be necessary to heal the wound. I talked it over with one of my favorite surgeons who was making early rounds that day. He agreed with me and commented that the patient needed to go back to surgery to close the wound but he did not want to get involved. That day, I watched for the patient's surgeon to make his daily rounds. I told him that I was concerned about the patient and I needed to discuss it further with him and my supervisor. He responded pleasantly, saying, "You do what you think is right."

I reported the patient case to my supervisor, who reported the case up the chain of command to her supervisor, the director of nursing, and the chief executive officer (CEO) of the hospital. The CEO discussed the case with the medical executive committee and they asked the original surgeon to take the patient back to surgery. The patient was taken back to surgery, healed well, and was discharged. The initial operating surgeon never spoke to me again but I felt I had taken the right action to advocate for the patient and provide safe care.

Patricia Kelly Vana, RN, MSN
Oak Lawn, Illinois

BOX 4.2 Developing Clinical Judgment

The nurse is working in the ED with a 20-year-old patient with a history of asthma, who was admitted with severe difficulty breathing and wheezing. The nurse obtains vital signs and finds the patient with a respiratory rate of 28, rapid and shallow, and a pulse oximetry of 91%. The patient's facial expression is stressed. The nurse places the patient on oxygen, and prepares to administer the prescribed breathing treatment as ordered. The nurse recognizes the duty of the caregivers to determine how to safely monitor the patient. The patient's clinical status and care must also be documented carefully to record interventions for this acute breathing problem and demonstrate high-quality, safe, patient care.

1. What **CUES** (Assessment) can the nurse assess?
2. What **HYPOTHESIS (Diagnosis)** will the nurse consider?
3. What **ACTION (Plan and Implement)** will be most effective for the nurse to take to meet the caregivers' duty in assuring the patient's safety in this situation?
4. How will the nurse evaluate the patient's **OUTCOME (Evaluation)** for the purpose of arriving at a satisfactory clinical outcome that meets the standard of care?

Responsibility for Prevention of Hospital-Acquired Infections

The nurse is obligated to conform to the standard of care to prevent patients from acquiring infections while hospitalized. A **hospital-acquired infection (HAI)** is an infection that a patient did not have at the time of admission but is acquired after being admitted to the hospital. Examples of HAIs include central line associated bloodstream infections (CLABSI), catheter-associated urinary tract infections (CAUTI), ventilator-associated pneumonia (VAP), and surgical site infections. Some courts have identified these as "hospital-induced infections." In determining any liability for HAI, courts will determine if the HAI occurrence is the result of general negligence of medical or nursing staff, considering if staff failed to take the care that an objectively reasonable person would have taken in the same circumstances. The court's determination of negligence in cases of HAI does not depend on the severity of the HAI. Rather, it depends on determining whether any act that may have caused the HAI was professional in nature or was merely a routine ministerial act. Ministerial acts are those acts performed by a reasonable person, in a prescribed manner, in obedience to an authority, without regard to one's own judgment or discretion.

The distinction between a professional act and a routine ministerial act is important. If the court is considering professional conduct, such as administering an intravenous medication, the court will call upon a healthcare expert to determine if the nurse was acting as a reasonable professional nurse would act. If the court is considering only a routine ministerial act, such as delivering a food tray to a patient, the court will allow the jury to determine whether the nurse was acting as a reasonable person would have done in the situation. The distinction between the two determines whether a healthcare expert is used by the court to comment on professional acts. Note that an expert is not needed to comment on routine ministerial acts.

Nurses are expected to adhere to hospital guidelines and practices they have been taught in their nursing education, and to use general common sense in order to avoid liability for the spread of infection to a patient. Some sample legal cases where the hospital was found liable for HAIs were when:

1. Instruments were not sterilized.
2. Physicians, nurses, or other workers were not properly supervised by administrators and physicians.

3. Infections were not diagnosed in a timely manner.
4. Informed consent was not obtained.
5. Policies were not followed.

HEALTH INSURANCE PORTABILITY AND ACCOUNTABILITY ACT OF 1996

Advances in technology have impacted the healthcare profession in many ways. One significant impact is the advent of electronic patient information. On one hand, technology has made it easier for patient information to be shared among healthcare professionals, which in turn has made it easier to diagnose and treat patients, but on the other hand, patient information may fall into the wrong hands or otherwise be misused, potentially causing damage or harm to the rights of patients. If patient information is misused, organizations, individuals, or other entities could discriminate against patients based upon their medical condition.

To address the issue of misuse, the **Health Insurance Portability and Accountability Act** (HIPAA) was passed in 1996, setting national standards for the protection of patient information. The Department of Health & Human Services (HHS) published the final rules implementing HIPAA in 2000 and 2002. These rules are applicable to health plans and healthcare providers who electronically transmit health information in connection with transactions for which HHS has adopted standards. Generally, these transactions concern billing for services or insurance coverage by hospitals, academic healthcare centers, physicians, and other healthcare providers who electronically transmit billing claims to a health plan. The major goal of HIPAA is to ensure individuals that their patient information will be protected, while at the same time, the free flow of information that is needed to provide the best care for the patient's health and well-being is promoted. HIPAA attempts to strike a balance that enables professionals to use patient information while it also protects patient privacy.

Regulation of Patient Information

HIPAA regulates the use and maintenance of patient information. Patient information includes any details about demographic data, an individual's past, present, or future physical or mental health or condition, the provision of healthcare to that individual, or the past, present, or future payment for the provision of healthcare to that individual. In order for the information to constitute protected health information, it must include identifier information that can be used to identify an individual. Identifier health information may include the name, address, birthdate, or social security number of the patient. There are ways to de-identify health information by removing specified identifiers such as name or address.

Permitted Uses of Patient Information by Health Insurance Portability and Accountability Act

HIPAA defines when patient information may be used and disclosed. HIPAA rules provide that a healthcare provider may not use or disclose protected patient information items except for (a) as the HIPAA rule permits (e.g., for treatment or payment), or (b) if the individual who is the subject of the information has authorized it in writing. Healthcare providers must rely on professional ethics and best judgment in deciding whether either item is applicable. Providers must also disclose protected health information to patients when patients specifically request access to it or to the HHS when it is undertaking a HIPAA compliance investigation.

Health Insurance Portability and Accountability Act Authorized Disclosure of Patient Information

A healthcare provider is required to turn over patient information to the patient upon request. Many times, a nurse may be faced with a request for patient information by a family member or another person other than the patient in question or another healthcare professional. HIPAA allows healthcare providers to treat a legally appointed personal representative the same as the individual patient with respect to information uses and disclosures. A **personal representative** is a person who is legally authorized to make healthcare decisions on an individual's behalf or to act for a deceased individual or an estate (such as acting under a power of attorney or as a guardian). However, a healthcare provider is not permitted to disclose patient information to others who are not a patient's personal representative. In situations with minors, the parents are considered to be personal representatives of the patient.

Health Insurance Portability and Accountability Act Penalties

The U.S. Health and Human Services Office for Civil Rights may impose a penalty on a healthcare provider for failure to comply with HIPAA. These penalties may vary and it depends on many factors that are relevant to the violation in question. The penalty ranges from $150 to $50,000 or more per HIPAA violation depending on the severity of the violation. A criminal penalty may also be involved and assessed against a person who knowingly obtains or discloses protected patient information. Such fines could be up to $50,000 as well as up to a 1-year imprisonment. If the HIPAA violation was a result of willful neglect and no effort was made to correct the violation within 30 days, the minimum fine is $50,000.

MEDICARE HOME HEALTH CERTIFICATION REQUIREMENTS

The exploding baby-boomer population has impacted many facets of American society, and the healthcare industry is no exception. Medical technology has contributed to the longer life span of individuals. Within nursing, one area that has gained additional growth is the home healthcare arena. **Home healthcare** is the provision of limited healthcare services by a nurse or other healthcare professional in the home of the patient. Although not exclusively, much of home healthcare is funded through the U.S. Centers for Medicare & Medicaid Services (Medicare), which covers individuals 65 years of age and older. Many nurses today provide services through a home healthcare agency. Within that industry, there are certain regulatory requirements that must be understood.

In order for an individual to be eligible for reimbursement for home healthcare services, an individual must meet certain Medicare Certification requirements. The requirements are summarized as follows:

1. Patient must have medical necessity.
2. Patient must be homebound.
3. A physician must certify and/or prescribe the need for home healthcare services.

If any person, nurse, and/or agency attempts to submit claims to Medicare for reimbursement for the provision of healthcare services to a patient that does not meet these three requirements, they may be subject to penalties and/or criminal prosecution.

Federal Anti-Kickback Statute

The **Federal Anti-Kickback Statute** is a law that prohibits the payment or receipt of any gift or remuneration in exchange for federal healthcare referrals to Medicare patients. Congress has determined that a compensation structure that rewards referring patients for the receipt of Medicare reimbursement is potentially abusive and would lead to fraud and waste within the Medicare program. The term "remuneration" is broad and includes anything of value, transferred either directly or indirectly in cash or gifts; this could include trips, meals, and tickets to events.

While the Federal Anti-Kickback Statute concerns any individual, the Stark Law relates strictly to physicians. The **Stark Law** prohibits a physician from making a Medicare or Medicaid referral to a healthcare provider or organization with whom the physician or their family member has a financial relationship. Similar to the Federal Anti-Kickback Statute, the Stark Law seeks to prevent potentially abusive circumstances whereby Medicare may be defrauded due to fraudulent physicians.

CASE STUDY

Dr. Thompson operates a thriving patient practice in Chicago. Many of his patients are over 65 years of age. Many of them suffer with chronic healthcare conditions but do not require hospitalization. Dr. Thompson started a home healthcare agency that is eligible to seek reimbursements from Medicare.

1. *Can Dr. Thompson legally refer a patient to his agency?*
2. *Would it be legal if Dr. Thompson limited his referrals only to patients in need of nonclinical home care services?*

Civil Monetary Penalties Law

In addition to the Federal Anti-Kickback Statute and the Stark Law, there is a Civil Monetary Penalties Law. This law states that a monetary penalty may be assessed against a person if they provide remuneration to a Medicare or Medicaid beneficiary when a person knows or should know that such action is likely to influence the beneficiary's selection of a particular provider, practitioner, or supplier. When evaluating whether a monetary penalty should be assessed, there is a three-prong test:

- Was there remuneration of an item or service to a Medicare or Medicaid beneficiary?
- Was it likely that the item or service influenced the beneficiary to select the provider?
- Did the provider know that the item or service was likely to influence the beneficiary's selection of the provider?

It is generally held that items of value of $10 or less are considered to be not subject to Civil Monetary Penalties Law. Those guilty of a Federal Anti-Kickback Statute violation may be convicted of a felony, assessed a $25,000 fine, or potentially given a 5-year prison sentence. For Civil Monetary Penalties Law violations, there may be a penalty of up to $10,000 for each violation.

Exclusions From Medicare, Medicaid, or Other Federal Healthcare Programs

The U.S. Department of Health and Human Services Office of the Inspector General has the authority to exclude certain individuals and entities from participation in the Medicare, Medicaid, or other federal healthcare programs. Being named an excluded individual or entity is a severe penalty. Organizations employing or contracting with an excluded individual are not eligible to be paid directly or indirectly by a federal healthcare program for any items or services provided by the excluded individual. Those individuals or providers found guilty of violating the Federal Anti-Kickback Statute or the federal Civil Monetary

Penalties Law may be excluded from the Medicare program. In addition, any provider who employs an excluded individual may be required to return to Medicare any revenue received that is attributable, directly or indirectly, to the excluded individual.

WHISTLEBLOWER CLAIMS

If a nurse notices patterns and suspects the hospital or healthcare facility is committing systematic illegal acts against their patients or against third-party payers, the nurse may consider filing a qui tam (another word for "whistleblower") claim. A **whistleblower claim** is a formal complaint that exposes or describes certain types of misconduct from a hospital or healthcare facility. Because some nurses may be afraid to take adverse action against their employer, many states have laws, which reward and protect nurses who bring successful whistleblower claims. whistleblower claims are good for several reasons: they encourage employers to follow the law; they protect nurses from having to decide whether they should break the law and harm their patients just to keep their jobs; and they protect the public from hospitals and practitioners violating laws. Because filing a whistleblower complaint is serious and life-changing, a nurse should first plan with an attorney before acting (Philipsen & Soeken, 2011). There are several types of whistleblower claims.

An example of a whistleblower claim is one in connection with the Medicare program. In 2020, the U.S. Department of Justice took severe measures against nursing homes who made "false claims" to the government, such as providing unnecessary and dangerous therapy treatments, billing for services not actually provided, and falsely certifying that their patients qualify for certain programs. In filing a whistleblower claim with the U.S. government, the nurse must satisfy the following three elements:

- There was a false claim.
- The false claim was presented to the United States for payment and approval of a claim.
- There was knowledge that the claim was false.

Another example of a whistleblower claim would be an action brought against a physician for knowingly filing a claim to Medicare for reimbursement for services the physician never performed. In order to file the whistleblower claim, the nurse does not need to have been harmed, meaning punished or fired for complaining about the false claim.

If a nurse is able to prevail on a whistleblower claim, the nurse will usually receive about 15% of the total damages or settlement as a personal reward. The nurse will also have their attorney fees paid by the court, so there will be no cost to the nurse for coming forward. In addition, if the nurse accrues additional costs such as losing one's job, and thus not having an income for a period of time, the court may award additional damages to the nurse to cover this loss. The American Nurses Association (ANA) encourages nurses considering whistleblowing to be sure they have adequate written documentation about any wrongdoing and they should seek the counsel of someone trusted outside of the situation.

INTERNATIONAL COUNCIL OF NURSES CODE OF ETHICS, THE AMERICAN NURSES ASSOCIATION CODE OF ETHICS, AND UNDERLYING PRINCIPLES

In addition to the laws that govern the practice of nursing, there are also ethical codes that nurses must observe in the performance of their duties. The International Council of Nurses (ICN) Code of Ethics (2012) states that the need for nursing is universal and that nurses have four fundamental responsibilities:

- Promote health.
- Prevent illness.
- Restore health.
- Alleviate suffering.

The ICN Code of Ethics also has four principal elements that outline the standards of ethical conduct. These elements of the ICN Code of Ethics are (a) nurses and people, (b) nurses and practice, (c) nurses and the profession, and (d) nurses and coworkers. The ICN Code of Ethics is available at https://www.icn.ch/sites/default/files/inline-files/2012_ICN_Codeofethicsfornurses_%20eng.pdf.

The ANA Code of Ethics (ANA, 2015) has been developed to provide an ethical framework for nurses. The ANA Code makes it clear that inherent in nursing is respect for human rights, including the right to life, to dignity, and to be treated with respect. The ANA Code of Ethics is divided into nine distinct provisions and their accompanying interpretive statements. View the ANA Code of Ethics at https://www.nursingworld.org/practice-policy/nursing-excellence/ethics/code-of-ethics-for-nurses/. Table 4.3 describes the underlying ethical principles and theories that influence the practice of nursing.

TABLE 4.3 ETHICAL THEORIES AND PRINCIPLES THAT INFLUENCE NURSING PRACTICE

ETHICAL THEORIES AND PRINCIPLES	DESCRIPTION	APPLICATION
Beneficence	Demonstrates compassion. Takes positive action to advocate for and help others. Desires to do good.	Applies principles of professional nursing ethics and human rights daily in patient care and professional situations. Helps older adult patients gain access to COVID-19 vaccine. Joins a hospital or community board of directors and advocates for quality patient care for all. Provides all patients, including the terminally ill, with evidence-based care and information. Becomes an advocate for patients in need of organ donations. Treats every patient with respect and courtesy. Gives needed pain medication as quickly as possible. Demonstrates ethical behaviors in practice. Suggests solutions when unethical behaviors are observed. Changes behavior based on self and situational awareness. Assumes accountability for working to resolve ethical dilemmas.

(continued)

TABLE 4.3 ETHICAL THEORIES AND PRINCIPLES THAT INFLUENCE NURSING PRACTICE (*continued*)

ETHICAL THEORIES AND PRINCIPLES	DESCRIPTION	APPLICATION
Nonmaleficence	Avoids harm or injury and is the core of nursing ethics.	Reflects on own actions and the consequences. Uses appropriate personal protective equipment when working with patients. Works within one's scope of practice. Never gives information or performs duties one is not qualified to do. Ensures that the patient is oriented when signing consent forms. Keeps patient areas clutter-free and safe from hazards. Performs procedures according to facility protocols. Never takes shortcuts. Confirms practice with an appropriate person when unsure. Reviews evidence-based care and maintains up-to-date education and skills.
Justice	Refers to an equal and fair distribution of resources, based on analysis of the benefits and the burdens of a decision. Implies that all citizens have an equal right to the goods distributed, regardless of what they have contributed or who they are.	Treats all patients ethically and equally, regardless of economic or social background. Learns the law and the facility's policies and procedures for reporting suspected abuse. Reports unethical behaviors when observed. Safeguards privacy, confidentiality, and autonomy in all interactions. Advocates for the individual's right to self-determination Analyzes current policies and practices in the context of an ethical framework. Models ethical behaviors in practice and leadership roles.

(continued)

TABLE 4.3 ETHICAL THEORIES AND PRINCIPLES THAT INFLUENCE NURSING PRACTICE (*continued*)

ETHICAL THEORIES AND PRINCIPLES	DESCRIPTION	APPLICATION
Autonomy	Respects another's right to self-determine a course of action. Supports independent decision-making.	Respects all patient choices and the individual's right to decision-making. Becomes familiar with federal and state laws and facility policies addressing autonomy and privacy, including HIPAA and the Patient Self Determination Act. Never releases patient information of any kind without a signed patient release. Does not discuss a patient with anyone who is not professionally involved in the patient's care.
Fidelity	Requires loyalty, fairness, truthfulness, advocacy, and dedication to patients. Involves an agreement to keep promises and keep commitments. Is based upon the virtue of caring.	Assures that contracts have been completed. Provides clear information to patients. Patients may only hear the "good news." Keeps promises to patients. Keeps patient information confidential.
Paternalism	Occurs when healthcare professionals make decisions about diagnosis, therapy, and prognosis for the patient. Is based upon the healthcare professional's belief about what is in the best interest of the patient.	Gives patients complete and accurate information about their diagnosis, therapy, and prognosis so they can make informed decisions. Doesn't withhold patient information in order to maintain power over the patient.
Relativism	Holds that morality is relative to the norms of one's culture.	States there are no absolute truths in ethics and that what is morally right or wrong varies from person to person or from society to society. Believes that variances in culture and society influence whether an act is moral.
Feminism	Holds that traditional ethical theorizing has undervalued women's moral experience and it therefore chooses to reimagine ethics through a holistic feminist approach	Asks how the action affects women, all persons, the family, and those depending upon one another (e.g., community).

(*continued*)

TABLE 4.3 ETHICAL THEORIES AND PRINCIPLES THAT INFLUENCE NURSING PRACTICE (*continued*)

ETHICAL THEORIES AND PRINCIPLES	DESCRIPTION	APPLICATION
Deontology	Judges the morality of an action based on the action's adherence to rules.	States that whether an action is ethical depends on the intentions behind the decisions rather than the outcomes that result.
Utilitarianism	Supports what is best for most people. States that the value of the act is determined by its usefulness, with the main emphasis on the outcome or consequences.	Examines what creates the most happiness for the most people.

Source: Data from American Association of Colleges of Nursing. (2021). *The Essentials: Core competencies for professional nursing education*. https://www.aacnnursing.org/Education-Resources/AACN-Essentials; American Nurses' Association. (2016). *Short definitions of ethical principles and theories familiar words, what do they mean?* https://www.happynclex.com/wp-content/uploads/2016/04/ANA-ethics-defi nitions-and-examples.pdf.

CURRENT LITERATURE

CITATION

NewsCAP: Nurses across varied settings were still experiencing significant shortages of PPE during July and August. (2020). *American Journal of Nursing, 120*(12), 16. https://doi.org/10.1097/01.NAJ.0000724188.76212.a4

DISCUSSION

Nurses across varied settings were still experiencing significant shortages of personal protective equipment (PPE) during July and August, 2020, at the height of the COVID-19 pandemic. In a survey conducted by the American Nurses Association, half of the 21,000 nurse respondents reported having treated a patient with or suspected of having COVID-19 in the previous 2 weeks. The percentage of nurses who experienced a shortage of PPE decreased slightly to 42% from 45% in May, with 16% reporting widespread shortages. While there were shortages of all types of PPE, N95 masks were in the shortest supply. Two-thirds of the nurses were required to reuse the N95 masks and more than half of the nurses reused the masks multiple times. In some cases, nurses wore used masks up to 2 weeks. Staff nurses and those working in long-term care or hospice reported the worst N95 mask shortages, placing nurses at risk.

IMPLICATIONS FOR PRACTICE

Nurses in all roles have an ethical imperative to advocate for disaster planning. By working to serve on hospital and nursing committees, including the hospital board of directors, nurses can ensure planning for current and future hospital supplies as part of their commitment to assure patient safety and their own safety in all conditions. Adequate inventory must always be kept so supplies can be obtained before they run out, as opposed to afterwards. If an adequate inventory process is not already in place, nurses must be proactive in creating it to assure nursing and patient safety even through disasters like the COVID-19 pandemic.

STEPS OF THE ETHICAL DECISION-MAKING PROCESS

When faced with ethical dilemmas, nurses working with the interprofessional team may use an ethical decision-making process as guidance. The steps of an ethical decision-making process, similar to the problem-solving process, are:

- Problem definition
- Data collection
- Data analysis
- Identification, exploration, and generation of possible solutions to the problem and the implications of each
- Selecting the best possible solution
- Performing the selected desired course of action to resolve the ethical dilemma
- Evaluating the results of the action

These steps identify the ethical decision making process. Nurses and interprofessional teams may add an organized approach to data collection and analysis to ensure that they are considering all points of view. Jonson et al. (2015) identified a broad four-box topic approach to illustrate four points of view to be considered when analyzing a clinical ethical problem (Table 4.4). Once the answers to the four-box questions are collected, they are analyzed together for a comprehensive view of an ethical problem. These answers serve as a broad guide to identify, explore, and generate possible solutions and consider the implications of each solution. This broad approach helps patients, families, and the interprofessional team work together to select the best possible solution and course of action to resolving ethical problems and evaluating the results of the action.

TABLE 4.4 SOME QUESTIONS USED WITH THE FOUR-BOX APPROACH TO EXPLORING CLINICAL ETHICAL PROBLEMS

MEDICAL INDICATIONS	PATIENT PREFERENCES	QUALITY OF LIFE	CONTEXTUAL FEATURES
What are the probabilities of success of various treatment options?	Has patient been informed of benefits and risks, understood this information, and given consent?	What are plans and rationale to forgo life-sustaining treatment?	What are the familial, social, institutional, financial, and legal features? Are there issues of public health and safety that affect the clinical decision?

Source: From Jonson, A., Siegler, M., & Winslade, W. (2015). *Clinical ethics: A practical approach to ethical decisions in clinical medicine* (8th ed.). McGraw-Hill Education.

Real World Interview

The Medical Center's Integrated Ethics Council (IEC) provides a standardized, comprehensive approach to ethics, provides oversight for ethical practices in our healthcare system, and provides guidance for our staff working with ethical dilemmas that include informed consent, advanced directives, and patient decision-making. The IEC is composed of an Ethics Leadership Council and an Ethics Sub-Council, which share responsibility for ensuring the Medical Center implements a standardized, comprehensive, and systematic approach to ethics in healthcare delivery. This approach to ethics is outlined in a Veterans Healthcare Administration (VHA) National Center for Ethics in Healthcare Directive. The Directive gives guidance to ethics councils in all Veterans Health Administration Medical Centers and sets policy and operational requirements for the IEC.

The IEC Leadership Council meets bimonthly with the Ethics Sub-Council meeting in the months that the Leadership Council does not meet. There does not have to be an ethical issue before either group in order for them to meet. The Ethics Leadership Council includes the nurse executive, medical department directors, nurse managers, and other clinical and nonclinical staff in senior positions throughout the medical center. The Ethics Leadership Council provides oversight to the Ethics Sub-Council. Some of the Ethics Leadership Council members, such as the integrated ethics program officer, the ethics consultant coordinator, and the preventive ethics coordinator, also hold leadership roles in the Ethics Sub-Council. Other members of both councils are nonsupervisory staff from many different departments, including nurses, physicians, social workers, psychologists, chaplains, educators, patient privacy staff, and business operations compliance staff.

The Ethics Leadership Council provides oversight and delegates responsibilities to the Ethics Sub-Council for two programs: Preventive Ethics and Ethics Consultation. The Preventive Ethics Program prevents gaps in ethics quality, tackles ethical concerns, and provides education on ethics topics. For example, the Preventive Ethics Program improved the Medical Center's system for ensuring that all patients have the opportunity to complete an advance directive. The program followed the Medical Center's standardized quality improvement approach to this, including a literature search and a benchmarking search of high-quality ethics programs at other healthcare facilities, to identify a strong ethical process for managing advance directives.

The Ethics Consultation Program, whose members have been trained to help with ethical uncertainty and conflicts in ethical values, provides ethics consultation and education to help all staff, patients, and families resolve ethical concerns when ethical uncertainty or a conflict of ethical values exists. For example, a nurse may be concerned about possible financial exploitation of a patient by a family member and brings the concern to the attention of the IEC. The IEC refers this concern to the Ethics Sub-Council's Consultation Program, which provides ethics consultation and education to help the nurse achieve the highest quality, most ethical outcome for the patient.

Both the IEC Leadership Council and the Ethics Sub-Council are responsible for role-modeling an ethical culture throughout the organization and demonstrating a commitment to resolving ethical issues in a transparent and nonthreatening manner. Members of both the IEC Leadership Council and the Ethics Sub-Council make rounds in the Medical Center weekly to solicit input from staff and patients and discuss recommendations for improvement in healthcare delivery based on their actual experiences at the Medical Center. These discussions with staff and patients may or may not be specifically about ethical issues but they may uncover ethical concerns. For example, these discussions may reveal privacy protection concerns related to how staff share information about special care needs for patients with behavioral issues. Both the IEC Leadership Council and the Ethics Sub-Council review these patient and staff discussions during their meetings. The Ethics Leadership Council ensures that staff are aware of follow-up actions being taken to improve the patient care experience in a weekly all-employee email message.

Nurses are important members of both the Ethics Leadership Council and the Ethics Sub-Council. Coatesville Veterans Administration Medical Center welcomes the participation of all staff in the IEC regardless of their level of experience. Nurses and all other members of the IEC receive training from the VHA National Center for Ethics in Healthcare. This VHA ethics training includes roles and functions of the IEC Leadership Council and the Ethics Sub-Council, understanding ethics quality, and how to use tools to improve ethical healthcare. This supports the development of an interprofessional team skilled in the identification, analysis, and improvement of ethics in healthcare.

Diane Gibson, MHA, RN, WCC
Performance Improvement Consultant
Preventive Ethics Coordinator, Coatesville Veterans Administration Medical Center, Coatesville, Pennsylvania

END-OF-CHAPTER RESOURCES

KEY CONCEPTS

1. The three branches of the United States (U.S.) federal government are the executive branch, the legislative branch, and the judicial branch.
2. The U.S. Department of Health and Human Services has many administrative agencies that influence laws surrounding many aspects of the healthcare delivery system, including payment of healthcare services, regulation of medical drugs and devices, vaccine programs, healthcare research, and patient safety.
3. There are many state and federal laws that govern the healthcare industry and influence and shape the practice of nursing.
4. Nurses are affected by both civil and criminal law.
5. Nurse practice acts vary by state but generally include a definition of the scope of nursing practice allowed in the state.
6. A person bringing a malpractice or negligence suit must prove the four elements of malpractice or negligence.
7. The four elements of malpractice or negligence are that (a) a duty of care was owed to the patient, (b) there was a breach in that duty, (c) any injury was proximately caused by the breach of duty, and (d) there were damages.
8. Nurses have a responsibility to follow hospital guidelines and physician's orders and assure patient safety.
9. Nurses follow the hospital chain of command to report any problems in patient care delivery.
10. Nurses have an independent responsibility to assure patient safety.
11. The HIPAA was passed in 1996 to set national standards for the use of patient information.
12. Medicare and other third-party payors affect the delivery of patient care.
13. There are specific Medicare Home Health Certification requirements.
14. Whistleblowers must develop thorough documentation of any patient care concerns.
15. The Federal Anti-Kickback Statute, the Stark Law, and the Civil Monetary Penalties Law seek to prevent potentially abusive circumstances whereby Medicare may be defrauded.
16. The International Council of Nurses Code of Ethics identifies four principal elements that outline the standards of ethical conduct for nurses. These responsibilities are promoting health, preventing illness, restoring health, and alleviating suffering.
17. The American Nurses Association Code of Ethics (ANA, 2015) is divided into nine distinct provisions and their accompanying interpretive statements.
18. Ethical principles and theories guide the practice of nursing (e.g., beneficence, justice, autonomy, fidelity, nonmaleficence, paternalism, utilitarianism).
19. When confronted with an ethical decision, nurses and interprofessional teams can use the ethical decision-making process and the four-box approach as strategies to develop a broad point of view to support ethical clinical decision-making.

CRITICAL DISCUSSION POINTS

1. What are the checks and balances in the United States federal government system?
2. What is the purpose of the Health Insurance Portability and Accountability Act?
3. What is the purpose of the Stark Law?

KEY TERMS

> Breach in duty
> Common law
> Duty of care
> Executive branch
> Federal Anti-Kickback Statute
> Health Insurance Portability and Accountability Act (HIPAA)
> Home healthcare
> Hospital-acquired infections
> Judicial branch
> Legislative branch
> Malpractice
> Negligence
> Nurse practice acts (NPAs)
> Personal representative
> Separation of powers
> Stark Law
> Statutory laws
> Whistleblower claim

REVIEW QUESTIONS

Answers to Review Questions appear in the Instructor's Manual. Qualified instructors should request the Instructor's Manual from textbook@springerpub.com.

1. A nurse is caring for a 62-year-old man with respiratory distress and acute renal injury following an IV pyelogram to investigate recurring infections. The prescriber orders vancomycin at double the regular dose. The nurse is concerned by the dose and by the patient's renal function. Which actions would be most appropriate to take? *Select all that apply*.
   - **A.** Discuss the order with the prescriber, clearly stating concerns related to safety.
   - **B.** Contact the pharmacist to discuss the order and confirm reasons for concern.
   - **C.** Report the prescriber to the nurse manager.
   - **D.** Notify the charge nurse of the order and the concerns and actions taken.
   - **E.** Put the order aside for the time being and hope the prescriber realizes the error.
2. The nurse is named in a civil lawsuit involving a patient who suffered a broken hip following a hospital fall and subsequently died from pneumonia. Which aspects will impact the outcome of the lawsuit? *Select all that apply*.
   - **A.** Whether nursing actions were in accordance with the state NPA.
   - **B.** Whether the nurse established a therapeutic relationship with the patient and family

C. Prior decisions made by courts related to negligence
D. The ability of the nurse to pay financial damages
E. Whether the nurse was covered by an individual malpractice insurance policy

3. The HIPAA protects which of the following?
   A. A patient's right to be insured regardless of employment status or ability to pay
   B. The confidentiality of certain protected health information
   C. The nurse's right to patient information related to health insurance
   D. The hospital's right to disclose protected health information

4. All of the following elements are necessary for a nurse to be found negligent in a court of law except which?
   A. A duty or obligation for the nurse to act in a particular way
   B. A breach of that duty or obligation
   C. The nurse's intention to be negligent
   D. Physical, emotional, or financial harm to the patient

5. A nurse fails to put the bedside rails up on a confused patient's bed. Subsequently, the patient falls and is injured. When there is a connection between the nurse omitting a duty and an injury occurring to a patient, this is an example of which of the following?
   A. Duty
   B. Breach
   C. Causation
   D. Damages

6. The nurse is notified by hospital administration that a patient's family is bringing a suit for damages against the surgeon, the nurses who cared for the patient, and the hospital for a patient who developed a CLABSI postoperatively. The infection resulted in a prolonged hospital stay and recovery. The nurse knows that for the family to be successful in the suit, which of the following must be proven? *Select all that apply.*
   A. The nurse had a duty to care for the patient in a way that would prevent infection.
   B. The patient had an extended stay in the hospital as a result of the infection that left him physically weak and debilitated for 2 years afterward, ultimately losing his job.
   C. The patient and family are angry that the patient suffered.
   D. The documentation in the nursing notes demonstrates the patient's central line dressing was not changed in accordance with national standards.
   E. The nurse only had 2 years of experience working in the surgical unit.

7. A healthcare provider has issued a do not resuscitate (DNR) order for the patient, a 55-year-old man with cancer. The nurse speaks with the patient and the patient clearly states he wishes to be resuscitated in the event that he stops breathing. What is the most appropriate course of action for the nurse to take?
   A. Ignore the patient's wishes because the healthcare provider wrote the DNR order.
   B. Consult the hospital's policies and procedures manual, speak to the healthcare provider, and discuss the matter with the nurse manager if the concern is not resolved.
   C. Attempt to talk the patient into agreeing to the DNR.
   D. Contact the medical licensing board to report the healthcare provider.

8. A healthcare provider has ordered the nurse to discharge Mr. Jones from the hospital despite a new temperature of 102 °F (38.8 °C). The provider refuses to talk with the nurse about the patient. In this situation, which of the following is an appropriate nursing action?
   - A. Administer an antipyretic medication and discharge the patient.
   - B. Discharge the patient with instructions to call 911 if he has any problems.
   - C. Do not discharge the patient until the nurse discusses the matter with the nurse manager and is satisfied regarding patient safety.
   - D. Discharge the patient and tell the patient to take Tylenol when he gets home.
9. The nurse is given a written order by a healthcare provider to administer an unusually large dose of pain medicine to a patient. In this situation, which of the following is an appropriate nursing action?
   - A. Administer the medication because a healthcare provider ordered it.
   - B. Refuse to administer the medication, and move on to care for another patient.
   - C. Speak with the healthcare provider about the concerns, and clarify with the provider or pharmacy whether the medication dose is accurate.
   - D. Select a dose that is appropriate and administer that dose.
10. Nurse Jones works at a home healthcare agency. After submitting her notes relating to visits with her patients, Nurse Jones observes other coworkers adding other visit note-like paperwork with what appears to be her signature (even though Nurse Jones did not prepare such notes). Nurse Jones learns that such behavior has occurred on several other patient files. Before commencing a whistleblower claim, whom should Nurse Jones notify?
   - A. An attorney
   - B. The coworkers who falsified the notes
   - C. The agency administrators
   - D. The local police department

REVIEW ACTIVITIES

1. Identify the ways in which nurses you observe in your clinical rotations discuss medication orders and treatments with healthcare providers. How do nurses address incorrect or questionable medication orders? Talk with the nurses you see about how they handle this situation.
2. Visit the NCSBN website for all state board of nursing NPAs at https://www.ncsbn.org/npa.htm. Choose your state from the drop-down list and review your NPA and rules. Discuss what you find there.

EXPLORING THE WEB

1. Visit https://qsen.org/publications/videos/the-lewis-blackman-story. Scroll down and click on Part Four: Disclosing Error and Accountability. Watch the video and answer the questions about nursing accountability.
2. Visit www.nso.com/risk-management/individuals?SelectedTabID=3722. Review the legal cases found there.

A robust set of instructor resources designed to supplement this text is located at **http://connect.springerpub.com/content/book/978-0-8261-6145-1.** Qualifying instructors may request access by emailing **textbook@springerpub.com.**

REFERENCES

American Association of Colleges of Nursing. (2021). The essentials: Core competencies for professional nursing education. https://www.aacnnursing.org/Education-Resources/AACN-Essentials

American Nurses Association. (2015). *The code of ethics for nurses with interpretive statements.* http://www.nursingworld.org/MainMenuCategories/EthicsStandards/CodeofEthicsforNurses/Code-of-Ethics-For-Nurses.html

International Council of Nurses. (2012). *The ICN code of ethics for nurses*. https://www.icn.ch/sites/default/files/inline-files/2012_ICN_Codeofethicsfornurses_%20eng.pdf

Jonson, A., Siegler, M., & Winslade, W. (2015). *Clinical ethics: A practical approach to ethical decisions in clinical medicine* (8th ed.). McGraw-Hill Education.

McGuire, C., & Mroczek, J. (2017). *Nurse malpractice*. National Center of Continuing Education. https://www.nursece.com/courses/99

Philipsen, N., & Soeken, D. (2011). Preparing to blow the whistle: *A Survival Guide for Nurses. The Journal for Nurse Practitioners, 7*(9), 740–746. https://doi.org/10.1016/j.nurpra.2011.07.006

Relias Media. (2016). *More nurses, hospitalists being sued for malpractice, studies say*. https://www.reliasmedia.com/articles/137567-more-nurses-hospitalists-being-sued-for-malpractice-studies-say

SUGGESTED READING

Aliakbari, F., Hammad, K., Bahrami, M., & Aein, F. (2015). Ethical and legal challenges associated with disaster nursing. *Nursing Ethics, 4*, 493–503. https://doi.org/10.1177/0969733014534877

Hammer, M. J. (2019). Beyond the helix: Ethical, legal, and social implications in genomics. *Seminars in Oncology Nursing, 35*(1), 93–106. https://doi.org/10.1016/j.soncn.2018.12.007

Miller, J. (2019). Ethical issues arising from marijuana use by nursing mothers in a changing legal and cultural context. *HEC Forum, 31*(1), 11–27. https://doi.org/10.1007/s10730-018-9368-1

Rubio-Navarro, A., Garcia-Capilla, D. J., Torralba-Madrid, M. J., & Rutty, J. (2019). Ethical, legal and professional accountability in emergency nursing practice: An ethnographic observational study. *International Emergency Nursing, 46*, 1. https://doi.org/10.1016/j.ienj.2019.05.003

Salehi, Z., Ghezeljeh, T. N., Hajibabaee, F., & Joolaee, S. (2020). Factors behind ethical dilemmas regarding physical restraint for critical care nurses. *Nursing Ethics, 27*(2), 598–608. https://doi.org/10.1177/0969733019858711

Schiller, C. J., Pesut, B., Roussel, J., & Greig, M. (2019). But it's legal, isn't it? Law and ethics in nursing practice related to medical assistance in dying. *Nursing Philosophy, 20*(4), e12277. https://doi.org/10.1111/nup.12277

CHAPTER 5

Delegation and Setting Priorities for Safe, High-Quality Patient Care

Danette Ver Woert and Ruth I. Hansten

"The secret of leadership is ... never to ask of others what you would not willingly do yourself."

–J. Donald Walters

Upon completion of this chapter, the reader should be able to:

1. Define delegation, responsibility, delegated responsibility, assignment, accountability, authority, and supervision.
2. Describe the Five Rights of Delegation.
3. Discuss the American Nurses Association (ANA) and the National Council of State Boards of Nursing (NCSBN) National Guidelines for Nursing Delegation
4. Review the nursing chain of command as it relates to delegation.
5. Apply the Scope of Nursing Practice Decision-Making Framework to nursing practice.
6. Describe communication factors influencing the delegation process.
7. Discuss delegation in community settings.
8. Discuss assignment sheets and patient handoff report.

CROSSWALK

This chapter addresses the following:

QSEN Competencies: Patient-Centered Care, Teamwork & Collaboration, Safety
The American Association of Colleges of Nursing (2021). *The Essentials: core competencies for professional nursing education* (2021).

Domain 2: Person-Centered Care
Domain 5: Quality and Safety
Domain 6: Interprofessional Partnerships

OPENING SCENARIO

Sylvia arrives at 0700 for her morning shift. She just completed her new graduate residency and she is excited about starting her new job. She is also a little nervous to be fully on her own. She had told the charge RN that she loves working on a team although she finds it a little uncomfortable to "tell people what to do." She is assigned a team of four patients. Two of the four patients need repositioning every 2 hours. After she receives bedside report from the night shift, Sylvia quickly becomes immersed in a patient's request for pain medicine and forgets about the every 2 hour repositioning schedules. At 1000, she realizes she has not made a plan for the day with her assigned nursing assistant and she has not repositioned her patients. Sylvia is new to healthcare and she is not used to giving a nursing assistant specific direction. She is also not used to the fast-paced environment of the medical-surgical floor.

1. What safety issues should Sylvia consider when planning her day?
2. How do those safety issues influence her communication with a nursing assistant?
3. What suggestions could the charge RN have for Sylvia in order to build her confidence level with "telling people what to do"?

INTRODUCTION

Nurses use many critical thinking skills each shift to plan and provide high-quality patient care. A nurse simultaneously prioritizes which patient to see first as well as deciding how to effectively communicate the plan of care to other team members. One of the important skills nurses must develop is delegation. In order to assure that all of the important tasks a nurse is responsible for during a shift are accomplished, a nurse must become comfortable and skilled in delegation. Nurses today must be willing and able to function interdependently on a highly skilled interprofessional healthcare team. The nurse uses their knowledge of the nursing scope of practice, their knowledge of the scope of practice of their teammates, and their knowledge of the emotional intelligence of both themself and others to effectively collaborate with patients, families, providers, and other members of the interprofessional healthcare team. **Emotional intelligence** includes reflection and analysis of emotion within self and others, as well as the ability to self-regulate emotions (Marquis & Huston, 2021). Delegation is needed in order to meet patient needs and provide appropriate care to each patient when they need it. Delegation is particularly important today for many reasons, including the nursing shortage, increases in patient acuity levels, increases in the older adult population, advances in healthcare technology, and ongoing cost containment requirements.

Nursing is a team sport and one nurse can't do it all. Without leveraging the power of delegation, nurses are overworked (Al-Moteri, 2020). Effective delegation and assignment can reduce overwork, help to reduce healthcare costs, increase positive patient outcomes, decrease patient length-of-stay, and enhance positive working relationships among members of the healthcare team. Working together is more efficient than working alone. It is also more fun!

This chapter provides an overview of delegation. Definitions of delegation, responsibility, delegated responsibility, assignment, accountability, authority, and supervision are provided. When a nurse delegates, they must consider the policies and procedures of their state's regulatory structures (i.e., their state board of nursing and their state nurse practice act [NPA]). They must also consider the National Guidelines for Nursing Delegation of Nursing Practice, the National Council of State Boards of Nursing (NCSBN) Five Rights of

Delegation, the American Nurses Association (ANA) and the NCSBN National Guidelines for Nursing Delegation, and the Scope of Nursing Practice Decision-Making Framework for nursing practice. The chapter discusses the nursing chain of command used if patient care problems arise and the use of good communication when delegating care in an agency and the community to achieve high-quality, safe patient care. The use of assignment sheets and patient handoff report is also discussed. In this chapter, the term "nurse" is used to indicate an RN registered nurse. When the chapter refers to an LPN/LVN (licensed practical nurse/licensed vocational nurse), they are identified as such (LPN/LVN). Unlicensed assistive personnel (UAP) consist of nurses' aides, certified nursing assistants, patient care technicians, or other position designations or titles within the work environment (NCSBN and ANA National Guidelines for Nursing Delegation, 2019).

DELEGATION

The ANA defines **delegation** as the "transfer of responsibility for the performance of a task from one individual to another while retaining accountability for the outcome" (ANA, 2014, p. 22). The ANA and NCSBN 2019 Joint Statement *National Guidelines for Nursing Delegation* states that, "The decision of whether or not to delegate or assign is based upon the RN's judgment concerning the condition of the patient, the competence of all members of the nursing team and the degree of supervision that will be required of the RN if a task is delegated" (NCSBN & ANA, 2019, p. 1). In an earlier document, the NCSBN explains that, "The licensed nurse must determine the needs of the patient and whether those needs are matched by the knowledge, skills, and abilities of the delegatee and can be performed safely by the delegatee" (NCSBN, 2016, p. 10). The licensed nurse cannot delegate nursing-specific activities such as clinical reasoning, nursing judgment, or critical decision-making. When making the decision to delegate an activity, the nurse must follow the Five Rights of Delegation, explored later in this chapter (NCSBN & ANA, 2019).

State Nurse Practice Acts

In the United States, each state and territory has its own unique NPA with associated rules and regulations. Two terms used by state NPAs regarding delegation are "delegating" and "assigning." Whether or not the RN is identified as "delegating" or "assigning" patient care is determined by the state in which the nurse practices. In some states, recent definitions of delegation and assignment by the NCSBN and ANA Joint Statement 2019 have been adopted, while other states use a former definition. For example, in one state an RN may be "delegating" a basic care task like vital signs to a UAP, whereas in another state using the 2019 NCSBN and ANA definition, the term used would be "assigning" vital signs because the task is within the basic education of a UAP in that state's regulations. Both "delegation" and "assignment" require that the RN would not delegate or assign any task that was not sanctioned by state regulations, agency policy, and procedure, or was beyond that delegate's ability or competence, and the team member's job description. When RNs are ensuring that delegated tasks are completed, their decision will not be dependent on whether the task is termed "delegation" or "assignment"; the same degree of direction and follow-up is required.

All RNs should familiarize themselves with their own NPA prior to delegating. It is the nurse's responsibility to know what their NPA says about delegating along with a clear understanding of the delegation policies of their employer. Each state determines the scope and limitations of nursing practice and may vary throughout the 50 states and territories. Each NPA must reflect the basic education required for RNs, LPN/LVNs, and UAP (Marquis & Huston, 2021). RNs must be able to quickly find and understand their state's

TABLE 5.1 NCSBN'S NURSE PRACTICE ACT (NPA) DATABASES

NCSBN's NPA Database	www.ncsbn.org/npa.htm, accessed October 17, 2020
NCSBN's Environmental Scan: A Portrait of Nursing and Health Care in 2020 and Beyond, Appendix A*	www.ncsbn.org/2020_JNREnvScan.pdf

* Appendix A lists various State Board of Nursing (BON) policy and position statements, as well as NPA provisional changes and amendments issued or revised by BONs from September 2018 through October 2019.

NCSBN, National Council of State Boards of Nursing

NPA. Use NCSBN's NPA website list to locate a specific state or territory's NPA and other applicable state rules and regulations (Table 5.1).

Delegation is a complex nursing skill. RNs must only delegate tasks that the delegatee is competent and trained to complete, within the state regulations, and approved by their workplace job descriptions. The delegatee has to agree to accept and complete the task and should express an understanding of desired outcomes (Hansten, 2020a, 2020b). When delegating tasks, the nurse retains authority for the decisions and outcomes associated with patient care. For the nurse to effectively delegate there must be a clear understanding of specific terms: responsibility, delegated responsibility, assignment, accountability, authority, and supervision.

Responsibility

Responsibility is the acceptance of overall accountability for the patient, even when tasks are delegated, although the delegate shares responsibility for the completed delegated activity, task, or procedure (NCSBN, 2019). Delegation is not complete until the person who receives the assignment accepts the responsibility for the delegation and agrees to complete it. Without this acceptance of responsibility, assignments cannot be delegated. Further, if a person does not have the knowledge, skill, experience, or willingness needed to complete an assignment, it is inappropriate to accept responsibility for the assignment. Nurses retain legal responsibility for informed consent, confidentiality, and delegation (Black, 2020).

Nurses make decisions daily affecting the well-being of their patients. Because they have access to personal information about patients and interact with them during stressful times, they are in a position of responsibility and trust. Nurses are trusted with sensitive patient information and therefore assume legal responsibility to handle patient information confidentially and ethically. Being fully informed will help nurses minimize risks related to these areas. When delegating patient care, the RN must ensure their nursing judgment is never being delegated and clearly communicate that the delegatee does not have the power to change or alter their delegated or assigned tasks (Anderson, 2018).

Delegated Responsibility

A **delegated responsibility** is the transfer of a nursing activity, task, or procedure from a nurse to another member of the healthcare team (NCSBN, 2019). The responsibilities considered for delegation must be in accordance with the state's/jurisdiction's laws and rules as well as organizational policies and procedures prior to the RN making a final decision to delegate. For example, a nurse knows that a UAP is trained and able to complete a blood glucose fingerstick reading. This task is listed in the job description of the UAP. The UAP has performed this task daily for nurses. In this example, the nurse is delegating the responsibility to complete the blood glucose reading. The UAP is expected to report the reading back to the nurse. The nurse does not delegate any further action by the UAP based on the blood glucose reading. If, at any point, the nurse does not feel delegation of a responsibility is appropriate, the nurse must complete the responsibility themself.

Assignment

Assignment involves the transfer of routine RN or LPN/LVN care activities and/or part of the routine functions of the UAP from one member of the healthcare team to another (NCSBN, 2019). When a nurse assigns a task to a UAP, the nurse is assigning a task that was included in the coursework of the delegatee's educational background (NSCBN, 2016). For example, when the nurse assigns a UAP the task of bathing a patient, the nurse is assigning tasks to the UAP that were included in the coursework of the delegatee's educational background. Note that in some states, UAP roles are expanding to include medication administration. Although the UAP has formal training in medication administration and is assigned the task, the nurse is responsible to appropriately delegate and supervise this process (NCSBN, 2016). For example, a nurse must ensure the UAP or LPN/LVN can demonstrate proper injection technique before giving a patient an injection (National Association of School Nurses [NASC], 2019; NSCBN, 2016; Shannon & Kubelka, 2013). The organization is responsible for developing competency checklists and continuing education for all staff regarding task competency.

Another example of an assignment is the LPN/LVN caring for a patient with Crohn's disease. The RN assigns the LPN/LVN to complete portions of the patient intake data form, monitor intake and output (I & O), administer medications, and take vital signs. These skills are taught in the LPN/LVN education program and, thus, are part of the LPN/LVN scope of practice.

There are exceptions when speaking to the basic educational preparation of a UAP. The tasks once believed to be performed only by an RN are now taught to UAPs in certain states' advanced UAP education programs. For example, in some states, UAPs identified as certified medication assistants (CMA) are given special training to pass oral medications and give injections. UAPs may also be identified as medical assistants (MA) in ambulatory settings. In ambulatory care settings in many states, physicians and nurses both delegate to and supervise UAPs who are identified as MA; they assist with office visit intake forms and may administer vaccinations or deliver standardized educational handouts to patients. Since there is a significant level of skill needed when administering medications or injections, employers and nurses will need to validate the UAP's competency. To validate competency, employers and nurses give skill tests, make observations, and document accordingly as needed.

Accountability

According to the ANA, **accountability** is to be answerable to self and others, based on the agreed upon standards of professional nursing ethics (ANA, 2015). An RN is accountable for their professional performance and the alignment of their actions with organization-specific and state-specific laws, as well as with their educational preparation (ANA, 2015). The nurse is also accountable for the quality of nursing care provided and for recognizing limits, knowledge, competency, and experience of delegatees (ANA, 2015). UAPs and LPN/LVNs are also accountable to the RN. Accountability for the act of delegating involves the appropriate choice of delegatee and selection of their delegated or assigned task. For example, a nurse might delegate a task to the UAP. If the nurse has not determined in advance that the UAP understands the delegated task and has the skills, knowledge, and judgment to complete the task, or the nurse does not supervise the completion of the delegated task and the UAP does not carry out the responsibility adequately, the nurse is accountable for this act of improper delegation.

Authority

Authority is the right to act or to command the action of others (NCSBN, 2019). In nursing, authority is inherent and is required for a nurse to appropriately provide patient care. The nurse must be able to make decisions regarding patient care. Without authority, the nurse will be unable to provide high-quality, safe patient-centered care. Authority is based on the state's/jurisdiction's NPA and guides the development of an organization's job description. If the nurse is in charge of a group of patients, the nurse must have the authority to act or command the action of others to coordinate care needed for optimal patient outcomes.

Supervision

Nurses are responsible to provide adequate and timely supervision to all delegatees. This entails following up with the delegate at the completion of the delegated activity (NCSBN, 2019). **Supervision** is the active process of directing, guiding, and influencing the outcome

CURRENT LITERATURE

CITATIONS

Hansten, R. (2020b, April 13). *Delegation/assignment/supervision in a pandemic*. LinkedIn. https://www.linkedin.com/pulse/delegationassignmentsupervision-pandemic-ruth-hansten-rn-mba-phd; Hansten, R. (2021, January 5). *Crisis/contingency standards of care COVID delegation & assignment*. LinkedIn. https://www.linkedin.com/pulse/crisiscontingency-standards-care-covid-delegation-ruth Hansten, R. (2021, January 14). *Delegation and assignment in COVID crisis, contingency, surge modes; Care delivery models* [Video]. YouTube. https://www.youtube.com/watch?v=V0d7Uiyvw3Y&t=103s

DISCUSSION

Delegation during a national emergency or pandemic setting requires flexibility of the entire healthcare team and an understanding of the changing federal and sometimes state-level rules regarding licensing, practice permits, AP scope of practice, and nursing education. A national emergency requires nurses to know the basics of delegation as well as how to safely accommodate the scope of practice of each member of the healthcare team in the midst of changing practice guidelines.

IMPLICATIONS FOR PRACTICE

During a national emergency or pandemic, nurses are likely to work with new, inexperienced nursing graduates and nurses who have been deployed from retirement. These new graduates and retired nurses require appropriately assigned tasks and additional technical support and communication regarding high-quality, safe nursing practice. The experienced nurse should use the nursing process to assess fellow nurses' understanding of the patient-care scenario and their ability to carry-out the task safely, as well as their ability to plan, implement, and evaluate patient care and use resources judiciously.

of an individual's performance of a task (Duffy & Fields, 2014). Supervision includes guidance or direction, oversight, evaluation, and follow-up by the RN for the accomplishment of a delegated nursing task. The delegatee is responsible for communicating patient information to the RN during the delegation (NCSBN, 2019).

Supervision involves initial and ongoing communication between the RN and the delegatee. The nurse monitors the quality of the work completed by the delegatee and provides appropriate and timely feedback to the delegatee based on performance and patient outcomes. On the other hand, the delegatee provides the RN with appropriate and timely communication about any problems encountered with the delegated task and any issues that may have arisen during completion of the task. Supervision is generally categorized as on site (the RN being physically present or immediately available while the activity is performed) or off site (the RN has the ability to provide direction through various means of written and verbal communication). When appropriate, an RN supervising care will provide clear directions to the interprofessional team.

NATIONAL GUIDELINES FOR NURSING DELEGATION

The NCSBN convened two groups of experts representing education, research, and practice in 2015. They developed a set of National Guidelines for Nursing Delegation that standardized the nursing delegation process in 2016 and 2019. These National Guidelines for Nursing Delegation are meant for RNs, although a large aspect of the guidelines addresses UAPs and UAP advanced roles. Many tasks or processes that were once exclusive to RNs and/or LPN/LVNs are now taught in advanced UAP programs. See Table 5.2 for nursing responsibilities commonly done by RNs, LPN/LVNs, UAPs, or UAPs with advanced certification. Review your state's NPA for complete details of your state's nursing responsibilities.

TABLE 5.2 NURSING RESPONSIBILITIES

TEAM MEMBERS	TASK AND PROCESSES*
RN	Utilizes the nursing process and completes the following: • patient assessment and analysis • nursing diagnosis/problem identification • planning with patient/family to review intended outcomes • implementation of patient care • evaluation of patient care Demonstrates leadership and assures safe, high-quality patient care and the best use of available personnel Delegates tasks following Five Rights of Delegation of Patient Care (i.e., right task, right circumstance, right person, right direction and communication, and right supervision and evaluation; Table 5.3) Assesses qualifications of AP Retains responsibility for all delegated patient care Supervises task completion, gives feedback to delegates Communicates with patients, families, and interprofessional team Plans/executes/evaluates patient education and health maintenance Completes patient transfers and future care planning Anticipates patient safety and care needs Nursing technical tasks: Examples: gives medications; administers IV fluids, blood, and blood products; maintains airway and central lines; completes dressings, treatments, and tube feedings; maintains chest tubes and drains; plans and executes pain control

(continued)

TABLE 5.2 NURSING RESPONSIBILITIES *(continued)*

TEAM MEMBERS	TASK AND PROCESSES*
LPN/LVN	Assists with nursing process, data gathering, and care planning process May or may not delegate and supervise AP, depending on state Communicates findings to supervising RN Provides standardized teaching as instructed by RN or provider Assists in adjustments to care plans Delivers hygienic care and nutrition assistance Completes intake and output data gathering, assists with toileting Assists with stable patient mobilization, turning, ambulation Recognizes patient safety needs and follows up Nursing technical tasks (e.g., gives oral and IM medications; monitors and hangs IV fluids; monitors central lines; completes dressings, treatments, and tube feedings; maintains airway; maintains chest tubes and drains; plans and executes pain control
UAP	Performs basic tasks of patient hygiene and linen change Delivers meals and feeds patients (special training needed for patients with dysphagia) Takes vital signs Gathers data for intake and output; does toileting and enemas Collects specimens Transfers, mobilizes, turns, and ambulates stable patients Prepares patient rooms Makes patient safety rounds In some states, does glucose finger sticks
UAP with Advanced Certification	In addition to basic AP role noted previously, AP can be certified in some states to do the following: Give oral medications Give insulin in home care, long-term care, or community settings Give ambulatory patient immunizations Provide student medications in schools Do basic patient teaching and give education in the community with pre-established written standards

AP, assistive personnel; IM, intramuscular; IV, intravenous; LPN/LVN, licensed practical nurse/licensed vocational nurse; UAP, unlicensed assistive personnel.

Note: Review your state's nurse practice act for complete details.

NATIONAL COUNCIL OF STATE BOARDS OF NURSING FIVE RIGHTS OF DELEGATION

The NCSBN Five Rights of Delegation (NCSBN & ANA, 2019) address the necessary components nurses must consider when delegating to any person on the healthcare team. The Five Rights of Delegation are the:

- right task
- right circumstance
- right person
- right direction and communication
- right supervision and evaluation

As RNs think through the possible tasks (right task) that might be assigned or delegated, they will simultaneously consider their clinical setting (right circumstance) and the

TABLE 5.3 THE FIVE RIGHTS OF DELEGATION

THE FIVE RIGHTS	DESCRIPTION
Right Task	The activity falls within the RN's job description or is included as part of the established written policies and procedures of the nursing practice setting. The facility needs to ensure the policies and procedures describe the expectations and limits of the task and provide any necessary competency training allowed by the NPA.
Right Circumstance	The health condition of the patient must be stable. If the patient's condition changes, the assigned person must communicate this change in the patient's circumstance to the RN. The RN must then reassess the situation and the appropriateness of the assignment.
Right Person	The RN along with the employer and the assigned staff person is responsible for ensuring that the assigned staff person possesses the appropriate skills and knowledge and is the right person to perform the activity.
Right Direction and Communication	Each delegation situation should be specific to the patient, the licensed nurse, and the person assigned. The RN is expected to communicate specific directions and instructions for the assigned activity to the selected right person. The right staff person, as part of two-way communication, should ask any clarifying questions. This two-way communication must identify any data that needs to be collected, the method for collecting the data, the time frame for reporting the results to the licensed nurse, and any additional information pertinent to the situation. The entrusted right staff person must understand the terms of the delegation or assignment and must agree to accept the delegation or assignment.
Right Supervision and Evaluation	The RN is responsible for monitoring and the right supervision of the assigned activity, following up with the assigned right person at the completion of the activity, and completing the right evaluation of the patient's outcomes. The assigned right person is responsible for communicating patient information to the RN during the delegated activity. The RN should be ready and available to intervene as necessary for patient safety. The RN must ensure that appropriate documentation of the activity is completed.

NPA, nurse practice act.

Source: National Council of State Boards of Nursing and American Nurses Association. (2019, April 29). *National Guidelines for Nursing Delegation.* https://www.ncsbn.org/NGND-PosPaper_06.pdf

individual patient's care plan, their needs, and their clinical stability (right circumstance) while matching the competencies and willingness of potential AP (right person). When the needs of the patient coincide with the skills, knowledge, and competency of AP and can be performed safely (right person), the RN will decide that delegation can occur. This decision is guided by the NCSBN Five Rights of Delegation (1995, 1996, 2016). RNs also consider how best to offer the initial instructions and directions and ongoing communication and supervision throughout the episode of patient care (right direction and communication and the right supervision and evaluation) so that the planned patient and healthcare team outcomes are achieved and reviewed carefully by the RN (Table 5.3).

BOX 5.1 Developing Clinical Judgment

The physical therapist (PT) is going to help the RN use a mechanical assist device to move a patient to a chair. The RN has not worked with this PT before. The RN and PT must work collaboratively to provide patient care. The RN and PT must both have a clear understanding of their professional scope of practice and the roles of other healthcare team members. Although the RN does not delegate to or assign to the PT, good teamwork uses principles similar to the Five Rights of Delegation.

1. What **CUES (Assessment)** can the RN assess?
2. What **HYPOTHESIS (Diagnosis)** will the RN weigh?
3. What **ACTION (Plan and Implement)** will be most effective for the RN to take to assure the patient's safety in this situation?
4. How will the RN evaluate the patient's **OUTCOME (Evaluation)** for the purpose of arriving at a satisfactory clinical outcome?

Throughout patient care delivery, the RN supervises LVN/LPN and AP delegatees, while following the Five Rights of Delegation. Note that delegation and assignment are important processes used to assure safe, high-quality patient care, whether there is one RN for one, two, five, 10, or 20 or more patients or whether the RN works with a school full of students or works with a large community caseload. One RN cannot deliver all the care needed for multiple patients. The RN must work together with the delegatees and use safe delegation and assignment practices, including the Five Rights of Delegation, to assure that all patients receive safe, high-quality care.

CASE STUDY

Jane, the charge nurse, has assigned Joo, a newly graduated nurse, to care for patients on the day shift with the assistance of a UAP. After receiving handoff report, Joo makes fast rounds on all his patients to assure their safety and delegates some of the morning care to the UAP. Then, Joo's phone starts ringing. Physical therapy, occupational therapy, the provider, and pharmacy are all trying to reach Joo. He talks to each of them and then begins to plan for completion of a complex wound-vac dressing change. Joo estimates it will take him about 45 minutes. He goes into the patient's room and begins setting up for the dressing change. The UAP comes to the door saying, "The patient in room 523 is requesting oxycodone." Apply Table 5.3 to this scenario.

1. *Identify the right task for Joo to assign.*
2. *Identify two of the right people to whom Joo can safely assign the right task.*
3. *Discuss the right direction, communication, supervision, and evaluation needed in this situation to maintain patient safety.*

Real World Interview

I had been an emergency room (ER) nurse for just over two and a half years when the COVID-19 virus pandemic began in my home state of Washington. While this situation came with many unknowns, I felt confident in our ER team's ability to work together in this situation, even if we didn't know what to expect or how to plan. During one of my shifts, I was floating throughout the ER and helping nurses with their various tasks, when I was called upon to admit a new patient arriving via ambulance. The patient was a middle-aged man complaining of shortness of breath, chills, cough, and chest pain. He reported he had stayed home with the hopes he'd get better and avoid the risks of going to the hospital during the virus outbreak. Per the current protocol with any viral-like symptomatic patients, I made sure to don full airborne personal protective equipment (PPE) before entering the room and completing the new patient's physical assessment.

In the fast-paced environment of the ER, RNs rely on teamwork with each other and the ER technicians (ER techs) or assistive personnel. As I entered the patient's room, the ER tech I was working with that day also donned PPE. Before I assessed the patient, I communicated with the ER tech about the priority tasks we needed to complete and the urgency of the situation. The ER tech began to address these tasks, starting with gathering a full set of vital signs, placing the patient on full cardiac monitoring, and tending to patient needs while I spoke with the ambulance medics. The ER tech informed me that the patient was febrile with a temperature in the 100s. This information along with the patient's tachycardia, tachypnea, and presentation suggested the need to call a "Code Sepsis" overhead. At our hospital, a "Code Sepsis" call triggers a slew of extra hands to assist the nurse and patient at the bedside of the room mentioned in the "Code Sepsis" call. An ER provider and two extra ER techs arrived quickly and checked in with me before entering the room. One ER tech spoke to me through the door and asked about what items he should bring with him in order to reduce trips in and out of the room and multiple PPE changes. Due to the pandemic, there was a national-wide shortage of PPE, so we were planning our trips into isolation rooms very carefully. A "Code Sepsis" requires quite a few nursing interventions. Each nursing intervention is enacted quickly in order to increase the likelihood of a better outcome for the patient. I asked the ER tech if he could gather blood culture supplies, ice to cool certain lab samples, and a COVID-19 test swab/tube, as none of these things were kept at the bedside. As he went to retrieve supplies, I asked the remaining ER tech to complete an EKG due to the patient's complaints of chest pain and shortness of breath. I completed the physical assessment and all aspects of the nursing process. I delegated tasks not associated with the nursing process, like gathering supplies, to the ER tech. It was so helpful that all of the ER techs knew exactly what a "Code Sepsis" meant and how to respond quickly as a team.

Caroline Lindberg
Emergency Room RN
Seattle, Washington

CHAIN OF COMMAND

The organization is responsible to provide sufficient staffing; an appropriate staffing mix; and ongoing education and competency support for all those involved in the delegation process in the organization and patient care team. The organization has a chain of command (Figure 5.1) that identifies organizational and nursing responsibilities. The bedside RN, including the new graduate RN, is accountable to the charge RN of the unit where they are working. The charge RN is accountable to the RN nurse manager, who is

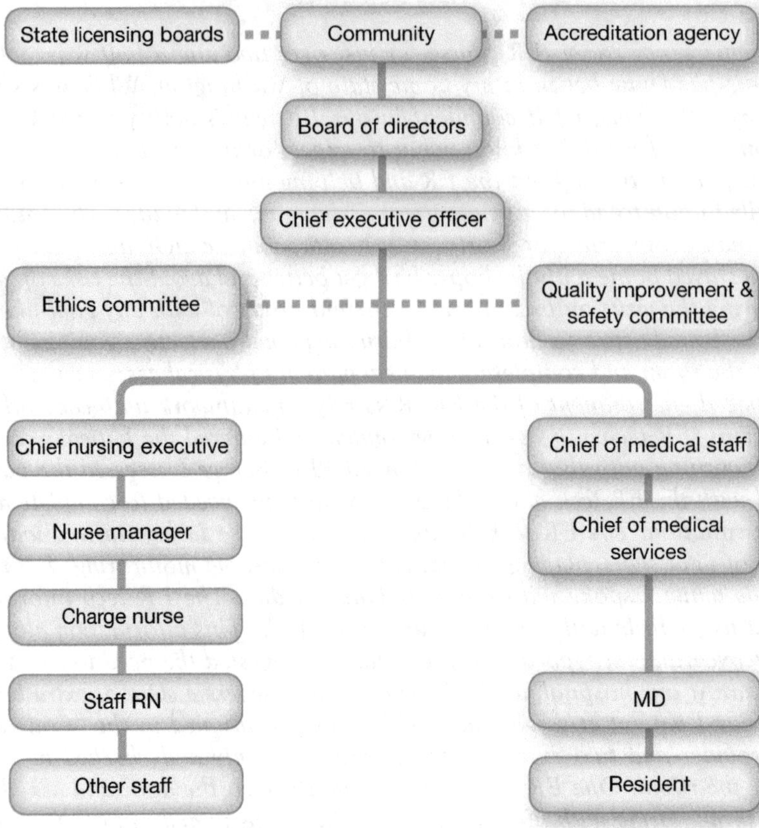

FIGURE 5.1 Organizational Chain of Command.

accountable to the chief nursing executive. The charge RN can delegate and assign tasks to staff RNs and other staff (e.g., LPN/LVN, UAP). The licensed staff RN most frequently seeks advice regarding delegation questions from the charge RN. If the charge RN needs additional support, they would communicate their concern to the unit's nurse manager. If the nurse manager is unavailable, emergency issues could also be communicated to a nursing house supervisor, and/or a hospital or nursing administrator on call. If needed, emergency issues could also be communicated to the chief nursing executive, who would communicate concerns to the chief executive officer, who could communicate any concerns to the board of directors.

AMERICAN NURSES ASSOCIATION AND NATIONAL COUNCIL OF STATE BOARDS OF NURSING NATIONAL GUIDELINES FOR NURSING DELEGATION

The ANA and NCSBN National Guidelines for Nursing Delegation (Figure 5.2) identifies responsibilities of the employer/nurse leader, the licensed nurse, and the delegatee for public protection. These guidelines highlight the need to communicate information about the delegation process and the delegatee competence level; the need for two-way communication and public protection; and the need for training and education.

Each of the persons identified in the three main sections of the ANA Nursing and NCSBN Delegation Guidelines (i.e., the employer/nurse leader, the licensed nurse, and

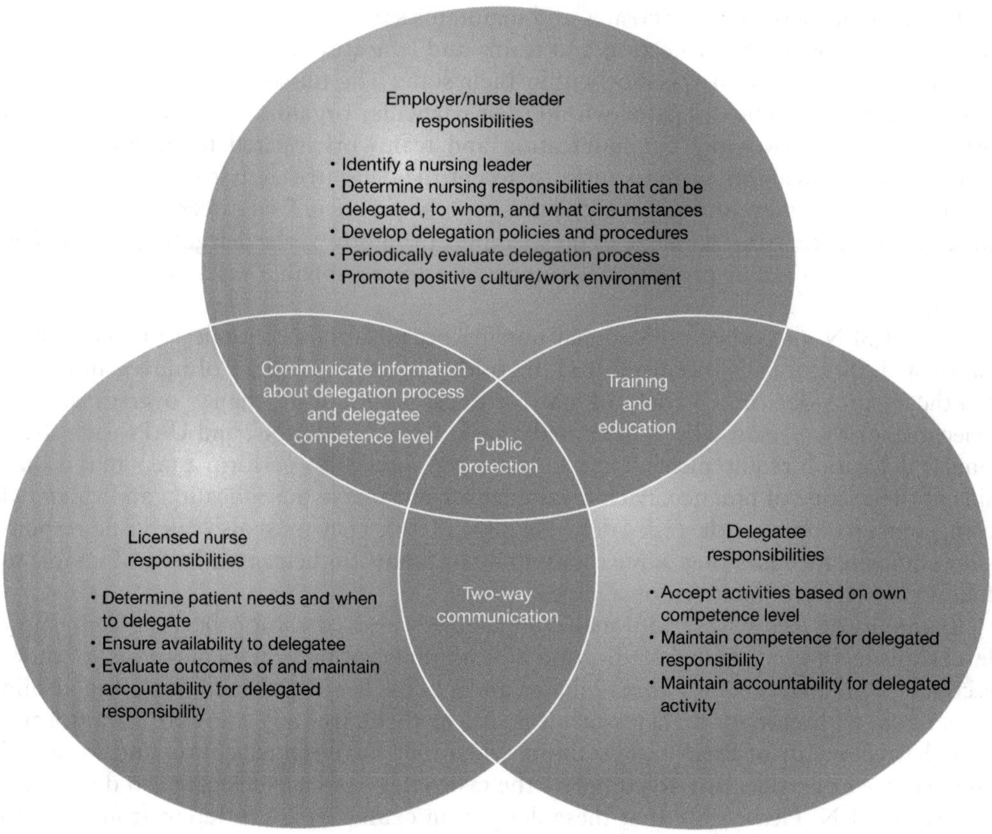

FIGURE 5.2 The American Nurses Association and National Council of State Boards of Nursing National Guidelines for Nursing Delegation.

Source: From National Council of State Boards of Nursing. (2016). Nursing guidelines for nursing delegation. *Journal of Nursing Regulation*, *7*(1), 5-12. http://www.ncsbn.org/NCSBN_Delegation_Guidelines.pdf

the delegatee) has have specific responsibilities they are expected to exercise for public protection. For example, the employer will identify a nurse leader who will determine nursing responsibilities that can be delegated, to whom, and under what circumstances. The employer/nurse leader will develop delegation policies and procedures; periodically evaluate the delegation process; and promote a positive culture and work environment. The employer/nurse leader will also communicate information about the delegation process and delegatee competence level to the RN, provide training and education, and public protection.

The licensed nurse responsibilities identified in the ANA and NCSBN Nursing Delegation Guidelines include determining patient needs and when to delegate; ensuring availability to delegatee; and evaluating outcomes of and maintaining accountability for delegated responsibility. The licensed nurse communicates information about the delegation process and delegatee competence level to the employer/nurse leader. The licensed nurse also assures public protection and maintains two-way communication with the delegatee.

The delegatee responsibilities identified in the ANA and NCSBN Nursing Delegation Guidelines are to accept activities based on their own competence level and maintain competence and accountability for delegated responsibility (ANA & NCSBN, 2019).

The nurse leader/employer creates and maintains safe policies and procedures related to delegation for public protection and trains and educates licensed nurses and delegatees regarding delegation specifics within their state. The nurse leader/employer ascertains what tasks can be delegated within their particular organizational roles. They also promote positive two-way communication and teamwork related to delegation. The delegatee's responsibilities are to agree to accept the delegated activity based on self-assessment of their current competency and scope of practice. Delegatees must complete the delegated activity or, if unable to do so, report promptly to the delegating nurse. They must continue to retain professional competence for reasonable tasks within their job description.

The NCSBN and other professional nursing organizations continue to explore delegation as healthcare advancements and the roles and responsibilities of nurses and other healthcare providers in a variety of state settings continuously change over time. As a delegatee, or the person who is delegated a task, RNs, LPN/LVNs, and UAPs each share similar delegation requirements. First, they are not allowed to perform a task that is outside of their scope of practice. Each team member must have the education and validated competence to complete the task safely (NCSBN, 2016). They must also safely and responsibly complete the tasks they agree they will do or report to their nurse leader if unable to follow through with their responsibilities.

Examples of APs with additional competencies and education beyond their entry level skills include a certified medication aide administrating oral medications, a school secretary administering an asthma inhaler, and a home health aide administering insulin to patients with chronic diabetes mellitus. All of them are only allowed to perform a task that is outside of their basic training when they have the education and validated competence or certification to complete the task safely and are delegated to do so by a supervising RN. Please note that these delegation examples are different from state to state.

SCOPE OF NURSING PRACTICE DECISION-MAKING FRAMEWORK

The Tri-Council for Nursing, consisting of an alliance between the American Association of Colleges of Nursing (AACN), the ANA, the American Organization for Nursing Leadership, the NCSBN, and the National League for Nursing (NLN), developed a Scope of Nursing Practice Decision-Making Framework (Figure 5.3) to assist nurses and their employers in determining the responsibilities a nurse can safely perform. A nurse may not delegate a task that is not within their own scope of practice. Nurses, whether novices or seasoned, are often confused about which procedures they can perform if ordered by a provider and nurses may be confused by regulation differences across state lines. Nurses should not rely on physicians or others to know more about the nursing scope of practice than the nurses themselves. Nurses must make their own practice decisions thoughtfully and with the state board's restrictions and patient safety in mind. While decisions to delegate patient care responsibilities are unique to different situations, the Scope of Nursing Practice Decision-Making Framework provides a safe, standardized decision-making process for nurses to navigate uncertain clinical situations (Ballard et al., 2016).

The Scope of Nursing Practice Decision-Making Framework can be applied to most patient care situations. This Framework can be used by all nurses with various types of education and roles in different settings.

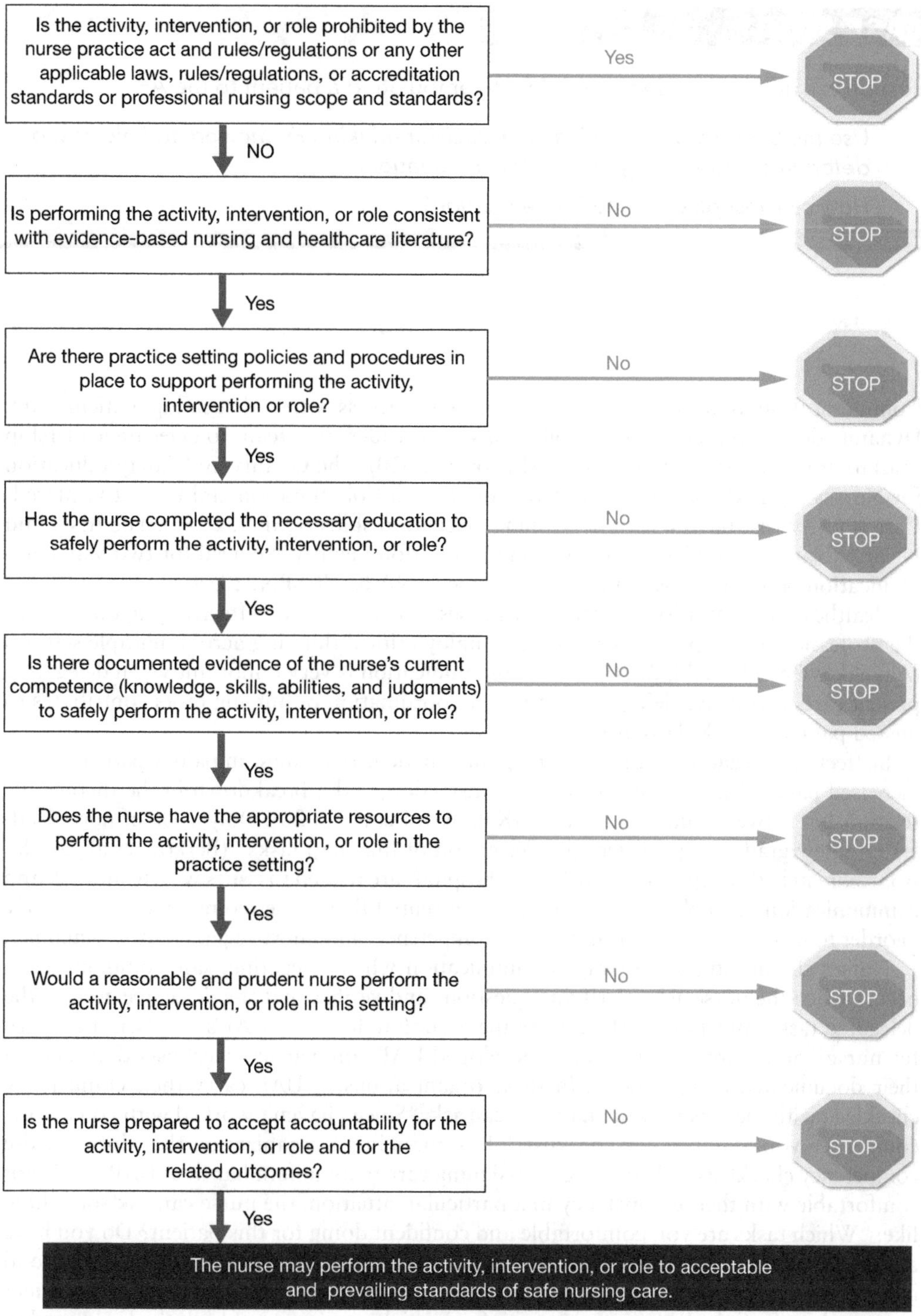

FIGURE 5.3 Scope of Nursing Practice Decision-Making Framework.

Source: From Ballard, K., Haagenson, D., Christiansen, L., Damgaard, G., Halstead, J. A., Jason, R. R., Joyner, J. C., O'Sullivan, A. M., Silvestre, J., Cahill, M., Radtke, B., & Alexander, M. (2016). Scope of Nursing Practice Decision-Making Framework. *Journal of Nursing Regulation, 7*(3), 19-21. https://doi.org/10.1016/S2155-8256(16)32316-X. Reprinted with permission.

CASE STUDY

Joseph is a new nurse. He must delegate ambulating a patient to the AP.

1. *Use the Scope of Nursing Practice Decision-Making Framework to help Joseph determine a safe delegation of the ambulation.*
2. *How can Joseph evaluate his delegation?*

COMMUNICATION FACTORS INFLUENCING THE DELEGATION PROCESS

Communication is a cornerstone to achieving success when delegating patient care. Dynamic delegation refers to the ability of senior leaders in a team to delegate leadership roles to more junior team members (Al-Moteri, 2020). The Quality and Safety Education for Nurses (QSEN) competencies of Teamwork and Collaboration and Patient-Centered-Care (PCC) assist the nurse in developing delegation skills (QSEN, 2017). The ANA and NCSBN National Guidelines for Nursing Delegation identify the need for two-way communication between the RN and the delegatee (ANA & NCSBN, 2019).

Healthcare organizations expect new nurses to communicate effectively upon entry to the profession and expect new nurses to employ critical thinking across multiple settings (Almekkawi & El Khalil, 2020). Good communication is very important when delegating patient care. Ineffective delegation and poor coordination of nursing tasks contributes to missed patient care (Kalankova et al., 2018).

Ineffective delegation contributes to poorer patient outcomes, impaired patient safety, increased patient falls, decreased patient satisfaction, and a breakdown in the therapeutic relationship between nurse and patient (Kalánková et al., 2020). Only 10% of nurse leaders rate new graduates proficient in "delegation of (nursing) tasks" (Berkow et al., 2008). Approximately three-quarters of deaths in hospitals are related to issues with teamwork and communication (Campbell et al., 2020). It is essential that nurses communicate effectively in order to increase delegation confidence, competence, and improve patient care outcomes.

Nurses should utilize two-way communication when delegating; safe communication occurs when the nurse asks clarifying questions and verifies that the delegatee accepts the delegated task (Anderson, 2018). Assessing an unfamiliar float UAP's ability is a concern for nurses. Some organizations have developed UAP competency checklists that identify their documented competencies. In these organizations, if UAP carry their competency checklists with them as they float, nurses can ask, "Since I haven't worked with you before, could I see your competency checklist?" If a nurse in an organization that does not use competency checklists is delegating or assigning care to an unfamiliar float UAP and is not comfortable with their competency in a particular situation, the nurse can ask something like: "Which tasks are you comfortable and confident doing for this patient? Do you have any concerns? Let's go through the steps of how you normally report to RNs about blood glucose results." Rounding with the float UAP and offering instructions with the patient present also offers the RN an opportunity for a quick assessment of both the UAP's understanding and the patient's condition. When questioning a UAP raises uncertainty in the nurse or the UAP, the nurse should observe and help the UAP in performing any tasks that could present a problem. This helps ensure patient safety.

Setting up times for the RN and UAP to regroup before and after breaks or mealtimes during the shift is a recommended method that contributes to ongoing UAP supervision and review of progress. Note there are times when the RN will want to share concerns about a UAP's performance and, as needed, with the unit's charge nurse or nurse manager. Use

BOX 5.2 Developing Clinical Judgment

A nurse working in the emergency department asks an AP if he wants to try to start an intravenous line (IV). The nurse knows the AP is graduating from an RN program in a few short months. Without hesitation, the AP agrees to start the IV.

1. What **CUES (Assessment)** can the nurse assess?
2. What **HYPOTHESIS (Diagnosis)** will the nurse weigh?
3. What **ACTION (Plan and Implement)** will be most effective for the nurse to take to assure the patient's safety in this situation?
4. How will the nurse evaluate the patient's **OUTCOME (Evaluation)** for the purpose of arriving at a satisfactory clinical outcome?

emotional intelligence to consider how it would feel if faced with the same assignment as the UAP. Communication between nurses and coworkers often involves nursing delegation. Offering positive feedback to an UAP such as, "I appreciate the way you spoke with the patient in Room 2345 to get him to ambulate twice this shift," goes a long way toward team building. "I will help you as soon as I can," and then following through with helping as soon as you can, is a way to acknowledge that all team members' responsibilities are important.

The RN also assures that all communication between the RN and the delegatee is culturally appropriate and that the person receiving it is treated respectfully. Evidence shows that the better the communication and collaborative relationship between the RN and the delegatee, the better the chance a positive outcome of the delegation process will ensue (Corazzini et al., 2013; Damgaard & Young, 2014; Young & Damgaard, 2015). Reviewing delegated responsibilities with the delegatee and allowing for questions for clarification must be welcomed by the nurse.

The RN should be available to the UAP for assistance and guidance in an ongoing manner. Under no circumstance is the RN permitted to delegate a responsibility that requires any form of clinical reasoning, nursing judgment, or critical decision-making. For example, when a RN delegates the responsibility of checking a patient's blood sugar every 2 hours and reporting the results to the RN, the delegation cannot include having the delegatee make a nursing judgment of what action to take when the patient's blood sugar is low.

DELEGATION IN COMMUNITY SETTINGS

Delegation occurs frequently in both acute care settings and community settings. The community-based nurse is responsible for a complex array of critical thinking and clinical judgment scenarios and must maximize the scope of their license as well as maximize the safe use of UAP. In any setting, the UAP's knowledge and level of competence impacts effective delegation. This knowledge and competency can be obtained from a formal educational program or from on-the-job training. Nurses must be aware of their state's NPA and the specifics of practicing in a community setting. In some states, different portions of the state law and regulations specify separate guidelines for community settings. These guidelines assist nurses and UAPs during planned, thorough supervision by RNs with detailed delegation instructions and forms. See Table 5.4, Standards for Delegation in Community Settings in Two States.

In some states, an RN can delegate the administration of certain medications in a school setting to UAPs such as secretaries, teachers, or other individuals. The ANA and NCSBN Five Rights of Delegation must be followed by the RN and the UAP (NCSBN & ANA, 2019). The knowledge the UAP gains from such things as an in-service training followed

TABLE 5.4 STANDARDS FOR DELEGATION IN COMMUNITY SETTINGS IN TWO STATES

STATE STANDARDS FOR DELEGATION IN COMMUNITY SETTINGS	SUMMARY
Oregon: Standards for Community-Based Care, Registered Nurses Delegation Process (accessed July 20, 2020). These standards provide guidance for nurses to delegate specific tasks of nursing care and teach administration of noninjectable medications to unlicensed persons. www.oregon.gov/osbn/Pages/laws-rules.aspx#39a94d10-65db-4cae-b1e7-abc493c8d4f0	These standards apply only in settings where an RN is not regularly scheduled and not available to provide direct supervision (e.g., local corrections facilities, juvenile detention facilities, youth corrections facilities, detoxification facilities, adult foster care facilities, residential care facilities, and training and treatment facilities).
Washington: Delegation of Blood Glucose Monitoring to Nursing Assistants or Health Care Aides in Community-Based Settings www.doh.wa.gov/Portals/1/Documents/6000/NCAO14.pdf	These standards state that it is within the scope of the RN to delegate the following to assistive personnel in the community: • Pierce the skin to get a blood sample to measure blood glucose to monitor treatment response and/or for administering medications for the treatment of diabetes. • Give insulin injections and non-insulin injections for the treatment of diabetes.

by a return demonstration for competency is tested. School nurses must comply with their state NPA and follow the NASC's Position on Delegation to UAPs in the school setting (NASC, 2019; Shannon & Kubelka, 2013).

Each school nurse must adhere to their state's NPA. Many State Boards of Nursing allow for some degree of delegation in the community setting to UAP. For example, administration of medicines for chronic diseases such as asthma can be delegated in many states. The decision to delegate is based on the application of the ANA and NCSBN Five Rights of Delegation (NCSBN & ANA, 2019; Shannon & Kubelka, 2013). Delegation of tasks in a school setting uses the same decision-making and mental processes as in a hospital setting. The same considerations are employed, including the nurse's guidance by the state's RN NPA; the State Board of Nursing; an organization's administration, policies and procedures; and the state's Scope of Practice for LPN/LVN and UAP.

There is significant variation between states in relation to LPN/LVNs being allowed to administer medication and blood transfusions, make comparative clinical judgments regarding normal and abnormal patient data, independently plan care, and provide patient education (Spector, 2005). However, there is agreement that in most states, LPN/LVNs do not independently develop a plan of care, make changes to a plan of care, or perform telephone triage (Spector, 2005). The RN must always be aware of their state's NPA. RNs cannot train front office staff to provide medical advice over the phone, as it requires assessment and critical thinking (Maningo & Panthofer, 2018). Also, for example, RNs must refer to their state NPA to verify if LPNs can initiate intravenous (IV) therapy in the clinic setting; however, note that a nurse cannot delegate IV therapy to a UAP under any circumstance (Maningo & Panthofer, 2018).

ASSIGNMENT SHEETS AND HANDOFF REPORT

At the start of each shift, the charge RN completes a patient assignment sheet (Table 5.5) to identify patients, their room numbers, and their needs for activities, tasks, or procedures.

TABLE 5.5 PATIENT ASSIGNMENT SHEET

RN'S ASSIGNED PATIENTS PATIENT ROOM AND PATIENT INFORMATION	PLANNED OUTCOMES FOR PATIENT TODAY: PATIENT/FAMILY WILL HAVE....	LONG-TERM OUTCOMES: PATIENT/FAMILY WILL....	AP TASKS: AP 0700-1900 (NOTE TIMING, ACCEPTABLE PARAMETERS, REPORTING MECHANISMS)	LPN TASKS: (LPN ARRIVES AT 1400 FOR SHIFT OVERLAP UNTIL 2330)	OTHER INTER-PROFESSIONAL TEAM MEMBERS	HIGH-RISK QUALITY/ SAFETY FACTORS & NOTES
Patient 101 85-year-old male fell at assisted living facility; Recent type 2 diabetes mellitus; Recently widowed; borderline renal; hypertension; Hip pinning today	Probable hip pinning today; Pain 3/10, which is acceptable according to the patient; blood pressure within normal limits; Blood glucose within normal limits	Probably plan to return to assisted living facility; Determine reason for fall; Offer grief counseling postop with at-home follow-up to check on ability to be alone and manage meds and blood glucose	Maintain safe fractured hip alignment; hygienic care prior to surgery; Check blood glucose, BP, and vital signs every 2 hours and report results; offer bedpan/urinal for toileting	Check surgery schedule and prepare patient room before planned patient arrival time; check with RN to plan for frequent vital signs, glucose monitoring	Social worker: Plan for home health; assessment of need for assisted living facility or home healthcare Physical therapy: Plan for assistance postop Nutritionist: Plan for diabetic diet	Postop: remains at risk for falls
Patient 102 54-year-old male Post-op day 1 bowel resection (no ostomy); High-risk skin breakdown; substance use disorder (alcohol)	Pain 4/10, which is acceptable according to the patient; Begin activity as tolerated; Urinate without catheter; Avoid alcohol; Check for alcohol withdrawal; Vital signs within normal limits	Decide on future plan for possible bowel cancer; Determine if patient lives alone; Plan rehab or treatment for substance abuse	Move/turn q 2h; First/dangle/ ambulate with RN; Report jittery, vision change, other signs of alcohol withdrawal; Toilet/urinal post retention catheter removal by RN; Watch skin carefully and report condition post bath; Report any vital signs beyond parameters asap	Assist with IV meds (RN refers to NPA and LPN job description); Assist AP with turning and coughing and deep breathing patient; See RN at 1400 for other tasks upon arrival	Wound care nurse referral, respiratory tech referral; social worker referral	Skin assessment: poor; High fall risk; High alcohol withdrawal risk

(continued)

TABLE 5.5 PATIENT ASSIGNMENT SHEET (*continued*)

RN'S ASSIGNED PATIENTS PATIENT ROOM AND PATIENT INFORMATION	PLANNED OUTCOMES FOR PATIENT TODAY: PATIENT/FAMILY WILL HAVE....	LONG-TERM OUTCOMES: PATIENT/FAMILY WILL....	AP TASKS: AP 0700-1900 (NOTE TIMING, ACCEPTABLE PARAMETERS, REPORTING MECHANISMS)	LPN TASKS: (LPN ARRIVES AT 1400 FOR SHIFT OVERLAP UNTIL 2330)	OTHER INTER-PROFESSIONAL TEAM MEMBERS	HIGH-RISK QUALITY/ SAFETY FACTORS & NOTES
Patient 103 35-year-old female, admitted for community-acquired pneumonia of unknown etiology	Identify cause of pneumonia; Breathe more comfortably without constant cough and shortness of breath; oxygen saturation above 97 with oxygen at 6 liters on nasal cannula; vital signs stable	Avoid intubation plan to quit smoking (no other risk factors)	Vital signs and ongoing pulse oximetry every 2 hours; Two-person assist due to shortness of breath; ask RN or LPN for assist with toileting; Oxygen on 6 liters per nasal cannula at all times	Assist AP with hygiene/ toileting of patient as needed for safety; Meds; vital signs every 2 hours and as instructed by RN	Respiratory tech; lab tests; public health & contact tracers	COVID risk; isolation; two-person assist due to shortness of breath
Patient 104 55-year-old female; new admit; rule out bowel obstruction- Status unknown; expected at 1400 post diagnostic tests; not yet admitted	Identify treatment plan and patient priorities	To be determined based on diagnosis	Check room cleaned, ready, and set up for NG drainage.	Assist RN with admission VS; Gather data for RN initial assessment and planning		

AP, assistive personnel; BP, blood pressure; LPN, licensed practical nurse; NG, nasogastric; NPA, nurse practice act; postop, postoperatively; VS, vital signs.

The assignment sheet also identifies which team member is responsible for which patients. The oncoming RN receives handoff report and discusses the status and needs of patients on the unit with the offgoing RN. The oncoming RN may make quick patient rounds on the unit to observe the patients' conditions. Then the oncoming RN provides initial direction to the team and makes a plan to supervise and evaluate the care being provided by nursing team members throughout the day. The RN also develops a plan to receive and give patient feedback to each other throughout the shift. The Five Rights of Delegation are referred to by the RN throughout the shift as different decisions are made in an ongoing manner for safe and effective patient care.

Handoff Reports

Handoff reports regarding patient status, needs, and safety occur any time a patient is transferred from one caregiver to another caregiver (e.g., patient transfers between shifts, patient transfers between departments or locations in a healthcare facility, and patient transfers between different healthcare facilities). Verbal communication regarding patients on a patient care unit often begins with the offgoing and oncoming RNs discussing the patients' needs. A verbal handoff report takes place from one nurse going off shift to the oncoming nurse to assure continuity of patient care. Accuracy of handoff reports is essential to patient safety.

During handoff report, the oncoming nurse often fills out a personal worksheet identifying patient status and needs or the nurse may receive a computer print-out of a "Nursing Brain" (**Exhibit 5.1**) for each of their patients. The "Nursing Brain" is a computerized worksheet that identifies patient care assignments on the unit for individual team members and patient priorities for the shift. The oncoming nurse may add information about each of their patients to the Nursing Brain during bedside handoff report from the offgoing nurse. Note that computer systems vary. Some computers do not print off a Nursing Brain, though they usually have important patient information available online for the nurse to refer to as they take handoff report or afterwards. In this case, the nurse will complete a personal information worksheet on each patient as they take handoff report. This personal information worksheet contains many of the elements seen in the Nursing Brain, specific to each patient. The worksheet serves as a reminder of patient needs to the nurse throughout the day.

Once the oncoming RN has received bedside handoff report and completed the Nursing Brain, the RN considers several factors (Box 5.3) and includes specific reporting guidelines,

EXHIBIT 5.1 NURSING BRAIN

Name Age/Gender Attending MD	Room # Allergies Diagnosis
PMH	VS, Pain
Neuro	IV, Skin
Card	Resp
GI/GU	Labs, Tests, Diagnostics
Plan (include specific reporting guidelines, timing for interventions, and deadlines for accomplishment of tasks)	

GI/GU, gastrointestinal/genitourinary; IV, intravenous; PMH, past medical history; VS, vital signs.

BOX 5.3 Factors Considered When Delegating or Assigning Patient Care

- number and acuity of patients
- priority patient needs
- number and type of staff
- state laws
- patient care standards
- accreditation regulations
- unit routines
- geography of nursing unit
- complexity of patient needs
- staff responsibilities
- environmental concerns
- lunch/break times
- all delegation policies
- organizational policies and procedures
- attitude and dependability of staff
- need for continuity of care by same staff
- need for fair work distribution among staff
- need of patient for isolation and/or protection
- need to protect patient and staff from injury
- skill, education, and competency of staff (i.e., RN, LPN/LVN, AP)

timing for patient interventions, and deadlines for accomplishment of patient care tasks when delegating them or assigning patient care.

The patient assignment sheet (Table 5.5) presented a simplified example of patient care assignments in an acute care setting. The offgoing and oncoming charge RNs may collaborate to determine which patient each RN will be responsible for. The assignment sheet will also identify what patient care the RN delegates or assigns to LPN/LVNs and UAPs. As always, RNs must consult their own state NPA act, state board advisory opinions, and NCSBN and ANA guidelines, along with the facility's job descriptions, patient care guidelines, and departmental staff competency checklists when delegating or assigning patient care.

Note that it is safe to delegate when the patient is stable, the task is within the delegate's job description, the nurse is able to teach and supervise as needed, and the nurse has a plan in place to monitor the patient's response (Alfaro-LeFevre, 2020). It is not safe to delegate complex assessment or clinical judgment, or if the outcome is unpredictable, or if there is an increased risk of harm to the patient (Alfaro-LeFevre, 2020). A nurse should start with the patient and family's desired outcomes in mind, thereby increasing the likelihood of a successful outcome (Hansten, 2019). Without clear communication between the nurse and patient, prioritization and delegation of tasks leads to frustration, inefficient use of time and resources, and wrong choices (Hansten, 2019).

APPLICATION OF THE FIVE RIGHTS OF DELEGATION

To best learn how to apply delegation and assignment concepts when working with an LPN and UAP, it is helpful for a student to practice applying the Five Rights of Delegation to a set of patients. In Table 5.5 the patient assignment sheet, an RN works a 12-hour shift with an UAP beginning at 0700. Another LPN/LVN is scheduled to arrive for an overlap shift at 1400 until 2330 due to busy admitting and discharge levels at those times on this particular medical-surgical unit.

Right Task and Right Circumstances

The RN first reviews the team's assigned patients and tasks and thinks through the right tasks and the right circumstances by reviewing staff job description and competencies, patients' needs, and desired outcomes for the shift. Is the patient stable? For RNs working in a setting outside a hospital, the "right circumstances" would include being certain that they are following the portion of their NPA that refers to rules about how to delegate and supervise in that setting.

Right Tasks Assigned to the Right Person Under the Right Circumstances Using the Right Direction and Communication

The RN then decides what are the right tasks that could be safely delegated or assigned to a competent and willing team member (right person). As each team member arrives for work, including the UAP who arrives at the same time as the RN at 0700 and the LPN/LVN who arrives for work at 1400, the RN reviews, are these the right circumstances? What are the patient needs and is the patient stable? If so, the RN is then able to deliver the right direction and the right communication to let each team member know time frames for what, how, and when a task should be done, and how and when to report their findings. As a continuous, ongoing process, the RN will apply the Five Rights throughout the shift, adjusting the workload for the additional person, the LPN/LVN, arriving at 1400.

The Right Supervision and Evaluation

The right supervision and evaluation is achieved by the RN making regular patient rounds and setting up a plan with the team to regroup and meet at time intervals throughout the shift and share information with each other. These meeting times to offer two-way feedback are often before and after assigned breaks and meals but will vary depending on the individual patient's needs. At these meeting times, the RN can offer feedback to the UAP and the LPN/LVN as to the results the RN has evaluated through observation and rounding and can receive an update about patient progress. The RN may also seek feedback about what the RN can do to improve patient outcomes and teamwork.

CURRENT LITERATURE

CITATION

Beeber, A. S., Zimmerman, S., Mitchell, C., & Reed, D. (2018). Staffing and service availability in assisted living: The importance of nurse delegation policies. *Journal of the American Geriatrics Society*, *66*(11), 2158–2166. https://doi.org/10.1111/jgs.15580

DISCUSSION

This article explores delegation policies in residential care and assisted living settings, with consideration given to residential care and assisted living characteristics, services, and staffing. Some states allow certified nursing assistants and certified unlicensed personnel to administer medications with off-site supervision and carefully designed safeguards in writing to guide the nurse and the AP. Other states allow personnel to help patients self-administer medications and may require more involved RN on-site supervision. States specify detailed rules and instructional documents for both the RN and AP that ensure patient safety even while off-site.

IMPLICATIONS FOR PRACTICE

Some states allow certified unlicensed personnel to perform medication administration in assisted living, home health, or other community settings. In other states, certified unlicensed personnel are allowed to accomplish other complex services such as review of the patient's subjective statements, data collection, blood sugar testing, cognitive surveys, and wound care. It is important to check the current state in which a nurse practices to view the state's NPA, rules, and advisory opinions.

END-OF-CHAPTER RESOURCES

KEY CONCEPTS

1. Delegation is a key aspect of providing high-quality nursing care. Delegation is used in both acute care and community health settings.
2. It is essential that nurses understand the terms "delegation," "responsibility," "delegated responsibility," "assignment," "accountability," "authority," and "supervision," as well as how to safely implement each term in the clinical setting.
3. Nurses bear the ultimate responsibility and accountability for delegated tasks.
4. Regulatory bodies define and clarify the scope of practice for RNs, LPN/LVNs, and UAPs.
5. Nurses have many resources for verifying their knowledge of delegation in any practice setting. The primary resources include the nurse's state-specific NPA, the NCSBN and ANA National Guidelines for Nursing Delegation, the NCSBN and ANA Five Rights of Delegation, the Scope of Nursing Practice Decision-Making Framework, and the nurses' organizational policies and procedures.
6. Delegation occurs at the one-on-one level between RNs and team members. Nurses must know their organization's delegation guidelines and the chain of command if they encounter an unresolved delegation-related issue. Nurses must know and use their organization's chain of command if they encounter an unresolved patient care problem.
7. High-quality communication and clear expectations are required for patient care teams to give and receive safely delegated tasks.
8. Assignment sheets and patient handoff report clarify patient care assignments.
9. The healthcare organization, nurses, and all members of the healthcare team are responsible for delivery and appropriate delegation of safe, high-quality patient care.
10. Nurses must be aware of their scope of practice, and should refer to their state-approved regulations in order to make high-quality clinical decisions in all agency and community settings.

CRITICAL DISCUSSION POINTS

1. What references should an RN refer to when moving to a new state and considering delegating to a UAP in a state other than their own?
2. During clinical experiences, what examples of assignment or delegation were observed between RN and UAPs?
3. Name two effective communication strategies an RN can use to enhance safe delegation.
4. Do any aspects of delegation feel uncomfortable (e.g., communication, asking others to "do work" because they are asked by an RN, supervising and monitoring, providing feedback, and so on)? If so, why?
5. An RN is working with a UAP they have not worked with before. What is a strategy for quickly assessing the competency of a UAP's skill set for a desired task?

KEY TERMS

- > Accountability
- > Assignment
- > Authority
- > Delegated responsibility
- > Delegation
- > Emotional intelligence
- > Responsibility
- > Supervision

REVIEW QUESTIONS

Answers to Review Questions appear in the Instructor's Manual. Qualified instructors should request the Instructor's Manual from textbook@springerpub.com.

1. Delegation and assignment are similar concepts about work allocation. Which of the following is NOT a correct statement? *Select all that apply.*
   A. Whether delegating or assigning, the delegatee must be competent to perform a specific task they are asked to complete.
   B. The nurse must always supervise the UAP when they delegate or assign.
   C. Delegation (as defined by the NCSBN) is allowing a delegatee to perform a specific nursing activity, task, or procedure that is beyond the delegatee's traditional role and not routinely performed.
   D. Delegation has been defined as allocating a task that is beyond the UAP's foundational educational training while assigning would be allocating those tasks that the UAP would have been taught in their school and as a basic part of their skill set.
   E. The nurse can delegate or assign tasks that state regulations allow, whether or not the organization's job descriptions allow those tasks.
2. The nurse is performing an assessment on a patient who is taking 400 mg of Naproxen for abdominal pain. Which task(s) or processes during the assessment can be delegated to a UAP?
   A. Review the results of the patient's hemoglobin and hematocrit.
   B. Collect and send a stool sample to the laboratory for guaiac testing.
   C. Auscultate the abdomen for bowel sounds.
   D. Call the patient's family to discuss plans for discharge.
3. Which of the following is a responsibility of the employer and/or nurse leader to create a professional culture for delegating and assigning nursing responsibilities to the UAP? *Select all that apply.*
   A. Making sure that specific competencies are checked off during orientation and training and appropriate skills are maintained by all personnel
   B. Establishing licensure guidelines for UAP
   C. Making certain that appropriate policies and procedures for delegation and assignment are in place
   D. Periodically reviewing policies and procedures related to delegation and assignment
   E. Helping the team create a care delivery model that encourages excellent teamwork and ongoing feedback and two-way communication

4. An RN would like to delegate or assign tasks to an LPN/LVN. Which of these tasks would most likely be listed in the LPN/LVN's job description and competency checklist? *Select all that apply.*
   A. Obtain vital signs and gather other patient intake information.
   B. Administer oral medications and injections.
   C. Assist the RN in developing the plan of care.
   D. Start blood products administration.
   E. Assist in teaching the patient using a previously developed standardized teaching plan.
   F. Insert a nasogastric tube.
5. The nurse assigned the UAP the responsibility to ambulate the patient to the bathroom. Halfway through the shift, the UAP has not yet completed this delegated task. What is the proper action the RN must take? *Select all that apply.*
   A. Ask the UAP about what she understood from the RN's beginning of shift team discussion and initial direction, for example, "Just to clarify, I could be mistaken; could we review our plan regarding your ambulating this patient?"
   B. Notify the next shift that the ambulation was not completed and that the next shift will have to ambulate the patient three times.
   C. Give feedback to the UAP about the importance of ambulation for this particular patient and develop a plan together to make sure the task is completed by the end of the shift, for example, "It is so important we figure out how to make sure Mrs. Jones is ambulated twice because she is at high risk for pneumonia and emboli. How can we get this done?"
   D. Document that the patient was unable to ambulate to the bathroom.
   E. Ambulate the patient without the UAP's help.
6. The nurse delegated to an LPN/LVN to disconnect an intravenous line from a patient once the infusion is complete. Which factors should the nurse consider prior to deciding to allocate this task to an LPN/LVN? *Select all that apply.*
   A. Right task
   B. Right circumstances
   C. Right person
   D. Right direction and communication
   E. Right supervision and evaluation
7. Accountability for nursing care means that which of the following are true? *Select all that apply.*
   A. The UAP has no license so they are not accountable, but the nurse is accountable.
   B. Every team member is accountable to the patient for the care they provide.
   C. Each team member must only accept assignments that they are competent to perform.
   D. The RN is accountable to follow professional standards.
   E. The RN is accountable to follow professional ethics.
   F. The RN is accountable for the nursing care of the team's patients.

8. Quality and Safety Education for Nurses (QSEN) has developed six key quality and safety elements to guide nursing practice. As discussed in the chapter, identify which of the following choices is considered the element of QSEN that applies to nurse delegation and assignment.
   A. Safety, teamwork and collaboration, and patient-centered care
   B. Quality improvement, safety, and student-centered learning
   C. Informatics, evidence-based practice, and strategic planning
   D. Professionalism, student-centered learning, and informatics
9. What steps would a nurse take to determine whether or not she can inject sterile normal saline into a chest tube, as ordered by the pulmonologist? The RN has not heard of nurses doing this procedure and is unsure what to do. Choose the best three immediate actions.
   A. Review the Scope of Nursing Practice Decision-Making Framework.
   B. Consult with the organization's policies regarding RNs injecting into chest tubes.
   C. Review the NPA for rules and advisory opinions.
   D. Call the State Board of Nursing and ask for an advisory opinion.
   E. Look on the Pulmonology Nursing Association website for advice.
   F. Make a phone call to the nursing union for help.
10. The physician in the RN's outpatient oncology clinic has asked a medical assistant (MA, an ambulatory care AP) to administer IV chemotherapy through a patient's preexisting central line port. The clinic RN plans to do the following to ensure the patient's safety. *Select all that apply.*
   A. The clinic RN will tell the physician that in this state the MA is delegated to and supervised by both the MD and the RN and this plan to delegate chemotherapy seems like unsafe delegation.
   B. Tell the MD that he will be reported to the clinic administrator by the clinic RN, if necessary.
   C. The clinic RN will teach the MA how to safely administer the prescribed drugs per port and observe the first infusion.
   D. The clinic RN will check the organization's job descriptions, competency checklists, and the state practice information (if any) related to permitted MA skills.
   E. The clinic RN will explain to the physician that there is in-depth continuing education training for nurses to give chemotherapy and the RN will refuse to allow the MA to administer chemotherapy and access central ports.
   F. The clinic RN will tell the MD that the plan to allow the MA to deliver the chemotherapy per port will be allowed to occur just this once since it is a very busy day.

REVIEW ACTIVITIES

1. Click on the link from QSEN to watch the Lewis Blackman story, https://qsen.org/publications/videos/the-lewis-blackman-story. What responsibilities could the nurses have assigned to a competent AP to allow more time to focus on the patient's vital signs, urine output trends, and listening to the family's concerns?
2. Interview three nurses on the unit where a student is currently doing a clinical rotation. Ask each nurse, "What task is entrusted to assistive personnel (AP) most often on this unit?" Write down their responses and compare the three nurses'

answers. Review the healthcare organization's policy and procedure for the responsibilities permitted to be assigned to AP.

What did the student nurse find?

3. Show two nursing instructors the Scope of Nursing Practice Decision-Making Framework in Figure 5.3. Ask each instructor how they implement this Framework in their practice. What were their responses?

EXPLORING THE WEB

1. Visit www.youtube.com. Type in "Delegating effectively NCSBN". Select the Popular Videos, Delegation & Nursing. Begin viewing one of over 100 videos on delegation.
2. Visit the Indiana Center for Evidence-Based Nursing Practice at www.ebnp.org. Hover over "About Us". Then click on "Evidence into Practice". Review two to three resources available that pertain to an area of nursing practice that is of interest.
3. Log in and register at Lippincott's, www.nursingcenter.com, to receive articles, continuing education, and information on topics such as quality, safety, and delegation.
4. Go to https://qsen.org/student-resources. Click on CDC—Public Health Quality Improvement Webinars. Click on CDC—Public Health Quality. Choose one or two interesting articles or multimedia resources and review them.
5. Go to https://qsen.org/student-resources. Click on National Association for Health Care Quality—Quality Certification and Education. Review one or two education resources available.
6. Review the LinkedIn Pulse information and the YouTube about Crisis Standards of Care During a Pandemic by Hansten. In what ways could this information help a student or novice deal with contingency plans for assignments during national emergencies? www.linkedin.com/pulse/crisiscontingency-standards-care-covid-delegation-ruth, and YouTube Crisis Standards of Care: www.youtube.com/watch?v=V0d7Uiyvw3Y&t=103s.

SPRINGER PUBLISHING CONNECT™

A robust set of instructor resources designed to supplement this text is located at **http://connect.springerpub.com/content/book/978-0-8261-6145-1.** Qualifying instructors may request access by emailing **textbook@springerpub.com.**

REFERENCES

Alfaro-LeFevre, R. (2020). *Critical thinking, clinical reasoning and clinical judgment: A practical approach* (7th ed.). W.B. Saunders.

AlMekkawi, M., & El Khalil, R. (2020). New graduate nurses' readiness to practice: A narrative literature review. *Health Professions Education, 6*(3), 304–316. https://doi.org/10.1016/j.hpe.2020.05.008

Al-Moteri, M. (2020). Entrustable professional activities in nursing: A concept analysis. *International Journal of Nursing Sciences, 7*(3), 277–284. https://doi.org/10.1016/j.ijnss.2020.06.009

American Association of Colleges of Nursing. (2020). *Draft essentials: Domains, descriptors, contextual statements, and competencies.* https://www.aacnnursing.org/Portals/42/Downloads/Essentials/DRAFT-Domains-Descriptors-Competencies-May-2020.pdf

American Nurses Association. (2015). *Code of ethics for nurses with interpretive statements.* https://www.nursingworld.org/DocumentVault/Ethics-1/Code-of-Ethics-for-Nurses.html

Anderson, A. (2018). Delegating as a new nurse. *American Journal of Nursing, 118*(12), 51–55. https://doi.org/10.1097/01.NAJ.0000549691.41080.6c

Ballard, K., Haagenson, D., Christiansen, L., Damgaard, G., Halstead, J. A, Jason, R. R., Joyner, J. C., O'Sullivan, A. M., Silvestre, J., Cahill, M., Radtke, B., & Alexander, M. (2016). Scope of Nursing Practice Decision-Making Framework. *Journal of Nursing Regulation, 7*(3), 19–21. https://doi.org/10.1016/S2155-8256(16)32316-X

Berkow, S., Virkstis, K., Stewart, J., & Conway, L. (2008). Assessing new graduate nurse performance. *Journal of Nursing Administration, 38*(11), 468–474. https://doi.org/10.1097/01.NNA.0000339477.50219.06

Black, B. P. (2020). *Professional nursing: Concepts & challenges* (9th ed.). Elsevier.

California Nurse Practice Act Standards of Competent Performance. California Code of Regulations 1443.5. https://www.rn.ca.gov/pdfs/regulations/npr-i-20.pdf

Campbell, A. R., Layne, D., Scott, E., & Wei, H. (2020). Interventions to promote the teamwork, delegation, and communication among registered nurses and nursing assistants: An integrative review. *Journal of Nursing Management*, 28(7), 1465–1472. https://doi.org/10.1111/jonm.13083

Corazzini, K. N., Anderson, R. A., Mueller, C., Hunt-McKinney, S., Day, L., & Porter, K. (2013). Understanding RN and LPN patterns of practice in nursing homes. *Journal of Nursing Regulation, 4*(1), 14–18. https://doi.org/10.1016/S2155-8256(15)30173-3

Cronenwett, L., Sherwood, G., Barnsteiner J., Disch, J., Johnson, J., Mitchell, P., Sullivan, D., & Warren, J. (2007). Quality and Safety Education for Nurses. *Nursing Outlook, 55*(3), 122–131. https://doi.org/10.1016/j.outlook.2007.02.006

Damgaard, G., & Young, L. (2014). Virtual nursing care for school children with diabetes. *Journal of Nursing Regulation, 4*(4), 15–24. https://doi.org/10.1016/S2155-8256(15)30106-X

Duffy, M., & Fields, S. (2014, August). *Delegation and you: When to delegate and to whom.* Nursesbooks.org

Hansten, R. (2019). Introductory chapter. In L. LaCharity, C. Kumagai, & B. Bartz (Eds.), *Prioritization, delegation and assignment* (4th ed.). Elsevier.

Hansten, R. (2020a). Delegation in the clinical setting. In J. Zerwekh & A. Garneau (Eds.), *Nursing today: Transitions and trends* (9th ed., pp 301–323). Elsevier.

Hansten, R. (2020b, April 13). *Delegation/assignment/supervision in a pandemic.* LinkedIn. https://www.linkedin.com/pulse/delegationassignmentsupervision-pandemic-ruth-hansten-rn-mba-phd

Kalánková, D., Bartoníčková, D., Žiaková, K., & Kurucová, R. (2020). Missed and rationed care: What do we know? Review of qualitative studies. *Ošetrovateľstvo: Teória, výskum, vzdelávanie [online], 10*(1), 18–23. https://www.osetrovatelstvo.eu/en/archive/2020-volume-10/number-1/missed-and-rationed-care-what-do-we-knowreview-of-qualitative-studies

Kalankova, D., Gurkova, E., Zelenikova, R., & Ziatova, K. (2018). Application of measuring tools in the assessment of the phenomenon of rationing/missed/unfinished care. *KONTAKT/Journal of Nursing and the Social Sciences Related to Health and Illness* (Kont.zsf.jcu.cz). https://doi.org/10.32725/kont.2018.001

Maningo, M., & Panthofer, M. (2018). Safety corner: Appropriate delegation in ambulatory care nursing practice. *AAACN Viewpoint, 40*(1), 14–15.

Marquis, B. L., & Huston, C. J. (2021). *Leadership roles and management functions in nursing: Theory & application* (10th ed.). Lippincott.

National Association of School Nurses. (2019). *Nursing delegation in the school setting* (Position Statement). Author. https://www.nasn.org/advocacy/professional-practice-documents/position-statements/ps-delegation

National Council of State Boards of Nursing. (2016). Nursing guidelines for nursing delegation. *Journal of Nursing Regulation,* 7(1), 5–12. https://www.ncsbn.org/NCSBN_Delegation_Guidelines.pdf

National Council of State Boards of Nursing and American Nurses Association. (2019, April 29). *National Guidelines for Nursing Delegation.* https://www.ncsbn.org/NGND-PosPaper_06.pdf

National Council of State Boards of Nursing. (2020). NCSBN's environmental scan: A portrait of nursing and health care in 2020 and beyond. *Journal of Nursing Regulation*, *10*(4 Suppl.), S1–S35. https://doi.org/10.1016/S2155-8256(20)30022-3

Shannon, R. A., & Kubelka, S. (2013). Reducing the risks of delegation use of procedure skills checklist for unlicensed assistive personnel in schools, Part 1. *NASN School Nurse, 28*(4), 178–181. https://doi.org/10.1177/1942602X13489886

Spector, N. (2005). *Practical nurse scope of practice white paper*. National Council of State Boards of Nursing.

Washington Administrative Code. WAC 246-840-010. https://app.leg.wa.gov/wac/default.aspx?cite=246-840-010

Young, L., & Damgaard, G. (2015). Transitioning the virtual nursing care for school children with diabetes study to a sustainable model of nursing care. *Journal of Nursing Regulation, 6*(2), 4–9. https://doi.org/10.1016/S2155-8256(15)30380-X

SUGGESTED READINGS

Diab, G., & Ehrahim, R. (2019). Factors leading to missed nursing care among nurses at selected hospitals. *American Journal of Nursing Research, 7*(2), 136–147. http://pubs.sciepub.com/ajnr/7/2/5/index.html

Hansten, R. (2021). Delegation, assignment, and supervision of patient care. In P. Kelly Vana & J. Tazbir (Eds.), *Kelly Vana's nursing leadership and management* (4th ed., pp. 456–489) Wiley-Blackwell.

Jarosz, L. (2020). Trends and challenges in regulating nursing practice: 10 years later. *Journal of Nursing Regulation, 11*(1), 12–20. https://doi.org/10.1016/S2155-8256(20)30055-7

Kalisch, B. J. (2011). The impact of RN-UAP relationships on quality and safety. *Nursing Management, 42*(9), 16–22. https://doi.org/10.1097/01.NUMA.0000403284.27249.a2

McCaughey, R. A., McCarthy, A. M., Maughan, E., Hein, M., Perkhounkova, Y., & Kelly, M. W. (2020). Emergency medication access and administration in schools: A focus on epinephrine, albuterol inhalers, and glucagon. *The Journal of School Nursing*. Advance online publication https://doi.org/10.1177/1059840520934185

McCloskey, R., Donovan, C., Stewart, C., & Donovon, A. (2015). How registered nurses, licensed practical nurses and resident assistants spend time in nursing homes: An observational study. *International Journal of Nursing Studies, 52*(9), 1475–1483. https://doi.org/10.1016/j.ijnurstu.2015.05.007

McMullen, T. L., Resnick, B., Chin-Hansen, J., Geiger-Brown, J. M., Miller, N., & Rubenstein, R. (2015). Certified nurse aide scope of practice: State-by-state differences in allowable delegated activities. *Journal of the American Medical Directors Association, 16*(1), 20–24. https://doi.org/10.1016/j.jamda.2014.07.003

Seibert, S. A. (2021). Learning delegation through role-play: A problem-based learning activity for nursing students. *Nursing Education Perspectives*, 42(6), E143–E144. https://doi.org/10.1097/01.NEP.0000000000000692

UNIT II

Quality and Safety Competencies

CHAPTER 6

Person-Centered Care

Elizabeth Riley and Jamie L. Jones

"And so, we see ourselves moving from physician-centered to person-centered, from transactional and episodic care to managed care by a team over time, from the idea of sick care to well-being. We're moving from care that's inaccessible and tied to bricks and mortar to care that's going to be convenient and available 24/7/365."

–Tony Tersigni, CEO, Ascension Health System, St. Louis, 2015

Upon completion of this chapter, the reader should be able to:

1. Describe a brief history of person-centered care (PCC).
2. Identify the characteristics of PCC.
3. Discuss the importance of organizational structures that enhance PCC.
4. Describe important components of effective communication to foster PCC.
5. Articulate how psychosocial factors of health affect patient decision-making and clinical outcomes.
6. List strategies to support patients' and caregivers' engagement in their care.
7. Discuss the importance of constructing a PCC plan for patients that incorporates psychosocial factors and the social determinants of health (SDoH).
8. Describe shared decision-making techniques and the use of patient decision aids to promote PCC.
9. Discuss discharge planning as a means of ensuring continuity of care.
10. List innovations for patients that facilitate PCC.
11. Describe legislation, such as the Patient Protection and Affordable Care Act (PPACA) that supports PCC.
12. Describe the use of PCC measures to monitor the quality of healthcare.
13. Explain the importance of measuring patient satisfaction and the impact on PCC.

CROSSWALK

This chapter addresses the following:

QSEN Competency: Patient-Centered Care

The American Association of Colleges of Nursing. (2021). *The essentials: Core competencies for professional nursing education.*

Domain 2: Person-Centered Care

OPENING SCENARIO

The nurse on a medical-surgical unit is caring for a patient named Mrs. Rodriguez. Mrs. Rodriguez is a 76-year-old patient who suffered a stroke. She is a widow whose children live an hour away and her most frequent visitor is the priest from her church.

The interprofessional team would like to discharge Mrs. Rodriguez within the next few days. She is still experiencing some motor deficits from her stroke that are affecting her ability to perform activities of daily living. She has been making small improvements using physical and occupational therapy. Each day, the interprofessional team completes rounds on the unit. As the contact point for Mrs. Rodriguez and her family, you have been directed by the charge nurse to communicate the discharge plan to the patient and family/designee.

1. In what ways can PCC be used by the nurse during interprofessional team rounds to ensure Mrs. Rodriguez is included in her care?
2. What information should the team convey to Mrs. Rodriguez to help her make an informed decision about her post-hospitalization care? How can the nurse facilitate the sharing of information?
3. What factors specific to Mrs. Rodriguez should the nurse ensure the team is aware of as final plans for discharge are being made?
4. How else can the nurse, as part of the interprofessional team, support an effective care transition for Mrs. Rodriguez?

INTRODUCTION

In this chapter, a brief history of person-centered care (PCC) is described, and the characteristics of PCC are identified. The importance of organizational structure to support PCC and effective communication are discussed. The way in which psychosocial factors affect patient decision-making and clinical outcomes is articulated. Strategies to support patients' and caregivers' engagement in their care are listed. The importance of constructing a PCC plan for patients with physical illness and injury that incorporates psychosocial factors and the social determinants of health (SDoH) is discussed. Discharge planning as a means of ensuring continuity of care is discussed. The use of shared decision-making techniques and patient decision aids to encourage PCC are described. Innovations that facilitate PCC are listed. The impact of legislation, such as the Patient Protection and Affordable Care Act (PPACA), in facilitating PPC is described. The use of PCC measures to monitor quality of healthcare is described. Finally, the way in which measurement of patient satisfaction impacts PCC and facility reimbursements is explained. This chapter focuses on strategies and practices that support a broad definition of PCC with the goal of improving patient safety and the quality of patient care, while providing strategies to help reduce barriers to PCC implementation.

A BRIEF HISTORY OF PERSON-CENTERED CARE

The American Association of Colleges of Nursing (AACN) defines **person-centered care** (PCC) as care that focuses "on the individual within multiple complicated contexts, including family and/or important others," and that is "holistic, just, respectful, compassionate, coordinated, evidence-based and developmentally appropriate" (2019, p. 11). The importance of fostering PCC for new graduate nurses is demonstrated by the AACN Vision for

Academic Nursing task force, which states that a nurse generalist should provide care across the life span and healthcare continuum (AACN, 2019). The Quality and Safety Education for Nurses (QSEN) Institute uses a similar term, "patient-centered care," which "recognizes the patient or designee as the source of control and full partner in providing compassionate and coordinated care based on respect for patient's preferences, values, and needs" (Cronenwett et al., 2007, p. 123). The QSEN competency for patient-centered care provides a structured guide for developing and assessing a nurse's ability to acknowledge the patient's and/or their designee's full authority over the patient's care (QSEN Institute, n.d.). This patient-centered care competency is illustrated in the Appendix and includes measures of knowledge, skills, and attitudes (KSAs) needed by nurses. The KSAs serve as curricular guidelines and they provide a framework for student nurses and practicing nurses who are seeking more meaningful ways to incorporate them into their own practice. The QSEN Institute provides many resources for partnering with patients, residents, and families for patient- and family-centered care.

While numerous terms are used for similar concepts that include holistic healthcare, Eklund et al. (2019) contend that PCC is more inclusive than other terms such as patient-centered care, through the consideration of and respect for all aspects of the patient's life. Other terms for PCC representing its evolution can be found in the literature, including "individualized care," "client-centered care," "resident-centered care," "family-centered care," "patient- and family-centered care," "patient-centered medicine," and even "client-centered therapy." These terms are often used interchangeably in the literature. While the terms may vary, the central concept of PCC remains as used and described throughout this chapter. PCC is utilized for all patients, in all settings, including patients with chronic and/or complex healthcare conditions in the hospital or at home, as well as with healthy people in a community who need healthcare support and disease prevention. Nurses and other members of the interprofessional healthcare team support the health of all persons in a community with unbiased, easily understood healthcare information, so they can maintain control of their own healthcare decisions.

The provision of healthcare has seen a paradigm shift that has been decades in the making. Prior to the 1960s, paternalistic healthcare decisions were often made by the physician and carried out by the nurse or a family caregiver, largely unopposed by patients. This paternalistic, physician-directed decision-making was perceived to be in the patient's best interest. Essentially, the physician decided on the plan of care based on their professional expertise with minimal, if any, input from patients or staff (Blodgett & Petsas Blodgett, 2021; Sánchez-Izquierdo et al., 2019).

However, studies have increasingly suggested that establishing meaningful, caring relationships and engaging in partnerships with patients and families can improve patient outcomes and staff satisfaction while decreasing healthcare utilization and costs (Jayadevappa et al., 2019; Poitras et al., 2018; Schierhorn, 2019). Therefore, many leaders in healthcare, such as the Institute of Medicine (renamed the National Academy of Medicine [NAM] in 2015), the Institute for Healthcare Improvement, the Agency for Healthcare Research and Quality (AHRQ), and TJC, among others, have pushed for the implementation of PCC to improve the quality and safety of healthcare in the United States.

This push has placed a nationwide focus on transforming communities and healthcare settings into accountable, safe environments that respect the unique needs and values of all persons, patients, and families. Departing from the days of paternalistic medicine, nurses and other members of the interprofessional team must not only be more inclusive of patients' and families' perspectives, needs, and preferences, they must support the health of all persons in the community, including patients and families with unbiased, easily understood healthcare information to promote informed decision-making in all settings. When PCC is fully implemented, interprofessional team members recognize

BOX 6.1 Core Concepts of Patient- and Family-Centered Care

Dignity and Respect: Healthcare practitioners listen to and honor patient and family perspectives and choices. Patient and family knowledge, values, beliefs, and cultural backgrounds are incorporated into the planning and delivery of care.

Information Sharing: Healthcare practitioners communicate and share complete and unbiased information with patients and families in ways that are affirming and useful. Patients and families receive timely, complete, and accurate information in order to effectively participate in care and decision-making.

Participation: Patients and families are encouraged and supported in participating in care and decision-making at the level they choose.

Collaboration: Patients, families, healthcare practitioners, and healthcare leaders collaborate in policy and program development, implementation, and evaluation; in research; in facility design; and in professional education, as well as in the delivery of care.

Source: Adapted from Johnson, B. H., & Abraham, M. R. (2012). *Partnering with patients, residents, and families: A resource for leaders of hospitals, ambulatory care settings, and long-term care communities*. Institute for Patient- and Family-Centered Care. https://www.ipfcc.org/about/pfcc.html

the patient and family as integral members of the interprofessional team without question, and encourage patients and families to be fully engaged at all levels of healthcare (Centers for Medicare and Medicaid Services [CMS], 2020). See Box 6.1 for some core concepts of patient- and family-centered care, which apply to the health of patients, residents, families, all leaders of hospitals, ambulatory care settings, and long-term care communities.

While this transformation from paternalistic, physician-directed care to PCC has been occurring for several decades, PCC is still not practiced consistently. There is no consensus on the definition of the concept of PCC, nor is there any agreement on which single term should be used to describe the concept. This lack of consensus has led to inconsistent application across communities and healthcare facilities, as different terms and definitions are used. Additionally, barriers and resistance to fully engage in PCC are still very much a reality (Sinaiko et al., 2019). Barriers to fully employing PCC include provider attitudes, beliefs, and training, as well as a lack of institutional support for PCC training, personal staff belief conflicts, or lack of staff engagement in PCC.

CHARACTERISTICS OF PERSON-CENTERED CARE

Central to PCC is the idea that all persons, families, and communities are full partners in control of their own health. It is important to note that the term "family" is used throughout this text to include any relative, partner, friend, neighbor, or community member the patient considers as a family member and should be included in patient care and decision-making according to patient preference (Institute for Patient- and Family-Centered Care, [n.d.]). Using PCC, nurses and other members of the interprofessional team can coordinate patient care services with compassion and respect, as they develop collaborative partnerships with the patient and family. The term PCC includes the person, family, and community with an emphasis on health for both hospitalized and nonhospitalized persons. Figure 6.1 visually demonstrates the connection and overlap of PCC with regard to the development of persons, families, and communities in various countries and

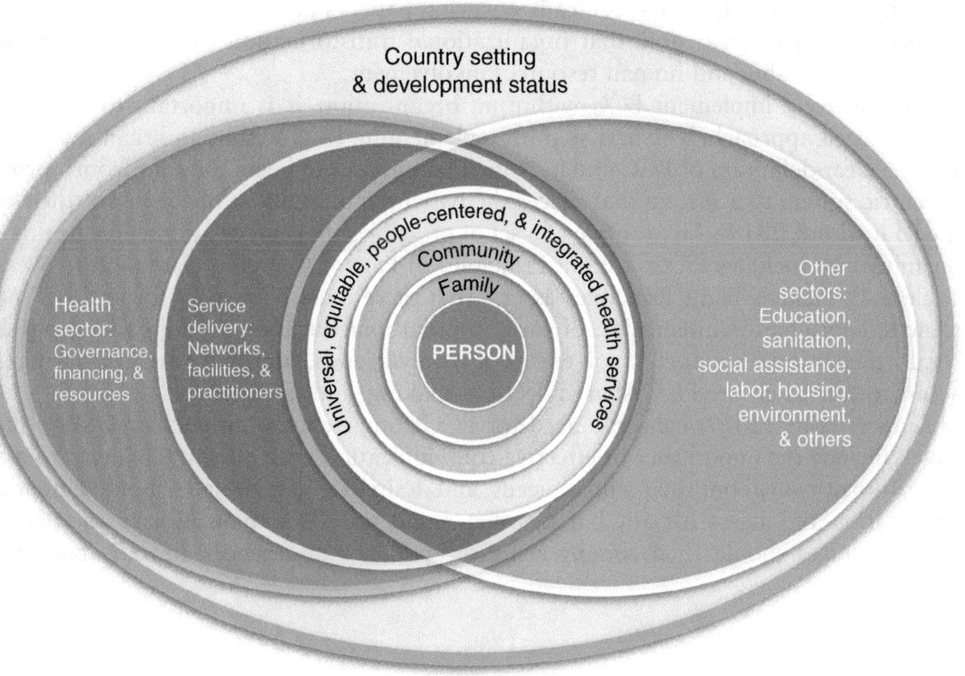

FIGURE 6.1 World Health Organization Framework on Integrated People-Centered Health Services.

Source: From World Health Organization. (2021). https://www.who.int/teams/integrated-health-services/clinical-services-and-systems/service-organizations-and-integration

settings and how these interact with the health sector, service delivery, and other sectors in education, sanitation, social assistance, environment, and others. The World Health Organization (WHO) uses the term "people-centered health services," which is defined as "an approach to care that consciously adopts the perspectives of individuals, families and communities, and sees them as participants as well as beneficiaries of trusted health systems that respond to their needs and preferences in humane and holistic ways" (WHO, n.d., para 4).

The National Academy of Medicine, as well as other national campaigns for quality care, have drawn attention to the necessity of maintaining safety, providing quality care, and keeping patients and families at the center of their care to meet their health needs. This national attention is intended to ensure all interprofessional team members are accountable for quality care through PCC services, careful monitoring of patient outcomes, and validation of improvement in patient health.

ORGANIZATIONAL STRUCTURES OF PATIENT-CENTERED CARE

Grant and Johnson (2019) posit that nurse leaders are in a unique position to lead organizational transformation to ensure care that is centered on the patient and family. This, they argue, can be carried out by ensuring PCC goals are included in organizational strategies. They begin this argument by stating the absolute need for PCC goals and commitment to PCC by healthcare facilities based on respect for patient self-determination (or the right to make decisions for oneself) and autonomy (the right to self-govern based on values). With these goals, they address the need for nurse leaders to accept the responsibility for the achievement of PCC by specifically ensuring patients are fully engaged in all aspects of their care. They also note that organizational transformation cannot occur without physician leadership and human resources involvement.

To effectively implement PCC within an organization, it is important to begin with an organized approach. The first step in implementing PCC within an organization is to adopt a clear definition of PCC and its principles in order to begin the shift from a provider-centric system to a system that places the patient and family at the center of their care (ECRI Institute, 2019). An example of a set of principles that can be adopted by healthcare organizations includes Picker's Eight Principles of Patient-Centered Care (Figure 6.2 and Table 6.1). Picker's Eight Principles asserts that there must be respect for patients' preferences, coordination/integration of care, information/education to the patient, physical comfort, emotional support, involvement of family/friends, continuity and transition, and access to care to ensure PCC, shared decision-making, and engagement.

Kuipers et al. (2019) echo the need for PCC competencies outlined by QSEN (n.d.), which include the importance of effective communication with allowing patients to articulate information about their values, needs, and desires for care. Nurses should gather this information and assess for any barriers that might impede actualization of the patient's wishes. Nurses should then communicate the patient's preferences and any barriers to

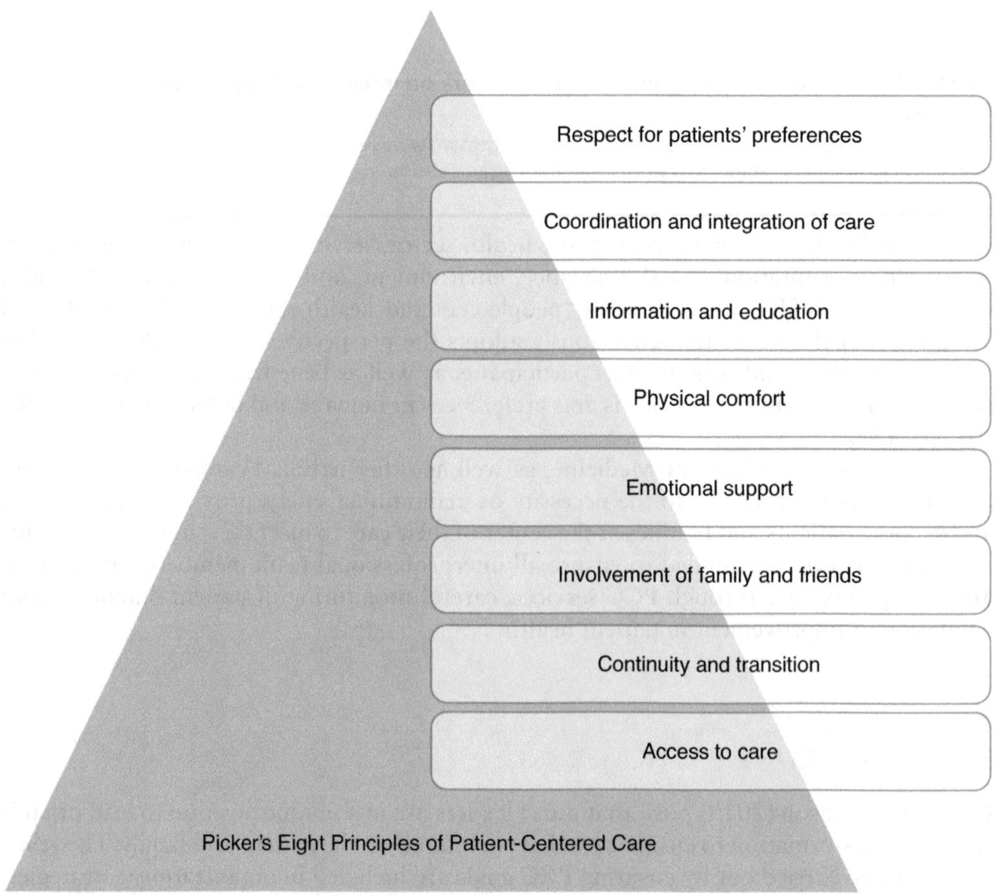

FIGURE 6.2 Picker's Eight Principles of Patient-Centered Care.

Source: From O'Neill, N. (2015). The eight principles of patient-centred care. *Oneview*. https://www.oneviewhealthcare.com/the-eight-principles-of-patient-centered-care. Reprinted with permission.

TABLE 6.1 PICKER'S PRINCIPLES OF PATIENT-CENTERED CARE WITH REAL-WORLD EXAMPLES

PICKER'S PRINCIPLES OF PATIENT-CENTERED CARE	EXAMPLE
Respect for patients' preferences - Include involving patients in decision-making, recognizing unique values/preferences, and treating each person with dignity, respect, and autonomy.	Educate new parents regarding the benefits and risks of circumcision while respecting their cultural and preferred preferences during the decision-making process; communicating to parents their right to autonomy.
Coordination/integration of care - Provide access and information regarding clinical care, ancillary services, and patient care as necessary to the patient in coordinated manner from the interprofessional team.	Organize patient care activities between the patient and multiple members of the interprofessional team (e.g., physical therapy, dietitian, and radiology).
Information/education - Communicate clinical status, progress, and tailored healthcare information to patient and chosen caregivers to facilitate autonomy and self-care.	Provide health education tailored to the patient's specific needs and health literacy levels and include family and/or chosen caregivers based upon patient's preference.
Physical comfort - Ensure an environment that nurtures and fosters the patient's individualized well-being based on their preferences and needs.	Assess and manage patient's pain, assistance with activities of daily living, and overall environment.
Emotional support - Evaluate and provide resources to alleviate patient anxiety regarding physical status, impact of illness on life, and financial concerns.	Request hospital chaplain or patient's preferred spiritual leader to visit a patient experiencing emotional distress.
Involvement of family/friends - The role of family and friends in the patient experience	Provide inclusive measures for caregiver(s), family, and/or friends through accommodations allowing involvement in decision-making at the level preferred by the patient and caregiver(s).
Continuity and transition - Coordinate plan of care and discharge with interprofessional team to ensure patient transitions to a realistic setting that will promote healing.	Collaborate with social work and case management to develop an individualized plan of care and appropriate discharge plan.
Access to care - Ensure ease of access for appointments, referrals, resources for transportation, and clear discharge instructions.	Ensure patient and caregiver understand discharge instructions and ask the patient about access to transportation for follow-up appointments.

Source: From Oneview – Picker Institute Europe. (2020). *The eight principles of patient-centered care*. https://www.oneviewhealthcare.com/the-eight-principles-of-patient-centered-care. Reprinted with permission.

the rest of the interprofessional team. Patient education should be provided based on the patient's assessed needs, not to sway the individual's choices, but to ensure fully informed decision-making. Patients should be empowered through the provision of knowledge and ability to negotiate with all members of the interprofessional team. Nurses are in a unique and effective position to provide patient education, support, and advocacy that facilitates patient engagement. While patient engagement is important, it is imperative to understand that many patients may be disinclined to participate in their own decision-making. In fact, some patients are reluctant to participate in their own care decisions due to culture, health literacy, education, and many other factors (Blumenthal-Barby, 2017). LeBlanc et al. (2019) performed a qualitative study that found that patients with terminal or advanced malignancies preferred to defer treatment decisions to their oncologist. It is important for nurses and other healthcare providers to consider the patient's preference for the level of decision-making they want to be involved in regarding their health status. Nurses and other members of the interprofessional team should discuss patient preferences regarding treatment decisions and provide patients with necessary information, while also following patients' wishes regarding decision-making.

Real World Interview

We have known for some time that patients' participation in their care is instrumental in their healing. More recently, we have seen how important their participation is in the success of the organization as well. By engaging patients as partners in the design of care delivery, including physical spaces, human interaction, and workflow, we can create care models and processes that benefit our patients. Too often, we become too focused on cost or efficiency and lose sight of the patient and their needs and desires. Families have a unique perspective on the patient, and their insight is invaluable in delivering appropriate care. As true partners in healthcare, we can achieve high reliability in both patient experience and quality care.

Trenda Ray, PhD, RN
Chief Nursing Officer
University of Arkansas for Medical Sciences, Little Rock, Arkansas

ROLE OF CUSTOMS IN PATIENT-CENTERED CARE

It is vital to understand that the implementation of PCC requires respect for unique customs held by all persons. These unique individual customs impact each person's decisions and can be influenced by many personal factors, including a person's health beliefs, health customs, ethnic customs, religious beliefs, dietary customs, and interpersonal customs (Table 6.2). Asking about and seeking to understand each person's customs is a cornerstone of ensuring PCC. Naughton (2018) supports the need to consider all aspects of a patient's value system and customs within the context of evidence-based healthcare. This allows all members of the interprofessional team and the patient an opportunity to establish a relationship based on respect, trust, equality, and shared responsibility. Naughton (2018) contends this ensures the successful intersection of science, compassion, and quality, which is key in the delivery of PCC.

CULTURAL COMPETENCE

Another key consideration to aid members of the interprofessional team with PCC strategies involves cultural competence. **Cultural competence** in healthcare has been defined by the American Hospital Association [AHA] as "the ability of systems to provide care to patients with diverse values, beliefs and behaviors, including the tailoring of healthcare delivery to meet patients' social, cultural, and linguistic needs" (AHA, n.d., para 1). Effective cultural competence can enhance PCC through decreasing safety errors, improving communication, and driving increased patient engagement and decision-making (AHRQ, 2019b). Several crucial factors related to education on cultural competence are included in Table 6.3, which are important to understanding how cultural features are constructed and how they relate to PCC and healthcare.

TABLE 6.2 INDIVIDUAL CUSTOMS AND BELIEFS THAT IMPACT PEOPLES' DECISIONS

Health Beliefs:	In some cultures, people believe that talking about a possible poor health outcome will cause that outcome to occur.
Health Customs:	In some cultures, family members customarily play a significant role in healthcare decision-making.
Ethnic Customs:	Differing roles of women and men in society may determine who makes decisions about accepting and following through with healthcare treatments.
Religious Beliefs:	Religious faith and spiritual beliefs may affect healthcare-seeking behavior and people's willingness to accept specific healthcare treatments or behavior changes.
Dietary Customs:	Disease-related dietary advice will be difficult to follow if it does not conform to the foods or cooking customs and methods used by the patient.
Interpersonal Customs:	Eye contact or physical touch will be expected in some cultures and inappropriate or offensive in others.

Source: From Agency for Healthcare Research and Quality. (2020). *Health literacy universal precautions toolkit* (2nd ed.). https://www.ahrq.gov/health-literacy/improve/precautions/tool10.html

TABLE 6.3 CONTENTS OF SESSIONS–EDUCATION ON CULTURAL COMPETENCE

NAME OF EACH SESSION	CONTENT OF THE SESSION
"What is culture?"	• Different cultural dimensions and how these dimensions occur in our everyday life and in healthcare.
"Culture in me"	• Significance of being aware of one's own cultural features in order to be able to understand others. How are our own cultural features constructed, and how are they seen in healthcare work? • Why are cultural 'facts' or assumptions not applicable in patient care? • Cultural pain. How do background and previous experiences affect pain interpretation? • Cultural "cage." *(that is, not seeing beyond one's own culture).* How does it regulate our behavior toward others?
"Communication"	• Personal space. How can it be communicated to others? • What are our own communication features and challenges? • How do cultural values affect our way of communicating? • What is good and understandable communication with patients from different cultural backgrounds? • What issues typically mess up or complicate the communication process?
"Meaning of communication"	• What is our own attitude toward spiritualism? What can different attitudes mean in a healthcare context? • Interaction between culture and religion. Does culture generate religion, or is it the other way around? • How can we value a patient's convictions and spirituality? • Introduction to a conversational model (opening model) that can be used to assess patients' spiritual needs

Source: Data from Kaihlanen, A. M., Hietapakka, L., & Heponiemi, T. (2019). Increasing cultural awareness: Qualitative study of nurses' perceptions about cultural competence training. *BMC Nursing, 18*(1), Article 38. https://doi.org/10.1186/s12912-019-0363-x

ADVOCACY

Serving as a healthcare advocate for all people in a community as well as for patients is another key hallmark of PCC and is an essential component of nursing and leadership. **Advocacy** refers to any activity that helps a person achieve and maintain good health as well as receive the "best" healthcare needed depending on the person's needs and wishes. Some hospitals have created patient advocate positions, which provide a means to increase the flow of information to patients and staff, address patient concerns, and provide emotional support to patients and families. A patient advocate can be supplied by the hospital or may be a friend or family member. Being a patient advocate does not require medical or healthcare training. The only requirement is that the advocate is someone the patient trusts and can effectively communicate with and for the patient as needed. Florence Nightingale emphasized nurses must keep the patient central to nursing care, an obligation that remains embodied in nursing's application of values such as beneficence and fidelity (Gaines, 2020). Beneficence is the principle of acting for the good and welfare of patients, while fidelity means remaining faithful to providing competent, safe care. Patient empowerment reflects a form of self-directed advocacy that enables and motivates patients to bring about changes and make decisions to manage and improve their health (Castro et al., 2016). Through a person-centered (PC) approach to advocacy and empowerment, improved communication and a partnership between the caregiver and the patient can increase the patient's autonomy and involvement in their own care (Berger et al., 2017).

BOX 6.2 Developing Clinical Judgment

Consider the following situation and identify the nurse's behaviors associated with promoting the patient's sense of control over her care. Mrs. Huong Nguyen, an 81-year-old female, is in a subacute rehabilitation facility recovering from a knee replacement. Mrs. Nguyen moved to the United States from Vietnam 10 years ago to be with her son and his family. Sue Williams is her primary nurse. Nurse Williams introduces herself and asks Mrs. Nguyen how she would like to be addressed. She also reviews with Mrs. Nguyen what she might expect from the rehabilitation program and how she might deal with the discomfort that could result from her therapy. Nurse Williams provides Mrs. Nguyen with choices of times for therapy and menus for meal choices. She answers all of Mrs. Nguyen's questions and provides her with the list of her therapies.

1. What behaviors did Nurse Williams exhibit that could support and encourage Mrs. Nguyen's sense of control over her care?
2. How could Nurse Williams assess Mrs. Nguyen's customs to incorporate PCC in the nurse–patient relationship?
3. What additional questions might Nurse Williams consider regarding culture and communication to better understand Mrs. Nguyen's perspective on healthcare practices?
4. What actions did Nurse Williams implement to ensure a PCC approach to advocacy? What are some additional actions she can take?
5. How could Nurse Williams evaluate Mrs. Nguyen's clinical progress in a way that includes PCC?

CASE STUDY

Anne Davis, a 72-year-old female, was admitted to the hospital due to knee pain, increasing agitation, difficulty sleeping, and intermittent confusion. The physician suspects that Mrs. Davis' recent knee replacement is infected, and diagnostic tests are underway. Benjamin, a nurse for 20 years, is assigned to care for Mrs. Davis, and he introduces himself during morning rounds. "Good morning, Mrs. Davis, I'm Benjamin, and I will be your nurse today." Mrs. Davis replies, "Oh great, a male nurse. You must not have been able to make it into medical school. I hope you know what you are doing. My knee is hurting, and I don't need someone who can't do their job." Mrs. Davis' undertones are obviously hostile and offensive.

1. *How might Benjamin have felt when listening to the hostile tones in Mrs. Davis' voice and remarks toward his competency?*
2. *How should Benjamin respond, while maintaining a respectful and open dialogue between him and the patient?*
3. *How can Benjamin assure PCC with the patient in this situation?*

COMMUNICATION AND PATIENT-CENTERED CARE

Effective communication is one of the key features of PCC. To communicate effectively, the nurse must be aware of how verbal and nonverbal components in the communication process create meaning (Figure 6.3). Communication includes deciding whether nonverbal communication (Table 6.4) is congruent with verbal communication. When verbal

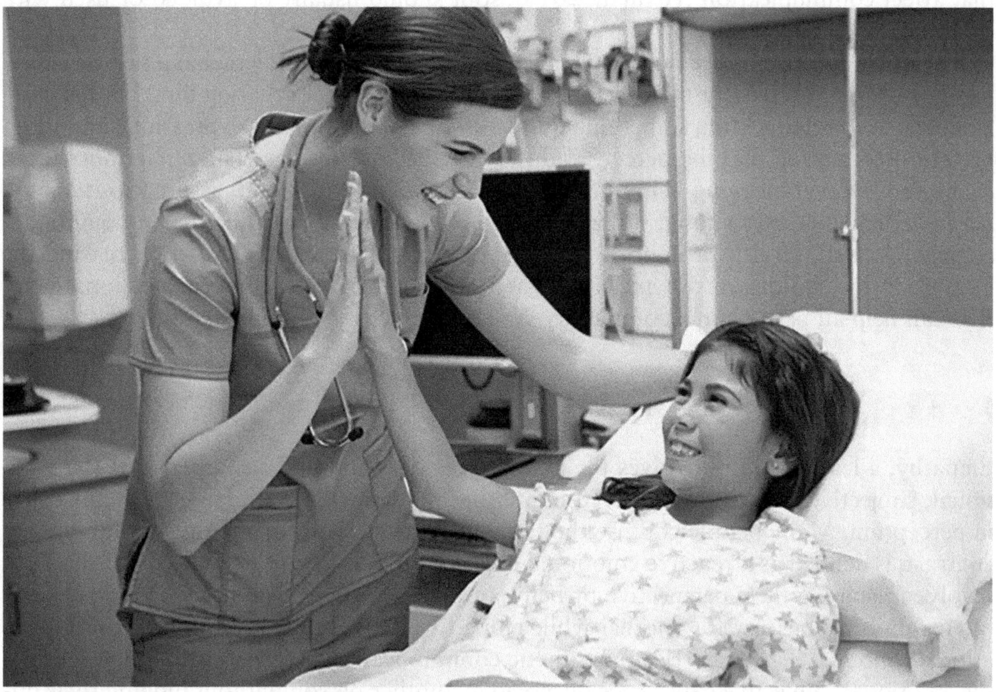

FIGURE 6.3 Nurse and Patient Interacting With Verbal and Nonverbal Communication.
Source: Courtesy of upsplash.com.

TABLE 6.4 EXAMPLES OF NONVERBAL BEHAVIOR

NONVERBAL BEHAVIOR	EXAMPLES
Eye movement and features	Either steady eye contact or inability to make eye contact; blinking, teary eyes opened or closed
Body position, movement, behavior, and stance	Tense, relaxed, jerky, fidgety, legs crossed, arms crossed, agitated, calm, use of hands, gestures
Facial expression	Grimaces, smiles, frowns, no expression or flat affect, exaggerated expression
Tone of voice	Mumbles, whispers, high pitched, quiet; rate of speech either speedy or slowed
Skin	Blushes, sweats, general pallor
General appearance	Appropriateness of dress for weather and/or event, neatness, accessories, stature

Source: Keutchafo, E. L. W., Kerr, J., & Jarvis, M. A. (2020). Evidence of nonverbal communication between nurses and older adults: A scoping review. *BMC Nursing, 19*(1), Article 53. https://doi.org/10.1186/s12912-020-00443-9

and nonverbal components of communication are incongruent, the speaker may be trying to convey thinly veiled disapproval or contempt by using sarcasm. Sarcasm is saying the opposite of what is true in an attempt at humor, or as a thinly veiled expression of disapproval or contempt. For example, a speaker may talk about something distasteful in a positive tone, which may indicate sarcasm. Sarcasm may be difficult to understand for those from various cultures, or for those with autism spectrum disorder or brain injuries that affect communication (Pexman, 2018), so it should usually be avoided or used with caution.

The nurse can also notice body language clues that may contradict what a person is saying. For example, a patient might verbally say that nothing is bothering him, but his body language is communicating something quite different. Additionally, expressions and interpretations of caring may be perceived differently across cultures. The nurse must work to discern the real meaning behind the patient's communication and assumptions should never be made. Nurses should utilize effective communication techniques in community settings, as well. Health promotion and prevention practices are vital to decreasing the burden on the healthcare system. Nurses are key members of the interprofessional team that can help all persons in a community via clear, effective communication.

EMPATHETIC COMMUNICATION

Empathy, a learned skill, involves the ability to understand and make sense of the emotional, subjective experience observed in another person without judging their difference in perception. Many people confuse the term "empathy" with "sympathy." **Sympathy**, by contrast, is defined as a reactive emotional concern or distress for another, and it does not involve imagining their perspective or being in their situation. In other words, sympathy often entails feeling pity for another while empathy involves imagining oneself in the situation of another (Jeffrey, 2016). **Empathetic communication** is the act of making sense of the emotional, subjective experience observed in another person without judging their difference in perception and understanding that their perceptions are guided by their feelings, values, and background. When using empathetic communication, the nurse has a genuine

TABLE 6.5 EMPATHETIC AND NONEMPATHETIC COMMUNICATION BEHAVIORS

EMPATHETIC COMMUNICATION	NONEMPATHETIC COMMUNICATION
Listens carefully and reflects back a summary of the patient's concerns	Interrupts patient with irrelevant information
Uses terms and vocabulary that is appropriate for the patient	Uses vocabulary that is either beneath the level of the patient or not understandable to the patient
Calls patient by patient's preferred name	Uses language that may be perceived as cajoling, patronizing, or demeaning, for example, honey
Uses respectful and professional language	Uses nonprofessional language
Asks patient what they need and responds promptly to those needs	Chastises patient
Provides helpful and informative information	Provides patient with inappropriate information
Solicits feedback from the patient	Asks questions at inappropriate times and gives patient advice inappropriately
Uses self-disclosure appropriately	Self-discloses inappropriately
Employs humor as appropriate	Preaches to the patient
Provides words of comfort when appropriate	Scolds the patient

Source: From Lorié, Á., Reinero, D. A., Phillips, M., Zhang, L., & Riess, H. (2017). Culture and nonverbal expressions of empathy in clinical settings: A systematic review. *Patient Education and Counseling, 100*(3), 411–424. https://doi.org/10.1016/j.pec.2016.09.018. Reprinted with permission.

sense of respect for the patient's and family's opinions, perceptions, and decisions. The use of empathetic communication can improve the nurse–patient relationship, as patients are more likely to divulge their thoughts and concerns if they feel that the person listening can understand their perspective without judgment and pity (Pehrson et al., 2019). Likewise, there are nonempathetic communication behaviors that hinder communication and thereby impede PCC. Table 6.5 lists a representative sample of empathetic and nonempathetic communication behaviors and may be applied to communication with both the patient and family members to foster the components of PCC.

INFLUENCE OF CULTURE AND LANGUAGE ON PATIENT-CENTERED CARE COMMUNICATION

Nurses and other members of the interprofessional team must also realize that expressions of caring can be perceived differently across cultures. For example, direct eye contact may be considered rude in some cultures, while it may show sincerity and respect in other cultures. Additionally, people in some cultures feel touch is an important aspect of caring and empathy, while in other cultures, touch is considered an invasion of space.

There are many factors that can affect the quality and clarity of communications and healthcare providers must be proactive in addressing any potential barriers to communication. For example, language barriers may be present. The use of interpreters can provide a safe space where patients can freely express their concerns and be understood through the interpreter, calming their fears and apprehensions in an unfamiliar situation and setting.

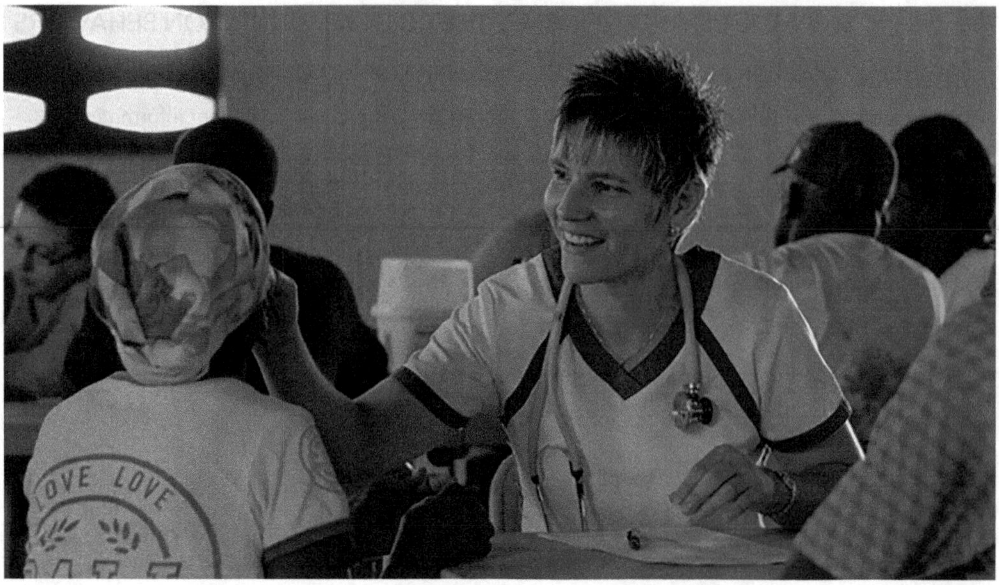

FIGURE 6.4 Healthcare Provider Interacting During Mission Trip With Patients of Diverse Cultures.
Source: Courtesy of upsplash.com.

While bilingual family members can be appropriately used for basic exchanges of information, communication of complex healthcare information will require the help of trained interpreters. Some hospitals or other healthcare facilities will have an interpreter on site for face-to-face interpretation, while others may use a service to interpret through the telephone or virtually. Healthcare providers can access trained interpreters through various certified telephonic and remote services, such as CTS Language Link, which can be accessed through its website at www.ctslanguagelink.com. The nurse should use interpreting services if a noticeable barrier to communication is present that could affect the delivery of PCC and education. Healthcare organizations receiving federal financial assistance are required to offer free, accessible language services by qualified translators and interpreters (Jacobs et al., 2018).

The nurse should follow the policies, procedures, and guidelines set forth by the specific unit and facility for appropriate interpreting services. For more information about providing language access services, please visit www.ncihc.org. Using a substitute interpreter or an unapproved online source is never appropriate for interpreting healthcare information to the patient and family. Effective communication utilizing PCC, even when done through an interpreter, provides an opportunity for a personal exchange between patient and all members of the interprofessional team that fosters clarity and an understanding of what is needed to continue the patient's care and includes the patient as an active partner in the recovery process. Patience and fortitude in understanding the patient's cultural norms and healthcare practices that are unique to the patient's culture must be demonstrated (Figure 6.4).

PATIENTS AND INTERPROFESSIONAL COMMUNICATION

Patients and their caregivers should be included in bedside report or interprofessional rounds. Having patients and their caregivers be a part of the report or rounding process allows them to hear all information being discussed and ask questions about any

CASE STUDY

Nurse Shondra is caring for a patient, James Jackson, with a severely low hemoglobin and red blood cell values. The physician has ordered one unit of packed red blood cells. Shondra finds that there is no signed patient consent for blood products on the patient's chart. Shondra approaches the patient to inform him of the new orders and states, "I noticed you did not have a signed consent form for blood products, so I am going to contact your physician to get that consent signed." Mr. Jackson glares at Shondra and states, "Oh no! You're not going to give me any of that blood. I've told everyone I don't want any blood, and no one listens to me. You know I'm a Jehovah's Witness, right? None of you know what's going on around here!"

1. *How can Nurse Shondra use PCC principles to help resolve this incongruence between Mr. Jackson's preferences and the physician's order for blood administration?*
2. *What empathetic communication techniques can Nurse Shondra use with Mr. Jackson to promote PCC?*

BOX 6.3 Developing Clinical Judgment

Nurse Tsosie is caring for Mrs. Aleksandra Kowalski, a patient recently diagnosed with diabetes. Mrs. Kowalski speaks English as a second language and is a recent immigrant to the United States. The patient can make her basic needs known but does not ask questions or speak unless prompted to do so. Nurse Tsosie has been unable to determine if this patient can self-inject her insulin. Mrs. Kowalski nods and smiles as Nurse Tsosie begins teaching her about insulin and her diagnosis.

1. What **CUES (Assessment)** can Nurse Tsosie assess to help with her clinical judgment of what to do next for Mrs. Kowalski?
2. What **HYPOTHESIS (Diagnosis)** will the nurse consider?
3. What **ACTION (Plan and Implement)** can Nurse Tsosie employ to help Mrs. Kowalski facilitate self-management?
4. What resources and/or services can Nurse Tsosie use to evaluate the **OUTCOME (Evaluation)** that ensures Mrs. Kowalski has understood the teaching?

information they do not understand or need clarified. This process fosters PCC, patient autonomy, and education. Care should be taken to ensure all verbal and nonverbal communication is person-centered, objective, congruent, nonthreatening, and nonjudgmental.

PSYCHOSOCIAL FACTORS ASSOCIATED WITH THE ROLE OF THE PATIENT

Understanding how a person's life is affected by illness is essential in understanding patient reactions and emotions. This level of understanding leads to the ability to take another's perspective and is a precursor to empathetic communication, the cornerstone of PCC (Jeffrey, 2016). Being a patient is a role that most people find challenging. This is because illness can impact a person's self-concept (Shpigelman & HaGani, 2019). For a better understanding of the impact of illness on the patient, all members of the interprofessional team need to understand self-concept and the impact illness has on how one perceives their self-concept. **Self-concept** is the conception an individual holds about their own traits, aptitudes, and unique characteristics (Shpigelman & HaGani, 2019).

CASE STUDY

Mary is a 28-year-old female in the prime of her life. She has completed her master's degree in education and is employed as a kindergarten teacher, which she absolutely loves. She has always been independent and hard-working. Mary developed generalized pain that progressively worsened over the course of 2 years. Her general energy level significantly decreased, and she could no longer concentrate for any length of time. After seeking medical care, Mary was diagnosed with fibromyalgia. Frustrated with her pain, lack of energy, and inability to concentrate, Mary was forced to give up her teaching job. She believes the fibromyalgia has affected her physically, professionally, and financially.

1. *How has chronic fibromyalgia affected Mary's perspective on her personal and professional life?*
2. *How can the nurse use the components of PCC to advocate for Mary?*
3. *Explore the web for support services that are available to Mary at home. What are some support services the nurse might share with Mary specific to her needs?*

STRATEGIES TO SUPPORT PATIENT-CENTERED CARE PRACTICE

The NAM's 2011 report titled *Health Care Comes Home: The Human Factors* brings PCC and human factors to the forefront of healthcare. The NAM report identifies specific aims to improve the quality and safety of healthcare. Among these aims, the PCC model has become a core component that ensures patient values and guides clinical decisions. NAM has also published several guidelines, such as developing a decision score to optimize treatment options and providing patients with decision-making tools, which discuss the use of research, informatics, and evidence-based strategies to promote personalized PCC (Kent et al., 2019). Through the PCC model, the healthcare industry is called upon to develop innovative strategies to support patients and caregivers in becoming greater participants in their healthcare. PCC outcomes research emphasizes decision-making between the patient and provider that is collaborative, mutual, and shared. Health literacy is one major factor grounded in informed decision-making. Thus, many innovative strategies exist to alleviate barriers to health literacy.

ALLEVIATING BARRIERS TO HEALTH LITERACY

Health literacy is the ability to read, write, and perform tasks related to health and health information (Nutbeam et al., 2018). Measurement of health literacy is a vital aspect to foster PCC because each person may require a different form of information and education for autonomy. Alleviating barriers to health literacy relate directly to the PCC components of information sharing and collaboration. A person's basic education and competencies in reading, writing, and mathematics are important components of their health literacy as well as skills such as listening and speaking. People with limited health literacy skills and knowledge do not have the same resources, ability, or competencies to achieve optimal health services as those who are health literate. Populations vulnerable to low levels of health literacy include ethnic minority groups, recent immigrants, older adults, individuals living with chronic diseases, and populations of people in poverty or lower socioeconomic class (Joszt, 2018).

Healthy People 2030 (Office of Disease Prevention and Health Promotion: Healthy People 2030, n.d.) has identified improving health literacy as one of its key goals in promoting healthy outcomes and enhancing quality of life. In the past, health literacy was considered a task of educators and viewed from the perspective of the patient's intellectual deficits. Today, health literacy is recognized as a healthcare system issue. Thus, the use of appropriate health literacy strategies is crucial for both hospitalized patients with simple and complex illnesses, and those persons within the community who need health promotion, disease prevention education, or who require care or education for complex healthcare issues at home.

Health literacy is promoted when nurses and the interprofessional team reinforce pertinent information with the patient through simple explanations that avoid medical jargon. Patients must understand their role and what they need to do to safely follow dietary and healthcare treatments. They must understand the importance of adhering to prescribed treatment plans and communicating with their provider when encountering difficulties. Patients who are well informed and more involved in their care experience better health outcomes (Centers for Disease Control and Prevention [CDC], n.d.-b).

Patient initiatives, such as Ask Me 3: Good Questions for Your Good Health (Institute for Healthcare Improvement [IHI], n.d.) and Questions Are the Answer (AHRQ, 2019b), are campaigns designed to encourage patients to ask questions of their providers, such as:

- What is my main problem?
- What do I need to do?
- Why is it important for me to do this?

More resources for health literacy can be found at www.cdc.gov/healthliteracy/learn/Resources.html.

CURRENT LITERATURE

CITATION

Loan, L. A., Parnell, T. A., Stichler, J. F., Boyle, D. K., Allen, P., VanFosson, C. A., & Barton, A. J. (2018). Call for action: Nurses must play a critical role to enhance health literacy. *Nursing Outlook, 66*(1), 97–100. https://doi.org/10.1016/j.outlook.2017.11.003

DISCUSSION

Patients with low health literacy may struggle with obtaining, understanding, and applying health information. Without a simple understanding of health issues, patients will struggle with feeling empowered, engaged, and active in their healthcare decisions. Strategies to help improve low health literacy include a PCC approach to improve communication between interprofessional team members and patients by providing information to patients in various formats and improving patient access to services.

IMPLICATIONS FOR PRACTICE

Nurses play a critical role in assessing and improving health literacy, especially for patients with complex chronic conditions. Research demonstrates a renewed call for health literacy promotion for patients including several of the following recommendations:

Related to nursing practice:

- Urge the global use of a health literacy universal precautions approach and advocate for assuming that all patients are at risk for not understanding health information (DeWalt et al., 2011; Koh et al., 2013);
- Integrate patient-centered nursing practice elements that maximize patient engagement and health literacy into interprofessional practice models;
- Assimilate patient-specific health literacy nursing diagnoses, nursing interventions, and patient predischarge self-management capabilities into the electronic medical record;
- Promote shame-free environments where health literacy can flourish (Brach et al., 2012; Rudd & Anderson, 2006);
- Use plain language and the teach-back method in all patient communications (Baker et al., 2011).

Related to healthcare systems:

- Promote organizational use of existing resources;
- Increase the use of health communication strategies, health information technology, and measures of patient post-encounter self-management competency to monitor and improve healthcare quality and population health outcomes, and to achieve health (U.S. Department of Health and Human Services, 2021);
- Develop goals, accountability, and financial incentives for professionals in all healthcare settings;
- Build a business case for recruiting and retaining a diverse workforce with health literacy expertise;
- Encourage and engage community partners to participate in the development and evaluation of health.

Related to partnerships:

- Collaborate with nursing and other healthcare organizations to integrate nursing models of care for health literacy into QSEN, Nursing Alliance for Quality Care, and other national healthcare initiatives to improve quality and patient safety;
- Encourage nurse educators and leaders to use the Health Literacy Tapestry conceptual model (Parnell, 2015);
- Urge TJC to evaluate successful incorporation of health literacy universal precautions;
- Advocate for funding to evaluate nursing and other health literacy programs in education, practice, and systems of care;
- Urge the American Nurses Credentialing Center to require evidence of health literacy initiatives and sustained achievements as a component of Magnet® recognition.

SHARED DECISION-MAKING

Shared decision-making is a collaborative process in which both the patient and interprofessional team members work together to agree on healthcare decisions that are aligned with the patient's health and life preferences (Kamal et al., 2018). Shared decision-making allows the patient to have a voice regarding their healthcare decisions and can enhance the patient's perceived value of healthcare (Kamal et al., 2018). Patients may be more likely to maintain continuity of care when they perceive the benefits of shared decision-making.

Numerous models for shared decision-making have been created and can be found in the literature. Bomhof-Roordink et al. (2019) performed a systematic review of 40 articles describing shared decision-making models, which can be further reviewed for more information. While there are differences in these models, the authors identified several common overlapping components (see the Current Literature box on page 196).

One such model by authors Elwyn et al. (2017) discusses the use of a Three-Talk Model of Shared Decision Making, which simplifies the shared decision-making process for patients and healthcare providers. The Three-Talk Model of Shared Decision Making identifies three steps to help providers with shared decision-making, focusing on the use of team collaboration, discussing options and alternatives in care, and providing information to help people make decisions based on individualized preferences. The first step refers to teamwork, which includes the provider, patient, and family working together to support goals. The second step is called option talk, which discusses alternatives for treatment with analysis of risk and comparison of options. The third step is called decision talk and relates to the patient's preferences regarding possible decisions for treatment or interventions. In all three steps, there is active listening, paying close attention, deliberation, and careful thinking regarding options for the decision (Figure 6.5).

BOX 6.4 Developing Clinical Judgment

Eleanor is a 32-year-old woman recently diagnosed with stage IV cervical cancer. She has learned that it has spread into her bladder and rectum, along with some local lymph nodes. The 5-year survival rate for individuals with this stage of cervical cancer is 17%. Eleanor is married, has three young children, and has a successful career in home design. Eleanor is having a very difficult time with her new diagnosis. She has been admitted to the hospital due to blood loss. The interprofessional team is preparing to discuss treatment plans with Eleanor.

1. How can the interprofessional team use the first step in the Three-Talk Model of Shared Decision Making, team talk (Figure 6.5), accessible at www.bmj.com/content/bmj/359/bmj.j4891.full.pdf, when approaching Eleanor to discuss her treatment options?
2. What behaviors could the interprofessional team exhibit that could support and encourage Eleanor's sense of control over her care?
3. In the second step of the Three-Talk Model of Shared Decision Making, option talk, what information is important to relay to Eleanor?
4. What questions should the interprofessional team ask Eleanor to help her arrive at an informed decision in the third step, decision talk, of the Three-Talk Model of Shared Decision Making?
5. What are some barriers to shared decision-making that the interprofessional team must consider?

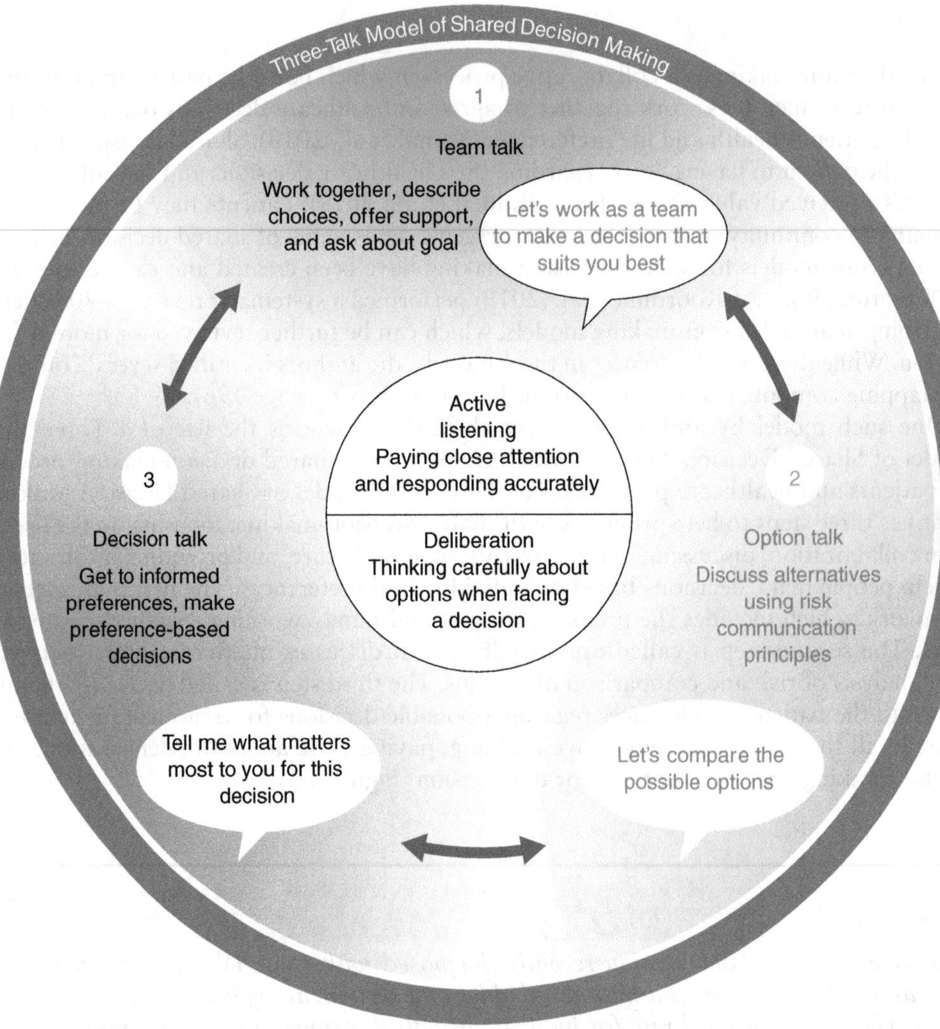

FIGURE 6.5 Three-Talk Model of Shared Decision Making.
Source: Bomhof-Roordink, H., Gärtner, F. R., Stiggelbout, A. M., & Pieterse, A. H. (2019). Key components of shared decision making models: A systematic review. *BMJ Open, 9*(12), e031763. https://doi.org/10.1136/bmjopen-2019-031763. Reprinted with permission.

CURRENT LITERATURE

CITATION

Bomhof-Roordink, H., Gärtner, F. R., Stiggelbout, A. M., & Pieterse, A. H. (2019). Key components of shared decision making models: A systematic review. *BMJ Open*, 9(12), e031763. https://doi.org/10.1136/bmjopen-2019-031763

DISCUSSION

Shared decision-making is an important part in the modern model of care which allows patients the ability to collaboratively make healthcare decisions with healthcare professionals. Shared decision-making is based on the thought that healthcare professionals are the experts on the medical evidence and patients are the experts on what matters most to them. As healthcare continues to modernize to a shared decision-making model, a clearer view of shared decision-making will emerge. The authors discuss an up-to-date overview of shared decision-making models and identify the major shared components found from a systematic review of 40 articles describing unique shared decision-making models.

IMPLICATIONS FOR PRACTICE

Based on this systematic review, several overlapping components were found in 40 shared decision-making models. The components included:

- Describe treatment options (88% frequency)
  - Benefits/risks
  - Feasibility
  - List options
  - Present evidence
- Make the decision (75% frequency)
  - Discuss decision
  - Make or explicitly defer decision
  - Patient retains ultimate authority over decision
  - Revisiting decision
- Patient preferences (65% frequency)
  - Patient concerns
  - Patient goals of care
  - Patient preferences
  - Patient values

Tailor information (65%), *deliberate (58%)*, *create choice awareness (55%)*, and *learn about the patient* (53%) were present in the majority of the models (27/40). Shared decision-making models may vary by healthcare setting and patient population. However, description of treatment options, with the patient retaining authority over the decision, and patient preferences play a large role in aiding patients with shared decision-making in the healthcare discipline. Nurses should have knowledge on these components while also understanding that the shared decision-making process will vary for each individual patient.

Conversely, a lack of shared decision-making can lead to worse patient-reported health outcomes, lower scores on quality indicators, and increased usage of emergent care instead of primary or preventive care (Hughes et al., 2018). Activities that enhance shared decision-making include training programs for interprofessional team members, educational materials for patients, email reminders, organizational policies, clinical guidelines, incentives, and assessment of organizational/patient culture (Légaré et al., 2018; Scholl et al., 2018).

PATIENT DECISION AIDS

Soliciting the patient's values, needs, and preferences is but one part of helping them in shared decision-making. **Patient decision aids** are defined by the International Patient Decision Aid Standards [IPDAS] Collaboration as "tools designed to help people participate in decision-making about healthcare options" (IPDAS, 2017, para. 1). One major

BOX 6.5 Five Steps for Implementing Patient Decision Aids

Step 1: Identify the decision.

Step 2: Find the patient decision aids.

Step 3: Identify barriers and explore ways to overcome them.

Step 4: Provide training.

Step 5: Monitor use and outcomes.

function of the IPDAS Collaboration involves maintaining and revising criteria used to evaluate the quality of patient decision aids since they are routinely created and developed by many different individuals and groups around the world (IPDAS, 2017). The IPDAS works with an interprofessional team of researchers, practitioners, and stakeholders to create standards for evaluating the quality of patient decision aids.

Patient decision aids can help patients make higher quality decisions, and can foster congruency in practice among multiple healthcare professionals. There are several resources for helping members of the interprofessional team effectively implement patient decision aids in the clinical setting. The Ottawa Hospital offers an implementation toolkit, which serves as a practical guide for using patient decision aids. The toolkit stresses the importance of implementing PCC while also recognizing that patients can struggle with decision-making. The toolkit also identifies the need for legislation to support decision-making (The Ottawa Hospital, 2020).

Patient decision aids have been found to improve decision quality and decision-making processes (Stacey et al., 2017). The Ottawa Hospital (2020) describes five steps that have been found effective in implementing and using patient decision aids via research and the Knowledge to Action Framework (see Box 6.5). Example decision aids for a multitude of health problems can be found at decisionaid.ohri.ca/azlist.html. Stacey et al. (2017) suggest that research is needed regarding patient decision aids and their effect

CASE STUDY

Charles Ellington, a 78-year-old male, presents to the clinic with long-term peripheral artery disease (PAD). He complains that the pain in his feet and legs are worse with exertion than 1 year ago. He reports that this change has impacted his quality of life, stating, "I am not able to take my short walks with my grandkids in the afternoons like before." He discusses lifestyle: he is not currently a smoker and takes a low-dose aspirin daily. Charles suffers from hypertension and takes lisinopril daily. The following questions involve the use of a patient decision aid (found here: www.healthwise.net/ohridecisionaid/Content/StdDocument.aspx?DOCHWID=ue4756)

1. ***Using the given patient decision aid, what are some important points to discuss with Charles regarding management and treatment of his PAD?***
2. ***How might the patient decision aid be used to discuss Charles' needs and preferences for management and treatment?***
3. ***How can the nurse support Charles' decision and ensure he has adequate information to make a decision?***

TABLE 6.6 WEBSITES WITH EXAMPLES OF PATIENT DECISION AIDS

WEBSITE	EXAMPLES OF PATIENT DECISION AIDS
decisionaid.ohri.ca	Decision aids for specific conditions or any decision The Ottawa Hospital
www.ahrq.gov/evidencenow/tools/decision-support.html	Toolkit to aid with integration of patient decision aids into primary care Agency for Healthcare Research and Quality (AHRQ)
https://patientdecisionaid.org	Patient decision aids University of Colorado, School of Medicine funded by the National Institutes on Aging and Patient-Centered Outcomes Research Institute
https://patient.info/decision-aids	Multitude of decision aids for various medical-surgical diseases and issues © Patient Platform Limited. * Registered in England and Wales
www.cincinnatichildrens.org/research/divisions/j/anderson-center/evidence-based-care/decision-aids	Pediatric-focused decision aids Cincinnati Children's Hospital Medical Center
http://careforyourmind.org/depression-decision-aid-update	Decision aids for mental health disorders and diseases Care for Your Mind, Families for Depression Awareness
https://carethatfits.org	Decision aids for various conditions and complications Mayo Clinic
www.healthit.gov/topic/safety/clinical-decision-support	Clinical decision support for use in healthcare organizations. HealthIT.gov Office of the National Coordinator for Health Information Technology (ONC)

on patients' confidence with decision-making, cost, resource use, adherence to selected treatment options, and regret. Patient decision aids often offer education about specific medical and surgical conditions, mental health, various treatments and medication, senior health, and so on, and often provide pros and cons of treatments typically suggested (https://patient.info/decision-aids). Websites that offer patient decision aids are a starting point for relevant discussion with patients and members of the interprofessional team (Table 6.6). More decision aids are available through the Mayo Clinic, AHRQ, and HealthITh.gov.

PERSON-CENTERED CARE AND THE SOCIAL DETERMINANTS OF HEALTH

The SDoH have been defined by the *Healthy People* 2030 Initiative as "conditions in the environments in which people are born, live, learn, work, play, worship, and age that affect a wide range of health, functioning, and quality-of-life outcomes and risks" (Office of Disease Prevention and Health Promotion, n.d., para 4). Nurses can incorporate strategies to help people maintain health and assess their SDoH by working with the community to promote PCC related to economic stability, social and community context, neighborhood and built environment, healthcare, and education (Table 6.7).

TABLE 6.7 LIST OF THE SOCIAL DETERMINANTS OF HEALTH WITH REAL-WORLD PERSON-CENTERED CARE EXAMPLES

SDOH	EXAMPLE
Economic Stability Employment Food insecurity Housing instability Poverty	Team of APRNs and RNs provide prenatal education, social work referrals, and housing/ food/employment assistance to women in the community who are pregnant and have insecure housing.
Neighborhood and Built Environment (Natural and Human-Made) Access to foods that support healthy eating patterns Crime and violence Environmental conditions Quality of housing	Nurse works with community to improve all people's access to health foods. Nurse provides anticipatory guidance regarding culinary and dietary choices to help patients reach healthy decisions about eating high-quality meals based on the specific disease, access to foods, and budgetary concerns.
Health and Healthcare Access to healthcare Access to primary care Health literacy	Nurse refers a patient who is newly diagnosed with HIV to resources to help them afford multiple medications that are an expense and burden.
Social and Community Context Civic participation Discrimination Incarceration Social cohesion	Psychiatric nurse provides incarcerated female offenders with psychosocial treatment modalities and substance abuse therapy to reduce, eliminate, or prevent drug or crime relapse.
Education Early childhood education and development Enrollment in higher education High school graduation Language and literacy	School nurse delivers ongoing health-related services to a student and helps students overcome obstacles to completing their high school graduation.

Source: From Office of Disease Prevention and Health Promotion. (n.d.). *Social determinants of health*. https://www.healthypeople.gov/2020/topics-objectives/topic/social-determinants-of-health

STRATEGIES TO ENHANCE TEAM-BASED APPROACH TO SOCIAL DETERMINANTS OF HEALTH

In 2018, the American Academy of Family Physicians [AAFP] published a report outlining strategies to enhance a team-based approach for addressing the SDoH in primary care (AAFP, 2018). The United States CDC provides several tools to aid members of the interprofessional team with implementing assessment and care of patients regarding their specific SDoH (CDC, n.d.-a). Awareness of SDoH is the first step for interprofessional team members. Communication and referral are key and the plan of care must reflect appropriate assessment and interventions for SDoH-related concerns. Table 6.8 provides resources to help nurses and all members of the interprofessional team enhance awareness and assessment of the SDoH.

DISCHARGE PLANNING AND PERSON-CENTERED CARE CONTINUITY

Fragmented patient care is a challenge for patients transitioning between care settings and increases the risk for avoidable hospitalizations (Mitchell et al., 2018). There is a call for

TABLE 6.8 RESOURCES TO HELP ENHANCE AWARENESS AND ASSESSMENT OF SOCIAL DETERMINANTS OF HEALTH

SOURCE	RESOURCE
Office of Disease Prevention and Health Promotion www.healthypeople.gov/2020/topics-objectives/topic/social-determinants-of-health	*Healthy People 2020*: Social Determinants of Health
American Academy of Family Physicians www.aafp.org/dam/AAFP/documents/patient_care/everyone_project/team-based-approach.pdf	Addressing Social Determinants of Health in Primary Care: Team-Based Approach for Advancing Health Equity Report
Centers for Disease Control and Prevention www.cdc.gov/socialdeterminants/tools/index.htm	Tools for Putting Social Determinants of Health Into Action

research on improved patient communication handoffs to avoid common mistakes that can occur during transitions in care (Gordon et al., 2018). Hospitals are implementing various PCC discharge planning initiatives and comprehensive programs, such as the Road to Home Program (Wilson-Smith et al., 2018) and Vancouver 3M Clinical Pathway (Wood et al., 2019) to facilitate safe patient discharges that will support patients in their transition from hospital to home and prevent unnecessary readmissions to the hospital (AHRQ, 2016). For example, the Vancouver 3M Clinical Pathway uses stringent inclusion/exclusion criteria for patients receiving a transfemoral transcatheter aortic valve replacement with a criteria-driven discharge plan. Programs like these provide toolkits with various interventions and practices that can help with successful PCC and discharge planning. Research shows there are five top strategies to consider implementing to decrease hospitalization readmissions (Kash et al., 2018; Box 6.6).

BOX 6.6 Five Top Strategies to Decrease Hospitalization Readmissions

Collaboration with clinical teams and community providers

- Working together with other clinical teams for effective discharge process for patients

Post-discharge home visits

- Physical visits by healthcare provider to patient's home

Telephone follow-up calls

- Follow-up monitoring telephone communication for patient self-care management and education post-discharge

Patient/family education

- Patient-directed education or coaching to increase patient/family's knowledge and involvement in care

Appropriate discharge planning

- Ensuring appropriate communication between interprofessional team and patient/patient's network; evaluating patient's/family's abilities for self-care

Source: Adapted from Kash, B. A., Baek, J., Cheon, O., Coleman, N. E., & Jones, S. L. (2018). Successful hospital readmission reduction initiatives: Top five strategies to consider implementing today. *Journal of Hospital Administration*, 7(6), 16–23. https://doi.org/10.5430/jha.v7n6p16

Real World Interview

As a nurse, your caring hands help heal patients. Your gentle words inspire patients to get well, and your tender heart touches many when a cure isn't meant to be. Most of us, at some point, entrust our life, or the lives of a loved one, to a team of clinicians, anchored by the compassionate, unfailing care of a nurse.

Research tells us that PCC goes hand-in-hand with safety and quality by contributing to better clinical outcomes and increased adherence with recommended treatments, leading to fewer complications and fewer hospitalizations. We know that PCC promotes partnerships and brings to light the voices of our patients by integrating their values, their individual experiences, and their personal perspectives to achieve better outcomes.

Are you embedding the tenets of PCC in the care of your patients—every person, every encounter, every time? Are you helping to create a safe environment by encouraging your patients to speak up? As a nurse, isn't this what you want for your own care and for that of your loved ones?

Julie Ginn Moretz, BS
Chief Experience Officer, Assistant Vice President
Patient- and Family-Centered Care, Augusta University Health, Augusta, Georgia

Despite using the previously noted strategies, discharge planning is complex and must be individualized to each patient using a PCC approach. The nurse should identify and provide potential supportive resources specific to patient needs. Better understanding the patient's unique wishes and needs allows for the discharge plan to be tailored to improve patient adherence to a mutually agreed upon plan of care.

PATIENT NAVIGATORS

A **patient navigator** is a clinical nursing staff member who is paired with a patient at the time of admission to support, educate, and facilitate the patient's interactions throughout their hospitalization, experience of care, treatment, and discharge from the hospital. Patient navigators coordinate PCC among many members of the interprofessional team. The patient navigator relationship is maintained until the patient is discharged. Several research studies have shown that the use of patient navigators leads to enhanced patient outcomes, especially for poor and underserved populations, with increased patient satisfaction and lowered healthcare costs and helps with connections to needed primary care services (Mailloux & Halesey, 2018; McBrien et al., 2018; Peart et al., 2018). Patient navigators are frequently used for patients who may experience barriers related to SDoH regarding management and access to appropriate health services.

CURRENT LITERATURE

CITATION

Mitchell, S. E., Laurens, V., Weigel, G. M., Hirschman, K. B., Scott, A. M., Nguyen, H. Q., Howard, J. M., Laird, L., Levine, C., Davis, T. C., Gass, B, Sbaid, E., Li, J., Williams, M. V., & Jack, B W. (2018). Care transitions from patient and caregiver perspectives. *The Annals of Family Medicine, 16*(3), 225–231. https://doi.org/10.1370/afm.2222

DISCUSSION

The transition from hospital to home can be a complex process for patients and caregivers. There is little research on the perspectives of patients and caregivers in transitioning home and the aspects of the process that are vital to them. Three desired outcomes and five desired care transition services emerged from qualitative focus groups and interviews with patients and caregivers regarding their experiences during care transitions. The three desired outcomes were for the patient to:

1. Feel cared for and cared about by healthcare providers,
2. Have unambiguous accountability from the healthcare system, and
3. Feel prepared and capable of implementing care plans.

The five desired care transition services were to have all staff:

1. Use empathetic language and gestures,
2. Anticipate the patient's and caregiver's needs to support self-care at home,
3. Receive collaborative discharge planning,
4. Provide actionable information, and
5. Provide uninterrupted care with minimal handoffs.

IMPLICATIONS FOR PRACTICE

Healthcare systems and interprofessional team members must provide patients with better preparation for discharge and care transitions. Effective communication strategies are key when educating patients and caregivers about their illness and available services. Patients and caregivers seek accountability, continuity of care, and caring attitudes from nurses and interprofessional team members during the patient's transition to home to promote a recovery that is individualized and based on PCC.

INNOVATIONS TO SUPPORT PERSON-CENTERED CARE

Several technologies exist that can help foster PCC, such as electronic health records (EHR), patient portals, and telemedicine (see Chapter 8 for more information). Additionally, the use of patient journals, patient-driven research (PDR), and online patient communities are innovations that may be beneficial in fostering PCC.

PATIENT JOURNALS

The Josie King Foundation has created a paper and electronic version of a patient care journal as a tool to help patients and their families record details of their care along with the questions to ask and important things to remember (Josie King Foundation, 2016). Hospitals can order these patient care journals to provide to patients and their families, or patients can request a care journal for themselves at the Josie King website found at https://josieking.org/jkf-tools/care-journals. This type of initiative drives PCC by empowering patients with a specific tool to facilitate active engagement in their own healthcare.

PATIENT-DRIVEN RESEARCH

PDR is an evolving phenomenon that began in the internet's earliest days. From access to online support groups to access to world-renowned healthcare centers, patients have access to an incredible amount of health information online that they can

BOX 6.7 Developing Clinical Judgment

Teresa is a 10-year-old patient diagnosed with juvenile diabetes. She has been hospitalized four times in the past year for complications related to diabetic diet noncompliance. Teresa is an only child who lives with her parents and maternal grandmother of Italian immigrant descent. Teresa and her family have been in America for 8 years; Teresa and her parents have mastered the English language, and Teresa has been a particularly good student. Her parents work on the assembly line at the same factory. Several interprofessional team members have counseled Teresa and her parents on the risks involved with diabetes and dietary noncompliance. Teresa and her parents understand the importance of following her prescribed diabetic diet. The nurse notices that Teresa's grandmother spends a great deal of time with her and appears quite agitated by the fact that her granddaughter is "not getting better." Her grandmother expresses concern to the nurse about Teresa being readmitted to the hospital yet again.

1. What **CUES (Assessment)** can the interprofessional team assess regarding this situation?
2. What **HYPOTHESIS (Diagnosis)** would the interprofessional team consider?
3. Within a PCC environment, how could the interprofessional team approach Teresa's grandmother?
4. How will the interprofessional team evaluate the patient's **OUTCOME (Evaluation)** related to knowledge deficit and Teresa's diabetic diet compliance?
5. How might the SDoH and health literacy play a role in Teresa's health and providing PCC?

now use to become an active member of the interprofessional team to promote PCC (www.pcori.org).

PDR also involves patients as participants in clinical outcomes, research questions, research data, and communities of scientific inquiry. PDR is an investigative process undertaken by the patient in conjunction with clinical leaders at special meetings, conferences, or at sign-ups to participate in research. These activities can help foster PCC by engaging and incorporating patients in understanding their illness, research opportunities, and treatment modalities. See Table 6.9 for examples of several organizations that support PDR.

TABLE 6.9 EXAMPLES OF ORGANIZATIONS THAT SUPPORT PATIENT-DRIVEN RESEARCH

SUPPORTING ORGANIZATIONS	WEBSITE
Patient-Centered Outcomes Research Institute	www.pcori.org/blog/textbook-example-patient-driven-research
National Opinion Research Center at the University of Chicago	www.norc.org/Research/Projects/Pages/patient-driven-research-community-learning-network-coordination-.aspx
Metastatic Prostate Cancer Project	https://mpcproject.org https://cancerdiscovery.aacrjournals.org/content/8/5/OF4
Rare UK Disease Study (RUDY)	https://ojrd.biomedcentral.com/articles/10.1186/s13023-016-0528-6

ONLINE E-PATIENT COMMUNITIES

Healthcare information online allows interested patients to be more informed about their choices and raises their level of expectations for quality care and safety when seeking healthcare services. Many online health communities exist, offering opportunities for patients to share experiences and learn about diseases and treatments. The term "**e-patient**" has been coined to identify this new trend of informed healthcare consumers who are equipped, enabled, empowered, and engaged in their health and healthcare decisions. Healthcare has responded to this trend through the development and diffusion of several online health communities. Research regarding the measurement of usage and usefulness of online health communities shows that the perceived usefulness, satisfaction, and continuance of use of them is determined by three variables external to the patient (social support, information quality, and quality in service provided; Wu, 2018). This research result adds to the growing body of evidence that patients need support from members of the interprofessional team and caregivers, as well as appropriate high-quality information pertinent to their health concerns, and quality in the service provided. See Table 6.10 for practices to address challenges that are unique to members of online patient communities.

LEGISLATION THAT SUPPORTS PATIENT-CENTERED CARE PRACTICES

The United States has initiated several legislative efforts to support PCC practices. These legislative efforts facilitate PCC by providing care that is collaborative, benefits the patient's interests, seeks to coordinate care between all members of the interprofessional team, and makes primary, secondary, and tertiary care accessible and affordable. Each of

TABLE 6.10 CHALLENGES AND PRACTICES TO ADDRESS CHALLENGES

CHALLENGES	PRACTICES TO ADDRESS CHALLENGES
Passion - Individuals may share or argue varying beliefs that may not be applicable to others.	Use of meaningful and positive semantics to ensure communication is appropriate and applicable to all members of the online community may be helpful.
Nonmedical Advice - Online community members may share experiences that may be taken by others as medical advice.	Use of instructive practices to question nonmedical advice or inaccurate advice can help patients ensure that members are cautioned regarding the risks of inaccurate advice.
Personal Information - Sharing information must be done carefully as to not violate privacy or the Health Insurance Portability and Accountability Act (HIPAA).	Persons should ensure shared information meets HIPAA guidelines; healthcare providers should encourage online members to use reflective techniques with healthcare information and begin building a personal health record (PHR).
Community Participation - Lack of participation from online community or engagement within members can hinder communication and relationships.	Encourage participants to build relationships and engage with other members of online patient community; ensure patients are still seeking follow-up appointments with healthcare provider and discussing treatment option findings from online community with healthcare provider.

Source: Data from Skousen, T., Safadi, H., Young, C., Karahanna, E., Safadi, S., & Chebib, F. (2020). Successful moderation in online patient communities: Inductive case study. *Journal of Medical Internet Research, 22*(3), e15983. http://www.jmir.org/2020/3/e15983

the legislative efforts discussed in the text that follows relates to PCC because they strategize how to appropriately provide PCC to patients needing care in various settings and with differing needs.

PATIENT PROTECTION AND AFFORDABLE CARE ACT

In March 2010, Congress passed the PPACA, which increases access to health insurance coverage, expands federal health insurance market requirements, and includes measures to improve the delivery and quality of care (www.innovations.cms.gov). PPACA is being implemented in several ways through new agency programs, grants, demonstration projects, and regulations. Under PPACA, the Centers for Medicare and Medicaid Innovation has been established to pilot payment and service delivery models driven by the need for quality PCC and fiscal responsibility (2020). The original PPACA included a tax penalty as an individual mandate for U.S. citizens who did not obtain health insurance. The purpose of the tax penalty mandate was to encourage more people to obtain health insurance for preventative care, as well as to keep PPACA premiums low. In 2017, legislation was passed that eliminated the tax penalty mandate for U.S. citizens who did not have health insurance. As of 2021, a Supreme Court hearing is pending to confirm the constitutionality of the PPACA based on the mandate individuals have to pay as a penalty tax for being uninsured. A resolution is not likely to occur until 2022 (Keith, 2019).

PATIENT-CENTERED MEDICAL HOME

The Patient-Centered Medical Home (PCMH) is a care delivery model whereby patient treatment is coordinated through their primary care physician to ensure patients receive the necessary care when and where they need it, in a manner the patient can understand. The objective is to have a centralized setting that facilitates partnerships between individual patients, their personal physicians, and, when appropriate, the patient's family. Care is facilitated by registries, information technology, health information exchanges, and other means to assure that patients get the indicated care when and where they need and want it in a culturally and linguistically appropriate manner (American College of Physicians, n.d.).

The use of the PCMH explicitly relates to PCC because it strategizes how providers and organizations can assess and incorporate a person's values and preferences into their care. As healthcare reformers seek to improve patient outcomes and reduce costs, the PCMH has become a major strategy in the transformation of primary care and the healthcare system in general (Jolles et al., 2019). The PCMH Model has many core functions and health interventions (Table 6.11) and can be adopted by any facility to offer the core functions of accessible, coordinated, high-quality, comprehensive, patient-centered care.

PATIENT-CENTERED PRIMARY CARE COLLABORATIVE

In 2006, the Patient-Centered Primary Care Collaborative (PCPCC) emerged after several large national employers sought the assistance of the American Academy of Family Physicians (AAFP) and other primary care physician groups to address the issue of a failing system of comprehensive primary care. The goals of the PCPCC were to enable improvements in patient–physician relations and develop a more effective and efficient model of care delivery. The PCPCC has taken a significant interest in the development and advocacy of the PCMH Model to ensure the delivery of only the highest standards of effective and efficient PCC (PCPCC, 2019).

TABLE 6.11 PATIENT-CENTERED MEDICAL HOME CARE FUNCTIONS AND HEALTH INTERVENTIONS

1. Accessible Care	• Offer enhanced options for access to in-person care o In-person care outside of traditional business hours o Schedule same day appointments • Facilitate and document remote access to health consultation/clinical advice o 24/7 Patient access to clinical advice o 24/7 On-call patient access to PCMH team • Create written processes and defined standards to facilitate patient access to their EHR o Online patient portals o Secure electronic messaging
2. Coordinated Care	• Create an infrastructure to exchange information via shared records o EHRs to access, document, and share patient data • Provide guidance to patients to navigate and cooperate within a team-based care approach o Tracking and follow-up for all tests and results, with identified time frames for notifying patients of results o Regular case review meetings with interprofessional team • Create explicit workforce agreements regarding division of labor o Dedicated care manager who is responsible for overall management of patient's care plan o Clear process for providing care management services
3. Committed to Quality Care	• Deliver care guided by evidence-based principles o Document clinic-wide improvement strategy with performance goals • Enable a system for decision support and education to facilitate use of evidence o Electronic prescribing o Evidence-based clinical decision-making tools • Track population health status and create mechanisms to encourage/achieve health promotion and prevention o Registry and risk stratification tools to assess health status and needs of the entire practice o Performance reports to track and compare results for the established population of patients in the practice • Monitor and measure care as delivered to assure adherence to evidence-based standards o Health home provider makes use of available HIT (health information technology) and accesses data through the regional health information organization/qualified entity
4. Comprehensive Care	• Identify needs and services on health continuum, including social and behavioral needs o Care plans that are longitudinal and meet patients' complex healthcare needs o Care plans that include community-based and other social support services • Establish sources of services and arrangements to deliver and document service delivery o Policies and procedures to support effective collaborations with community-based resources o Screening strategy for mental health, substance use, and developmental conditions with documentation of onsite and local referral resources

(continued)

TABLE 6.11 PATIENT-CENTERED MEDICAL HOME CARE FUNCTIONS AND HEALTH INTERVENTIONS *(continued)*

5. Patient-Centered Care	• Assess patient values, needs, and preferences o Written materials published in primary language of the community o Providers or telephone trained interpreters speak a patient and family's language of choice • Take patient values and preferences into account to design and deliver care o Care plan identifies family members and other supports involved in the patient's care o PCMH-related communication tools • Foster relationship-based care vs. impersonal care with an orientation to whole person care o Patient-centered care planning to engage patients in their care o Peer supports, support groups, and self-care programs to engage patients in their care • Educate and support patients in learning to manage their own care and fully participate in care decisions o Strategies for patient/family's participation in a healthcare decision using informed and shared decision-making o Individualized care plan for patients includes complex medical and social concerns

EHR, electronic health record; PCMH, patient-centered medical home.

Source: From Jolles, M. P., Lengnick-Hall, R., & Mittman, B. S. (2019). Core functions and forms of complex health interventions: A patient-centered medical home illustration. *Journal of General Internal Medicine, 34*(6), 1032–1038. https://doi.org/10.1007/s11606-018-4818-7

MEDICAID HEALTH HOMES

The PPACA also provides financial incentives to states for the development of Medicaid Health Homes (CMS, 2021b). Health Homes, provided to Medicaid beneficiaries with chronic health needs, are designed to be PCC models that enable access to and coordination of comprehensive medical, behavioral health, and long-term healthcare services and supports needed by Medicaid beneficiaries with chronic health needs.

The Medicaid Health Homes Model is different from the PCMH Model because Medicaid Health Homes focus on comprehensive care for patients with multiple chronic conditions needing secondary and tertiary care and it is managed by CMS rather than by the patient's primary care provider. The Medicaid Health Home supports the CMS's approach to improving healthcare by improving the patient's care experience, improving the health of populations, and reducing the costs of healthcare (CMS, 2021b). Medicaid Health Homes do not occur in a physical home but they connect Medicaid beneficiaries with resources to assist with finding a healthcare provider, mental health assistance, substance abuse clinic, medication assistance and education, housing assistance, social services, and community programs.

Nurses may work or partner with state, national, or stakeholder-driven organizations in the role of linking eligible patients with Medicaid Health Homes in their area. The implementation of Medicaid Health Homes is expected to reduce emergency room use, reduce hospital admissions and readmissions, reduce healthcare costs, and help patients become less reliant on long-term facilities while improving overall patient satisfaction and quality outcomes (Medicaid.gov, n.d.).

PERSON-CENTERED CARE MEASURES TO MONITOR QUALITY HEALTHCARE

Monitoring quality improvement (QI) and measuring patient satisfaction are important to evaluate the effectiveness of PCC delivery. Nurses should use information from hospital quality indicators and patient satisfaction surveys to guide their evidence-based care. By incorporating both this evidence and the patient's preferences, nurses can foster PCC that promotes safety, quality, and individualized care. A summary of strategies for QI, surveys to measure patient satisfaction, and measures of quality outcomes as they relate to PCC is discussed in the text that follows.

STRATEGY FOR QUALITY IMPROVEMENT IN HEALTHCARE

The secretary of the United States Department of Health and Human Services (USDHHS) has established a National Strategy for Quality Improvement in Healthcare in conjunction with AHRQ to set priorities that guide the nation to increase access to high-quality, person- and family-centered, affordable healthcare for all Americans (AHRQ, 2016; Table 6.12).

TABLE 6.12 NATIONAL STRATEGY FOR QUALITY IMPROVEMENT IN HEALTHCARE

PRIORITY	ACTIONS
1. **Patient Safety:** Making care safer by reducing the harm caused in the delivery of care	Exercise relentless efforts to reduce risk for injury from care. Aim for ZERO harm to patients. Create healthcare systems that reliably provide high-quality care.
2. **Patient- and Family-Centered Care:** Ensuring that each person and family are engaged as partners in their care	Give patients and families an active role in their care. Adapt care to individual and family situations, cultures, languages, disabilities, and health literacy levels.
3. **Care Coordination:** Promoting effective communication and coordination of care	Develop processes and use technology to provide seamless care, that is, electronic health record (EHR), e-prescribing, telemedicine. Eliminate healthcare gaps and duplication of care. Use effective care models to facilitate coordination and communication across the continuum of care.
4. **Effective Prevention and Treatment:** Promoting effective prevention and treatment practices for the leading causes of mortality, starting with cardiovascular disease	Practice key interventions for cardiovascular disease, that is, ABCS–aspirin, blood pressure control, cholesterol reduction, and smoking cessation
5. **Healthy Living:** Working with communities to promote wide use of best practices to enable healthy living	Create strong partnerships between local healthcare providers, public health professionals, and individuals. Provide clinical preventive services and increase adoption of evidence-based interventions.
6. **Care Affordability:** Making quality care more affordable for individuals, families, employers, and governments by developing and spreading new healthcare delivery models	Ensure the right care is provided at the right time for the right patient. Reduce healthcare-acquired conditions. Reform payment structures, reduce waste. Establish health insurance exchanges to improve cost of insurance for individuals and small businesses.

Source: From Agency for Healthcare Research and Quality. (2016). *2015 national healthcare quality and disparities report and 5th anniversary update on the national quality strategy* [AHRQ Publication No. 16-0015]. Author. https://www.ahrq.gov/research/findings/nhqrdr/nhqdr15/priorities.html

PATIENT SATISFACTION

Tangible, measurable patient outcomes, such as infection rates, are an important indicator of the quality of care patients have received. However, patient satisfaction with the care that has been provided is now also recognized as another quality indicator. Patient satisfaction provides powerful feedback about PCC and how respected and valued a patient felt as well as how engaged the patient was in the development of their plan of care. Medicare, Medicaid, and private insurance companies place a financial value on patient satisfaction through incentive payments to acute care hospitals based on meeting quality patient satisfaction scores compared to other facilities and showing baseline improvement within a facility (CMS, 2021a).

The goal to keep the patient's preferences, values, and needs paramount starts with a healthcare culture focused on the specific intention of asking for the patient's voice, honoring it, and ensuring that it is respected. The nurse has several roles with patient satisfaction related to communication, education, comfort, and anticipatory guidance (Lotfi et al., 2019). Several PCC examples include the nurse discussing the plan of care with the patient and family, assessing the patient's physical comfort, and seeking out opportunities to meet special needs of patients. Many agencies provide PCC resources to help patients and institutions (Tables 6.13 and 6.14).

PATIENT SATISFACTION SURVEYS

Two surveys are used most often in hospitals to monitor patient satisfaction (i.e., the Hospital Consumer Assessment of Health Care Providers and Systems [HCAHPS] Survey and the Press Ganey Survey). These two surveys measure patient satisfaction within the hospital as well as in comparison to other hospitals.

TABLE 6.13 AGENCIES THAT PROVIDE PERSON-CENTERED CARE RESOURCES FOR PATIENTS AND INSTITUTIONS

AGENCY	PCC RESOURCE
Institute for Healthcare Improvement, www.ihi.org/resources/Pages/Tools/PatientCenteredCareImprovementGuide.aspx	Patient-Centered Care Improvement Guide
Institute for Patient- and Family-Centered Care, www.ipfcc.org/resources/Patient-Centered-Care-The-Road-Ahead.pdf	Booklet, Patient Centered Care, The Road Ahead, The Picker Institute,
National Academy of Medicine, www.healthaffairs.org/doi/10.1377/hlthaff.2020.02204	Article, Vital Directions for Health and Health Care: Priorities for 2021, including: • Health costs and financing, • Early childhood and maternal health, • Mental health and addiction, • Better health and healthcare for older adults, and • Infectious disease threats.
Planetree International, https://planetree.org/planetree-certification-criteria	Discussion of nonprofit organization that offers PCC consulting services to support a healthcare organization at any of the stages of Planetree Certification Criteria.

TABLE 6.14 PLANETREE INTERNATIONAL'S PERSON-CENTERED CARE HOSPITAL CERTIFICATION PROGRAM ELEMENTS

Create organizational structure that promotes engagement	• Develop interprofessional PCC oversight group • Use team-based model to guide PCC implementation • Foster communication between stakeholders and partnerships between leadership, and staff • Engage staff in PCC and incorporate into job descriptions, performance evaluation systems, recognition programs, and new hire screening • Minimize barriers to incorporating PCC
Connect values, strategies, and action	• Connect goals and objectives to PCC and to the mission/vision of organization • Ensure leadership and staff participate in experiences to connect concepts of PCC to care provided • Create partnerships with community institutions to address the SDoH

Implement practices that promote partnership	• Incorporate communication practices to promote active involvement of patients/families:
	  • Utilize shift-to-shift communication
	  • Foster interdepartmental/interprofessional communication
	  • Communicate across levels of care
	  • Participate in care planning conferences
	  • Provide discharge planning and education based on patient-preferred learning styles, cultures, and literacy levels

Know what matters	• Incorporate patient goals into care planning and shared decision-making • Support staff with emotional and grief support, health promotion, and decision-making capability functional to role
Use evidence to drive improvement	• Measure data on: O Clinical quality performance O Patient safety O Patient experience of care O Staff engagement, satisfaction, and experience O Organizational indicators of efficiency and excellence

PCC, person-centered care, SDoH, social determinants of health.

Source: Data from Planetree. (2018). *Planetree certification criteria*. https://planetree.org/planetree-certification-criteria

In 2005, the National Quality Forum, a national organization of healthcare stakeholders, consumer organizations, public and private purchasers, physicians, nurses, hospitals, accreditation/certification bodies, supporting industries, healthcare researchers, and QI organizations, endorsed the HCAHPS (pronounced H-CAPS) survey (Exhibit 6.1). The intent of this HCAHPS survey is to provide a standard instrument to be used by hospitals across the nation to measure patients' satisfaction with their hospital experience. The HCAHPS survey asks a core set of standardized questions to assess patient satisfaction with their care by members of the interprofessional team, responsiveness of hospital staff, pain management, communication about medicines, cleanliness, and quietness of the hospital environment. These standardized questions allow valid comparisons of patient care experience at hospitals locally, regionally, and nationally. Use of the HCAHPS survey, the Press Ganey Survey, and measurements of patient outcomes are currently being used as

EXHIBIT 6.1 SAMPLE OF HOSPITAL CONSUMER ASSESSMENT OF HEALTH CARE PROVIDERS AND SYSTEMS SURVEY QUESTIONS

	ANSWER OPTIONS
During this hospital stay, how often did nurses treat you with courtesy and respect?	1. Never 2. Sometimes 3. Usually 4. Always
During this hospital stay, how often did doctors listen carefully to you?	1. Never 2. Sometimes 3. Usually 4. Always
Before giving you any new medicine, how often did hospital staff tell you what the medicine was for?	1. Never 2. Sometimes 3. Usually 4. Always
During this hospital stay, did doctors, nurses, or other hospital staff talk with you about whether you would have the help you needed when you left the hospital?	1. Yes 2. No
During this hospital stay, staff took my preferences and those of my family or caregiver into account in deciding what my healthcare needs would be when I left.	1. Strongly disagree 2. Disagree 3. Agree 4. Strongly agree
When I left the hospital, I had a good understanding of the things I was responsible for in managing my health.	1. Strongly disagree 2. Disagree 3. Agree 4. Strongly agree

Source: Centers for Medicare and Medicaid Services. (2021). *HCAHPS survey*. https://hcahpsonline.org/globalassets/hcahps/survey-instruments/mail/effective-december-1-2021-and-forward-discharges/2021_survey-instruments_english_mail_updateda.pdf

indicators of quality care to reward or withhold Medicare payments. The HCAHPS survey is focused on three areas:

1. The patients' perception of care that allows objective and meaningful comparisons of hospitals on topics important to patients.
2. Public reporting of results, which provides an incentive for hospitals to improve the quality of care.
3. Public reporting, which also enhances accountability in healthcare by increasing transparency of the quality of the care provided (HCAHPS, 2021).

Since 2008, the HCAHPS survey patient satisfaction scores have been available to the public on the CMS Hospital Compare website that can be found at www.medicare.gov/HomeHealthCompare/search.aspx. Exhibit 6.2 has a sample of the HCAHPS survey questions.

Press Ganey is another survey used to gauge patient satisfaction Exhibit 6.2. The Press Ganey survey includes the HCAHPS survey questions to provide a comprehensive assessment of what the patient experienced and felt while hospitalized, collecting both objective and subjective data. Hospitals are not required to use the Press Ganey survey. While the HCAHPS survey focuses on measuring "how often a service is provided," the Press Ganey survey aims to capture how well that service was delivered and perceived by the patient.

EXHIBIT 6.2 SAMPLE OF PRESS GANEY SURVEY

QUESTIONS	ANSWER OPTIONS
1. Friendliness/courtesy of the care provider	1. Very Poor 2. Poor 3. Fair 4. Good 5. Very Good
2. Explanation the care provider gave about your problem or condition	1. Very Poor 2. Poor 3. Fair 4. Good 5. Very Good
3. Concern the care provider showed for your questions or worries	1. Very Poor 2. Poor 3. Fair 4. Good 5. Very Good
4. Care provider's efforts to include you in decisions about your treatment	1. Very Poor 2. Poor 3. Fair 4. Good 5. Very Good
5. Information the care provider gave you about medications (if any)	1. Very Poor 2. Poor 3. Fair 4. Good 5. Very Good
6. Instructions the care provider gave you about follow-up care (if any)	1. Very Poor 2. Poor 3. Fair 4. Good 5. Very Good
7. Degree to which care provider talked with you using words you could understand	1. Very Poor 2. Poor 3. Fair 4. Good 5. Very Good
8. Amount of time the care provider spent with you	1. Very Poor 2. Poor 3. Fair 4. Good 5. Very Good
9. Instructions the care provider gave you about follow-up care (if any)	1. Very Poor 2. Poor 3. Fair 4. Good 5. Very Good

For more information, see https://www.wakehealth.edu/About-Us/Quality-and-Awards/Quality-and-Safety-Measures/Patient-Experience/About-the-Press-Ganey-Patient-Experience-Survey

END-OF-CHAPTER RESOURCES

KEY CONCEPTS

1. PCC is an inclusive process that promotes the paradigm shift from physician-directed care to the needs, preferences, customs, and values of each person related to their healthcare decisions and wellness.
2. PCC involves recognizing the patient's control over their healthcare decisions and advocating for coordinated care that respects the patient's preferences, values, and needs.
3. Several structures exist to aid organizations with PCC, such as Picker's Eight Principles of Patient-Centered Care, QSEN PCC competency, and the WHO Framework for PCC.
4. Empathetic communication is the ability to communicate with someone else from their vantage point based on their feelings, values, and perspectives. Utilizing these feelings, values, and perspectives based on the patient's needs, wants, and culture help to facilitate effective communication and planning for healthcare decisions that match the patient's desires.
5. The nurse must include the assessment and inclusion of the patient's self-concept and cultural considerations during the care planning and decision-making process.
6. Health literacy, cultural competence, and shared decision-making are all helpful strategies that can help to support both patients' and caregivers' engagement in healthcare decisions.
7. Shared decision-making is a collaborative process that involves providing the patient with information at an understandable level regarding the risks and benefits of all available treatments to facilitate a patient-driven decision.
8. Patient decision aids are tools that healthcare providers can use to help guide patients in informed decision-making by providing them with all available options and relevant information.
9. Assessment measures must be in place for healthcare providers to properly ask questions regarding the SDoH. Healthcare providers must effectively communicate and initiate referrals, and the care plan must reflect assessment and interventions for SDoH-related concerns.
10. Discharge planning begins upon admission and involves the use of patient education, patient navigators, advocacy, and involving patients and caregivers in healthcare decisions. Appropriate, individualized discharge planning is paramount to decreasing rehospitalizations, ensuring positive patient outcomes, and managing reimbursements for facilities and hospitals.
11. Innovations that may be used to enhance the patient experience include patient journals, patient-driven research, online patient communities, and telemedicine. As technology continues to grow, the various strategies used in healthcare must evolve to fit each patient's needs.
12. PCC is highly affected by legislative efforts regarding insurance, medical reimbursement, and restrictions to healthcare. Currently, the PPACA facilitates PCC. However, the individual tax mandate and credibility of the PPACA is currently under review by the Supreme Court regarding if it will be overturned. Only time will tell what the outcome of this situation will be. Healthcare providers and clinicians must continue to evolve their practice based on legislative changes.

13. The National Strategy for Quality Improvement in Health Care, in conjunction with AHRQ, is the organization which sets priorities that guide the nation to increase access to high-quality PCC.
14. Several measurements are used for reimbursement based on patient outcomes and satisfaction and include HCAHPS and Press Ganey. Positive patient outcomes and experiences are now vital for hospitals to ensure appropriate reimbursement for healthcare services to effectively manage the facility.

CRITICAL DISCUSSION POINTS

1. What factors are a part of PCC, and who is involved in PCC strategies? How might stakeholders be involved in PCC?
2. What key communication techniques can nurses use to care for patients from diverse backgrounds?
3. What is one key strategy related to patient education that nurses can use to support PCC? Discuss how the strategy may be used.
4. How can government organizations empower nurses and the interprofessional team to foster PCC?
5. What are some important strategies learned from the chapter that each member of the interprofessional team could use to foster PCC?
6. How are patient outcomes and patient satisfaction used to measure PCC within facilities?

KEY TERMS

> Advocacy
> Cultural competence
> E-patient
> Empathetic communication
> Empathy
> Health literacy
> Patient decision aids
> Patient navigator
> Person-centered care
> Self-concept
> Shared decision-making
> Sympathy

REVIEW QUESTIONS

Answers to Review Questions appear in the Instructor's Manual. Qualified instructors should request the Instructor's Manual from textbook@springerpub.com.

1. A nurse will attend a seminar discussing the topic of including patients and their families and significant others in healthcare decision-making at an interprofessional healthcare conference. What will most likely be the primary topic of the seminar?

   A. Primary care

   B. Medical Homes

   C. Interprofessional team approach

   D. Person-centered care

2. The nurse wants to use a person-centered approach to perform patient care. Which of the following best describes the nurse's approach?

A. Developing friendships with patients as a means of providing better care
B. Creating an environment of coworkers committed to helping each other
C. Providing care through the eyes of the patient
D. Understanding the nurse's role within the interprofessional team

3. The nurse is preparing to review discharge instructions with a patient. The nurse instructs the patient regarding medications and wound care for her foot. During the nurse's evaluation of patient learning, which of the following indicates the patient understands the discharge instructions?

A. The patient signs the discharge instruction sheet.
B. When asked by the nurse, the patient denies any questions or concerns.
C. The patient asks for new prescriptions for the pharmacy.
D. The nurse observes the patient changing the dressing on her foot wound.

4. When rounding, the nurse discovers that a patient in isolation has soiled the bed. Upon inquiry, the patient indicated that he did not want to bother the nurse because she was busy. How can the nurse most effectively communicate that she is available to the patient?

A. Remind the patient frequently to use the call bell.
B. Ensure that all the patient's needs have been met before leaving the patient's room, avoid appearing rushed, and let the patient know when the nurse will return.
C. Go in and out of patients' rooms to ensure the patients are aware that the nurse is available.
D. Educate the patient to call the front desk when necessary.

5. The nurse is caring for a patient who has multiple chronic conditions and has been hospitalized twice in the last month. The patient has a complex medication regimen, limited family support, and admits to having missed his last two physician appointments because he did not have transportation. What is the benefit of a referral to a Health Home for this patient?

A. Referrals always lower rehospitalization rates.
B. Complex cases are not managed through home health.
C. Home care services will enhance patient satisfaction.
D. Comprehensive care management enables access to and coordination of care.

6. A nurse is reviewing discharge instructions with a patient. The patient asks the nurse about a cardiac medication he forgot to list upon admission. Which action by the nurse is most appropriate when reviewing discharge medications?

A. Explain to the patient that he should follow up with his primary physician within 7 days to review the medication regimen.
B. Contact the physician to relay the discrepancy and receive direction regarding the discharge instructions before discharge.
C. Instruct the patient to take only the medications listed on the discharge instructions.
D. Advise the patient to continue taking the medication until he sees his primary physician.

7. A patient newly diagnosed with breast cancer is asking in-depth questions about her diagnosis and is sharing what she has found online that has worked for other patients. The nurse recognizes that this patient represents a growing number of informed healthcare consumers. Which intervention by the nurse demonstrates support for the patient's involvement in her care? *Select all that apply.*

   A. Caution the patient about inaccurate information that may be available on the internet.

   B. Instruct the patient to discuss her findings and potential treatment options with the medical provider.

   C. Advise the patient to begin building a personal health record (PHR).

   D. Explain to the patient the importance of regular checkups to identify any changes in condition.

   E. Encourage the patient to seek out natural remedies to replace some of her medical care.

8. Which of the following actions demonstrates an understanding of the nurse's role with patient satisfaction? *Select all that apply.*

   A. The nurse discusses the plan of care with the patient and family.

   B. The nurse asks about the patient's comfort with the room temperature and desire for a meal.

   C. At the change of shift, the nurse makes rounds with the oncoming nurse and introduces the new nurse to the patient.

   D. The nurse obtains permission for the patient's pet to visit after the nurse overhears the patient express that she misses her dog and is afraid she will not see it again.

   E. The nurse tells the patient to fill out the patient survey she will receive after discharge and make sure to rate her experience as excellent if the nurse met her needs.

9. A non-English-speaking patient arrives in the emergency department and is noted to be crying quietly. Which of the following is the most important action for the nurse to consider in initially providing care for this patient?

   A. Expressions and interpretations of caring may be perceived differently across cultures.

   B. Therapeutic touch is a universal communication of caring.

   C. Cultural competence includes looking patients in the eye and communicating in their language even if through an interpreter.

   D. Nurses should not consider the patient's cultural beliefs when providing care.

10. The nurse manager in the surgical step-down unit at a large metropolitan hospital would like to evaluate the perceived effectiveness of pain management for prior patients on the unit. Which measure would best assist the nurse manager in understanding past patients' satisfaction?

    A. Home health compare data

    B. Value-based performance data

    C. HCAHPS data

    D. Sentinel event reports

REVIEW ACTIVITIES

1. During post-conference, identify any of your patient care strategies that incorporate the QSEN PCC competencies in the Appendix to enhance communication and patient care.
2. Reflect upon a past clinical/patient care experience and describe the facilitators and barriers to communication with the interprofessional team using Tables 6.3 and 6.4.
3. Using Picker's Eight Principles of Patient Centered Care in Figure 6.2, describe methods that you could use to foster person-centered care with future patients.

EXPLORING THE WEB

1. Using the QSEN PCC competency (knowledge, skills, and attitudes) in the Appendix, describe the attributes of PCC. Discuss how hospital administrations can support nurses, and healthcare providers to collaborate and provide PCC in acute and long-term care facilities.
2. Explore the web for professional sites:
   - Future of Nursing; Robert Wood Johnson Foundation, NAM at https://campaignforaction.org/resource/future-nursing-iom-report. Identify two goals of the Future of Nursing in relation to PCC.
   - Future of Nursing; Campaign for Action, NAM at https://campaignforaction.org/wp-content/uploads/2019/07/r2_CCNA-0029_2019-Dashboard-Indicator-Updates_1-29-20.pdf. Review the data for the seven corresponding indicators from the Future of Nursing dashboard, which shows an evaluation of the efforts to implement the NAM recommendations.
3. Explore websites offering patient decision-making tools in Table 6.8. List the pros and cons of one of the tools.

REFERENCES

Agency for Healthcare Research and Quality. (2016). *2015 national healthcare quality and disparities report and 5th anniversary update on the national quality strategy* [AHRQ Publication No. 16-0015]. Author. https://www.ahrq.gov/research/findings/nhqrdr/nhqdr15/priorities.html

Agency for Healthcare Research and Quality. (2019a). *Cultural competence and patient safety.* https://psnet.ahrq.gov/perspective/cultural-competence-and-patient-safety#_ednref1

Agency for Healthcare Research and Quality. (2019b). Tips & tools: Questions are the answer. https://www.ahrq.gov/patients-consumers/patient-involvement/ask-your-doctor/tips-and-tools/index.html

American Academy of Family Physicians. (2018). *Addressing social determinants of health in primary care: Team-based approach for advancing health equity.* https://www.aafp.org/dam/AAFP/documents/patient_care/everyone_project/team-based-approach.pdf

American Association of Colleges of Nursing. (2019). *AACN'S vision for academic nursing.* https://www.aacnnursing.org/Portals/42/News/White-Papers/Vision-Academic-Nursing.pdf

American College of Physicians. (n.d.). *The patient centered medical home & specialty physicians.* https://www.acponline.org/practice-resources/business-resources/payment/delivery-and-payment-models/patient-centered-medical-home/understanding-the-patient-centered-medical-home/the-patient-centered-medical-home-specialty-physicians

American Hospital Association. (n.d.). *Becoming a culturally competent health care organization.* https://www.aha.org/ahahret-guides/2013-06-18-becoming-culturally-competent-health-care-organization

Baker, Julie A. (2011). And the winner is: How principles of cognitive science resolve the plain language debate. University of Missouri-Kansas City Law Review, Forthcoming, Suffolk University Law School Research Paper No. 11-33, Available at SSRN: https://ssrn.com/abstract=1915300

Berger, Z. D., Boss, E. F., & Beach, M. S. (2017). Communication behaviors and patient autonomy in hospital care: A qualitative study. *Patient Education and Counseling, 100*(8), 1473–1481. https://doi.org/10.1016/j.pec.2017.03.006

Blodgett, T., & Petsas Blodgett, N. (2021). Patient-centered care. In P. Kelly Vana & J. Tazbir (Eds.), *Kelly Vana's nursing leadership and management* (4th ed., pp. 206–229). Wiley.

Blumenthal-Barby, J. S. (2017). 'That's the doctor's job': Overcoming patient reluctance to be involved in medical decision making. *Patient Education and Counseling, 100*(1), 14–17. https://doi.org/10.1016/j.pec.2016.07.010

Bomhof-Roordink, H., Gärtner, F. R., Stiggelbout, A. M., & Pieterse, A. H. (2019). Key components of shared decision making models: A systematic review. *BMJ Open, 9*(12), e031763. https://doi.org/10.1136/bmjopen-2019-031763

Brach, C., Keller, D., Hernandez, L. M., Baur, C., Parker, R., Dreyer, B., ... & Schillinger, D. (2012). Ten attributes of health literate health care organizations. *NAM Perspectives.* https://nam.edu/wp-content/uploads/2015/06/BPH_Ten_HLit_Attributes.pdf

Castro, E. M., Van Regenmortel, T., Vanhaecht, K., Sermeus, W., & Van Hecke, A. (2016). Patient empowerment, patient participation and patient-centeredness in hospital care: A concept analysis based on a literature review. *Patient Education and Counseling, 99*(12), 1923–1939. https://doi.org/10.1016/j.pec.2016.07.026

Centers for Disease Control and Prevention. (n.d.-a). *Tools for putting social determinants of health into action.* https://www.cdc.gov/socialdeterminants/tools/index.htm

Centers for Disease Control and Prevention. (n.d.-b). *Understanding health literacy.* https://www.cdc.gov/healthliteracy/learn/Understanding.html

Centers for Medicare and Medicaid Services. (2020). *Centers for Medicare and Medicaid innovation.* http://www.innovations.cms.gov

Centers for Medicare and Medicaid Services. (2021a). *Hospital quality initiative.* https://www.cms.gov/Medicare/Quality-Initiatives-Patient-Assessment-Instruments/HospitalQualityInits/index?redirect=/hospitalqualityinits/30_hospitalhcahps.asp

Centers for Medicare and Medicaid Services. (2021b). *Medicaid health homes: An overview.* https://www.medicaid.gov/state-resource-center/medicaid-state-technical-assistance/health-home-information-resource-center/downloads/hh-overview-fact-sheet.pdf

Cronenwett, L., Sherwood, G., Barnsteiner, J., Disch, J., Johnson, J., Mitchell, P., Sullivan, D. T., & Warren, J. (2007). Quality and Safety Education for Nurses. *Nursing Outlook, 55*(3), 122–131. https://doi.org/10.1016/j.outlook.2007.02.006

Department of Health and Human Services. (2012). *Plain writing act compliance report.* https://www.hhs.gov/sites/default/files/hhs-2021-plain-writing-act-compliance-rpt.pdf

DeWalt, D. A., Broucksou, K. A., Hawk, V., Brach, C., Hink, A., Rudd, R., & Callahan, L. (2011). Developing and testing the health literacy universal precautions toolkit. *Nursing outlook, 59*(2), 85–94.

ECRI Institute. (2019, May 21). Patient-centered care in acute care. *Healthcare Risk Control.* https://www.ecri.org/components/HRC/Pages/RiskQual7.aspx#

Eklund, J. H., Holmström, I. K., Kumlin, T., Kaminsky, E., Skoglund, K., Höglander, J., Sundler, A., Conden, E., & Merenius, M. S. (2019). "Same or different?" A review of reviews of person-centred and patient-centred care. *Patient Education and Counseling, 102*(1), 3–11. https://doi.org/10.1016/j.pec.2018.08.029

Elwyn, G., Durand, M. A., Song, J., Aarts, J., Barr, P. J., Berger, Z., Cochran, N., Frosch, D., Galasiński, D., Gulbrandsen, P., Han, P. K. J., Härter, M., Kinnersley, P., Lloyd, A., Mishra, M., Perestelo-Perez, L., Scholl, I., Tomori, K., Trevena, L., ... Van der Weijden, T. (2017). A three-talk model for shared decision making: Multistage consultation process. *BMJ, 359*, j4891. https://doi.org/10.1136/bmj.j4891

Gaines, K. (2020, September 4). *What is the nursing code of ethics?* Nurse. https://nurse.org/education/nursing-code-of-ethics

Gordon, M., Hill, E., Stojan, J. N., & Daniel, M. (2018). Educational interventions to improve handover in health care: An updated systematic review. *Academic Medicine, 93*(8), 1234–1244. https://doi.org/10.1097/ACM.0000000000002236

Grant, S. M., & Johnson, B. H. (2019). Advancing the practice of patient- and family-centered care: *The central role of nursing leadership. Nurse Leader, 17*(4), 325–330. https://doi.org/10.1016/j.mnl.2019.05.009

Hospital Consumer Assessment of Healthcare Providers and Systems. (2021). *CAHPS hospital survey*. https://hcahpsonline.org

Hughes, T. M., Merath, K., Chen, Q., Sun, S., Palmer, E., Idrees, J. J., Okunrintemi, V., Squires, M., Beal, E. W., & Pawlik, T. M. (2018). Association of shared decision-making on patient-reported health outcomes and healthcare utilization. *The American Journal of Surgery, 216*(1), 7–12. https://doi.org/10.1016/j.amjsurg.2018.01.011

Institute for Healthcare Improvement. (n.d.). *Ask me 3: Good questions for your good health*. http://www.ihi.org/resources/Pages/Tools/Ask-Me-3-Good-Questions-for-Your-Good-Health.aspx

Institute for Patient- and Family-Centered Care. (n.d.). *Project background: Patient- and family-centered care defined.* https://www.ipfcc.org/bestpractices/sustainable-partnerships/background/pfcc-defined.html

International Patient Decision Aid Standards Collaboration. (2017). *Home page*. http://ipdas.ohri.ca/what.html

Jacobs, B., Ryan, A. M., Henrichs, K. S., & Weiss, B. D. (2018). Medical interpreters in outpatient practice. *The Annals of Family Medicine*, *16*(1), 70–76. https://doi.org/10.1370/afm.2154

Jayadevappa, R., Chhatre, S., Gallo, J. J., Wittink, M., Morales, K. H., Lee, D. I., Guzzo, T. J., Vapiwala, N., Wong, Y.-N., Newman, D. K., Van Arsdalen, K., Malkowicz, S. B., Schwartz, J. S., & Van Arsdalen, K. (2019). Patient-centered preference assessment to improve satisfaction with care among patients with localized prostate cancer: A randomized controlled trial. *Journal of Clinical Oncology*, *37*(12), 964–973. https://doi.org/10.1200/JCO.18.01091

Jeffrey, D. (2016). Empathy, sympathy and compassion in healthcare: Is there a problem? Is there a difference? Does it matter? *Journal of the Royal Society of Medicine, 109*(12), 446–452. https://doi.org/10.1177/0141076816680120

Jolles, M. P., Lengnick-Hall, R., & Mittman, B. S. (2019). Core functions and forms of complex health interventions: A patient-centered medical home illustration. *Journal of General Internal Medicine, 34*(6), 1032–1038. https://doi.org/10.1007/s11606-018-4818-7

Josie King Foundation. (2016). *Josie King Foundation: Creating a culture of patient safety, together*. http://www.josieking.org

Joszt, L. (2018). 5 vulnerable populations in healthcare. *American Journal of Managed Care*. https://www.ajmc.com/view/5-vulnerable-populations-in-healthcare

Kamal, R. N., Lindsay, S. E., & Eppler, S. L. (2018). Patients should define value in health care: A conceptual framework. *The Journal of Hand Surgery, 43*(11), 1030–1034. https://doi.org/10.1016/j.jhsa.2018.03.036

Kash, B. A., Baek, J., Cheon, O., Coleman, N. E., & Jones, S. L. (2018). Successful hospital readmission reduction initiatives: Top five strategies to consider implementing today. *Journal of Hospital Administration*, *7*(6), 16–23. https://doi.org/10.5430/jha.v7n6p16

Keith, K. (2019). *Trump administration asks court to strike down entire ACA.* https://www.healthaffairs.org/do/10.1377/hblog20190326.572950/full/

Kent, D., Paulus, J., Ahmen, M., & Whicher, D. (Eds.). (2019). *Caring for the individual patient: Understanding heterogenous treatment effects.* National Academy of Medicine. https://nam.edu/wp-content/uploads/2019/08/Caring-for-the-Individual-Patient-prepub.pdf

Koh, H. K., Brach, C., Harris, L. M., & Parchman, M. L. (2013). A proposed 'health literate care model' would constitute a systems approach to improving patients' engagement in care. *Health affairs, 32*(2), 357–367.

Kuipers, S. J., Cramm, J. M., & Nieboer, A. P. (2019). The importance of patient-centered care and co-creation of care for satisfaction with care and physical and social well-being of patients with multi-morbidity in the primary care setting. *BMC Health Services Research, 19*(1), 13. https://doi.org/10.1186/s12913-018-3818-y

LeBlanc, T. W., Baile, W. F., Eggly, S., Bylund, C. L., Kurtin, S., Khurana, M., Najdi, R., Blaedel, J., Wolf, J. L., & Fonseca, R. (2019). Review of the patient-centered communication landscape in multiple myeloma and other hematologic malignancies. *Patient Education and Counseling, 102*(9), 1602–1612. https://doi.org/10.1016/j.pec.2019.04.028

Légaré, F., Adekpedjou, R., Stacey, D., Turcotte, S., Kryworuchko, J., Graham, I. D., Lyddiatt, A., Politi, M. C., Thomson, R., Elwyn, G., & Donner-Banzhoff, N. (2018). Interventions for increasing the use of shared decision making by healthcare professionals. *Cochrane Database of Systematic Reviews*, (7), Article CD006732. https://doi.org/10.1002/14651858.CD006732.pub4

Lotfi, M., Zamanzadeh, V., Valizadeh, L., & Khajehgoodari, M. (2019). Assessment of nurse–patient communication and patient satisfaction from nursing care. *Nursing Open*, *6*(3), 1189–1196. https://doi.org/10.1002/nop2.316

Mailloux, C., & Halesey, E. (2018). Patient navigators as essential members of the healthcare team: A review of the literature. *Journal of Nursing & Patient Care, 3*(1), 1–5. https://doi.org/10.4172/2573-4571.1000122

McBrien, K. A., Ivers, N., Barnieh, L., Bailey, J. J., Lorenzetti, D. L., Nicholas, D., Tonelli, M., Hemmelgarn, B., Lewanczuk, Edwards, A., Braun, T., & Manns, B. (2018). Patient navigators for people with chronic disease: A systematic review. *PLoS One, 13*(2), 1–33. https://doi.org/10.1371/journal.pone.0191980

Medicaid.gov. (n.d.). Health homes. https://www.medicaid.gov/medicaid/long-term-services-supports/health-homes/index.html

Mitchell, S. E., Laurens, V., Weigel, G. M., Hirschman, K. B., Scott, A. M., Nguyen, H. Q., Howard, J. M., Laird, L., Levine, C., Davis, T. C., Gass, B, Sbaid, E., Li, J., Williams, M. V., & Jack, B W. (2018). Care transitions from patient and caregiver perspectives. *The Annals of Family Medicine*, *16*(3), 225–231. https://doi.org/10.1370/afm.2222

Naughton, C. A. (2018). Patient-centered communication. *Pharmacy,* *6*(18), 1–8. https://doi.org/10.3390/pharmacy6010018

Nutbeam, D., McGill, B., & Premkumar, P. (2018). Improving health literacy in community populations: A review of progress. *Health Promotion International, 33*(5), 901–911. https://doi.org/10.1093/heapro/dax015

Office of Disease Prevention and Health Promotion. (n.d.). *Social determinants of health*. https://www.healthypeople.gov/2020/topics-objectives/topic/social-determinants-of-health

Office of Disease Prevention and Health Promotion: Healthy People 2030. (n.d.). *Social determinants of health*. https://health.gov/healthypeople/objectives-and-data/social-determinants-health

The Ottawa Hospital. (2020). *Implementation toolkit*. https://decisionaid.ohri.ca/implement.html

Parnell, T. A. (2014). Health literacy in nursing: Providing person-centered care. Springer Publishing Company.

Patient-Centered Primary Care Collaborative. (2019). *PMCH and primary care spend: A different kind of investment*. https://www.pcpcc.org/resource/pcmh-and-primary-care-spend-different-kind-investment

Peart, A., Lewis, V., Brown, T., & Russell, G. (2018). Patient navigators facilitating access to primary care: A scoping review. *BMJ Open, 8*(3), 1–12. https://doi.org/10.1136/bmjopen-2017-019252

Pehrson, C., Banerjee, S. C., Manna, R., Johnson Shen, M., Hammonds, S., Coyle, N., Krueger, C. A., Maloney, E., Zaider, T., & Bylund, C. L. (2019). Responding empathically to patients: Development, implementation, and evaluation of a communication skills training module for oncology nurses. *Patient Education and Counseling, 99*(4), 610–616. https://doi.org/10.1016/j.pec.2015.11.021

Pexman, P. M. (2018). How do we understand sarcasm? *Frontiers for Young Minds, 6*(56), 1–8. https://doi.org/10.3389/frym.2018.00056

Poitras, M. E., Maltais, M. E., Bestard-Denommé, L., Stewart, M., & Fortin, M. (2018). What are the effective elements in patient-centered and multimorbidity care? A scoping review. *BMC Health Services Research, 18*(1), 446. https://doi.org/10.1186/s12913-018-3213-8

Rudd, R. E., & Anderson, J. E. (2006). The health literacy environment of hospitals and health centers. Partners for action: Making your healthcare facility literacy-friendly. *National Center for the Study of Adult Learning and Literacy (NCSALL).* https://cdn1.sph.harvard.edu/wp-content/uploads/sites/135/2012/09/healthliteracyenvironment.pdf

Sánchez-Izquierdo, M., Santacreu, M., Olmos, R., & Fernández-Ballesteros, R. (2019). A training intervention to reduce paternalistic care and promote autonomy: A preliminary study. *Clinical Interventions in Aging, 14*, 1515. https://doi.org/10.2147/CIA.S213644

Schierhorn, C. (2019). *Joint Commission resources, AIA co-publish book championing patient-centered design and construction.* https://www.jointcommission.org/resources/news-and-multimedia/blogs/dateline-tjc/2019/11/joint-commission-resources-aia-copublish-book-championing-patientcentered-design-and-construction

Scholl, I., LaRussa, A., Hahlweg, P., Kobrin, S., & Elwyn, G. (2018). Organizational-and system-level characteristics that influence implementation of shared decision-making and strategies to address them—a scoping review. *Implementation Science, 13*(1), 40. https://doi.org/10.1186/s13012-018-0731-z

Shpigelman, C., & HaGani, N. (2019). The impact of disability type and visibility on self-concept and body image: Implications for mental health nursing. *Journal of Psychiatric and Mental Health Nursing, 26*(3-4), 77–86. https://doi.org/10.1111/jpm.12513

Sinaiko, A. D., Szumigalski, K., Eastman, D., & Chien, A. T. (2019). *Delivery of patient centered care in the U.S. health care system: What is standing in its way?* Robert Wood Johnson Foundation. https://www.academyhealth.org/sites/default/files/deliverypatientcenteredcare_august2019.pdf

Stacey, D., Légaré, F., & Lewis, K. B. (2017). Patient decision aids to engage adults in treatment or screening decisions. *JAMA, 318*(7), 657–658. https://doi.org/10.1001/jama.2017.10289

Wilson-Smith, M. G., Sachse, K., & Perry, M. T. (2018). Road to Home Program: A performance improvement initiative to increase family and nurse satisfaction with the discharge education process for newly diagnosed pediatric oncology patients. *Journal of Pediatric Oncology Nursing, 35*(5), 368–374. https://doi.org/10.1177/1043454218767872

Wood, D. A., Lauck, S. B., Cairns, J. A., Humphries, K. H., Cook, R., Welsh, R., & Blanke, P. (2019). The Vancouver 3M (Multidisciplinary, Multimodality, But Minimalist) clinical pathway facilitates safe next-day discharge home at low-, medium-, and high-volume transfemoral transcatheter aortic valve replacement centers: The 3M TAVR study. *JACC: Cardiovascular Interventions, 12*(5), 459–469. https://www.jacc.org/doi/full/10.1016/j.jcin.2018.12.020

World Health Organization. (n.d.). Service organizations and integration. https://www.who.int/teams/integrated-health-services/clinical-services-and-systems/service-organizations-and-integration

Wu, B. (2018). Patient continued use of online health care communities: Web mining of patient-doctor communication. *Journal of Medical Internet Research, 20*(4), e126. https://doi.org/10.2196/jmir.9127

SUGGESTED READING

Centers for Disease Control and Prevention. (n.d.). *Health literacy resources.* https://www.cdc.gov/healthliteracy/learn/Resources.html

Centers for Medicare and Medicaid. (2021). *The hospital value-based purchasing (VBP) program.* https://www.cms.gov/Medicare/Quality-Initiatives-Patient-Assessment-Instruments/Value-Based-Programs/HVBP/Hospital-Value-Based-Purchasing

Graham, I. D., Logan, J., Harrison, M. B., Straus, S. E., Tetroe, J., Caswell, W., & Robinson, N. (2006). Lost in knowledge translation: Time for a map? *Journal of Continuing Education in the Health Professions*, *26*(1), 13–24. https://doi.org/10.1002/chp.47

Institute for Healthcare Improvement. (n.d.). *Person- and family-centered care.* http://www.ihi.org/Topics/PFCC/Pages/default.aspx

Institute of Medicine. (2001). *Crossing the quality chasm: A new health system for the 21st century.* National Academies Press. https://doi.org/10.17226/10027

Institute for Patient- and Family-Centered Care. (n.d.). *Home page.* https://www.ipfcc.org

Légaré, F., Stacey, D., Turcotte, S., Cossi, M. J., Kryworuchko, J., Graham, I. D., Lyddiatt, A., Politi, M. C., Thomson, R., Elwyn, G., & Donner-Banzhoff, N. (2014). Interventions for improving the adoption of shared decision making by healthcare professionals. *Cochrane Database of Systematic Reviews,* (9), Article CD006732. https://doi.org/10.1002/14651858.CD006732.pub3

Légaré F., Turcotte, S., Stacey, D., Ratté, S., Kryworuchko, J., & Graham, I. D. (2012). Patients' perceptions of sharing in decisions: A systematic review of interventions to enhance shared decision making in routine clinical practice. *The Patient-Patient-Centered Outcomes Research, 5*(1), 1–19. https://doi.org/10.2165/11592180-000000000-00000.

Logan, J., Harrison, M. B., Graham, I. D., Dunn, K., & Bissonnette, J. (1999). Evidence-based pressure-ulcer practice: The Ottawa Model of Research Use. *Canadian Journal of Nursing Research Archive, 31*(1), 37–52. https://cjnr.archive.mcgill.ca/article/view/1507

Murray, M. A., Stacey, D., Wilson, K. G., & O'Connor, A. M. (2010). Skills training to support patients considering place of end-of-life care: A randomized control trial. *Journal of Palliative Care*, *26*(2), 112–121. https://doi.org/10.1177/082585971002600207

Nathan, S., Fiore, L. L., Saunders, S., Vilbrun-Bruno PA-C, S. O., Hinrichs, K. L., Ruopp, M. D., Wershof Scwartz, A., & Moye, J. (2019). My life, my story: Teaching patient centered care competencies for older adults through life story work. *Gerontology & Geriatrics Education.* Advance online publication. https://doi.org/10.1080/02701960.2019.1665038

O'Connor, A. M., Wennberg, J. E., Legare, F., Llewellyn-Thomas, H. A., Moulton, B. W., Sepucha, K. R., Sodano, A. G., & King, J. S. (2007). Toward the 'tipping point': Decision aids and informed patient choice. *Health Affairs*, *26*(3), 716–725. https://doi.org/10.1377/hlthaff.26.3.716

The Ottawa Hospital. (2020). *Patient decision aids.* decisionaid.ohri.ca/azlist.html

Patient-Centered Outcomes Research Institute. (2012). *Patient-centered outcomes research definition: Response to public input.* https://www.pcori.org/assets/PCOR-Definition-Revised-Draft-and-Responses-to-Input.pdf

Patient Platform Unlimited. (2020). *All topics.* https://patient.info/decision-aids

Planetree International. (2020). *Creating a standard of person-centered care.* https://planetree.org/how-we-help

Ploeg, J., Ireland, S., Cziraki, K., Northwood, M., Zecevic, A. A., Davies, B., Murray, M. A., & Higuchi, K. (2018). A sustainability oriented and mentored approach to implementing a fall prevention guideline in acute care over 2 years. *SAGE Open Nursing.* https://doi.org/10.1177/2377960818775433

QSEN Institute. (n.d). QSEN competencies. https://qsen.org/competencies/pre-licensure-ksas/#patient-centered_care

Registered Nurses Association of Ontario. (2015). *RNAO best practice guideline: Person- and family-centred care.* Registered Nurses Association of Ontario.

Roach, A., & Hooke, S. (2019). An academic-practice partnership: Fostering collaboration and improving care across settings. *Nurse Educator, 44*(2), 98–101. https://doi.org/10.1097/NNE.0000000000000557

Stacey, D., Chambers, S. K., Jacobsen, M. J., & Dunn, J. (2008). Overcoming barriers to cancer-helpline professionals providing decision support for callers: An implementation study. *Oncology Nursing Forum, 35*(6), 961–969. https://doi.org/10.1188/08.ONF.961-969

Stacey, D., Higuchi, K. A., Menard, P., Davies, B., Graham, I. D., & O'Connor, A. M. (2009). Integrating patient decision support in an undergraduate nursing curriculum: An implementation project. *International Journal of Nursing Education Scholarship*, *6*, Article10. https://doi.org/10.2202/1548-923X.1741

Stacey, D., Pomey, M. P., O'Connor, A. M., & Graham, I. D. (2006). Adoption and sustainability of decision support for patients facing health decisions: An implementation case study in nursing. *Implementation Science*, *1*, 17. https://doi.org/10.1186/1748-5908-1-17

Wennberg, J. E. (2002). Unwarranted variations in healthcare delivery: Implications for academic medical centres. *BMJ*, *325*(7370), 961–964. https://doi.org/10.1136/bmj.325.7370.961

CHAPTER 7

Interprofessional Teamwork and Collaboration

Gerry Altmiller

"It's less of a thing to do ... and more of a way to be."

–Unknown QSEN Conference Participant, 2007

Upon completion of this chapter, the reader should be able to:

1. Define the term "interprofessional team."
2. Identify the role and core competencies for interprofessional healthcare teams.
3. Analyze the evolution of nursing's role on interprofessional teams.
4. Discuss strategies for maximizing team effectiveness.
5. Identify the characteristics of effective interprofessional teams.
6. Describe the Team*STEPPS* program and strategies for effective communication.
7. Describe how informatics supports the interprofessional team's ability to more efficiently and effectively solve problems.
8. Examine how constructive feedback and reflection contribute to improving patient outcomes.
9. Explore strategies the nurse can implement to include the patient as a partner on the interprofessional team.
10. Apply strategies and techniques to overcome barriers to teamwork, as well as manage conflict and difficult communication, to maximize effective interprofessional communication.

CROSSWALK

This chapter addresses the following:

QSEN Competency: Teamwork and Collaboration

The American Association of Colleges of Nursing. (2021). *The essentials: Core competencies for professional nursing education.*

Domain 6: Interprofessional Partnerships

OPENING SCENARIO

A patient's wife and son tell the nurse they are concerned about their husband and father's care. The son states he is worried about his father's lack of energy since having a colectomy for diverticulitis. He believes his father has not been out of bed for 2 days. The wife voices concern that her husband has not begun to eat and has diabetes. They ask to speak to the people in charge of the patient's care.

1. What does the nurse know about the members of the interprofessional team caring for the patient?
2. How will the nurse bring the patient's immediate problems to the appropriate team member's attention?
3. How will the nurse convey the wife and son's concerns to the interprofessional team?
4. How can the interprofessional team work together to address this patient's needs?

INTRODUCTION

Caring for patients, especially in an acute-care setting, is becoming increasingly complex. Underlying chronic health conditions and advancing age can complicate even the most routine situations. It is clear that no one person can safely address all of an individual patient's needs. Providing high-quality care requires an interprofessional team of people working together, each contributing their individual expertise to ensure the well-being of the patient. To be safe and effective, patient care requires the coordinated services of many people, some not even directly involved with the patient, yet all focused on one thing, a positive outcome and experience for the patient and family.

This chapter describes what an interprofessional team is and discusses the characteristics that make a team most effective. It describes the importance of recognizing the patient and family as an integral part of the interprofessional team and how the role of the team is not to dictate care but instead support the patient and family in achieving an optimal patient outcome. Strategies for how best to include the patient as a partner in care are presented. This chapter highlights resources that can be utilized as well as strategies that individuals and institutions can implement to create an environment where effective interprofessional communication supports patient safety and improves the overall quality of the care provided to patients.

With the increasing emphasis on healthcare quality and safety, techniques to improve communication between interprofessional healthcare team members continue to be of great importance. Tools, techniques, and strategies for communication aimed at facilitating patient safety and quality of care are described, including the use of reflection by the nurse and other members of the interprofessional healthcare team as a means of improving patient outcomes. Team*STEPPS* is presented as a national initiative to improve team communications in healthcare, enabling interprofessional healthcare teams to better communicate with each other and promote situational awareness and patient safety. Strategies to create and develop effective team functioning are discussed in this chapter. Lastly, this chapter discusses how informatics and the many resources available through the internet contribute to effective teamwork by making information readily available so that team members can exchange ideas to solve problems.

As the person that spends the greatest amount of time with the patient, the nurse holds a key position on the healthcare team, providing constant assessment and monitoring, contributing to the plan of care, delivering nursing interventions, and providing that vital link between the patient, the patient's family, and the other members of the healthcare team. Skilled communication between the nurse and other members of the interprofessional healthcare team is essential to ensure the exchange of clear and concise information, which allows the team to react quickly to changing conditions, evaluate progress, and appropriately meet patients' needs with safe high-quality care.

WHAT IS AN INTERPROFESSIONAL TEAM?

A team is a group of individuals who work together for a common goal. In healthcare, the interprofessional team consists of people who have a stake or interest in and contribute to the well-being of the patient. An interprofessional team not only includes those directly involved in the patient's physical care such as the physicians, nurses, and family members, but it also includes those who provide support services such as pharmacists, social workers, dieticians, and those from departments such as housekeeping, radiology, the laboratory, transport services, and physical and occupational therapy. It is important to recognize the valuable contribution that all these interprofessional team members make to the patient's care.

ROLE AND CORE COMPETENCIES OF INTERPROFESSIONAL TEAMS

The most recent update of the Interprofessional Education Collaborative (IPEC) Core Competencies (2016) describes expectations for collaborative practice among and between individuals from various disciplines as the basis for providing safe, high-quality, accessible, patient-centered care. The four core competencies (Table 7.1) are scaffolded by 10 subcompetencies focused on shared values and ethics, 10 subcompetencies focused on roles and responsibilities of team members, eight subcompetencies addressing communication practices, and 11 subcompetencies designed to guide team relationships and the process of teamwork itself.

TABLE 7.1 INTERPROFESSIONAL EDUCATION COLLABORATIVE CORE COMPETENCIES, 2016

Competency 1	Work with individuals of other professions to maintain a climate of mutual respect and shared values. (Values/Ethics for Interprofessional Practice)
Competency 2	Use the knowledge of one's own role and those of other professions to appropriately assess and address the healthcare needs of patients and to promote and advance the health of populations. (Roles/Responsibilities)
Competency 3	Communicate with patients, families, communities, and professionals in health and other fields in a responsive and responsible manner that supports a team approach to the promotion and maintenance of health and the prevention and treatment of disease. (Interprofessional Communication)
Competency 4	Apply relationship-building values and the principles of team dynamics to perform effectively in different team roles to plan, deliver, and evaluate patient/population-centered care and population health programs and policies that are safe, timely, efficient, effective, and equitable. (Teams and Teamwork)

Source: From Interprofessional Education Collaborative. (2016). *Core competencies for interprofessional collaborative practice: 2016 update.* Interprofessional Education Collaborative. https://ipec.memberclicks.net/assets/2016-Update.pdf
Reprinted with permission.

Using the IPEC core competencies as a foundation in teaching health profession students guides the education process in a way that is relevant to all disciplines that might contribute to the work of the healthcare team. Moving away from teaching in the silos of specific disciplines and moving toward teaching in a way that increases understanding about the roles of different healthcare disciplines creates opportunities to better coordinate care that impacts the patient and engages students of different professions in interactive learning with each other.

NURSING'S EVOLVING ROLE ON INTERPROFESSIONAL TEAMS

Nursing's role has evolved into one of **collaboration** with other healthcare professionals, working cooperatively together, sharing responsibilities, and solving problems. Included in this collaboration is the patient and family who should be at the center of the interprofessional healthcare team and have input with all interactions and decisions in order to align the team's goals with the patient's goals. With this person-centered approach, the interprofessional team acknowledges patient preferences, individual health values, and priorities because without the patient, there would be no need for the team. Like patients, nurses have not always been considered members of the interprofessional healthcare team; traditionally, they have taken direction from hospital administrators and physicians rather than directly contributing to a collaborative plan of care. Historically, nurses were charged with direct patient care and focused mostly on providing patient hygiene under the direction of the physician. Differences in educational requirements prevented even routine tasks such as obtaining a patient's blood pressure from being delegated to the nurse. Nurses did not have a role in advocating for the patient and physicians did not confer with nurses regarding any aspect of the patient's care. The interprofessional relationship was strictly one of orders being dictated by the physician team member and orders being carried out by the nursing team member.

Gender issues have also contributed to the lack of interprofessional collaboration or the ability to effectively work together. In the past, males traditionally assumed the physician role while nurses have primarily been female. Much has changed in recent decades with both males and females assuming roles as physicians and nurses, independent of gender. Females still dominate the nursing profession with the U.S. Department of Labor reporting that in 2019, males made up only 11% of the nursing workforce (U.S. Department of Labor, 2020). In comparison, females were reported to make up 40% of the physician and surgeon workforce (U.S. Department of Labor, 2020).

Economic issues have also contributed to the lack of interprofessional collaboration. Nurses represent the largest segment of the hospital-based employee workforce and are paid as hourly workers by the healthcare system. Physicians have been community based and have managed their practice as a business, directly billing their patients and the insurance companies. Expanding roles for nurses have created opportunities for hospital-based nurses and for advanced practice nurses to bill directly for services. RNs and advanced practice nurses have increased their education, which is helping to bridge the gap between nurses and physicians. More standardized prelicensure education requirements for nurses have resulted in a bedside nurse who is able to assess, plan, implement, and evaluate care provided to patients, making the nurse a valuable team member.

Nursing knowledge is based on science combined with the art of caring for the individual needs of patients. Nursing brings a holistic perspective to patient care. The connection of the nurse to the patient and family through close and continued interaction allows nurses to understand and advocate for patient concerns and needs regardless of their practice level. Nurses can build rapport between patients and the team and facilitate collaboration between the interprofessional healthcare disciplines involved in the patient's care. Nurses' knowledge of the patient experience allows them to identify subtle changes

BOX 7.1 The Future of Nursing Four Key Recommendations

1. Nurses should practice to the full extent of their education.
2. Nurses should achieve higher levels of education through an improved education system that promotes seamless academic progression.
3. Nurses should be full partners with physicians and other healthcare professionals in the redesign of healthcare.
4. Better data collection and information infrastructure are necessary for effective workforce planning and policy making.

Source: From Institute of Medicine. (2011). *The future of nursing: Leading change, advancing health*. National Academies Press. https://doi.org/10.17226/12956

in the patient's condition and act quickly to prevent complications of illness. The ability of the nurse to function proactively helps to reduce unnecessary costs to hospitals as well as improve patient satisfaction and outcomes.

Nurses need to recognize the value of this perspective and acknowledge the positive impact they have on patient outcomes. It is important that nurses articulate both the value of this positive effect on patient satisfaction and the financial benefit that nurses bring to the institutions they serve in order to enhance their role as contributing team members and to advance the profession of nursing.

Recognizing the value of nursing, the Institute of Medicine (IOM), now known as the National Academy of Medicine, in collaboration with the Robert Wood Johnson Foundation (RWJF), published its report, *The Future of Nursing: Leading Change, Advancing Health* (IOM, 2011). This report identified the barriers that prevent nurses from being able to respond to the rapidly changing healthcare system. It also validated the important role that nurses play in the delivery of seamless, high-quality, affordable healthcare to all. The four key recommendations from the report were focused on the role that nursing should have in providing care (Box 7.1).

Advancing Healthcare Through Improved Education

Although educational differences exist among interprofessional team members, it is important to recognize that each team member brings a perspective to the team that represents specialized knowledge from their discipline. For physicians, the educational requirements include a baccalaureate degree with an additional 4 years of medical school, followed by a year of internship in clinical practice and 2 years of residency. Medical specialization adds additional years of training and fellowship. For nurses, there are varied levels of educational requirements for entry into practice. These include a 3-year diploma school education, a 2-year associate degree education, and a 4-year baccalaureate degree education as well as master's and doctor of nursing practice (DNP) completion programs. Other healthcare disciplines have varied educational degree requirements as well. No matter the educational requirements, each healthcare discipline needs to be able to collaborate with others to provide the highest quality care for the patient.

To support the appreciation of each healthcare discipline's perspective, expertise, and values, many programs now include an integration of interprofessional education as part of their curriculum. **Interprofessional education** is the opportunity for multiple healthcare disciplines to learn together in the same environment simultaneously, gaining a greater understanding for each discipline's role and contributions. A common example of this is medical and nursing students taking an ethics class together or participating in a communication exercise as part of an orientation program. While coordinating interprofessional education is challenging, the National League for Nursing (NLN) provides a toolkit to support effective interprofessional education experiences in nursing education (NLN, 2016).

STRATEGIES FOR MAXIMIZING EFFECTIVE INTERPROFESSIONAL TEAMS

The changing socialization of physicians and nurses as well as other disciplines has allowed for the formation of interprofessional teams that not only care for patients but also tackle some of the toughest problems facing healthcare today. In part, this change has come from changes in traditional gender roles as well as the attainment of baccalaureate, master's, and DNP degrees by more and more nurses. Working together, physicians and nurses have developed work processes to address quality and safety on all levels of patient care.

One process, the **root cause analysis** (RCA), is conducted by the interprofessional team to systematically investigate serious adverse events and errors to identify the root cause and contributing factors that led to error, patient injury, or a negative outcome so that those factors can be mitigated and future adverse events prevented. An RCA identifies mechanisms within the healthcare system that allowed for the error or near miss to occur. A **near miss** is an event that could have resulted in an error but was caught in time before it reached the patient. The investigative process allows for individual growth and development as team members learn about causes for errors. Additionally, the process provides the basis for change within the healthcare system policy and procedures to prevent similar events in the future. The RCA discovers the root of a problem by not stopping at the first answer it arrives at for an event's cause, but instead delving deeper into why the problem occurred, asking questions until there are no more questions to ask. See Chapter 10 for an example.

Rapid Response Teams

A strategy that brings interprofessional teams together to focus on emergent problems and find immediate solutions to help patients in the hospital setting is the **rapid response team** (RRT). An RRT includes specific healthcare professionals with specialized skills, who can mobilize and deliver immediate patient assessment and intervention if needed at the patient's bedside any time of day or night, 7 days a week, at the beginning signs of deterioration in the patient's health status. The RRT is separate from a "code" or resuscitation team that is also composed of specialized interprofessional team members who would respond to cardiac and/or respiratory arrest. The concept of the RRT was created in 2012 based on recommendations by the Institute for Healthcare Improvement (IHI) with the intention of preventing deaths outside of the ICU (IHI, n.d.). RRTs may be structured differently within institutions, but most RRTs consist of a physician, critical care nurse, and respiratory therapist, along with other designated interprofessional members, as needed. Expert communication skills are required by RRT members because the patient's safety and well-being depend on the rapid and accurate exchange of pertinent and clear information between team members coming together in a concerted effort to aid the patient. RRTs support an institution's nurses by providing access to immediate assistance for any patient whose condition is rapidly changing. RRTs may be summoned to a patient's bedside by anyone, including family members. Providing RRT support allows for early intervention at the first sign of deterioration in patients, before they become critically ill or experience a cardiac or respiratory arrest.

Teams Coordinating Care to Reduce Risks

Nowhere is interprofessional teamwork and collaboration more important than in providing required healthcare to patients in need. Although all members of the interprofessional

CASE STUDY

The nurse is caring for a patient admitted the previous night with exacerbation of chronic heart failure. The patient was stabilized with treatment that included bedrest, IV diuretic therapy, oxygen by 40% mask, and continuous monitoring with telemetry and pulse oximetry. When answering the patient's call bell on the evening shift, the nurse notices the patient is breathing rapidly and appears anxious. The patient states he is having difficulty breathing. The nurse places the patient in a full Fowler's position and auscultates the lungs to find rales halfway up the back. The nurse stat pages the patient's physician and carefully monitors the patient, watching an increasing respiratory rate and decreasing pulse oximetry reading. After waiting 10 minutes with no answer, the nurse calls an RRT.

1. ***What aspects of this situation support the decision to call an RRT?***
2. ***What expectation might the nurse have about the team members that may respond and the care that might be rendered?***

healthcare team possess specific expertise that would benefit the patient, if they were unable to coordinate those skills and connect vital services together, the patient would not have the best possible outcome. Team members must work together to provide coordinated care to achieve the best results.

Patients are at greater risk during transitions between care. **Handoff** is a term used to describe the communication method that the interprofessional team uses to transfer patient care information to one another between shifts or between patient care units or facilities. In healthcare, poor outcomes occur when there are breakdowns in communication, poor teamwork, or inefficient communication "handoffs" that create situations where information is missing, which can lead to errors. Effective interprofessional teams involved in direct patient care have common goals of high quality and safety, and ensuring that information about the patient is communicated accurately and completely to support those goals during transitions of care.

Interprofessional teams in healthcare can also be focused on more long-term projects. These interprofessional teams may be assembled to address anything from quality improvement (QI) processes to planning for the future of the healthcare institution. Although the work of these types of interprofessional teams may seem slower and more deliberate, the principles that guide them are the same as teams that respond to patient emergencies. For example, a long-term goal of a hospital might be to increase the number of baccalaureate-prepared RNs over the next 10 years. Collaboration between hospital administration, finance department leaders, nursing leadership, and broad representation from nursing staff, all using effective teamwork and communication skills, would be needed to conduct the same steps of assessment, definition of the problem, goal setting, implementation, and evaluation, all of which are part of the nursing process.

CHARACTERISTICS OF EFFECTIVE INTERPROFESSIONAL HEALTHCARE TEAMS

Effective interprofessional teams are able to think reflectively about the situation at hand considering past experiences, contemplate options from all perspectives, and deliberate the options in an atmosphere of mutual respect. In high-functioning, successful interprofessional teams, members can voice concerns and opinions, creating a group dynamic where all members contribute and share in the decision-making. Clear, focused communication and respectful negotiation decrease the potential for misunderstandings and promote camaraderie among the team members.

Accountability and Stages of Team Development

"Forming," "storming," "norming," and "performing" are terms used to describe the stages experienced by teams as they progress from formation to functioning as high-performance teams (Tuckman, 1965). The forming stage is generally a short phase when team members are introduced and objectives are established. As the team moves into the storming stage, team roles become clarified and processes as well as structures for the team are established. It is within this process that the details of the approach being used to accomplish the goals or assignment are decided upon. The workload of the task becomes clear during this storming phase and can overwhelm the team members. Conflicts may arise and members build relationships with other team members as they work through conflict resolution. In this storming stage, teams will fail if work processes and team relationships have not been well established.

In the norming stage, team members develop a stronger commitment to the team's goals and assume responsibility for the team's progress. Individuals show leadership in specific areas and team members come to respect each other's roles. As members become socialized as a team, they are able to provide constructive feedback to each other. It is important to note that teams can pass back and forth between the storming and norming stages as new tasks are assigned to the team. The performing stage is realized through achievement of the team's shared vision of the goal. At this point, teamwork feels easier and members can for the most part join and leave the team without affecting the team's performance. The progress achieved from the members' hard work establishes the team as a high-performance team. When the work of the team is complete, "adjourning" is the term used to describe the phase of dismantling the team so that members are free to move on to other projects (Tuckman, 1965).

CASE STUDY

The manager of a critical care unit wants to implement self-scheduling among his 80-member staff. He appoints two staff members from the night shift, two staff members from the day shift, one assistant manager, and one nurse aide to a committee with the goal of developing rules to guide the self-scheduling process. The committee is scheduled to meet weekly until all self-scheduling rules are developed and the processes can be put in place. Immediately, tensions run high in the committee as there is disagreement about the number of Fridays that must be worked by each staff member and the number of weekends that must be worked in a 6-week schedule. Through negotiation, agreement is reached on the committee regarding these issues. Just when they believe that they have all issues resolved, there is disagreement among the committee members regarding the number of schedule changes management can make to accommodate unit needs. This is a very heated topic and the negotiation for this continues for 3 weeks. Eventually, it is resolved with agreement by all. It is decided that the scheduling committee will remain intact, assist with the transition for staff, and manage the scheduling process. Committee members will work together to cover the unit needs.

1. *What team stage is identified as the team begins to work to resolve the number of Fridays and weekends that will be required by each staff?*
2. *What team stage is identified when the committee decides to remain intact to assist with the transition and manage the scheduling process?*

BOX 7.2 Developing Clinical Judgment

The nurse is caring for a patient admitted through the emergency department with new-onset dyspnea. She is 5 days post hysterectomy and has been on bedrest while at home. While in the treatment room, the patient states she needs to use the bathroom. The nurse wants to delegate this task to the assistive personnel while maintaining the patient's safety.

1. What **CUES (Assessment)** might the nurse identify and consider in this situation?
2. What **HYPOTHESIS (Diagnosis)** will the nurse consider based on the available information?
3. What **ACTION (Plan and Implement)** or instruction can the nurse give the assistive personnel to accomplish the task while meeting the patient's safety needs?
4. How will the nurse evaluate the OUTCOME (Evaluation) of the delegated task?

Delegation

Willingness to assist colleagues is pivotal to interprofessional teamwork and collaboration. Teamwork requires that members can effectively delegate work to each other. In patient care, it is essential that delegated tasks are within the scope of practice of the individual to whom the task is being delegated. For example, inserting an indwelling urinary catheter could be delegated by a nurse to another nurse. It could not be delegated to a nursing assistant. When delegating, the nurse employs the following steps: assess and plan; communicate what needs to be done; ensure availability to assist and support; and finally, evaluate effectiveness and give feedback (National Council of State Boards of Nursing and American Nurses Association, 2019).

With all delegation, clear communication of what needs to be done and confirmation of understanding from the individual being delegated to is essential to ensure patient safety. The nurse, who is delegating, needs to provide an opportunity for clarification and questions. If an outcome does not meet expectations, the nurse should lead the discussion with those involved to identify reasons for the unexpected outcome and determine what could be learned from the experience to improve care and to ensure a successful outcome in the future. Chapter 5 contains more on delegation.

Crew Resource Management

Crew resource management (CRM) refers to educating individuals who work in high-stress systems where the human aspect of operations can create an increased potential for error. Originating in the aviation industry for the cockpit crew, CRM develops communication, leadership, and decision-making safety strategies to combat the potential for human error that is inherent in high-stress systems and its devastating effects. The healthcare industry shares an interest in interprofessional teamwork and clear communication with the aviation industry to prevent catastrophic events. Healthcare has applied many CRM strategies to the daily interactions and continuous QI processes of the interprofessional healthcare team. CRM communication, leadership, and decision-making safety strategies focus on cognitive and interpersonal skills to promote situational awareness.

Situational awareness is having the right information at the right time alongside the ability to analyze that information to appropriately and effectively take action. Having this awareness allows for all team members to be aware of and attentive to the facts in any given situation. The vehicle for this attentiveness is effective communication between interprofessional healthcare team members.

TEAM*STEPPS*

Within healthcare, Team*STEPPS* is a program developed to provide training for effective communication techniques similar to those promoted by CRM. The program is designed to teach interprofessional teams how to communicate with each other to promote situational awareness and patient safety. Specifically, Team*STEPPS* is

- a powerful solution for improving patient safety within an organization
- an evidence-based teamwork system to improve communication and teamwork skills among healthcare professionals
- a source for ready-to-use materials and a training curriculum to successfully integrate teamwork principles into all areas of the healthcare system
- scientifically rooted in more than 20 years of research and lessons from the application of teamwork principles (Agency for Healthcare Research and Quality [AHRQ], n.d.)

Developed in collaboration with the Department of Defense, the AHRQ initiated Team*STEPPS* to augment the effort and abilities of interprofessional teams to ensure the highest patient outcomes within healthcare institutions and systems. By focusing on a three-phased process of team development, the program optimizes resources within a team, provides a framework for resolving conflict and enhancing communications, and provides the basis to effectively address potential barriers to effective patient safety and quality care.

AHRQ lists the three phases of Team*STEPPS* as (a) assessment; (b) planning, training, and implementation; and (c) sustainment. Assessment involves pretraining evaluation to determine the willingness and capacity of an organization to change. Within this phase of the process, an interprofessional team is established that is made up of a cross-section of healthcare leaders and professionals from within the organization itself. This phase also involves conducting a comprehensive site assessment to identify areas of weakness and needs relative to teamwork. From this assessment, the second phase of Team*STEPPS* is initiated; a training program is developed to effectively overcome the deficiencies of the team as well as maximize its strengths. Once this education has occurred, the third and final phase of sustaining what has been gained begins. The long-range goal of the third phase is to maintain and continually improve teamwork efforts throughout the organization. Through coaching, feedback, and reinforcement of strategies taught, teamwork and communication skills can be continually reinforced and built upon as opportunities for improvement in clinical and administrative situations throughout the organization.

Situation, Background, Assessment, and Recommendation

SBAR, an acronym for the words "situation," "background," "assessment," and "recommendation," is a framework for communication utilized in many healthcare settings (AHRQ, n.d.). It was developed by the military and is now applied to healthcare as a means to relay significant information regarding a patient's condition or to be used as patients' care is communicated and handed off from one caregiver to another. Following a structured communication framework helps to ensure that all pertinent information is included and details are not accidentally omitted (Table 7.2). In this way, it improves team communications and prevents errors.

Additional Techniques for Effective Communication Within Interprofessional Teams

Clear and open communication among team members allows ideas to be shared and counteracts the potential for human errors of judgment. Techniques such as cross-monitoring

TABLE 7.2 SITUATION, BACKGROUND, ASSESSMENT, AND RECOMMENDATION

SBAR	MEANING	EXAMPLE
S	Situation: Describe what is happening with the patient	Doctor, I am calling about Mrs. Smith, your patient admitted yesterday to room 304 with respiratory distress.
B	Background: Explain the background of the patient's circumstances	She was comfortable during the evening after being placed on 2 L oxygen by nasal cannula and receiving 20 mg of furosemide (Lasix) intravenously, but is now complaining of shortness of breath.
A	Assessment: Identify what data you have regarding the situation	Her respiratory rate is 28. Pulse is 110/min and her oximetry measures 91%. She has crackles in the lower third of her lung fields bilaterally. She is laboring to breathe.
R	Recommendation: Identify what you think needs to be done to correct the situation	I think she may need her furosemide (Lasix) dose increased.

Source: From Agency for Healthcare Research and Quality. (n.d.). *TeamSTEPPS™ fundamentals course: Module 1. Introduction: Instructor's slides*. https://www.ahrq.gov/teamstepps/instructor/fundamentals/module1/igintro.html

require that team members listen carefully to the details being communicated and provide correction for the team if needed. **Cross-monitoring** is the process of monitoring the actions of other team members for the purpose of sharing the workload and reducing or avoiding errors (AHRQ, n.d.). An example of this technique can occur during grand rounds where interventions are discussed by a group of physicians, nurses, pharmacists, and other healthcare providers. Decisions verbally agreed upon can sometimes be missed as orders are articulated for the patient. A nurse asking for clarification of an order they recall differently is an example of cross-monitoring to prevent errors.

Other communication techniques can be used to bring attention to patient situations. A callout is used to communicate important information to the entire team simultaneously (AHRQ, n.d.). In a callout, the team member would callout to others for assistance. For example, during a resuscitation effort, also known as a code, a nurse monitoring the patient's blood pressure might assertively state the changing status to the medical resident. Typically, the callout is then followed by a check back, which is where the receiver repeats back the information to verify it was received accurately so the receiver can then provide an appropriate response. In this example, the resident might acknowledge the callout and ask for medication to be given to stabilize the patient's blood pressure. Check back requires the receiver verbally acknowledge the message to provide opportunity for correction if it has been inaccurately interpreted.

The two-challenge rule states that if an individual does not believe that their first attempt to bring attention to a concerning patient situation has been successful, the individual is obligated to take a second attempt to make the problem known to others on the team (AHRQ, n.d.). The two-challenge rule is designed for situations when a team member's input is ignored purposely. It is the obligation of that team member to bring it forward again to make sure it is not ignored. An example of the two-challenge rule is when a nurse tells a physician about a concern they have for the patient, such as a low urine output, and the physician does not address it for one reason or another. The nurse is obligated to bring it forward again.

Another tool that can be used to advocate for a patient is CUS, which is an acronym for the words "concerned," "uncomfortable," and "safety" (AHRQ, n.d.). Frequently, nurses are expected to advocate for their patients, but they may not know how to do so. CUS is a tool that assists the nurse in taking an assertive stance to do what the nurse believes is needed for the patient. For example, in the case of a larger than recommended dose of medication being ordered for a patient, the nurse may approach the ordering provider and state, "I'm *concerned* with the dose that has been ordered. I am *uncomfortable* giving such a large dose to this patient because of her renal condition. I don't think it is *safe*."

The time-out is a safety strategy that is mandated in the operating room (OR) and procedure suites by The Joint Commission (TJC) to help ensure patient safety (TJC, n.d.). Time-outs can also be initiated during any procedure at the bedside. The time-out is a structured process for everyone on the interprofessional team in the room to stop what they are doing and review situational information to ensure that the correct patient is having the correct procedure done to the correct site. The time-out requires that everyone stop their work and devote their attention to the patient information review.

Another safety strategy that interprofessional teams employ is the use of safety huddles. Safety huddles allow those caring for the patient to review pertinent information and the plan of care. It is similar to a team huddle used in sports and ensures everyone is aware and working toward the same goals for the patient. An example of when a huddle would facilitate effective, coordinated care is when there is a rapid change in a patient's status. Responding to the patient's rapidly changing condition would best be handled with a focused, coordinated approach by as many interprofessional team members as possible.

All of the aforementioned communication strategies are developed by the AHRQ which provides reference videos for clinicians, administrators, and educators demonstrating Team*STEPPS* tools, strategies, and techniques at its website, www.ahrq.gov/professionals/education/curriculum-tools/teamstepps/instructor/videos/index.html (Table 7.3).

Another way that team members can work to prevent errors is by reporting them to other members of the healthcare team. Timely reporting of errors and near misses, also known as close calls where an error could have occurred but was stopped before it caused harm, provides an opportunity for the team to learn from them. In most cases, errors and

TABLE 7.3 AVAILABLE TOPICS FOR REFERENCE AND EDUCATION ON AGENCY FOR HEALTHCARE RESEARCH AND QUALITY TEAM*STEPPS* WEBSITE

SBAR	Provides a standardized framework for communication, that is, *situation, background, assessment*, and *recommendation*.
Cross-monitoring	Involves listening to other team members to identify correct and incorrect information. This allows the team to self-correct healthcare errors before they occur.
Callout	Asks for help from other team members.
Two-challenge rule	Obligates team members to make a second attempt to have a concern heard when their first attempt to bring attention to a concern is not acknowledged.
CUS	Advocacy strategy using the words "concerned," "uncomfortable," and "safety."
Check back/read back	Verbally calling out and repeating back information to confirm it is understood correctly.
Handoff	Transferring responsibility for a patient's care from one unit to another or from one individual to another.

CUS, concerned, uncomfortable, and safety; SBAR, *situation, background, assessment, and recommendation.*

Source: From Agency for Healthcare Research and Quality. (n.d.). *TeamSTEPPS™ fundamentals course: Module 1. Introduction: Instructor's slides.* https://www.ahrq.gov/teamstepps/instructor/fundamentals/module1/igintro.html

BOX 7.3 Developing Clinical Judgment

During morning assessment, the nurse identifies that Mr. John Smith, room 304, admitted for infection, has hives covering most of his back, a finding that was not reported during the patient handoff at change of shift. The nurse assesses the patient further and notes no other patient complaints or symptoms. In reviewing the patient's documentation from the previous 24 hours, the nurse finds no mention of hives. Considering causes of hives, the nurse reviews the medication list and identifies that the patient had an antibiotic added to his treatment regimen 12 hours ago.

1. What **CUES (Assessment)** might the nurse identify in this situation?
2. What **HYPOTHESIS (Diagnosis)** will the nurse consider based on the available information?
3. What safety strategy **ACTION (Plan and Implement)** would be most effective for the nurse to use to advocate for the patient in this situation?
4. How will the nurse evaluate the effectiveness of actions taken and the patient's **OUTCOME (Evaluation)**?

near misses are not the result of a single person's actions. They are often the result of a failure within a healthcare system. By reporting all errors or near misses, the need for an RCA can be evaluated more completely and effectively and actions can be taken to ensure the same situation does not put patients or staff at risk in the future.

USE OF INFORMATICS FOR EFFECTIVE PROBLEM-SOLVING

Minimizing the potential for errors is the goal of everyone on the healthcare team. Participating in behaviors that guard against error and protect patients is a fundamental part of daily healthcare practice. There are many available web resources for information funded by government agencies and national healthcare organizations that are designed to improve teamwork and collaboration, prevent error, promote patient safety, and improve the quality of the care that patients receive. Nurses, as well as other team members, can access these resources to learn about strategies that address quality and safety as a way to improve their practice and keep patients safe from errors (Table 7.4).

TABLE 7.4 WEB RESOURCES FOR TEAMWORK AND COLLABORATION, ERROR PREVENTION, PATIENT SAFETY, AND QUALITY IMPROVEMENT

RESOURCE	WEBSITE ADDRESS
Team*STEPPS* Videos	www.ahrq.gov/professionals/education/curriculum-tools/teamstepps/instructor/videos/index.html
Patient Safety Network	psnet.ahrq.gov
The National Database of Nursing Quality Indicators	nursingandndnqi.weebly.com/ndnqi-indicators.html
ISMP	www.ismp.org
The Future of Nursing Report	www.nationalacademies.org/hmd/Reports/2010/The-Future-of-Nursing-Leading-Change-Advancing-Health.aspx
QSEN	www.qsen.org
The Joint Commission	www.jointcommission.org

ISMP, Institute for Safe Medication Practices; QSEN, Quality and Safety Education for Nurses.

Auditing Patient Care and Outcomes

Teams can work together to conduct audits and other organizational studies that measure quality, safety, and patient outcomes. The results of audits frequently serve as a catalyst for QI. Collecting and analyzing data regarding patient care practices and patient outcomes allows the team to document differences between the actual system's performance and the goals of the organization. By documenting differences, changes can be made to narrow the gap between the two and improve team performance for quality of care and patient safety.

CONSTRUCTIVE FEEDBACK AND REFLECTION'S IMPACT ON IMPROVEMENT

All members of the interprofessional healthcare team have an obligation to improve patient care processes and outcomes by focusing on communication and QI. **Debriefing** is the process of reviewing performance effectiveness following challenging patient care situations. Utilizing strategies such as debriefing allows the interprofessional team to evaluate the effectiveness of their communication and teamwork and to identify areas where improvement is possible. It is during debriefing that constructive feedback is given and received. All team members should feel comfortable to participate in this process. Individuals may differ in how they provide feedback to peers, but Clynes and Raftery (2008) established early on a model that holds true today, that feedback, whether positive or negative, should always be an unbiased reflection of what occurred, opening the door to a discussion of evidence-based practice. Constructive feedback should carefully detail events as they occurred and avoid opinion.

Constructive feedback recounts events, offering options for improvement. One of the only systematic reviews on constructive feedback was done by Hattie and Timperley (2007) who found that feedback is most effective when focused on a task, a process used, or on self-regulation, because that focus contributes to learning; feedback focused on the individual is less effective because it does not increase learning. For instance, feedback such as "It was wise to gather your supplies before you went into the patient's room" focuses on the task. Feedback such as "Your explanation to the patient before you began allowed the patient to trust you" focuses on the healthcare process. Feedback such as "It is good that you realized you broke sterile technique and changed your gloves" focuses on self-monitoring. These types of constructive feedback support knowledge development. Feedback such as "You did a good job" focuses on the individual and is least effective because it does not add to one's understanding of what aspects of their practice were effective and "a good job."

Although it is difficult to give and receive unflattering feedback, team members must understand that feedback is essential for growth. Feedback is the mechanism that triggers reflection and allows one to make continual adjustments in practice. Receiving feedback is often a catalyst for change and should be viewed as an opportunity for growth. When receiving feedback that is perceived as negative, the individual is challenged to consider the validity of the comments made; particularly important is to consider whether the same feedback has been provided previously by other sources. If, after consideration, feedback received is perceived as inaccurate, the individual can ask for examples of poor performance and focus on improvement, seeking advice from the person providing the feedback for how they feel improvement can be achieved.

Reflection

Communication and interprofessional teamwork skills are a huge part of the protection from injury and complications that nurses provide for patients. These skills are important not only when interacting with patients and healthcare team members to solve problems but also when nurses reflect on patient care events and discuss ways to improve outcomes. Providing feedback to team members allows the team to identify strengths and weaknesses, make changes to the healthcare system, and adjust practice for individual growth and development.

Self-evaluation of one's communication and decision-making is a crucial element of professional growth and strengthens one's ability to contribute to the team's decisions by employing strong clinical judgment. As discussed earlier in the chapter, reflection supports confidence in decision-making and provides an opportunity for the individual to consider their interactions with others and determine what actions enhanced a positive outcome and what actions worked against it. Reflecting on clinical situations and the resulting outcomes allows team members to make appropriate changes to improve practice.

Developing Clinical Judgment to Think Like a Nurse

Clinical judgment models help to explain how nurses develop skill and expertise in patient care so they can think like a nurse. One of the most widely accepted frameworks is Tanner's Clinical Judgment Model (2006) which describes clinical judgment as being developed through experiences, followed by reflection to enhance critical thinking skills. Once a nurse has a clinical experience, interprets the outcome, and reflects on it, that thinking becomes part of the nurse's repertoire for making judgments about future experiences. Clinical judgment skills continue to develop throughout one's career and are enhanced by team strategies of situational awareness and mindfulness. **Mindfulness** in its simplest context implies staying focused on the situation, seeing the significance of early and weak signals in the patient's condition, and having the ability to take strong and decisive action to prevent harm (Weick & Sutcliffe, 2001).

Tanner's Clinical Judgment Model (2006) stems from review of approximately 200 studies focused on the nurses' development of clinical judgment. From her review, Tanner concluded that:

- Clinical judgments are more influenced by what nurses bring to the situation than the objective data about the situation at hand.
- Sound clinical judgment rests to some degree on knowing the patient and their typical pattern of responses, as well as an engagement with the patient and their concerns.
- Clinical judgments are influenced by the context in which the situation occurs and the culture of the nursing care unit.
- Nurses use a variety of reasoning patterns alone or in combination.
- Reflection on practice is often triggered by a breakdown in clinical judgment and is critical for the development of clinical knowledge and improvement in clinical reasoning (Tanner, 2006).

CURRENT LITERATURE

CITATION

Hovland, C. A., Whitford, M., & Niederriter J. (2018). Interprofessional education: Insights from a cohort of nursing students. *Journal for Nurses in Professional Development, 34*(4), 219–225. https://doi.org/10.1097/NND.0000000000000466

DISCUSSION

Interprofessional education (IPE) remains elusive in many nursing education programs although it has been identified by the IOM as a core competency for all healthcare professionals (Greiner & Knebel, 2003). Nurses, like most health profession students, are educated within their own schools learning a discipline-focused curriculum with little crossover occurring with other health professions. Learning experiences that include interprofessional simulation provide an opportunity for nursing students to learn about other professions and understand their contribution to the patient's care, interact and communicate with students from other disciplines, and prepare for the realities of practice. Role-playing through simulation in IPE creates a shared understanding of the teamwork and communication skills required to provide comprehensive care. This study explored nursing students' experiences with an IPE simulation experience.

IMPLICATIONS FOR PRACTICE

Nursing students gained an understanding for other healthcare professions' work and appreciated the benefits of interprofessional collaboration. Additionally, they identified the importance of communication with the patient, the family, and team members in providing safe and effective care. The experience seemed to bolster self confidence in the nursing students, gave them an opportunity to experience "real life" learning, and allowed them to experience collaborative team strategies such as participating in team huddle. IPE simulations are important to nursing education because they provide nursing students the opportunity to understand the nursing scope of practice, increase knowledge of other healthcare professions, validate their own nursing skills, and enhance their communication with patients, families, and other professionals.

STRATEGIES TO INCLUDE THE PATIENT AS PARTNER

Communication between the healthcare team, the patient, and the patient's family during times of stress and illness can be challenging but it is essential to safety and a key factor in patient satisfaction. Patients and families look to the nurse to provide a personal connection with the team. In addition, many patients and families look to the nurse as a source of information. The nurse should use language that is understandable to the patient and provide person-centered information that allows the patient to assume a role of partnership rather than dependency. The nurse plays a pivotal role in including the patient, providing explanations, and providing access for the patient to communicate with other members of the interprofessional team. To promote the patient's partnership with the interprofessional healthcare team, the nurse can create connections for the patient to other members of the team, such as providing information regarding when the physician usually makes rounds. The nurse can encourage the patient and family to write down their questions for the physician and put the questions in the chart so that the physician may address them.

OVERCOMING BARRIERS TO EFFECTIVE COMMUNICATION AND TEAMWORK

The nurse must possess strong communication skills to contribute to effective team functioning. Communication is the interactive process of exchanging information. Effective communication is clear, precise, and concise, with no ambiguities. Safety is enhanced when the communication sender uses the proper terminology and provides an opportunity for clarification. Ideally, in response, the receiver of the communication acknowledges the message as heard and understood.

Many barriers can interfere with communication, such as knowledge gaps, education levels, culture, language barriers, or stress. It is important for nurses to develop strategies to identify and overcome these barriers. Nonverbal cues, such as facial expression, eye contact, and body posturing, may signal a message from another, but when safety is a priority such as it is in healthcare, interpreting nonverbal cues only is not an acceptable technique for communicating. Any perception one develops from nonverbal communication must be verified verbally to maintain a safe environment.

Effective communication is essential to maintaining a safe and protected environment for patients. Ineffective communication continues to be identified as the root cause for many sentinel events reported to TJC (2019), which explains why improving communication is a safety priority for the next decade. Students and nurses who are new to practice may find team interaction intimidating for several reasons, including that they do not clearly understand the culture of healthcare communication, they have known knowledge gaps, and they have not yet gained enough experience in the healthcare setting from which they can draw understanding. Quality and safety in patient care are strongly influenced by the ability of the healthcare team to communicate clearly without uncertainty, in a timely manner, and to contribute to the healthcare team's productive, efficient approach to patient care. Recognizing what information needs to be communicated to which individuals on the team and in what time frame is essential to developing effective communication skills so regularly scheduled meetings of key team members will help to ensure effective communication. Team huddles are an effective example of this practice.

Real World Interview

In the OR, no one can work as an individual. Everyone must be part of the team to promote patient safety and positive patient outcomes; it is the culture and the team effort starts from the minute we meet the patient. As soon as the patient comes to the preoperative area, the nurse anesthetist, OR nurse, and preoperative nurse perform a "triple check," which is a review of all of the patient's records and information. This allows all team members to communicate and identify any concerns regarding the patient's surgery. Even the transferring of a patient from a stretcher or hospital bed to the OR table is a team effort with open communication to ensure the patient's safety. Every member is encouraged to be an active part of the team effort and communicate openly. The time-out procedure is a great example of teamwork and communication in the OR. Everyone must stop what they are doing and be attentive to the exchange of information to ensure the patient's safety. There is a lot of camaraderie in the OR because of the high stress associated with the work we do. Each member of the team contributes a vital service that supports the care of the patient. The nurse anesthetist has to be a calming force in the room to instill confidence in the rest of the team. As an advanced practice nurse of anesthesia, I feel valued as a team member. It motivates me to communicate with everyone, go above and beyond what is required, and take pride in what I do.

Daniel Boucot
Rancocas Anesthesia Associates
Thomas Jefferson Health System, Washington Township, NJ Division

BOX 7.4 Developing Clinical Judgment

The nurse is caring for a patient with an extensive burn injury that is scheduled for skin grafting at the end of the week. The patient's white blood cell count is 3.8 mm^3. The patient is ordered a regular diet with a calorie requirement of 3,500 calories daily. His 24-hour calorie count from yesterday totals 1,800 calories.

1. *What* **CUES (Assessment)** *might the nurse identify in this situation?*
2. *What* **HYPOTHESIS (Diagnosis)** *will the nurse consider based on the available information?*
3. *Which members of the interprofessional team would have the expertise to address the patient's needs through* **ACTION (Plan and Implement)**?
4. *How can the interprofessional team work together to meet the patient's* **OUTCOME (Evaluation)** *of nutritional needs?*

Strategies for Communication in Difficult Situations

Challenging patient care situations such as patient resuscitations, difficult patient procedures, rapid response efforts, or end-of-life events require extreme attention and clarity. Unnecessary conversation should cease during these situations and all communication should focus on the situation at hand without distractions. To ensure patient safety at these times, communication senders and receivers should continually verify their communication using check-backs. For example, during a difficult labor and delivery, the physician might assertively request many urgent medications and interventions. In this chaotic and unnerving situation, it is essential that the nurse and other healthcare professionals verify what orders and instructions are being understood and followed by repeating them to those giving the orders.

Documentation must be clear and accurate during these times so as to provide a written account of events. It is during these stressful patient care situations that communication with patients and families can sometimes be overlooked. This can be avoided by including the patient in decision-making whenever possible and appointing someone on the team to provide updates to the family. Family presence at patient resuscitations is becoming more commonplace. Institutions that support this practice designate a member of the team, frequently a nurse, to support the family and explain the interventions and actions of the healthcare team's efforts. Supporting the family during such a high-stress, high-stakes event requires skillful communication that is clear, accurate, and compassionate.

Managing Conflict

It is vital to patient safety that the lines of communication remain open among all those involved in the patient's care. When there is disruption in the smooth flow of communication among team members, it is important to address it promptly before it becomes a more prolonged barrier to communication. Destructive events such as physicians who will not respond to being paged, nurses who are resistant to carrying out legitimate orders, or pharmacists who do not move quickly to fill STAT or urgent prescriptions create difficult communications among healthcare providers that can negatively impact patient care but there are strategies the nurse can use to resolve these communication challenges (Table 7.5). Team members must be vigilant in fulfilling their ethical duty to work together for the patient's well-being.

TABLE 7.5 STRATEGIES FOR DIFFICULT COMMUNICATIONS

HEALTHCARE PROVIDER	COMMUNICATION ISSUE	THE NURSE'S BEST COMMUNICATION APPROACH
Physician	Not answering page	Call physician's office or overhead page to solve immediate problem; later discuss with physician that the patient's needs are the primary concern and give the reason for the page.
Physician	Speaking in an angry condescending manner	Maintain calm and keep focus on the patient; state your primary concern is to solve the patient's immediate need. Identify the patient's need clearly and succinctly using SBAR format.
Pharmacist	Not filling STAT orders quickly	Maintain calm and explain patient's immediate need.
Unlicensed assistive personnel	Not following through with delegated duties	Explore reasons for why duties were not completed. If needed, make adjustment to workload. Develop plan for future communication regarding delegated duties.
Nurse	Rolls eyes and sighs during report; indicates irritation with you	Respond in civil tone, stating that you sense there is something the nurse wants to say and that you learn when people are direct. Ask nurse to please be direct with their concerns.
Nurse	Does not provide assistance when needed	Explore reasons for lack of assistance; be quick to volunteer to help others to set example and model appropriate behavior.
Nurse	Resistant to carrying out legitimate orders	Explore concerns related to orders; develop plan. Offer assistance to peers when able.

SBAR, situation, background, assessment, and recommendation.

Negative or difficult communication in the work environment can come from patients, families, physicians, other nurses, or any person involved in the operations of the institution. Physicians who yell, do not answer calls, and display disrespect and condescension toward colleagues make it uncomfortable to practice. Miscommunications between the interprofessional team can put patients at risk. Stressed patients, families, and/or staff can act out frustrations and aggression. It is important that all members of the interprofessional team respect the expertise of each individual, giving each the power to speak up and provide input in decision-making with the team.

Horizontal Violence

One of the most troubling conflicts for nurses is nurse-to-nurse aggression, known as lateral violence or horizontal violence. Horizontal violence is uncivil behavior toward colleagues that causes injury to the dignity of another (Bloom, 2019). It can manifest in many ways that include subtle actions like making faces or raising eyebrows in response to comments, to more serious behaviors of withholding information that interferes with a colleague's ability to perform professionally or purposely making oneself unavailable to help. Newer vehicles for lateral violence include social media and public humiliation. Nurses can experience physical (loss of sleep, weight loss, irritable bowel syndrome) and/or psychological (depression, anxiety, and loss of confidence) symptoms as a result of lateral violence (Bloom, 2019). Along with injuring the individual nurse, lateral violence can interfere with continuity of care, put patients at risk, and be detrimental to institutions that provide care.

Conflicts and negative behaviors place patients at risk because they cause distraction, preventing the nurse from functioning at their best. Nurses have an obligation to report behaviors that compromise patient safety or the well-being of coworkers to their supervisor or someone else in authority who can adequately address the problem. If left unresolved, conflicts can keep nurses from communicating patient concerns to providers, from asking questions when they are unsure, and from asking for help when critical situations arise.

Nurses can experience hostile work conditions from peers, physicians, patients, or patient families. In these situations, bringing the discussion back to the patient's needs takes the focus off any perceived power struggle and helps everyone to refocus on the priorities at hand. Nurses can enlist the support of more senior colleagues when conflicts arise with team members. Other useful neutralizing techniques include listening attentively to others and demonstrating concern. Nurses can reduce negative situations by identifying people who are receptive to their questions and are willing to serve as resources. It is important for nurses to set the example by ending conversations where coworkers are being discussed in a negative manner.

New-to-practice nurses are more vulnerable to horizontal violence and hostile work conditions due to their lack of experience. Addressing these conditions as soon as possible frequently puts an end to it. However, it is important not to be confrontational in one's approach. An effective tactic against horizontal violence is to develop **de-escalation** strategies for these encounters, which can decrease the intensity and stress of the situation. Griffin (2004) developed de-escalation strategies all nurses can use regardless of level of experience. When confronted with nonverbal innuendos such as eyebrow raising, rolling of eyes, and long sighs by peers, one can be direct and say, "I sense that there is something that you want to say to me. I learn best when people are direct. It's okay if you are direct with me." This type of response directly addresses the horizontal violence in a civil manner without aggression. It indicates to the violator that their body language is perceived as negative and that it is preferable for the recipient to discuss the reason for it rather than ignore it. It should be said in earnest and not with anger to de-escalate the situation and open the lines of communication. Griffin and Clark (2014) developed a method that combines this direct process with team training skills for use when de-escalation strategies alone are not successful. They suggest using the CUS acronym, stating, "I'm concerned with the way you are speaking to me, I'm uncomfortable with where this conversation is going, and I don't think it is safe for us to continue." Using this strategy allows the exchange to end in a civil manner before it escalates further.

Those in leadership positions have a crucial role in creating a workplace environment where horizontal violence and hostile communications are not tolerated. Leaders need to set the standard for realistic expectations regarding workload so that their staff can meet those expectations and have a sense of accomplishment and satisfaction with their work and their work environment rather than feeling discouraged. Nursing leaders within the organization have an obligation to their direct care nurses to establish policies that discourage horizontal violence and help staff feel comfortable in confronting such behavior without fear of retaliation.

Communicating With Preceptors

Preceptors are experienced nurses who provide orientation and support to new-to-practice nurses as they learn the roles and responsibilities of a new job. Preceptors have increased responsibilities of caring for patients while providing instruction to new nurses. They are frequently chosen for this important role because of their expertise in caring for patients and because they exemplify professional behaviors. New-to-practice nurses rely heavily on their preceptors to guide them in learning how to communicate with other team members and become a productive member of the healthcare team. Communicating with team members requires that nurses maintain a professional presence and act with confidence.

During the orientation period, communication can be intimidating for the new nurse. It is difficult to feel like a valued member of the team when one is not sure about what to anticipate next. It can be a stressful time for both the preceptor and the orientee, particularly during high-stress patient care situations. To diffuse tense communication, an honest and open exchange between the preceptor and the orientee at a quiet moment later will provide an opportunity to clarify concerns and reach an understanding about expectations. The new nurse can open the discussion by identifying their desire to learn and understand the situation. New nurses need to maintain realistic expectations regarding their knowledge base and expertise and seek feedback that will help them develop skill and effective clinical judgment. Accepting that they have knowledge gaps will allow the new nurse to ask questions without injury to self-esteem. Collaboration skills improve as the nurse develops a better understanding of the work expectation and unit routine.

Cognitive Rehearsal

It is most important to continually promote an environment of respect and collaboration. Nurses must challenge themselves to use respectful negotiation when disagreements occur between members of the healthcare team and to remain civil in the face of incivility as part of their professional development. Cognitive rehearsal is one strategy that the nurse can use when confronted with incivility from a coworker or another person. Cognitive rehearsal is a prepared response that one practices ahead of time that would address a negative comment or situation in a civil manner. It allows one to not react emotionally but to pause and respond with a rehearsed, intellectually driven, civil response. For instance, if a coworker harshly criticizes the speed with which a nurse completes a task, rather than react emotionally and become hurt and angry, the nurse might respond by saying, "This is different from how I learned. Can you help me to understand how you complete it so quickly?"

As mentioned earlier, reflection and the ability to gain insight into one's actions can facilitate powerful, effective change. Specifically, reflecting on one's ability to communicate with colleagues and other members of the interprofessional team provides an opportunity to consider behaviors that build consensus among colleagues and behaviors that create barriers to communication and interfere with safe patient care. To guide reflection, one can ask oneself, "What went well?" "What could have gone better?" "What could I have done to improve this situation?" These questions will help to bring clarity to where improvement is possible.

Communicating With Hospital and Nursing Leadership

Hospital and nursing leadership have a significant influence on how teams function. Leaders can set the tone for communication, role model effective conflict management, and create and foster an environment that facilitates safety and quality care. Nurse managers, preceptors, and other leaders within the healthcare organization can support new-to-practice nurses by providing effective feedback. Nurses can approach leaders to facilitate needed change when a chain of command authority is needed. Most leaders continually assess their environment as well as the people that report to them to determine if adequate support is provided for their subordinates to do their jobs. However, leaders can miss

Real World Interview

I started my nursing career in critical care 6 months before the COVID-19 pandemic. I had just finished my new graduate residency program a couple weeks before my hospital encountered its first coronavirus patient. Even though I had completed the extensive orientation program, I still struggled to find confidence as a new nurse. I was often comparing my knowledge and clinical skills to that of nurses who worked on my unit for years or even decades. These insecurities soon faded when even the most experienced nurses and providers were overwhelmed and unfamiliar with the treatment modalities for COVID-19. We were all facing the same learning curve. Nurses who had precepted me 1-month prior would sometimes come to me with questions about the new policies and procedures we were to follow. Everyone came together to support one another. Staff from all over the hospital assumed different roles to create a more cohesive team. Speech pathologists became supply runners for the units. Physical therapists were trained to assist respiratory therapists and nurses to re-position and prone intubated patients. Among all of the craziness there was a strong sense of community between members of our care team. I was especially proud to be a nurse, especially a new nurse during this time. As stressful as it was, I feel I gained invaluable experience that will guide the rest of my career.

Amanda de Vera, RN
The Valley Hospital, Ridgewood, New Jersey

CASE STUDY

The new nurse and a senior colleague are assigned to the same patient room. The new nurse is caring for the patient in Bed B and the senior colleague is caring for the patient in Bed A. While in the room, the new nurse notices that the patient in Bed A is sleeping. On the bedside table, there is a filled medication syringe and an empty vial labeled heparin, 10,000 units/mL. Knowing this is unsafe, the new nurse carries the medication syringe and heparin out to the nurse's station and states to the senior colleague, "These were on the bedside table." The senior colleague takes them and states, "Yes, I have to remember to give the heparin to him when he wakes up" and returns them to the patient's bedside table.

1. *What standard is the senior colleague violating?*
2. *Recognizing that the senior colleague did not react to the implied concern for the patient's safety and the standard of practice, what communication strategy could the new nurse implement to maintain this patient's safety?*
3. *How can new nurses address practice concerns like this from an organization's point of view to prevent this type of practice?*

subtle signs of trouble or inefficiency. In that case, nurses must take it upon themselves to approach the leader to ask for help. Effective communication and team building help ensure the message for requesting help or clarification will be heard.

The responsibility of the nurse manager to serve as a role model for team building and collaboration cannot be understated. The nurse manager will be the leader that direct care nurses will have the greatest amount of interaction with, making it essential that they demonstrate active listening and partnership in solving problems. Engagement is supported by feedback that builds rather than tears down so skills in delivering and receiving constructive feedback need to be demonstrated by the nurse manager so that others can emulate them. Behaviors that demonstrate respect and collegiality will build and sustain a civil work environment and set the expectation for the interprofessional team.

Interprofessional teamwork and collaboration are essential to ensure quality healthcare for patients and maintain safety. Nurses are valued members of the interprofessional healthcare team. Nurses' contribution to the patient's care include knowledgeable assessments, reflective thinking, effective planning, thoughtful interventions based on evidence-based practice, and careful evaluation of care. Nurses' communication skills play a pivotal role in team building. Nurses who communicate concerns and address problems enhance their ability to prevent errors, achieve positive patient outcomes and patient satisfaction, and improve the system in which they work.

END-OF-CHAPTER RESOURCES

KEY CONCEPTS

1. An interprofessional healthcare team consists of people who have a stake or interest in and contribute to the well-being of the patient, for example, physicians; nurses; family members; and those who provide support services, such as pharmacists, social workers, dietitians, and those from departments such as housekeeping, radiology, the laboratory, transport services, and physical and occupational therapy.
2. The IPEC core competencies describe expectations for collaborative practice among and between disciplines in healthcare, forming a foundation for how each might contribute to the work of the healthcare team and effectively coordinate care (Table 7.1).
3. Recognizing the value of nursing, the IOM, now known as the National Academy of Medicine, in collaboration with the RWJF, published its report, *The Future of Nursing: Leading Change, Advancing Health* (IOM, 2011). The four key recommendations from the report were focused on the role that nursing should have in providing care (Box 7.1).
4. A rapid response team (RRT) is a team that includes specific healthcare professionals with specialized skills, who can mobilize and deliver immediate patient assessment and intervention if needed at the patient's bedside any time of day or night, 7 days a week at the beginning signs of deterioration in the patient's health status.
5. Root cause analysis (RCA) discovers the root of an error by not stopping at the first answer it arrives at for its cause, but by delving deeper into why the error occurred, asking questions until there are no more questions to ask so that causes for error can be identified and prevented in the future.
6. In healthcare, poor outcomes occur when there are breakdowns in communication, poor teamwork, or inefficient communication "handoffs" that create situations that can lead to errors.
7. "Forming," "storming," "norming," and "performing" are terms used to describe the stages experienced by teams as they progress from formation to functioning as high-performance teams (Tuckman, 1965).
8. When delegating, the nurse employs the following steps: assess and plan; communicate what needs to be done; ensure availability to assist and support; and, finally, evaluate effectiveness.
9. Originating in the aviation industry for the cockpit crew, crew resource management (CRM) develops communication, leadership, and decision-making safety strategies to combat the potential for human error that is inherent in high-stress systems and prevent its devastating effects.
10. Situational awareness is having the right information at the right time alongside the ability to analyze that information to appropriately and effectively take action. The vehicle for this attentiveness is effective communication between interprofessional healthcare team members.
11. Team*STEPPS* is a program designed to teach interprofessional teams how to communicate with each other to promote situational awareness and patient safety (AHRQ, n.d.).
12. Situation, background, assessment, and recommendation (SBAR; AHRQ, n.d.) was developed by the military and is now applied to healthcare as a means to relay significant information regarding a patient's condition or to be used as patients' care is communicated and handed-off from one caregiver to another (Table 7.2).

13. Time-outs are required structured work-stops for everyone in the room to stop and ensure that the correct patient is having the correct procedure done to the correct site as a way to prevent wrong-site surgeries.
14. Safety huddles provide semi-structured opportunities for those caring for the patient to review pertinent information and the plan of care.
15. Cross-monitoring; callout; two-challenge rule; concerned, uncomfortable, and safety (CUS); check-back/read-back, and handoff are developed by the AHRQ, which provides reference videos for clinicians, administrators, and educators demonstrating Team*STEPPS* tools, strategies, and techniques at its website, www.ahrq.gov/professionals/education/curriculum-tools/teamstepps/instructor/videos/index.html (Table 7.3).
16. Timely reporting of errors and near misses, also known as close calls, where an error could have occurred but was stopped before it caused harm provides an opportunity for the team to learn from them. In most cases, errors and near misses are often the result of a failure within a healthcare system.
17. There are many available web resources funded by government agencies and national healthcare organizations that are designed to improve teamwork and collaboration, prevent error, promote patient safety, and improve the quality of the care that patients receive (Table 7.4).
18. Debriefing is the process of reviewing performance effectiveness following challenging patient care situations.
19. Feedback, whether positive or negative, should always be an unbiased reflection of what occurred, opening the door to a discussion of evidence-based practice. Constructive feedback should carefully detail events as they occurred and avoid opinion.
20. Teams can work together to conduct audits and other organizational studies that measure quality, safety, and patient outcomes, which can have a significant impact on the process of quality improvement (QI).
21. Providing feedback to team members allows the team to identify strengths and weaknesses, make changes to the healthcare system, and adjust practice for individual growth and development.
22. Self-evaluation of one's communication and decision-making is a crucial element of professional growth and strengthens one's ability to contribute to the team's decisions by employing strong clinical judgment.
23. Tanner's Model of Thinking Like a Nurse (2006) demonstrates how clinical judgment is developed through reflection, enhancing critical thinking skills.
24. Mindfulness implies staying focused with the ability to see the significance of early and weak signals as well as to take strong and decisive action to prevent harm (Weick & Sutcliffe, 2001).
25. Communication between the healthcare team, the patient, and the patient's family during times of stress and illness can be challenging but it is essential to safety and a key factor in patient satisfaction.
26. Many barriers can interfere with communication, such as knowledge gaps, education levels, culture, language barriers, or stress. It is important for nurses to develop strategies to identify and overcome these barriers.

27. Effective communication is essential to maintaining a safe and protected environment for patients. Ineffective communication continues to be identified as the root cause for many sentinel events reported to The Joint Commission (2016).
28. Destructive events such as physicians who will not respond to pages, nurses who are resistant to carrying out legitimate orders, or pharmacists who do not move quickly to fill STAT prescriptions create difficult communications among healthcare providers that can negatively impact patient care (Table 7.5).
29. Horizontal violence, also known as lateral violence, is nurse-to-nurse aggression. New-to-practice nurses are more vulnerable to horizontal violence and hostile work conditions in the healthcare environment due to their lack of experience.
30. Reflection and the ability to gain insight into one's one actions can facilitate powerful, effective change.
31. Hospital and nursing leadership have a significant influence on how teams function.

CRITICAL DISCUSSION POINTS

1. During your last clinical experience, what examples of interprofessional teamwork and collaboration did you see?
2. What interprofessional teamwork and collaboration resources are available to nurses within the nursing unit or department of nursing in your practice setting? How are nurses involved in interprofessional teamwork and collaboration in the health system?
3. How are patients, families, nurses, and other healthcare professionals included in daily interprofessional rounds at your practice setting? Do you see examples of collaborative practice?
4. At your clinical site, how do the nurses feel about the culture of interprofessional teamwork and collaboration within their work environment?
5. If a nurse has an idea that will improve the interprofessional teamwork and collaboration regarding patient care delivery, where would they take that idea to share it?

KEY TERMS

> Collaboration
> Cross-monitoring
> Debriefing
> De-escalation strategies
> Handoff
> Interprofessional education
> Mindfulness
> Near miss
> Rapid response teams
> Root cause analysis
> Situational awareness

REVIEW QUESTIONS

Answers to Review Questions appear in the Instructor's Manual. Qualified instructors should request the Instructor's Manual from textbook@springerpub.com.

1. A nurse receives a telephone order from a physician for specific x-ray tests. The nurse established the identity of the patient involved and the name of the ordering physician. Which action should the nurse take next to ensure patient safety?
   A. Write the order on the order sheet in the chart.
   B. Repeat what the physician says and then write it down on the order sheet.
   C. Ask the physician to directly place the order with the radiology department.
   D. Write the order on the order sheet and then perform a read-back to the physician to verify the order is accurate.
2. The charge nurse is teaching the staff about RRT that will be initiated at the hospital to better meet the needs of patients. Which instructions should be included to describe how nurses should utilize the RRT? *Select all that apply.*
   A. Use the RRT when you need support for a medical-surgical patient whose status is deteriorating so that you can prevent a cardiac or respiratory arrest.
   B. Call an RRT to rapidly move a patient through the hospital system at the time of transfer.
   C. Initiate an RRT to notify the attending physician of the client's deteriorating status.
   D. Deploy the RRT to provide immediate assistance to patients in the intensive care unit.
   E. An RRT can be initiated any time of day or night by anyone, even the patient's family, to address a health concern.
3. The nurse is transferring a patient from the ICU to the step-down patient care unit. When the ICU nurse calls report to the receiving unit, what is the best way for the nurse to provide the handoff information?
   A. Systems, background, assessment, requirements
   B. Situation, background, assessment, recommendations
   C. Systems, background, activities, recommendations
   D. Situation, behaviors, activities, requirements
4. The nurse pages a physician due to the patient's change in status. When the physician calls the unit, the physician yells at the nurse for interrupting a procedure. Which of the following would be the nurse's best approach in responding to the physician?
   A. Tell the physician that he will be reported to the nursing supervisor.
   B. Tell the physician that the call is important and does not warrant being yelled at.
   C. Refocus the communication on the patient and the reason for the call.
   D. Apologize for interrupting the procedure and page the physician's partner.

5. The nurse is caring for a patient who is a paraplegic after an automobile accident. The patient is not eating and refuses to participate in rehabilitation activities. The mother of the patient asks the nurse to intervene. Which actions by the nurse would be most effective?

A. Assemble the interdisciplinary team caring for the patient to discuss a plan of care.
B. Discuss options with the patient for modifying the daily schedule.
C. Tell the patient he must eat and participate in rehabilitation to improve.
D. Encourage the family to bring food from home that the patient enjoys.
E. Assure the mother that all patients experience this reaction.

6. Following a serious medication error that resulted in patient injury, a nurse is assigned to a team assembled to investigate the cause. Which process would be the best method for determining how the error occurred and how similar errors can be prevented in the future?

A. Root cause analysis
B. Debriefing
C. Six Sigma
D. Crew resource management

7. The nurse on the oncology unit cares for a patient who frequently comments that she would like better pain control through the night. The nurse tells the patient that a note will be placed on the front of the patient's chart alerting the physician in case the nurse misses the physician during patient rounds. Which collaborative processes could the nurse use to ensure the patient's needs are met? *Select all that apply.*

A. Nursing rounds
B. Team huddle
C. Debriefing
D. Root cause analysis
E. Including the patient in bedside shift report

8. A patient's family is angry about their family member's deteriorating condition and tells the nurse that they are not satisfied with the patient's care. Which of the following actions by the nurse would be most appropriate? *Select all that apply.*

A. Notify the charge nurse of the family's dissatisfaction.
B. Explain to the family that the patient's condition is complex and that the patient is receiving appropriate care.
C. Convey understanding and notify members of the healthcare team so that a family meeting with the team can be provided.
D. Ask the family members why they feel the care is not satisfactory.
E. Describe to the family what actions are being taken with the current plan of care.

9. During a patient resuscitation, the team leader yells at the nurse for not having the appropriate medications at the ready for administration. Feeling hurt, the nurse seeks support from a nurse colleague regarding the incident. Which would be the most appropriate action by the nurse colleague?

A. Conduct a root cause analysis of the incident.
B. Explain that the incident occurred during a stressful experience.
C. Pull the team together for a post-resuscitation debriefing.
D. Instruct the nurse to use the CUS technique to confront the team leader.

10. The nurse draws up hydromorphone 2 mg instead of morphine 2 mg for a patient experiencing pain. Realizing the error before administering the medication, the nurse discards the hydromorphone with a witness and administers the correct medication to the patient. Afterward, which actions by the nurse will be most effective in preventing similar events in the future? *Select all that apply.*

A. Explain what happened to the patient and family.

B. Report the near-miss medication error so that it can be examined for a root cause.

C. Discuss the event at a staff meeting and elicit the feedback of peers.

D. Participate in a debriefing to discuss sound-alike medications used on the unit.

E. Describe the error at grand rounds.

REVIEW ACTIVITIES

1. At noon, Mrs. Joan Smith calls the nurse into the room and complains of shortness of breath. Mrs. Smith was admitted 1 day prior for pulmonary edema and has been treated with nasal oxygen at 4 liters, and furosemide (Lasix) 40 mg IV every 12 hours (8 a.m. and 8 p.m.). The nurse determines that the patient's respiratory rate is 30, the pulse oximetry reading is 91%, and auscultation of the lungs reveals crackles midway to the clavicles. Using the SBAR technique, provide report to the physician regarding the patient's condition.
2. The nurse believes the dose of vancomycin ordered for a patient is too high and may be dangerous for the patient to receive because of a reported creatinine of 1.9 mg/dL. What communication strategy would the nurse implement to alert the prescribing physician? How would it be implemented?
3. The nurse receives a critical lab result via telephone from the laboratory. What safety strategy should the nurse implement to ensure safety regarding the lab value? How would this be implemented?

EXPLORING THE WEB

1. Giving and Receiving Constructive Feedback. Review this 18-minute narrated presentation to learn how to give and to receive constructive feedback to improve practice and build teamwork: qsen.org/giving-and-receiving-constructive-feedback/

   Discussion: This is a narrated presentation focused on helping students to understand the importance of learning to give and to receive constructive feedback. Key points include understanding constructive feedback's role in QI and patient safety, and learning to view constructive feedback as an opportunity for improvement. Students may listen to it online, at home, or in the classroom with a faculty member. The presentation can be loaded into Electronic Course Frameworks and assigned. If assigned as an out of class activity, faculty can have students blog or post in discussions about what they gained from the presentation.
2. Access qsen.org and find the Teamwork and Collaboration Competency. Review the knowledge, skill, and attitude that embody the competency. Then go to the Publication tab and review the various articles, toolkits, and other resources. Do you find something that could help you with a current group of people/classmates/colleagues you are working with?

3. Review and access the websites listed in Table 7.4. What do you identify as the consistent theme or focus of all of these websites? What strategies do you see on these websites that would enhance teamwork?

REFERENCES

Agency for Healthcare Research and Quality. (n.d.). *TeamSTEPPS™ fundamentals course: Module 1. Introduction: Instructor's slides*. https://www.ahrq.gov/teamstepps/instructor/fundamentals/module1/igintro.html

Bloom, E. M. (2019). Horizontal violence among nurses: Experiences, responses, and job performance. *Nursing Forum, 54*, 77–83. https://doi.org/10.1111/nuf.12300

Clynes, M. P., & Raftery, S. E. C. (2008). Feedback: An essential element of student learning in clinical practice. *Nurse Education in Practice*, *8*, 405–411. https://doi.org/10.1016/j.nepr.2008.02.003

Greiner, A. C., & Knebel, E. (Eds.). (2003). *Health professions education: A bridge to quality*. National Academies Press. https://www.ncbi.nlm.nih.gov/books/NBK221528

Griffin, M. (2004). Teaching cognitive rehearsal as a shield for lateral violence: An intervention for newly licensed nurses. *The Journal of Continuing Education in Nursing*, *3*(6), 257–263. https://doi.org/10.3928/0022-0124-20041101-07

Griffin, M., & Clark, C. (2014). Revisiting cognitive rehearsal as an intervention against incivility and lateral violence in nursing: 10 years later. *Journal of Continuing Education in Nursing*, *45*(12), 535–542. https://doi.org/10.3928/00220124-20141122-02

Hattie, J., & Timperley, H. (2007). The power of feedback. *Review of Educational Research*, *77*(1), 81–112. https://doi.org/10.3102/003465430298487

Institute for Healthcare Improvement. (n.d.). *Rapid response teams*. Retrieved from http://www.ihi.org/explore/RapidResponseTeams/Pages/default.aspx

Institute of Medicine. (2011). *The future of nursing: Leading change, advancing health*. National Academies Press. https://doi.org/10.17226/12956

Interprofessional Education Collaborative. (2016). *Core competencies for interprofessional collaborative practice: 2016 update*. Interprofessional Education Collaborative. https://ipec.memberclicks.net/assets/2016-Update.pdf

National Council of State Boards of Nursing and American Nurses Association. (2019). *National guidelines for nursing delegation: Position paper*. https://www.ncsbn.org/NGND-PosPaper_06.pdf

National League for Nursing. (2016). *Guide to effective interprofessional education experiences in nursing education*. http://www.nln.org/docs/default-source/default-document-library/ipe-toolkit-krk-012716.pdf?sfvrsn=6

Tanner, C. A. (2006). Thinking like a nurse: A research based model of clinical judgment in nursing. *Journal of Nursing Education*, *4*(6), 204–211. https://doi.org/10.3928/01484834-20060601-04

The Joint Commission. (n.d.). *The universal protocol for preventing wrong site, wrong procedure, and wrong person surgery™: Guidance for health care professionals*. http://www.jointcommission.org/assets/1/18/UP_Poster.pdf

The Joint Commission. (2019). *Summary data of sentinel events reviewed by The Joint Commission*. https://www.jointcommission.org/-/media/tjc/documents/resources/patient-safety-topics/sentinel-event/summary-2q-2019.pdf

Tuckman, B. (1965). Developmental sequence in small groups. *Psychological Bulletin*, *63*(6), 384–399. https://doi.org/10.1037/h0022100

Unknown participant. (2007, June). *Quality and Safety Education for Nurses (QSEN) collaboration*.

U.S. Department of Labor. (2020). *Labor force statistics from the current population survey.* https://www.bls.gov/cps/cpsaat11.htm

Weick, K. E., & Sutcliffe, K. M. (2001). *Managing the unexpected.* Jossey-Bass.

SUGGESTED READINGS

Altmiller, G. (2012). The role of constructive feedback in patient safety and continuous quality improvement. *Nursing Clinics of North America*, *47*(3), 365–374. http://doi.org/10.1016/j.cnur.2012.05.002

American Nurses Association. (2015). *Code of ethics for nurses with interpretive statements.* http://nursingworld.org/MainMenuCategories/EthicsStandards/CodeofEthicsforNurses/Code-of-ethics.pdf

Callaway, C., Cunningham, C., Grover, S., Steele, K. R., McGlynn, A., & Sribanditmongko, V. (2018). Patient handoff processes: Implementation and effects of bedside handoffs, the teach-back method, and discharge bundles on an inpatient oncology unit. *Clinical Journal of Oncology Nursing, 22*(4), 421–428. https://doi.org/10.1188/18.CJON.421-428

Clark, C. (2019). Fostering a culture of civility and respect in nursing. *Journal of Nursing Regulation, 10*(1), 44–52. https://doi.org/10.1016/S2155-8256(19)30082-1

Cronenwett, L., Sherwood, G., Barnsteiner, J., Disch, J., Johnson, J., Mitchell, P., & Warren, J. (2007). Quality and Safety Education for Nurses. *Nursing Outlook*, *55*(3), 112–131. http://doi.org/10.1016/j.outlook.2007.02.006

Granitto, M., Linenfelser, P., Hursey, R., Parsons, M., & Norton, C. (2020). Empowering nurses to activate the rapid response team. *Nursing, 50*(6), 52–57. https://doi.org/10.1097/01.NURSE.0000662356.08413.90

Greiner, A. C., & Knebel, E. (Eds.). (2003). *Health professions education: A bridge to quality.* National Academies Press. https://www.ncbi.nlm.nih.gov/books/NBK221528

Lim, F., & Pajarillo, E. J. Y. (2016). Standardized handoff report form in clinical nursing education: An educational tool for patient safety and quality of care. *Nurse Education Today*, *37*(3), 3–7. http://doi.org/10.1016/j.nedt.2015.10.026

McNeill, M. M., Archer, S., Remsburg, D., Storer, J., & Rudman, H. (2019). Rapid response team–quality champion register nurse: Observations and perceptions. *Journal of Nursing Care Quality, 34*(4), 325–329. https://doi.org/10.1097/NCQ.0000000000000393

CHAPTER 8

Informatics

Beth A. Vottero

"The biggest waste in the healthcare system is not unnecessary treatment or duplicated test results; it is that we collect data and never use it again."

–*Chris Lehmann, MD, Vanderbilt University professor of pediatrics and biomedical informatics*

Upon completion of this chapter, the reader should be able to:

1. Define nursing informatics.
2. Identify the sciences that contribute to nursing informatics.
3. Explore the data, information, knowledge, and wisdom framework that guides nursing informatics.
4. Describe the benefits and limitations of technologies used in healthcare and their impact on safety and quality.
5. Identify key elements of an electronic medical record and electronic health record that support safe patient care.
6. Differentiate between the concepts of privacy, confidentiality and security in relation to patient data and information.
7. Examine the impact of regulations on nursing informatics.
8. Explain the role telehealth plays in the care of the homebound or rurally located patients.
9. Describe how to evaluate the quality of health-related content on websites and applications.
10. Explain technology initiatives that support the delivery of safe patient care such as clinical decision support systems and clinical alerts.

CROSSWALK

This chapter addresses the following:

QSEN Competency: Informatics

The American Association of Colleges of Nursing. (2021). *The essentials: Core competencies for professional nursing education.*

Domain 8: Informatics and Healthcare Technologies

OPENING SCENARIO

A patient is discharged from the hospital after a thyroidectomy and, during the discharge process, was given a code to access the hospital's web-based patient portal. At home, the patient logs into the hospital website and accesses the patient portal. The patient can view messages from the hospital and physician, lab results, test results, medication record, and follow-up appointments. While reviewing test results, the patient notices that the pathology report from the thyroidectomy stated papillary carcinoma. The patient did not know what this result meant and performed a web search for the topic. The patient was not informed that the pathology identified cancer while in the hospital and called the physician for clarification.

- *What is the benefit of a patient portal?*
- *What information should be accessible through a patient portal?*
- *What types of policies and procedures should be in place for patient portals?*

INTRODUCTION

Nursing informatics is an evolving specialty field in nursing. This growth is due in part to the expanding capacity of technology leading to breakthroughs in supporting communication and improving analytics. Healthcare has embraced the known abilities and the potential of technology in supporting high-quality, safe patient care nationwide. While still a new specialty, nursing informatics has grown to become a critical asset within healthcare organizations.

This chapter defines nursing informatics and the data, information, knowledge, and wisdom model that guides nursing informatics as a specialty as well as presents the sciences contributing to nursing informatics: computer science, cognitive science, and nursing science. The electronic medical record (EMR) and electronic health record (EHR) are explored through the lens of collecting and synthesizing patient data and information at the point of care. The role of technologies in hospitals and other healthcare systems is explored. In addition to inpatient examples of nursing informatics, the role telehealth plays in outpatient care is discussed. Health information technology designed to support the delivery of high-quality patient care is explored. Federal laws that protect identifiable information are detailed, providing differentiation between the concepts of privacy, confidentiality, and security. Lastly, the effects of technology on communication and telehealth are explored.

NURSING INFORMATICS DEFINED

While informatics is simply the science of collecting, managing, and retrieving information, **nursing informatics** is "the specialty that integrates nursing science with multiple information and analytical sciences to identify, define, manage, and communicate data, information, knowledge, and wisdom in nursing practice" (American Nurses Association [ANA], 2015, p. 1–2). Quality and Safety Education for Nurses (QSEN) describes informatics as the use of "Information and technology to communicate, manage knowledge, mitigate error, and support decision making" (Cronenwett et al., 2007, p. 197). Newly licensed nurses are expected to possess informatics knowledge, skills and attitudes that reflect the ability of the nurse to competently provide high-quality, safe patient-centered care in a technology-rich nursing care environment (Cronenwett et al., 2007).

Information and analytical sciences that make up nursing informatics include, but are not limited to, computer science, cognitive science, social science, communication science, and library science (ANA, 2015). Each of the sciences brings important elements to nursing informatics (Table 8.1). Each of these sciences contribute to how technology is used for patient care delivery through a different viewpoint, yet all of them are essential to nursing informatics.

METASTRUCTURE OF NURSING INFORMATICS

The guiding structure for nursing informatics, also known as the metastructure, was built upon the way nurses interact and use clinical information systems. In the ANA description, "data, information, knowledge, and wisdom" form the metastructure, which increases in complexity as work increases in interactions and interrelationships (2015). Both the sciences and the metastructure form the framework for understanding nursing informatics. Figure 8.1 is an illustration of how the concepts of data, information, knowledge, and wisdom form the metastructure for nursing informatics.

TABLE 8.1 SCIENCES CONTRIBUTING TO NURSING INFORMATICS

SCIENCE	CONTRIBUTION TO NURSING INFORMATICS
Computer Science	Design of computer hardware or software systems such as the electronic health or medical record, including how data is collected and stored and how people interact with the computer.
Cognitive Science	Examination of how humans process information. Computer systems are designed with decision supports, providing trended data, or reminders at the point of care.
Social Science	Investigation of the interactions among humans. How healthcare professionals interact with patients, specifically the dynamic between the patient and healthcare provider at the point of care.
Communication Science	Communication of data and information using technology. Health professionals using computer messaging of patient information using messaging systems.
Library Science	Collection, storage, and retrieval of articles. Healthcare professionals accessing the best available evidence to direct interventions to improve patient outcomes.

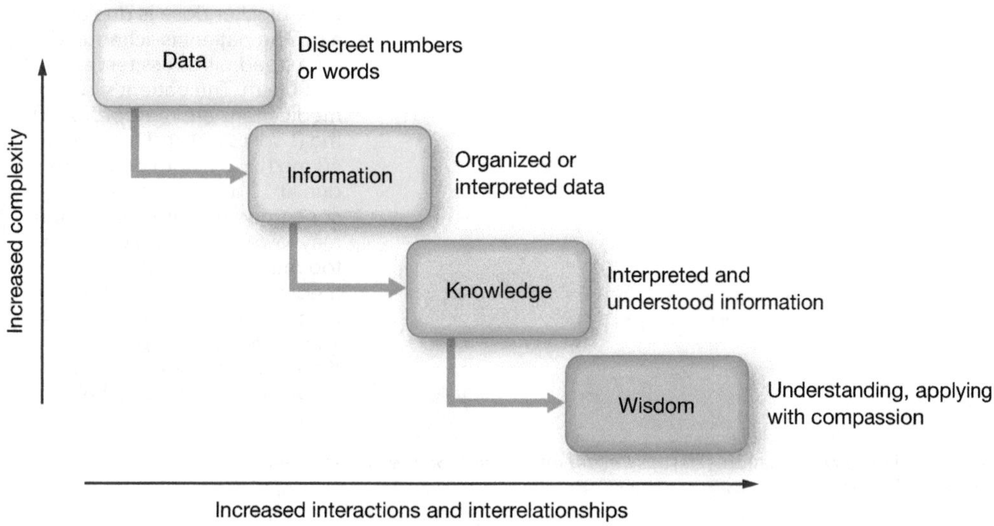

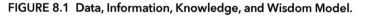

FIGURE 8.1 Data, Information, Knowledge, and Wisdom Model.

The ANA Scope and Standards for Nursing Informatics Practice describe what constitutes each component of the metastructure (Table 8.2).

TABLE 8.2 DATA TO WISDOM METASTRUCTURE COMPONENTS

METASTRUCTURE ELEMENT	DESCRIPTION	EXAMPLE
Data	Discreet points collected and described objectively without interpretation from a variety of sources and includes numbers or words	Data collected for one point in time during an assessment includes: Heart rate: 76 Blood pressure: 118/64 Respiratory rate: 18 Mental state: alert and oriented Eye and hair color: brown eyes, blonde hair
Information	Data that have been organized, structured, and interpreted	Heart rate assessment findings collected over the entire hospitalization that are trended using a graph to show highs and lows in the data
Knowledge	Synthesized information so that relationships are identified and formalized	Heart rate and blood pressure findings for the morning assessment prior to a beta-blocker dose, then looking at the same assessment findings 4 hours after the medication dose to see if it had an effect on heart rate and blood pressure findings. Includes reviewing the same information from previous mornings to see the effect.
Wisdom	The appropriate use of knowledge to manage and solve individual patient problems with consideration for how and when to apply knowledge to complex patient problems	Heart rate is 62 and blood pressure is 104/58 at 9 a.m. The trends over the past 2 days for both vitals show that medications do lower both the heart rate and blood pressure within 1 hour of taking the dose. The beta-blocker dose is due at 10 a.m. The patient is scheduled for a treadmill stress test at 11:00 a.m. The patient's 10 a.m. medications are metoprolol 50 mg (Lopressor) and furosemide 40 mg (Lasix). Both doses are due at 10 a.m. The nurse is concerned that the medications may lower the blood pressure too much and that the medications may also affect the treadmill stress test results. The nurse calls the physician to discuss concerns and ask if the medications should be held until after the test.

American Nurses Association. (2015). *Nursing informatics: Scope and standards of practice* (2nd ed.). Nursebooks.org.

BOX 8.1 Developing Clinical Judgment

Denise is a new nurse on a medical-surgical unit. She is just beginning to become comfortable providing nursing care to her assigned patients. She starts her day by receiving shift report on each of her patients. The shift report is delivered at the bedside allowing Denise to introduce herself and start a plan of care for the day with input from the patient. After report, she looks up the patient's laboratory results in the computer, noting both normal and abnormal findings as well as trends in the data. Denise then completes a thorough nursing assessment on each patient and documents her findings in the electronic documentation record. Today Denise is providing nursing care for a 63-year-old man admitted 2 days ago with heart failure and diabetes. Today the vital signs are blood pressure 90/54, heart rate 82, and respirations of 20. She knows the patient is due for a dose of Lopressor 50 mg PO and Lasix 80 mg PO.

Denise reviewed the EMR and noted the following findings.

	YESTERDAY 6 A.M.	YESTERDAY 11 A.M.	YESTERDAY 4 P.M.	YESTERDAY 10 P.M.	TODAY 6 A.M.	TODAY 10 A.M.	TODAY 4 P.M.
Glucose	148	104	298	423	116	312	469
B-Type Natriuretic Peptide (BTNP)	620				280		
Potassium (K+)	3.2				4.2		

Denise looked at the patient's medications including the following information:

- Lasix 80 mg PO BID at home. Lasix 80 mg IVP given yesterday.
- Levemir 72u SQ BID at home. The same dose is resumed while the patient is in the hospital.
- Lopressor 50 mg BID at home. The same dose is resumed while the patient is in the hospital.

Vital signs charted on the patient and medications given over the past 2 days included:

	YESTERDAY 6 A.M.	YESTERDAY 12 P.M.	YESTERDAY 6 P.M.	TODAY 12 A.M.	TODAY 6 A.M.	TODAY 12 P.M.	TODAY 6 P.M.
Blood Pressure	88/52 Lopressor 50 mg Levemir 72u Lasix 80 mg IVP	112/80	96/58 Lopressor 50 mg Levemir 72u Lasix 80 mg PO	102/62	102/84 Lopressor 50 mg Levemir 72u Lasix 80 mg PO	124/78	90/54
Heart Rate	88	72	74	72	90	96	78
Respirations	20	18	18	16	16	18	18

Answer the following questions based on the given data.

1. What **CUES (Assessment)** can the nurse decipher from the given information?
2. What **HYPOTHESIS (Diagnosis)** or hypotheses can the nurse consider?
3. What **ACTION (Plan and Implement)** will be most effective for the nurse to take to assure the patient's safety in this situation?
4. How will the nurse evaluate the patient's **OUTCOME (Evaluation)** to determine if a satisfactory clinical outcome is achieved?

BID, twice a day; IVP, ; PO, orally; SQ, subcutaneously.

ELECTRONIC MEDICAL RECORDS AND ELECTRONIC HEALTH RECORDS

The Health Care Information Management and Systems Society (HIMSS) discriminates between the two electronic types of records. An **electronic medical record** (EMR) is a legal record of what happened to a patient during one care encounter at a healthcare organization (ONC, n.d.-e). For example, an EMR includes data from one hospital stay, one physician's visit, or one instance of accessing healthcare. The EMR is confined to one point in time or range of dates. In contrast, an **electronic health record** (EHR) is a longitudinal electronic record of patient health information generated by one or more encounters in any care delivery setting (ONC, n.d.-e). Included in this record are patient demographics, provider progress notes, health problems, medication lists, vital signs, the patient's past medical history, past or current immunizations, laboratory data, and radiology reports. In order for an EHR to exist, there must be an EMR in place that captures data from the healthcare encounter. The EHR has the ability to generate a complete record of a clinical patient encounter, as well as supporting other care-related activities including evidence-based decision support, quality management, and outcomes reporting.

EHRs will form the basis of the National Health Information Network (NHIN), which is a plan that will enable the exchange of patient information electronically from one healthcare provider to another healthcare provider. NHIN will allow the healthcare provider to access previous information such as the patient's disease history, the list of medications, the known allergies, and the prior test results. The electronic exchange of patient information will eliminate delays that occur when paper records must be copied and sent to another provider. The NHIN will also help exchange patient information between healthcare providers and public health authorities. For example, submission of reports to government vaccination registries and the reporting of communicable diseases will be done from the EHR. The reports will be done at the same time care is provided (in real time) so agencies charged with protecting the health of the public will be able to act quickly. If a particular lot of a vaccine is recalled, health authorities will know which patients to contact. If a virulent strain of a virus occurs, such as the 2020 Coronavirus pandemic, health authorities can issue public health warnings and close some public places to prevent further spread of the disease. The electronic information exchange within NHIN must protect patient privacy and the content of the data. Healthcare providers have a legal and ethical duty to maintain the confidentiality of patient information. For patient safety, data cannot be altered in any way. For example, information regarding a medication must maintain the same name, dose, frequency, and route of administration as it is being transmitted to another provider. No one should be able to capture the data enroute and change it.

The Department of Health and Human Services predicts that the NHIN will enhance the quality of care by reducing healthcare errors (especially those related to medications), eliminating the need for duplicate testing, thus subjecting the patient to less risk and reducing delays that occur from lack of information. If the efficiency and effectiveness of care is improved, the costs of providing care should be reduced.

HISTORICAL BASIS FOR ELECTRONIC HEALTH RECORDS

Although work in the informatics discipline started many decades ago, a landmark 1991 report by the Institute of Medicine (IOM) brought national attention to the topic of informatics. The report titled *The Computer-Based Patient Record: An Essential Technology for Health Care* stated it was time for the healthcare industry to catch up with other industries regarding its use of information technology (IOM, 1997).

CASE STUDY

A 65-year-old man comes to the emergency department via ambulance after being in a car accident. He is currently unresponsive and has no family members present. He does have a wallet and identification and his car has out of state plates. Without a medical record of past history, medications, test results, or previous medical diagnoses, it is difficult to know how to treat the patient. At this hospital they do have links to a national EHR database. By entering his name and birthdate, the healthcare team can see that the patient has a history of an ischemic stroke and is on Coumadin. The patient also has diabetes and a history of heart failure. The healthcare provider can review the patient's current medications, previous test results, past history, and assessment findings.

1. *How does having access to a patient's previous medical records improve patient care?*
2. *Why is the EHR not currently used widely in the United States?*
3. *Create a concept map with the patient at the center that shows how an EHR can impact the delivery of safe, high-quality patient care.*

At the time of the report, the banking industry already used highly sophisticated electronic information systems with the ability to exchange information between banks and with banking customers with relative ease. Other industries such as the airlines also had initiated advanced electronic information systems that included the ability to make reservations and do flight scheduling. The airlines had access to information about all the passengers on each plane, the names of the staff members, and other important details about each flight. With electronic patient records, information could be more easily exchanged in real time (i.e., as it is happening) among healthcare providers, with legible records, and documentation done at the point of care. Care could be streamlined with more efficient methods of data collection, and computer programs could be written to improve safety issues such as medication interactions.

Progress on implementing electronic patient records has been slow, in part because of concerns for patient privacy and the perceived lack of funding for information technology. A 2001 report titled *Crossing the Quality Chasm: A New Health System for the 21st Century* devoted an entire chapter to information technology (Committee on Quality of Health Care in America, 2001). Among the recommended changes for healthcare technology were:

- computerized provider order entry (CPOE) with automated reminder systems to improve compliance with clinical practice guidelines
- computer-assisted diagnosis
- computer-assisted patient management
- computer-assisted patient education
- computerized clinical decision support systems (Committee on Quality of Health Care in America, 2001, p. 164)

To effectively address this list of recommended changes, the computer system should be used as a tool to alert the healthcare provider to problems with the patient; to remind the provider about clinical practice guidelines, allergies, or potential adverse effects of drug combinations; to help the provider arrive at an accurate diagnosis and an effective treatment plan; and to present educational information to patients either by an onsite computer or via the internet.

Real World Interview

Clinical informatics is a field that works with data and technology to improve patient care and promote patient safety. As a clinical informatics nurse, I have been involved in many projects to improve patient care and outcomes. One of those was the Adult Malnutrition project to improve patient health, decrease length of stay in the hospital, and decrease readmission rates. Our team was composed of a senior dietitian, several physicians, a clinical researcher, nursing leaders, and clinical informatics. The group knew from the literature that an estimated 30% to 50% of patients being admitted to the hospital had some component of malnutrition. As part of the work, it was my role to find a way using the EMR to identify which patients were at risk for malnutrition on admission and have the EMR initiate interventions without additional burden to the clinician. To accomplish this, a validated screening tool was added to the EMR to be done during the admission process. When the patient was identified as at risk, the EMR automatically dropped a consult to the dietitian and an oral supplement order was placed if the patient had an active diet order. Oral supplement therapy was started on average 36 hours earlier using the EMR vs waiting for a clinician to place an order. Through this work, our team decreased the patient length of stay by 26%, decreased readmission rates for these patients 29%, decreased pressure ulcer rates, and saved our organization almost 5 million dollars in 6 months.

Maureen Dziadosz, BSN

Director Clinical Informatics-Illinois

Advocate Aurora Healthcare

DEVELOPING ELECTRONIC HEALTH RECORDS

The Office of the National Coordinator for Health Information Technology (ONC) is charged with leading efforts to support nationwide health information exchange and to improve care (ONC, n.d.-a). The office is located within the Office of the Secretary for the Department of Health and Human Services (DHHS). ONC is responsible for national efforts and implementation of advanced health information technology and the electronic exchange of health information (ONC, n.d.-a). A major initiative founded by ONC is the Safety Assurance Factors for EHR Resilience (SAFER). SAFER is a collection of recommended practices for optimizing safety and safe use of EHRs. These include:

- Foundational Guides (organizational responsibilities, high priority practices)
- Infrastructure Guides (contingency planning, system configuration, and system interfaces)
- Clinical Process Guides (patient identification, computerized order entry, decision support, results reporting and communication)

Each guide contains a checklist of recommended practices to be used by healthcare facilities as a self-assessment. The guides are intended to address safety concerns as the landscape of EHRs frequently changes.

A 2011 IOM report titled *Health IT and Patient Safety: Building Safer Systems for Better Care* identified a series of characteristics that computer software developers should use to make electronic information systems easier for the healthcare professional to use. The following sections include the primary characteristics and explanation that is still the guidance for current electronic information systems (Committee on Patient Safety and Health Information Technology, 2012, p. 62).

Native, Accurate, Reliable, and Timely Data

The Committee's work clearly focused on increasing the efficiency and efficacy of computer and electronic information systems to aid and augment the work of the clinician and healthcare professional. For example, "native data" are information entered directly into the electronic computer system such as vital signs entered by a nurse, whereas imported data would include data coming from another electronic information system such as the electronic laboratory information system. In most healthcare organizations, laboratory tests are done on a completely different electronic system specific to the laboratory within the organization or by a laboratory outside the organization. For the data to be considered "accurate and reliable," the data could not have been changed in any way. Within this requirement, assurance is needed that no one is able to hack into the computer system and/or alter the data.

The Committee also recognized the importance of "timely" data. Data is timely if it is available as soon as they are created. For example, laboratory test results are needed immediately for patients in critical-care units such as intensive care. Once a blood chemistry test such as the serum level of potassium is completed, the information must be relayed to the healthcare provider immediately, especially if it is abnormal. If the potassium level in a patient is very low, intravenous administration of potassium would probably be necessary (low potassium levels may cause the patient's heart to beat irregularly). Quality care depends on having the results as soon as possible so interventions can be taken as the patient's condition warrants. A laboratory result sent 2 weeks after the blood chemistry was drawn is irrelevant when caring for the intensive care patient.

Easy to Use

An electronic record system must be easy to learn and easy to use so that it is streamlined into the current workflow for healthcare providers. The way information is entered and used in the electronic system should match the way the provider works. For example, a provider might have a standard set of questions to ask a patient with diabetes. The electronic record system should have the same set of questions in the same order so the provider can easily add the patient's answers as they are given. In some cases, a checklist of probable answers can be listed in the electronic patient record so all the provider has to do is check off the applicable answer. Ideally, providers should be able to customize the electronic record system to match the way they do their work.

Intuitive Displays

Intuitive data displays are those that present the information in a form that is understandable and easy to use at the point of care. For example, a nurse might want to see the blood pressure readings displayed in a table, whereas a physician might prefer that same information be displayed on a graph. If either the physician or the nurse wants to change the display format, it should be easy to toggle or change between the table and the graph. The master electronic information system will need to know what device the user has, so that the information will be properly displayed. Some information such as graphs can easily be read on a personal computer (PC) screen but may not be easily adapted to small displays such as on a smartphone.

Navigation

Another characteristic the Committee suggested was that EHRs be easy to "navigate." Navigation refers to the way the computer user moves from one part of the electronic patient record to the next part. For example, if a nurse wants to look first at patient assessment data and then look at the care plan data, it should be easy to make that move in the patient's electronic record. This is usually done through a navigation bar that may be on the side of the screen or across the top of the screen.

Evidence at the Point of Care

Evidence at the point of care refers to accessibility of scientific evidence at the bedside or in the examination room. The availability of this evidence to aid with decision-making is critical to providing quality care. For example, a wound care nurse who is treating a Stage IV pressure injury may want to see the best available evidence in full text from the National Library of Medicine. The nurse should be able to access those articles at the patient's bedside without having to go to the organization's library. This process is known as knowledge utilization, a method of bringing evidence to the bedside. Informatics is uniquely positioned to provide this knowledge utilization feature. Another means of providing evidence at the point of care is to base interventions on the best available evidence. Ideally, when the nurse selects an intervention, an option for viewing the evidence that supports the intervention is displayed. The convenience of having the best available evidence supporting patient care interventions at the point of care is the optimal scenario. While the current technology to support evidence-based nursing care at the bedside is not fully optimized for this feature, there is a push toward making this a reality. This is one way that electronic documentation can facilitate the use of evidence at the point of care.

Enhance Workflow

Electronic information systems transform data into information that is meaningful for the user. A simple example of the electronic transformation of data into information is the list of deposits and withdrawals made to a bank account. The transactions of deposits and withdrawals are the data. When those transactions result in an addition and/or subtraction of the money in the account, the data is processed electronically. The information is the balance in the bank account. The balance information guides the owner of the bank account in managing finances. Likewise, in healthcare when information is combined with experience and understanding, it becomes knowledge that can be used to make informed decisions (ANA, 2015). Knowledge becomes wisdom when it is compared to current understanding and experience, then externalized as an action.

Limit Inefficiencies

Electronic information systems should introduce efficiencies in the way work is done so no new physical or cognitive demands will be placed on the nurse. For example, a nurse should not have to travel to a separate computer or be required to be in a library to access scientific literature. Likewise, it is important not to make the nurse's work any more mentally demanding than it already is. Rather than create a delay in patient care, new electronic technologies should enhance patient care efficiently for all involved. Information in healthcare is expanding exponentially, and although healthcare providers are highly educated, no one provider can be expected to know everything. For example, point-of-care technology provides reliable information to fill the knowledge gap of providers at the time they need it most—while they are interacting with the patient.

Exchange of Information

Since patients are often treated across many different healthcare organizations, it should be quick and easy to obtain information from another organization. The coordination of the access and exchange of patient information occurs through the establishment of **health information exchanges** (HIEs), where a patient's vital health data is shared electronically on both a regional and national level (ONC, n.d.-b). HIEs usually operate on a regional level such as by cities or counties since most health information is shared between local healthcare providers. HIEs are not-for-profit organizations formed by a variety of vested healthcare professionals from healthcare organizations, institutions, and practices. At the regional level, these HIEs are referred to as regional health information organizations (RHIOs). When health information is shared over a longer distance, it is shared between HIEs. Thus, information about a patient in Syracuse, New York, can be shared with providers in Los Angeles, California. Patients have a choice to sign an authorization to have their information shared or can opt out of the HIE if they do not want their information shared.

IMPORTANT LEGISLATION IMPACTING PATIENT SAFETY

The reports of the IOM inform Congress about important legislation needed to bring about change in health informatics. As a result, several fundamental laws have been passed to advance the health informatics agenda. These laws include:

- the Health Insurance Portability and Accountability Act (HIPAA, 1996), which contains important provisions for privacy and security of health information (Pub. L. 104–191, August 21, 1996, 110 Stat. 1936).
- the Health Information Technology for Economic and Clinical Health (HITECH) Act (2009), which was part of the American Recovery and Reinvestment Act of 2009 (ARRA; Pub. L. 111–5). The HITECH Act provided billions of dollars of federal money in the form of grants to advance widespread use of health information technology.
- the Patient Protection and Affordable Care Act (PPACA) of 2010 (Public Law 111–148), often called the Affordable Care Act (ACA). The PPACA provides ongoing funding for health information technology (111th Congress, 2010).

Health Insurance Portability and Accountability Act

The **Heath Insurance Portability and Accountability Act** (HIPAA) of 1996 is a federal law requiring healthcare providers to use several privacy protections for patients and their records (Office for Civil Rights, n.d.-b). HIPAA protects an individual's identifiable health information that is in oral, written, and/or electronic form. HIPAA also requires that each healthcare facility have a designated privacy officer. There are two aspects to HIPAA, information privacy and security of private health information.

Information Privacy

Information privacy is the patient's right to limit the amount of personal healthcare information accessible to and known by others (HIPAA, 1996). Within this right of patients, providers are mandated to maintain confidentiality. Confidentiality is the duty the provider has to hold patient information private. Although the patient's right to information privacy is not stated in the U.S. Constitution, various court cases such as *Griswold v. Connecticut* (1965) interpreted sections of the Bill of Rights (the first 10 amendments to the U.S. Constitution) as giving the patient this right. In particular, the fourth amendment to the U.S. Constitution, which protects against unreasonable search and seizure of papers and effects, is thought to provide information privacy. Attention to privacy is extremely important because if patients think their privacy will not be protected, they will be reluctant to share information needed to provide quality care. An excellent online resource for staff training on privacy is available from the National Institutes of Health (NIH). Courses relevant for the new or novice nurse include the NIH Information Security Awareness Course and the NIH Privacy Awareness Course. Users can take the course on the website https://irtsectraining.nih.gov/publicUser.aspx and receive a certificate of completion.

CASE STUDY

Devon is a nurse working on a medical-surgical unit that was converted to a unit devoted to caring for COVID-19 patients who require hospitalization but do not require intensive care. During one of his shifts, Devon provided care for a patient who was beginning to show signs of respiratory distress. The physician decided to try turning the patient to a prone position (lying on the stomach). The respiratory technician placed the patient on high-flow oxygen. The healthcare team was trying to avert having to intubate the patient. Devon belonged to a Facebook group devoted to nursing care of the COVID-19 patient across the globe. After reading the posts, he decided to post the following question to the group:

I have a 63-year-old patient with COVID. She was healthy prior to this and worked at the Starbucks on the corner of Clark and Addison streets as a full-time barista. If you were ever near there, you would remember her as always smiling and happy to help. We are trying to avoid intubation with her so we placed her in the prone position. She is still having difficulty breathing and we are unsure what to do next. Does anyone have any suggestions?

1. ***Did Devon violate the patient's privacy by posting the question on the private Facebook group? Provide a rationale for your response.***
2. ***How does posting questions on a Facebook group that is private in order to find out what works for other healthcare providers pose confidentiality problems?***
3. ***Revise Devon's post so that it does not violate the patient's confidentiality.***

Security

HIPAA requires that healthcare organizations have specific measures in place to safeguard a patient's health information. First, there must be access controls in place such as passwords and pin numbers to limit unauthorized access to sensitive patient information. Second, health organizations must encrypt patient health information, meaning information cannot be read or understood unless the person is authorized and has a decryption key. Most times, the decryption key is linked to the person's password or pin number. **Security** is the set of protections placed on a computer system to prohibit unauthorized access and to prevent any loss or distortion of the data (HIPAA, 1996). HIPAA also requires that security measures be in place in an organization and that there is a designated security officer. The NIH training website (http://irtsectraining.nih.gov/publicUser0.aspx) also offers a course to the public on the topic of computer security.

The Health Information Technology for Economic and Clinical Health Act

The **HITECH Act** is a federal law that provides money to healthcare providers, institutions, and organizations to encourage the use of EHRs (ONC, 2019). However, the federal government also wanted to make sure its money was wisely spent. It will only give providers enhanced payments if they use certified EHRs. In addition, the provider must show the EHR is being used in a meaningful way. To assist providers in determining if their use of the EHR met the federal expectation, the Centers for Medicare and Medicaid (CMS) of the U.S. Department of Health and Human Services developed criteria showing Meaningful Use.

As new healthcare legislation is enacted, both HITECH and Meaningful Use are being integrated into the newer laws. This does not mean that the objectives of each Act are no longer relevant; they are still required of healthcare organizations and providers, just found within other regulations. The Medicare Access and CHIP Reauthorization Act (MACRA) of 2015 includes requirements from the EHR Merit-Based Incentive Payment System, or MIPS, began in January of 2017 and includes requirements for reimbursement and payment based on the quality of care provided, resource use, clinical practice improvement activities, and Meaningful Use of certified EHR technology. Both MACRA and MIPS replace certain initiatives set by the EHR Incentive Program (Meaningful Use) and HITECH so that organizations working toward meeting the requirements can continue moving forward without an interruption in requirements.

Meaningful Use

In 2011, the CMS initiated a program called the EHR Incentive Program, also known as Meaningful Use. **Meaningful Use** was an initiative designed to encourage the use of EHRs by using data collected in the clinical setting such as hospitals, clinics, or physician offices, to improve patient care outcomes (ONC, n.d.-c). It was an incentive program from CMS that provided reimbursements based on the ability of health organizations to meet specific criteria: data capture and sharing, advanced clinical processes based on data, and improved patient outcomes. The Meaningful Use initiative was beneficial in forcing healthcare providers and organizations to adopt and integrate EHRs in the care provision setting. While the EHR Incentive Program ended in 2016, the initiatives from the program are still required for reimbursement from CMS. Major outcomes from the initiative include using electronically captured health data to improve quality of care processes and patient outcomes, clinical decision supports (CDS), e-prescribing, and improving patient engagement in healthcare decisions through patient portals.

Standards for Interoperability

Interoperability is an agreed-upon standard of communication between hardware and software companies that allows for the effective exchange of patient information between various health information systems (Healthcare Information Management and Systems Society, 2013). The ONC is responsible for laying the foundation for connectivity and interoperability of health information technology (ONC, n.d.-d). ONC is guided by the 21st Century Cures Act, where the term 'interoperability,' with respect to health information technology, enables the secure exchange of electronic health information; allows for complete access, exchange, and use of all electronically accessible health information for authorized use; and does not block information (DHHS, 2020).

Interoperability is critical to making health records accessible across the care environments. HITECH and Meaningful Use both rely on systems to be interoperable in order for the regulations to work. For example, different hospitals use different EMR vendors; however, with interoperability standards in place, these various EMRs are able to exchange patient information seamlessly and accurately. The telephone system is an excellent example of interoperability. Regardless of the type of phone used or the service vendor selected, anyone is able to communicate via phone. That is because all the phone makers and all the service providers adhere to a common set of standards. The same level of interoperability is needed for the computer exchange of health information.

Many computer standards are currently available to facilitate communication between different health information systems and even more standards are under development. Policies, procedures, and development of standards for health information systems is coordinated by the American National Standards Institute (ANSI; http://ansi.org) and its Healthcare Information Technology Standards Panel (HITSP; www.hitsp.org). Standards development groups include representatives from government, the healthcare industry, and health informatics system vendors.

HEALTH-RELATED WEBSITES

A growing number of consumers use the internet as a handy way to access health-related information. Some health-related internet sites provide high-quality information to help consumers understand health problems, make informed health decisions, and provide insights about healthcare expectations. While the information is convenient and generally accessible, most health-related information on the internet is not monitored for quality. The average consumer generally may not have the knowledge to judge the quality of the source or the health information found on the internet. This raises concerns about the type of information available to guide consumer health decisions.

An expectation of nurses is that they have the knowledge to guide patients toward accessing the best quality health-related websites available on the internet. There are several types of website evaluation tools available with varying levels of reliability and validity. One widely recognized website evaluation tool specific to health-related sites was developed by the Health on the Net Foundation (HON). HON is a nonprofit, nongovernmental and international foundation that developed a set of criteria to judge the quality of health information available on the internet. There are a set of eight principles for evaluating a health website. If the content of the website meets the standards, they are considered HON certified and can display the HON logo on their website. To note, the user can click on the symbol and see how the website meets the criteria. The criteria are:

1. Authority: The qualifications of the authors or contributors are clearly stated.
2. Complementarity: A statement is included on the website that states the information is not meant to replace the advice of a healthcare provider.
3. Privacy: Confidentiality of personal information.
4. Information: Information is marked with date of last modification and external references.
5. Justification: Claims made on the website have supporting justification.
6. Contact: Website contact information is clearly stated.
7. Disclosure: All funding sources are clearly described.
8. Advertising: Website clearly discloses advertising sources and funding as well as differentiates between advertising and website content (Health on the Net, 2017).

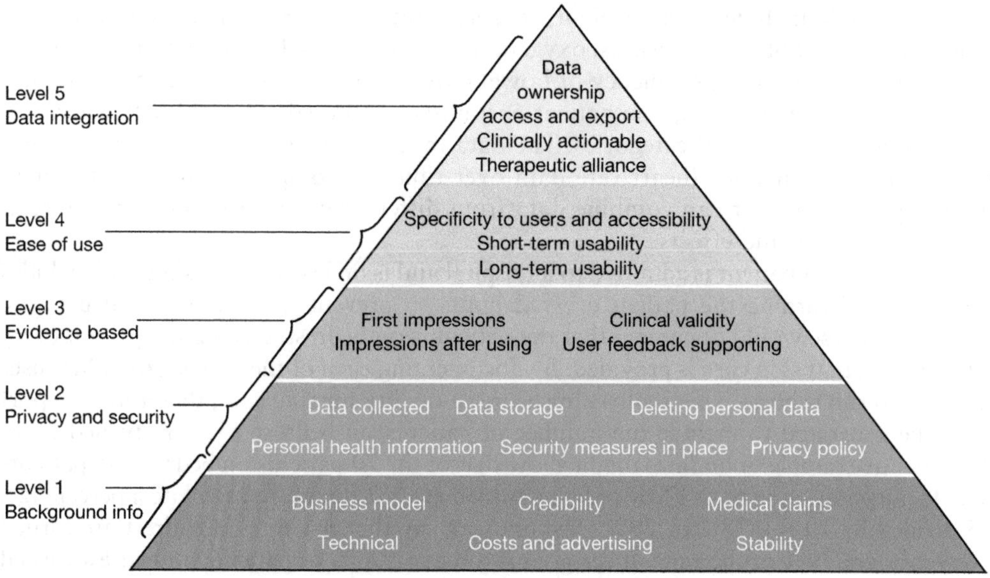

FIGURE 8.2 Hierarchal List of Mobile App Characteristics.

Source: From Henson, P., David, G., Albright, K., & Torous, J. (2019, June). Deriving a practical framework for the evaluation of health apps. *The Lancet: Digital Health, 1*(2), E52–E54. https://doi.org/10.1016/S2589-7500(19)30013-5. Reprinted with permission.

Healthcare applications have also gained popularity with mHealth (mobile health information). Criteria for appraising the quality of health-related applications is varied in the literature with almost all agreeing upon certain characteristics. While using a structured and standardized approach to appraising mobile health applications is critical to ensuring patients are guided to appropriate information, a challenge remains regarding the best health application for the individual person. Characteristics such as technology literacy, accessibility, treatment goals, and patient preferences are all important factors in selecting an appropriate health application (Henson et al., 2019). Figure 8.2 depicts the hierarchal list of Mhealth app characteristics, where the lowest level must be met in order to move to a higher level. Nurses should be familiar with the need to appraise health-related websites and mobile applications to guide patients in selecting appropriate electronic medical information.

TECHNOLOGY INITIATIVES FOR SAFE PATIENT CARE

Healthcare technologies rapidly evolve as developers find opportunities to assist the healthcare provider's ability to provide safe patient care in a variety of settings. Additionally, the level of sophistication for these technologies is growing exponentially. The following technologies have emerged as leading the way in how they support high-quality, safe patient care.

Data Capture to Improve Quality

Data is continuously captured during patient care encounters through patient assessments and documentation of interventions. Using this data to improve healthcare processes is a key part of Meaningful Use. Data captured during one patient care encounter could include height, weight, age, heart rate, blood pressure, respiratory rate, lung sounds, level of consciousness, oxygenation, orientation, level of activity, ability to ambulate, color of urine, frequency of bowel movements, and so on. This vast amount of data accumulated during one patient encounter is entered into an EMR where the data is placed into logical categories. The data in the categories can be extracted into trends within a category (heart rate data over time) or compared against other data using reports. A report can combine data from different categories to determine relationships or cause and effects.

For example, a patient is admitted to a hospital and is on bedrest. Nursing care includes skin care and turning the patient every 2 hours to prevent hospital-acquired pressure ulcers. The nurse would document that the patient is on bedrest, turning the patient every 2 hours, and that skin care is provided. By documenting each of these tasks, the EMR uses the data to run reports. This is also a measure of quality nursing care; therefore, a report could be generated to include the number of patients on bedrest who are turned every 2 hours. An example of findings might show that of the 70 patients on bedrest, 55 patients had documentation in their EMR of being turned every 2 hours. To calculate a percentage, 55 divided by 70 is 0.786, or 79%. The unit can say that patients on bedrest are turned every 2 hours 79% of the time. If the goal is to have 100% of patients on bedrest turned every 2 hours, then the data indicates that a problem exists. This same measure can occur every month to give a trended report of compliance. This is an example of the nursing informatics data to wisdom metastructure.

Clinical Decision Support Systems

A **clinical decision support system** (CDSS) is an integrated database of clinical and scientific information to aid healthcare professionals in providing care (Agency for Healthcare Research and Quality [AHRQ], 2019a). The CDSS is designed to look at a set of data and then lead the user through a decision-making process; for example, asking the user a set of questions that narrow possible choices to one choice that is the most effective. A CDSS might be used to arrive at a correct diagnosis or it might be used to determine the most effective treatment plan for the patient. CDS can take the form of alerts, alarms, hard stops (the nurse is unable to continue charting until a specific item is addressed), clinical guidelines, order sets and clinically relevant evidence to support decisions. For example, a doctor might be treating a patient who is a recovering drug addict with postoperative pain. By using the CDSS on the hospital's health information system, the provider is able to enter assessment data and confounding factors such as opiate addiction to decide the best alternative medication to prescribe.

Another example involves a hospital that collects data on patient falls per month. Upon admission and once a day afterwards, every patient receives a fall risk assessment. When using the fall risk assessment tool, the results are categorized into low, medium, or high-risk for falls. The hospital has a set group of interventions for patients who score at either the medium or high-risk categories. To meet Stage 1 of Meaningful Use, the hospital would integrate the interventions with the fall risk assessment. When the nurse completes a patient fall risk assessment in the electronic documentation system and the finding is high-risk, it triggers specific interventions based on the best available evidence that automatically appears in the EMR. The nurse must select the interventions in place for the patient before moving forward with the electronic charting. This form of CDS not only reminds the nurse of evidence-based interventions needed for the patient, but also requires implementing the evidence-based interventions before continuing with charting.

CURRENT LITERATURE

CITATION

Van de Velde, S., Heselmans, A., Delvaux, N., Brand, L., Marco-Ruiz, L., Spitaels, D., Cloetens, H., Kortteisto, T., Roshanov, P., Kunnamo, I., Aertgeerts, B., Vandvik, P. O., & Flottorp, S. (2018). A systematic review of trials evaluating success factors of interventions with computerised clinical decision support. *Implementation Science, 13*, Article 114. https://doi.org/10.1186/s13012-018-0790-1

DISCUSSION

This systematic review included 66 studies regarding a CDS to improve adherence to recommended practice. Small to large improvements in how well practitioners adhered to recommended practice were found, with the greatest compliance noted when the CDS automatically generated practice recommendations based on responses to assessment questions. Moderate compliance was noted when additional patient-specific data was entered into the computer system and when the system generated patient-specific recommendations. Adherence to practice recommendations improved slightly when the CDS interventions were combined with strategies that were professional-oriented (interventions) and patient-oriented (patient education). Providing CDS directly to patients electronically did demonstrate moderate impact on adherence to recommendation. There is limited evidence on the impact on patient outcomes due to the lack of research.

IMPLICATIONS FOR PRACTICE

Many factors have an influence on the success of CDS interventions. A CDS may be more effective when the advice is generated automatically and displayed on-screen. Additionally, when the advice and suggestions are more patient-specific there is a greater likelihood of adherence to recommendations. When CDS interventions are combined with other strategies there is an increased likelihood of adherence. Finally, providing CDS directly to patients electronically may also positively affect adherence.

E-Prescribing

An objective of Meaningful Use included e-Prescribing by clinicians in both the hospital and clinical setting. Whenever the letter "e" precedes a word it means "electronic." The goals of e-Prescribing were to reduce redundancies, prevent errors in transcription, and increase efficiencies in medication acquisition and sharing of medications across all care settings. To achieve this goal, a nation-wide computerized sharing of medication data among all pharmacies, healthcare organizations, and clinics was established. This allowed the sharing of medication information across all healthcare settings. Once data sharing was in place, all healthcare providers in all settings had to use e-Prescribing in order to capture all medications.

For example, a patient provides a home medication list upon admission to the hospital. During the course of the hospitalization, some medications are discontinued, new medications are added, and doses may be changed. Upon discharge, the medication list may look completely different than when the patient was admitted. The hospital physician uses e-Prescribing to order all medications from the patient's pharmacy they used at home. The new medication list is sent electronically to the pharmacy so that the new medications can be prepared. Additionally, the new medication list is also electronically stored and sent to all the patient's physicians. After discharge, the patient will see their primary and specialty physicians. During each physician visit, the new medication list is available for review or revision based on the patient's health needs. The seamless sharing of medications helps facilitate consistent and patient-centered care during every healthcare encounter.

Patient Portals

In 2019 the MyHealthEData initiative was established, also called the Interoperability and Patient Access final rule (CMS-9115-F). This rule required health providers to share health information gathered during encounters with the patient (CMS, 2020). One major impact of this legislation was to allow patient access to their personal health data by creating **patient portals** that allow patients timely access to health data and education (CMS, 2020). This initiative empowers patients to make informed decisions about healthcare when armed with knowledge about their specific healthcare needs. EMR vendors, along with healthcare organizations, are required to allow patients to access their health encounter information electronically to make these informed healthcare decisions.

For example, a patient sees an orthopedic physician about knee pain. The physician orders an MRI diagnostic test. During the appointment, the nurse asks the patient to sign up for the patient portal, explaining that the patient can access health information through the portal. The patient signs up for the portal and establishes a login and password. The patient has the MRI the next week and is scheduled to see the physician in 2 weeks. A day after the MRI the patient receives an email from the patient portal system that a new test is available to view. The patient accesses the patient portal and is able to review the MRI report. When the patient attends the appointment with the physician the patient is able to discuss MRI findings and ask questions based on the report.

TECHNOLOGIES AND INFORMATION SYSTEMS IN HOSPITALS

Hospitals have various information systems that feed into the EMR designed to support healthcare safety and quality of patient care. Among the most common information systems of importance to nursing staff are messaging/communication technology, CPOE, barcode medication administration (BCMA), and radiofrequency identification (RFID).

Communication Technologies

In almost every hospital or patient care setting, nurses carry assigned phones on their person. The phones are linked to the hospital phone system to facilitate communication between the nurse and other care providers as well as the unit secretary, the patient, and other hospital departments. The intent of the phone is to facilitate direct communication with the nurse and to eliminate delays in communication and miscommunication about issues of relevance to patient care. For example, a nurse may receive a notice of an abnormal lab value. The nurse can then directly notify the physician for any changes in orders. The nurse may also need to communicate with another department such as dietary. If a postoperative patient is able to tolerate liquids, the nurse could inform dietary to increase the diet to soft foods immediately.

While intending to facilitate communication, the phones may pose complications. For example, suppose a nurse is hanging a new intravenous medication for a patient when the phone rings. The phone ringing distracts the nurse from the current task, requiring the nurse to attend to the phone call. Upon returning to the intravenous medication, the nurse must recall what was being done prior to the phone call. This interruption caused a distraction which may result in a delay of care or committing a medication error.

Another form of technology that facilitates communication includes the EMR. Most EMR systems have an area for notes from the interprofessional team about care of a patient. This form of communication enhances patient care by sharing information among the healthcare workers who need it at the point of care. For example, a nurse can access dietary education, physical therapy, and respiratory therapy notes on a patient. Having this information available at the point of care helps the nurse identify any gaps in care or additional education needed.

Computerized Physician Order Entry

A **computerized physician (provider) order entry** is considered any system that allows the physician to directly transmit an order electronically to a recipient (AHRQ, 2019b). The CPOE is a software component of an EMR that allows the clinician to enter patient care orders directly into the computer system, thus eliminating any illegibility problems that can potentially occur with handwritten orders. Patient orders can be entered from any location so there is no longer a need for verbal orders or telephone orders. In addition, the CPOE will issue alerts about various aspects of the patient's condition. For example, the CPOE might alert the clinician to a low heart rate currently being experienced by a patient. The CPOE will also check orders against the hospital formulary to determine if a medication is stocked by the hospital pharmacy and then it will check known allergies, medication–medication interactions, and appropriate dosages of medication. Delays in care are avoided because orders for laboratory tests are immediately transmitted to the lab, medication orders are immediately transmitted to the pharmacy, and blood transfusion orders are immediately transmitted to the blood bank.

Bar-Code Medication Administration

Bar-code medication administration (BCMA) links the electronic medication administration record (eMAR) with medication-specific identification in the form of bar codes. BCMA receives orders from the CPOE system, which prints bar-coded labels that contain the patient's identification number (usually the patient's healthcare record number). BCMAs may also print the specifics of the medication order (i.e., name of the medication and dose). The patient identification bar-code label is then attached to the medication sent from the pharmacy to the nursing unit. Before the nurse administers the medication, the bar code on the patient's wrist bracelet is scanned and the bar code on the medication packet is scanned. The computer system will check to make sure that the packet contains the right medication for the patient and that the medication is being given according to the clinician's order. In order for BCMA to work, there must be interoperability between smart pumps, scanners, and the EMR (Joseph et al., 2020). The ability of these systems to exchange data and information is critical to the success of the BCMA.

Radio Frequency Identification

Radio frequency identification (RFID) is technology that uses radio waves to transfer data from an electronic tag to an object for the purpose of identifying and tracking the object (Seckman et al., 2017). The use of RFID tags in healthcare has evolved over the years. An early example involved a simple wrist band with an embedded chip worn by high-risk populations such as patients with Alzheimer's disease. Emerging examples include handwashing monitoring of nurses. RFID-embedded tags worn by nurses can detect when the nurse has washed their hands by a sensor at the sink detecting the RFID badge. The sensor can also note the time spent on handwashing at the sink.

RFID chips are used in surgical sponges to determine if any sponges are left in the patient at the end of the surgical procedure. This RFID technology ensures the patient will not have to return to surgery to remove a missed sponge (Lazzarro et al., 2017). It also protects the healthcare facility from liability and unnecessary costs. In 2008, the CMS determined it would no longer pay for higher costs of hospitalization associated with events such as objects left in an operative wound. Surgical sponge RFID chips help healthcare facilities meet the goal of zero sponges left postsurgery.

Technology in Direct Patient Care

Electrophysiological monitoring technology collects vital signs and other related data such as heart rhythms about the patient and immediately sends them to the EHR to give the clinician faster access to the data. The EHR can also issue clinical alerts to the clinician. The alerts might be present when the clinician signs on to the EHR or the EHR might send an electronic page, an email message, or a phone call to the clinician. The EHR systems eliminate the transcription errors that occur when vital signs data is handwritten and then later documented in the record.

A recent evolution of technology in direct patient care is the use of smartphones and smartwatches. The smartwatch can monitor blood oxygenation levels and heart rate and record a basic electrocardiogram. All of these pieces of data are recorded by a smartwatch that shares the data with a smartphone. The smartphone can take the data and provide trends that can be shared with a healthcare provider.

Smart Healthcare Devices

The miniaturization of computer chips allows their use in a number of healthcare devices. These devices are called smart devices because they are able to monitor certain parameters about a patient and transmit that information to the healthcare provider. In some cases, the smart devices are programmed to take corrective action when problems occur. An implantable cardioverter defibrillator (ICD) is one example. If the patient experiences ventricular tachycardia or ventricular fibrillation, the smart device will immediately evaluate the situation and deliver an electric impulse to the heart. If the heart rhythm does not convert to an acceptable level, the smart device will deliver another, stronger impulse (National Heart, Lung, and Blood Institute, n.d.). These smart devices save lives because they can identify and/or treat abnormal conditions much faster than the healthcare provider can.

Other common devices with smart technology include infusion pumps and implantable insulin pumps. Smart pumps are intravenous pumps in the clinical setting that are programmed with a library database of intravenous medications (Institute for Safe Medication Practices, 2020). Each medication has hard limits (cannot program the pump to deliver more than a specified range) and soft limits (an alert is given when a range of medication dose is reached but the pump will continue to deliver the medication). When used correctly, smart pumps have shown to reduce medication errors (Institute for Safe Medication Practices, 2020).

In each case, a computer processor is an essential component of the smart device. The use of smart devices will continue to expand with the advent of nanotechnology. According to the National Nanotechnology Initiative (Thomson, 2020), a nanometer is one billionth the size of a meter. It describes nanotechnology as the science involved with understanding, manipulating, and manufacturing materials of this small size. This will make it possible to have extremely small computer processors for smart devices and controlled delivery of medications.

Alarm Fatigue

Although automatic EHR alerts within hospitals can be very helpful, care should be taken in the electronic system design and implementation to make sure the physicians and the nursing staff are not receiving too many alerts. Otherwise, a problem known as alarm fatigue can occur. Alarm fatigue happens when the nurse becomes desensitized to the alarm because of the high volume of alarms that occur in the clinical setting that results in staff ignoring the alerts (Lewis & Oster, 2019). Staff may try to turn the alerts off and they can become increasingly annoyed with the system. The actual users of the electronic system should determine which alerts will be the most beneficial to them. For example, in a cardiac ICU, the interprofessional team may determine cardiac parameters they want alarms for, such as heart rates decreasing or increasing by 10%. The presence or absence of an alert does not relieve the nurse or the providers of the duty to provide quality care. Alerts are only tools. The responsibility to deliver quality care remains with the healthcare professional rather than the device.

CASE STUDY

Cheryl is a nurse on a medical-surgical unit. During her shift, the patient in room 302's intravenous (IV) smart pump alarmed for an obstruction in the line. Cheryl repositioned the patient's arm and was checking the IV site for patency when her phone rang. The call was from a physician asking questions about a patient in room 303. She continued to check the IV site while answering the question. She started to leave the room when the IV pump began to alarm again and as she turned to go back in the room, another one of her patients turned their call light on. As she began working on the IV pump alarm, her phone rang again with an order for a stat medication for the patient in room 302. Cheryl adjusted the IV pump, answered the patient's questions, and explained that she would return with the medication. In the medication room, Cheryl began removing medications when her phone rang. It was about the status of her patient in room 304. As Cheryl answered the questions and withdrew the medications, she suddenly realized that she could hear the IV pump alarm going off again as well as call light alerts. She forgot to answer the call light and couldn't remember hearing the alert as she walked to the medication room.

1. *What is the significance of having multiple alarm interruptions on nursing care and patient safety?*
2. *What can the nurse do to counteract alarm fatigue?*
3. *Develop a plan for identifying alarm fatigue and strategies to counteract this problem.*

TELEHEALTH

The Health Resources and Services Administration (HRSA) of the U.S. Department of Health and Human Services defines **telehealth** as the use of electronic information and communications technologies to support and facilitate clinical and population-based healthcare, patient health education, and health administration from long-distances (n.d.). Technologies include videoconferencing, the internet, image sharing, streaming media, and wireless communications. Telehealth programs experienced a rapid growth and spread during 2020 with the COVID-19 pandemic. The pandemic uncovered the potential of telehealth to provide healthcare services to homebound individuals and families.

The Office for Civil Rights (OCR) within the Department of Health and Human Services (HHS) is charged with enforcing regulations issued under HIPAA and HITECH. This is specifically important to telehealth, where personal health information is transmitted electronically between a patient and the provider. The OCR issued revised rulings and guidance regarding a Notification of Enforcement Discretion for telehealth. This guidance allows a healthcare provider to use "audio or video communication technology to provide telehealth to patients ... [using] any non-public facing remote communication product that is available to communicate with patients" (Office for Civil Rights, n.d.-a, para .4). The OCR instituted enforcement discretion to not impose penalties for noncompliance with HIPAA rules when healthcare is provided in good faith using telehealth during the COVID-19 public health emergency. Of interest, a healthcare provider under this regulation includes physicians as well as advanced practice nurses.

Telehealth uses some type of computer or communication device at both the sending end and the receiving end of the communication. Cameras and microphones may also be used to send pictures and sound. Technology allows a patient's home to serve as an extension of the healthcare facility in that it removes time and distance barriers in the provision of healthcare services. The typical telehealth scenario has nurses interacting with patients over telephone systems. The patients are usually in their homes and they may have home monitoring equipment connected to their phone lines. This monitoring equipment is used to gather data on the patient such as blood pressure, pulse oximetry, blood glucose, and weight. Originally, only telephones with landlines were used but now it is possible to use mobile devices such as cellular phones, satellite phones, phones connected over television cable systems, and the internet.

Some telehealth devices prompt the patient at a certain time of the day to obtain specified data for transmittal to the healthcare provider. For example, the patient may attach a blood pressure cuff to their arm, press a button, and then wait while the cuff inflates. The monitoring device records the blood pressure and transmits it over phone lines to the nurse who usually works for a home care agency. A pulse oximeter is attached to the patient's finger and, again, the data is transmitted to the nurse. For patients with conditions such as congestive heart failure, it is important to check the patient's weight to determine if they are retaining fluid. Thus, a scale may also be attached to the monitoring device. Patient data may be transmitted through cables attached to the home monitoring station or the data may be transmitted wirelessly to the station.

On the receiving end, a nurse uses a telehealth computer workstation to monitor the data coming in from the patient. The telehealth computer software will provide alerts if any information falls outside the parameters set for that patient. The nurse will usually phone the patient after the data arrives to discuss how the patient is feeling and to see if there are any problems that need to be addressed. If the nurse is unable to reach the patient, the nurse may contact family members and/or call 911 to check on the patient. The home health agency may also send a nurse to the patient's home.

One of the many benefits of telehealth use is among patients with chronic diseases. For example, identification of small changes that may signify a problem before it becomes life-threatening is critical. Telehealth can draw prompt attention to the patient's healthcare status to decrease their risk of exacerbation of the disease. Telehealth can improve patient outcomes and can be delivered at a lower cost than home healthcare. Along with reducing the burden on patients to travel to receive healthcare there are other benefits of telehealth such as increased patient independence, increased collaboration with other community organizations, and increased opportunities for nurses to provide education to patients and families.

CURRENT LITERATURE

CITATION

Kaplan, B. (2020). Revisiting health information technology ethical, legal, and social issues and evaluation: Telehealth/Telemedicine and COVID-19. *International Journal of Medical Informatics, 143*. https://doi.org/10.1016/j.ijmedinf.2020.104239

DISCUSSION

The COVID-19 pandemic highlighted the need for telehealth and telemedicine services, to allow patients to receive advice and care services from a distance. In the preceding years, scholars examined the legal and social issues of distanced care. A more recent review conducted during the pandemic identified four primary concerns of telehealth and telemedicine: quality of care, access, consent, and privacy. Additionally, emerging concerns included usability, tailoring care to the patient, training, commercialization, licensing, and liability. Infrastructure needs of interoperability, data access, cybersecurity, and informatics supports also emerged since the pandemic. This article provides guidance for future research on areas of importance for telehealth and telemedicine.

IMPLICATIONS FOR PRACTICE

The COVID-19 pandemic highlighted the importance of telehealth/telemedicine for providing a mechanism to access healthcare from home. Guidance on the use of telehealth/telemedicine is critical to the successful implementation of this technology. An exploration of interactions between caregivers and patients, including a focus on the social, legal, and ethical effects, especially during a pandemic where there is acceptance of this technology, is critical to developing evidence-based guidelines for use of telehealth.

END-OF-CHAPTER RESOURCES

KEY CONCEPTS

1. Nursing informatics is defined as a specialty that integrates different sciences to identify, define, manage, and communicate data, information, knowledge, and wisdom in nursing practice.
2. The sciences that contribute to nursing informatics include computer science, cognitive science, social science, communication science, and library science.
3. The metastructure guiding nursing informatics involves how data becomes information, information becomes knowledge, and knowledge becomes wisdom.
4. Key elements of an electronic medical record (EMR) and electronic health record (EHR) include timely data, ease of use, intuitive displays, clear navigation, point of care evidence, enhanced workflow, limits in inefficiencies, and assistance with exchange of information.
5. Users need to be aware of the benefits and limitations of healthcare technologies and their impact on patient safety.
6. The HIPAA, HITECH, and Meaningful Use regulations on privacy and security apply to EMRs and EHRs. Nurses have a duty to protect patient privacy and to secure private health information.
7. There are standardized tools available to appraise the quality of health-related content on websites and applications.
8. Many evolving technology initiatives are available that support the delivery of safe patient care such as clinical decision support systems and clinical alerts.
9. Telehealth has emerged as a critical part of healthcare delivery for more than just the care of the homebound or rurally located patients.

CRITICAL DISCUSSION POINTS

1. Consider a recent clinical experience. Describe how the data, information, knowledge, and wisdom framework were used in practice (e.g., technology supported gathering and communicating data, transformed data to information, helped the nurse take the information and use knowledge in patient care, and how technology did or could help the nurse use wisdom when providing care).
2. Discuss the use of the EHR and the EMR when providing patient care. Explain how each might facilitate the delivery of safe patient care.
3. Patient portals are becoming mainstream for communicating with patients in the community setting. What are the benefits and drawbacks of using patient portals for nurses? For patients? For providers (e.g., physician)? Ask if you can access the patient portal during your next clinical experience.
4. Access the Why Not the Best website at www.whynotthebest.org. Compare two different hospitals on the key indicators provided. What does the data tell you about the outcomes from care provided in the selected area? Does the website provide a clear picture of patient care outcomes? If yes, why? If no, what is missing?

KEY TERMS

- Bar-code medication administration
- Clinical decision support system
- Computerized physician (provider) order entry
- Electronic health record
- Electronic medical record
- Health information exchanges
- Health Information Portability and Accountability Act (HIPAA)
- HITECH
- Information privacy
- Interoperability
- Meaningful Use
- Nursing informatics
- Patient portals
- Radio frequency identification
- Security
- Telehealth

REVIEW QUESTIONS

Answers to Review Questions appear in the Instructor's Manual. Qualified instructors should request the Instructor's Manual from textbook@springerpub.com.

1. The nurse is caring for a patient and preparing to administer scheduled medications. Which of the following represents a benefit of using informatics technology with regard to medication administration?
   A. Automated medication systems alleviate the need for cross-checking allergies.
   B. Using automated medication systems prevents medication errors.
   C. Automated medication systems provide decision-making aids that alert the nurse to potential problems.
   D. Automated medication administration systems prevent the nurse from administering the wrong medication.
2. The nurse uses the EMR to review key components of the patient's health. What most directly impacts the nurse's ability to effectively use the EMR? *Select all that apply.*
   A. The functional design of the EMR system as described by the manufacturer
   B. Institutional guidelines on using the EMR
   C. The national guidelines for every nurse using an EMR system
   D. The state and federal initiatives mandating the use of EMR systems
   E. Local policies and training on the EMR
3. The facility is using a newly implemented EMR for patient care. The nurses have expressed some frustrations with the high volume of system alerts that are generated throughout the day. Which of the following demonstrates the most appropriate response to excessive alerts by the nurse?
   A. Turn alerts off so they do not slow down the data processing capability.
   B. Report excessive alerts to the software designer.
   C. Collaborate with the nurse informaticist in the institution to make necessary adjustments.
   D. Just ignore the alerts and they will eventually go away.

4. The nurse wants to decrease the rate of medication errors for patients and advocates for use of a CPOE system. Which of the following best indicates the benefit of CPOE systems?

A. Eliminates the need for the nurse to decipher illegible handwriting
B. Assists the nurse in receiving verbal orders from the providers
C. Eliminates the need for the nurse to chart
D. Takes the guesswork out of knowing when to call the provider

5. A patient presents to the ambulatory surgery clinic for scheduled rhinoplasty. During the admission interview, the patient notes a history of an allergic reaction to an antibiotic medication 3 years prior. The patient states that she does not know the name of the drug. Which of the following actions is best for the nurse to take?

A. Call the surgeon and share that the patient's allergy history remains incomplete.
B. Ask the patient to describe what the pills looked like.
C. Consult the patient's EHR.
D. Chart that the patient has an allergy to antibiotics.

6. A nurse on the cardiac unit overhears the licensed practical nurse (LPN) explain to a coworker how to check the status of patients in the labor and delivery unit even though the computer system should not provide this access. Where does the responsibility for system security reside to guard against this type of access?

A. With the nurse who will maintain patient privacy and avoid HIPAA violations
B. With the nurse informaticist who will make certain the EMR maintains confidentiality
C. With the federal government who will make sure no laws are violated
D. With the designated security officer who will make sure the entire system is secure

7. One feature of some EMR is decision-making pop ups. For example, the nurse will be alerted to the patient's medication allergies when administering medications. Which of the following best describes the potential workplace benefit for the nurse?

A. It is time saving and eliminates the need to ask the patient about allergies.
B. It establishes safer medication withdrawal and administration practices
C. It provides a double check opportunity for the nurse to remember to ask the patient.
D. It helps with communication. It eliminates cross-checking with pharmacy.
E. It is cost-effective and reduces the time the nurse spends in transcribing medications.

8. The nurse is preparing a patient for discharge. Which of the following represents the nurse's most effective application of the information technology at the bedside?

A. Accessing the best available evidence in preparation to answer the patient's questions upon discharge
B. Using the computer to print a list of websites that may be of interest to the patient
C. Posting the patient's questions to a social media website and compiling the response for the patient
D. Referring the patient to his healthcare provider so the provider can answer the patient's questions

9. The nurse is monitoring the telehealth computer and notices that the patient's pulse oximetry reading drops below 90%, which is the predetermined action criteria for this patient. Which of the following depicts the most appropriate next step the nurse should take?
   A. Call the patient's family and alert them to administer oxygen immediately.
   B. Call 911 to send emergency responders to the home.
   C. Call the patient and assess how the patient is feeling and what is currently happening.
   D. Call the primary care provider to obtain treatment orders.
10. Nurses need to increase awareness of the implementation of technology and informatics in patient care. Which of the following best represents a collaborative effort to ensure best practices in nursing informatics?
   A. HIPAA
   B. TIGER
   C. VISTA
   D. EHR

QUALITY AND SAFETY EDUCATION FOR NURSES ACTIVITIES

1. A self-paced module that illustrates the professional responsibilities inherent in informatics: http://qsen.org/heath-informatics-and-technology-professional-responsibilities/
2. Electronic health record case studies: http://qsen.org/effectively-using-ehrs-with-interdisciplinary-teams-improving-health-quality-of-care/

REVIEW ACTIVITIES

1. Search the web for position descriptions for a nurse informaticist. Consider the education requirements, position description, and required experience. Compare your findings with other classmates. What similarities did you find? What differences?
2. Form groups of three to five students. Create a brochure that helps explain the patient portal to a patient or family member. Consider the literacy level, understanding, knowledge, and prior experience of your patient population. Present your brochure to the class.
3. Go to Health on the Net (www.healthonnet.org/HONcode/Conduct.html). Review the HON code of conduct for health-related websites. Select a website or a health-related application and examine the content based on the HON principles. Select a website or application that does not currently have HON certification (can typically be seen at the bottom of the webpage by the HON Code symbol found on the website). What suggestions can you give to improve the website or application? Does the HON Code work for applications as well as it works for websites? How would you evaluate the quality of health-related information on an application?

EXPLORING THE WEB

1. Visit the HealthIT Buzz Blog at www.healthit.gov/buzz-blog. This blog is run by the Office of the National Coordinator for Health Information Technology (ONC). It contains blogs on the latest topics in health informatics. Follow the links to read three blogs. Be prepared to participate in a class discussion on these topics.

2. Visit the ONC's YouTube channel at www.youtube.com/user/HHSONC. Watch five videos about patients and their experiences with health information technology. Most videos are only 2 to 3 minutes long.
3. Prepare a list of five benefits that patients might experience as a result of the implementation of this health information technology. Draft a one-page, double-sided, trifold brochure that could be given to patients to educate them on the topic. Title the brochure "Health IT and You." Insert photos or graphics as you think appropriate.

REFERENCES

111th Congress. (2010). Public Law No: 111-148. H.R.3590. https://www.congress.gov/bill/111th-congress/house-bill/3590/text

Agency for Healthcare Research and Quality. (2019a). *Clinical decision support systems*. https://psnet.ahrq.gov/primer/clinical-decision-support-systems

Agency for Healthcare Research and Quality. (2019b). *Computerized provider order entry*. https://psnet.ahrq.gov/primers/primer/6/computerized-provider-order-entry

American Nurses Association. (2015). *Nursing informatics: Scope and standards of practice* (2nd ed.). Nursebooks.org.

American Recovery and Reinvestment Act of 2009 (ARRA) (Pub. L. 111–5).

Centers for Medicare and Medicaid Services. (2008). *Medicare and Medicaid move aggressively to encourage greater patient safety in hospitals and reduce never events*. https://www.cms.gov/newsroom/press-releases/medicare-and-medicaid-move-aggressively-encourage-greater-patient-safety-hospitals-and-reduce-never

Centers for Medicare and Medicaid Services. (2020). Medicare and Medicaid Programs; Patient Protection and Affordable Care Act; Interoperability and Patient Access for Medicare Advantage Organization and Medicaid Managed Care Plans, State Medicaid Agencies, CHIP Agencies and CHIP Managed Care Entities, Issuers of Qualified Health Plans on the Federally-Facilitated Exchanges, and Health Care Providers (CMS-9115-F). https://www.federalregister.gov/documents/2020/05/01/2020-05050/medicare-and-medicaid-programs-patient-protection-and-affordable-care-act-interoperability-and

Committee on Patient Safety and Health Information Technology. (2012). *Health IT and patient safety: Building safer systems for better care*. National Academies Press. https://doi.org/10.17226/13269

Committee on Quality of Health Care in America. (2001). *Crossing the quality chasm: A new health system for the 21st century*. National Academies Press. https://doi.org/10.17226/10027

Cronenwett, L., Sherwood, G., Barnsteiner J., Disch, J., Johnson, J., Mitchell, P., Sullivan, D., & Warren, J. (2007). Quality and Safety Education for Nurses. *Nursing Outlook*, *55*(3), 122–131. https://doi.org/10.1016/j.outlook.2007.02.006

Dick, R. S., Steen, E. B. & Detmer, D. E. (Eds.). (1997). *The computer based patient record: An essential technology for health care*. National Academies Press. https://www.ncbi.nlm.nih.gov/books/NBK233047

Department of Health and Human Services. (2020). *21st Century Cures Act: Interoperability, information blocking, and the ONC health IT certification program*. https://www.federalregister.gov/documents/2020/05/01/2020-07419/21st-century-cures-act-interoperability-information-blocking-and-the-onc-health-it-certification

Griswold v. Connecticut, 381 U.S. 479, (1965).

Healthcare Information Management and Systems Society. (2013). *HIMSS dictionary of healthcare information technology terms* (3rd ed.). Author.

Health Information Technology for Economic and Clinical Health Act (HITECH Act) (Pub. L. 111 5, div. A, title XIII, div. B, title IV, February 17, 2009, 123 Stat. 226, 467 [42 U.S.C. 300jj et seq.; 17901 et seq.]).

Health Insurance Portability and Accountability Act. (1996). (Pub. L. 104–191).

Health on the Net. (2017). *The commitment to reliable health and medical information on the internet*. https://www.hon.ch/HONcode/Patients/Visitor/visitor.html#accreditation

Health Resources Services Administration. (n.d.). *Office for the Advancement of Telehealth*. https://www.hrsa.gov/rural-health/telehealth

Henson, P., David, G., Albright, K., & Torous, J. (2019, June). Deriving a practical framework for the evaluation of health apps. *The Lancet: Digital Health, 1*(2), E52–E54. https://doi.org/10.1016/S2589-7500(19)30013-5

Institute for Safe Medication Practices. (2020). *ISMP issues revised and expanded guidelines for the safe use of smart infusion pumps*. https://www.ismp.org/news/ismp-issues-revised-and-expanded-guidelines-safe-use-smart-infusion-pumps

Joseph, R., Lee, S. W., Anderson, S. V., & Morrisette, M. J. (2020). Impact of interoperability of smart infusion pumps and an electronic medical record in critical care. *American Journal of Health-System Pharmacy*, 77(15), 1231–1236. https://doi.org/10.1093/ajhp/zxaa164

Lewis, C., & Oster, C. (2019). Research outcomes of implementing CEASE. *Dimensions of Critical Care Nursing, 38*(3), 160–173. https://doi.org/10.1097/DCC.0000000000000357

National Heart, Lung, and Blood Institute. (n.d.). *What is an implantable cardioverter defibrillator?* https://www.nhlbi.nih.gov/health-topics/defibrillators

Office for Civil Rights. (n.d.-a). Notification of enforcement discretion for telehealth remote communications during the COVID-19 nationwide public health emergency. https://www.hhs.gov/hipaa/for-professionals/special-topics/emergency-preparedness/notification-enforcement-discretion-telehealth/index.html

Office for Civil Rights. (n.d.-b). *Summary of the HIPAA security rule*. https://www.hhs.gov/hipaa/for-professionals/security/laws-regulations/index.html

The Office of the National Coordinator for Health Information Technology. (n.d.-a). *About ONC*. https://www.healthit.gov/topic/about-onc

The Office of the National Coordinator for Health Information Technology. (n.d.-b). *Health information exchange*. https://www.healthit.gov/topic/health-it-and-health-information-exchange-basics/health-information-exchange

The Office of the National Coordinator for Health Information Technology. (n.d.-c). *Meaningful use*. https://www.healthit.gov/topic/meaningful-use-and-macra/meaningful-use

The Office of the National Coordinator for Health Information Technology. (n.d.-d). *Promoting interoperability*. https://www.healthit.gov/topic/meaningful-use-and-macra/promoting-interoperability

The Office of the National Coordinator for Health Information Technology. (n.d.-e). *What are the differences between electronic medical records, electronic health records, and personal health records?* https://www.healthit.gov/faq/what-are-differences-between-electronic-medical-records-electronic-health-records-and-personal

The Office of the National Coordinator for Health Information Technology. (2009). *HITECH Act enforcement interim final rule*. https://www.hhs.gov/hipaa/for-professionals/special-topics/hitech-act-enforcement-interim-final-rule/index.html

Thomson, E. A. (2020). *A new platform for controlled delivery of key nanoscale drugs and more*. https://news.mit.edu/2020/new-platform-for-controlled-nanoscale-drug-delivery-0828

Patient Protection and Affordable Care Act (PPACA) of 2010 (Public Law 111–148).

Seckman, C., Bauer, A., Moser, T., & Paaske, S. (2017). *The benefits and barriers to RFID technology in healthcare*. https://www.himss.org/resources/benefits-and-barriers-rfid-technology-healthcare.

SUGGESTED READING

Thompson, B. W., & Skiba, D. J. (2008). Informatics in the nursing curriculum: A national survey of nursing informatics requirements in nursing curricula. *Nursing Education Perspectives, 29*(5), 312–317.

LaTour, K. M., & Maki, S. M. (Eds.). (2010). *Health information management concepts, principles and practice* (3rd ed.). American Health Information Management Association.

Murphy, J. (2011). Nursing informatics: Engaging patients and families in eHealth. *Nursing Economic$, 29*(6), 339–341.

The Office of the National Coordinator for Health Information Technology. (n.d.). *Clinical decision support*. https://www.healthit.gov/policy-researchers-implementers/clinical-decision-support-cds

The Office of the National Coordinator for Health Information Technology. (n.d.). *EHR incentives and certifications*. http://www.healthit.gov/providers-professionals/meaningful-use-definition-objectives

Schaaf, J., Sedlmayr, M., Schaefer, J., & Storf, H. (2020). Diagnosis of rare diseases: A scoping review of clinical decision support systems. *Orphanet Journal of Rare Diseases, 15*, Article 263. https://doi.org/10.1186/s13023-020-01536-z

CHAPTER 9

Evidence-Based Nursing Practice

Beth A. Vottero

"As more knowledge is generated through research, and as the ability to transmit information via such media as the internet or direct broadcast increases, all professionals in all fields will come under increasing pressure to show that they are abreast of current knowledge, and that they exhibit this through delivering services that are in line with the most recent and rigorous evidence."

–Alan Pearson, 2014.

Upon completion of this chapter, the reader should be able to:

1. Define evidence-based practice (EBP).
2. Explain what is meant by "best available evidence."
3. Craft a searchable population, intervention, comparison, and outcome (PICO) question.
4. Identify high-quality electronic databases and online resources for basic literature searches.
5. Create a basic search strategy to find the best available evidence.
6. Describe the significance of a hierarchy of types of evidence that inform an evidence-based practice project.
7. Appraise the quality of evidence using appropriate appraisal tools.
8. Explore how clinical expertise is determined.
9. Explain the significance of including patient preferences for EBP.
10. Describe the nurse's role in EBP.

CROSSWALK

This chapter addresses the following:

QSEN Competency: Evidence-Based Practice

The American Association of Colleges of Nursing. (2021). *The essentials: Core competencies for professional nursing education.*

Domain 1: Knowledge for Nursing Practice
Domain 2: Person-Centered Care
Domain 4: Scholarship for the Nursing Discipline

OPENING SCENARIO

You are the nurse representative for a medical-surgical unit on the nursing practice committee. At the quarterly meeting, the chair of the committee presented data on the rise in the number of patient falls throughout the hospital. The chair provided all committee members with an evidence-based fall prevention program that was created by nurses in the hospital quality department. You know that your unit director presented the patient fall data at the monthly unit meeting that showed patient falls have increased by 20% since the same time last year. The nursing practice committee was asked to take the evidence-based fall prevention interventions back to the units for implementation. You bring the fall prevention program to your unit and explain the changes required to patient care. One nurse asks how this program is evidence-based practice if it only addresses the evidence and not the patient preferences or nurse's clinical expertise. How would you respond?

INTRODUCTION

In 2011, the Institute of Medicine (IOM) set a target that, "*. . . by the year 2020, ninety percent of clinical decisions will be supported by accurate, timely, and up-to-date clinical information, and will reflect the best available evidence*" (2011). This prompted a national imperative that healthcare professionals and healthcare institutions set a goal to use the best available evidence throughout the healthcare delivery process. Since then, healthcare organizations are certainly focusing on bringing evidence to the bedside. This was an ambitious target that required healthcare workers to not only develop skills for evidence-based practice, but also demonstrate knowledge about the steps in the process. These steps include:

- identifying a clinical problem;
- asking a searchable question based on a clinical problem;
- searching the literature for the best available evidence;
- appraising the quality of the evidence;
- determining the level of the evidence based on a hierarchy;
- synthesizing the best available evidence into guidance for clinical practice;
- implementing the best available evidence into healthcare practice;
- evaluating the outcomes from the change; and
- sustaining the change.

This chapter will define and explore evidence-based nursing practice. It will examine the three concepts embedded in evidence-based nursing practice: best available evidence, nursing judgment, and patient preferences. This chapter will examine what best available evidence is and how to find this evidence. An overview of how to craft a searchable question and find the best available evidence by using appropriate high-quality databases will be presented. Search strategies including the use of keywords, subject headings, Boolean operators, and other search techniques are described. The role of nurses in evidence-based practice projects is detailed. It will also explore database tools for appraising the quality of the evidence and hierarchies that identify the level of evidence types.

DEFINITION OF EVIDENCE-BASED PRACTICE

Over the past four decades, the science of nursing has evolved into a research-based practice. While nursing interventions have always been based on research, the introduction of **evidence-based practice** (EBP) has revolutionized the science aspect of nursing. The first definition of EBP initiated this change, "... integrating individual clinical expertise with the best available external clinical evidence from systematic research" (Sackett et al., 1996, p. 971). This definition provided the basis for subsequent initiatives such as Quality and Safety Education for Nurses (QSEN). QSEN adapted the definition of EBP to include best available evidence and patient engagement, defining EBP as, "... the delivery of optimal health care through the integration of best current evidence, clinical expertise and patient/family values" (QSEN, 2012).

At first glance, EBP does not appear to be complicated. It is when the definition is deconstructed and the elements are examined that the complexity becomes apparent. One begins to see how each part contributes to the bigger picture. Best available evidence, clinical expertise, and patient preferences all affect the way evidence is used to make clinical decisions about patient care (Figure 9.1). The busy bedside nurse cannot possibly research the evidence on every clinical problem, nor can the nurse always access the best available evidence. This can create a gap between what the evidence says should be done and what

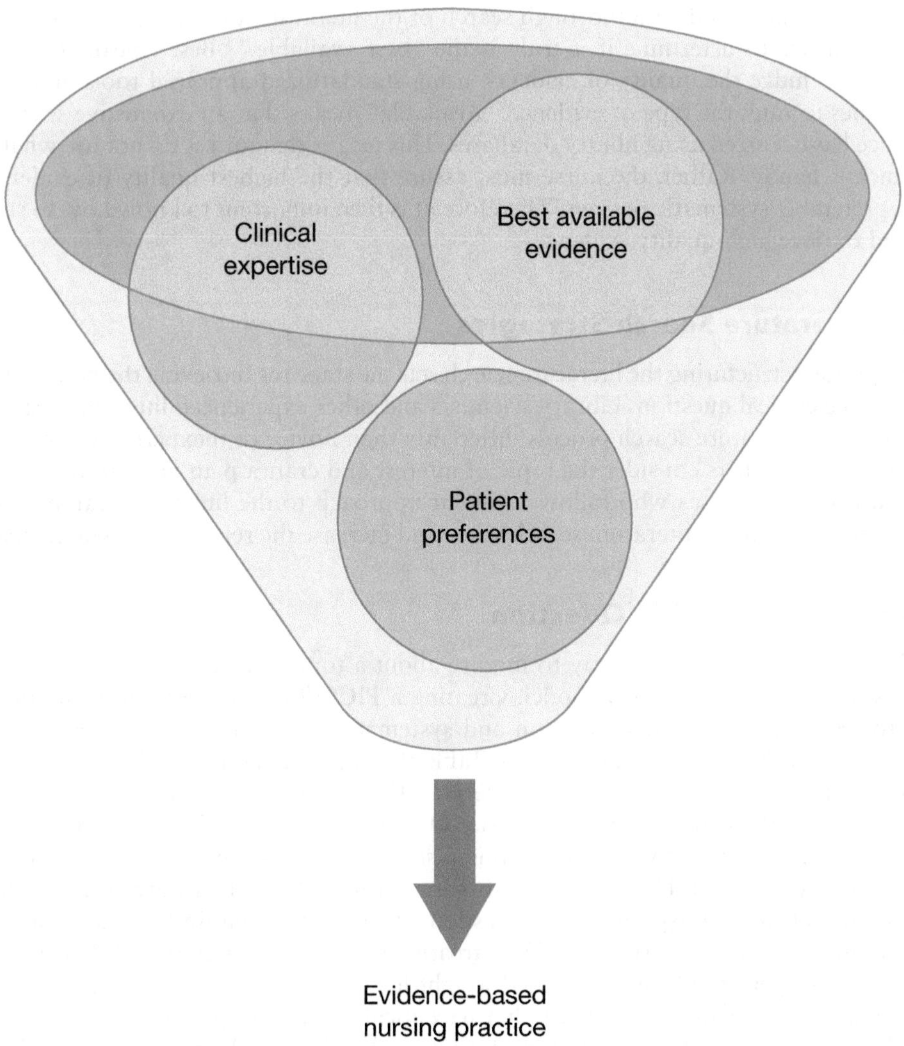

FIGURE 9.1 Evidence-Based Nursing Practice Model.

is actually done in practice. In response to the growing need for evidence, the emphasis of EBP is to bring updated and synthesized best available evidence to the busy direct care nurse.

A common mistake regarding EBP is approaching a project with the belief that EBP focuses solely on the use of evidence and forgetting to include patient preferences and values and clinical expertise. This is not the intent of EBP. In addition to the best available evidence, it is important to recognize that clinical expertise and patient preferences are equally important in the provision of evidence-based, optimal care. Each component of the EBP model should be explored and integrated into practice by nurses and other healthcare providers. The following investigates each part of the model separately to illustrate why each part is interdependent on each other.

BEST AVAILABLE EVIDENCE

The largest component of EBP requires the best available evidence to inform appropriate patient care clinical decisions. The term "**best available evidence**" implies that someone (or some group) must conduct a thorough search of the literature and then judge the quality of the evidence to determine if it truly is the "best available." "Best" means that there is a need to judge the quality of evidence using standardized appraisal tools and to use hierarchies to rank the type of evidence. "Available" means that an exhaustive search for evidence has occurred using library databases. This means that nurses do not use whatever evidence is handy. Rather, the nurse must assure that the highest quality of evidence is used, preferably systematic reviews. Therefore, it is then important to know how to search for and retrieve high-quality evidence.

Basic Literature Search Strategies

Appropriately structuring the literature search sets the stage for retrieving the best evidence that fits the clinical question. Library scientists and other experienced literature searchers approach the literature search process differently than novice or inexperienced searchers. Experienced searchers consider the topic of interest and craft a plan prior to beginning a literature search. Nurses who follow a similar approach to the literature search process can decrease the time a literature search takes and increase the relevancy of search results.

Crafting a Searchable Question

A slightly more sophisticated way to inquire about a topic is to develop a clinical question using the PICO or PICOT model. Creating a **PICO/PICOT** question is an effective way to generate a searchable question and systematically identify and retrieve relevant nursing and healthcare published papers. Table 9.1 explains the PICO elements. The "P" represents the patient or population of interest, "I" represents the intervention of interest, "C" represents the comparison of interest, "O" represents the desired outcome of interest, and "T" represents time. When crafting a searchable question, the "T", or time, may not always be included. Using a PICO question ensures that a literature search remains organized and that all aspects of the question are addressed within the search strategy. An example of a PICO question is, "Does treatment of patients with type 2 diabetes with weight loss surgery result in maintained weight loss of 20 pounds or more compared to traditional patient management with pharmaceuticals, diet, and exercise?"

When developing a PICO question, consider related and relevant synonyms. A synonym for weight loss surgery could be gastric bypass surgery. A synonym for body weight could be body mass index (BMI). Creating a list of synonyms and related terms will help

TABLE 9.1 PICO MODEL

ELEMENT	DESCRIPTION	EXAMPLE
(P) Patient/ Population of interest	Describes "who." The more precise the description is, the more specific the search results will be	Patients with type 2 diabetes or older adult female patients with type 2 diabetes who have no co-morbidities
(I) Intervention of interest	Describes "what." The more precise the description is the more specific the search results will be	Weight loss surgery or bariatric weight loss surgery using a non-invasive approach with a sleeve
(C) Comparison	Describes the intervention of interest (may or may not need a comparison)	Compared to management with pharmaceuticals, diet, and exercise
(O) Outcome	Describes the desired outcome	Maintain weight loss of 20 pounds or more

Source: Data from Hopp, L., & Rittenmeyer, L. (2020). *Introduction to evidence-based practice: A practical guide for nursing. 2nd Ed.* Philadelphia, PA: F.A. Davis; Stillwell, S.B., Fineout-Overholt, E., Melnyk, B.M., & Williamson, K.M. (2010, March) Evidence-based practice, step by step: asking the clinical question: a key step in evidence-based practice. *American Journal of Nursing, 110*(3), 58–61. doi: 10.1097/01.NAJ.0000368959.11129.79

to capture literature that uses any of the related terms. While this may broaden the search results, it will also capture relevant literature that might have otherwise been missed.

Deciding Where to Search

After drafting a PICO question, the next step is to consider where to find the best sources of evidence. While nursing information is found within a variety of sources, the best available evidence primarily comes from peer-reviewed articles in scholarly journals, professional association reports, white papers, and clinical practice guidelines (CPGs). Since the nursing profession favors scholarly peer-reviewed journal articles and professionally published information, this chapter will focus on high-quality electronic databases and online tools. The best type of database depends on the clinical question being asked. Most nurses need access to one or two **full-text databases** in order to find the best available evidence to answer their clinical question. Depending on an institution's subscriptions, bibliographic databases and full-text databases might be connected. This means that citations and abstracts in a bibliographic database could be linked to the fulltext of an article available in another full-text database. Additionally, it is critical to take the time to email or meet with a librarian or library scientist if one is available to ensure that all available information is accessed.

Electronic Databases for Searching the Literature

There are two main types of electronic databases: bibliographic databases or indices (as they are often called) and full-text databases. **Bibliographic databases** provide a basic record, or citation, for an article and often include an abstract or brief summary of the article. Bibliographic databases do not necessarily contain the complete text of the article itself. **MEDLINE** is the U.S. National Library of Medicine's (NLM's) bibliographic database, indexing thousands of journals in the fields of medicine, nursing, dentistry, veterinary medicine, healthcare systems, and the preclinical sciences. **The Cumulative Index to Nursing and Allied Health Literature** (**CINAHL**) is another bibliographic database which indexes thousands of journals in the fields of nursing, biomedicine, alternative/complementary medicine, consumer health and numerous allied health fields. CINAHL's name contains the word "index," which is a clue that not everything within the database is available in full text. The ability to access the fulltext of an item found in a bibliographic database depends on the institutional subscription. Bibliographic databases like MEDLINE and CINAHL are very important for EBP because they allow the user to search a wide range of relevant literature without limiting the results only to articles the user can access in full text.

MEDLINE requires paid subscription access through companies including OVID and EBSCO. The MEDLINE search screen, search capabilities, and access to the full-text content of the 25+ million citations varies by subscription. MEDLINE, MEDLINE Complete, and MEDLINE with Full Text can each be purchased as a subscription through an institution. Most of the same citations contained within MEDLINE can also be accessed through PubMed (www.ncbi.nlm.nih.gov/pubmed). **PubMed** provides free internet access to MEDLINE citations and abstracts. Though PubMed provides limited access to full-text articles, it is an excellent resource for those who do not have subscription access to electronic databases through their college, university, hospital, or organization. Table 9.2 provides basic information about select electronic databases and search engines for literature searching. This is not intended to be an exhaustive list; rather, it is a snapshot of some of the most commonly used resources available.

TABLE 9.2 SELECT ELECTRONIC DATABASES AND SEARCH ENGINES

ELECTRONIC DATABASES	
Cumulative Index to Nursing and Allied Health Literature (CINAHL), www.ebscohost.com/nursing/products/cinahl-databases, is a bibliographic database that indexes the contents of nursing and allied health publications. CINAHL is nursing-focused, making it essential for nursing literature searches.	**MEDLINE,** http://ovid.com/site/catalog/databases/901.jsp, is the United States. National Library of Medicine (NLM) database of journal articles related to biomedicine. The NLM is a component of the National Institutes of Health. Literature from the life sciences and biomedicine dates back to 1809. PubMed is the NLM's free publicly available version of MEDLINE.
The Cochrane Library, www.cochrane.org, is a full-text database of systematic reviews on clinical topics designed to help practitioners make healthcare decisions since 1993.	**The National Center for Biotechnology Information (NCBI),** www.ncbi.nlm.nih.gov, is a resource of biomedical literature from MEDLINE, life science journals, and online books.
Joanna Briggs Institute (JBI) EBP Database, https://joannabriggs.org/, is similar to the Cochrane Library. The JBI EBP database provides systematic reviews, best practice information sheets, evidence summaries, and evidence-based recommended practices.	**PsycINFO,** www.apa.org/pubs/databases/psycinfo/index.aspx, is a bibliographic database of peer-reviewed literature in the fields of mental health and the behavioral sciences. References for books, book chapters, and dissertations are included along with journal article citations and fulltext.
Embase, www.elsevier.com/online-tools/embase, is a bibliographic database indexing peer-reviewed literature in the biomedical and pharmaceutical sciences. Embase contains more than 1,800 journal titles not indexed by MEDLINE, Google, or Google Scholar.	**PubMed,** www.ncbi.nlm.nih.gov/pubmed/, is the National Library of Medicine's (NLM) free publicly available version of MEDLINE. PubMed provides access to 25+ million citations found within MEDLINE and in some cases links to the fulltext available for free from publishers or funding organizations.
SEARCH ENGINES	
Google, www.google.com, is a general search engine to find basic and preliminary general information about a topic or research question.	**Google Scholar,** http://scholar.google.com, is a separate Google search engine focused on retrieving scholarly literature. It is very important to avoid situations where a search engine is the only tool used during a literature search.

Point of Care Databases

There are a variety of patient care information tools that the nurse can access online at the bedside to provide immediate information for patient diagnosis, treatments, and procedures. Patient care tools can be divided into two types: point-of-care databases (Table 9.3) and **practice guidelines** (Box 9.1). Both provide objective, evidence-based information to assist healthcare practitioners in clinical decision-making. Like electronic databases, most point-of-care databases are only available by subscription. **Point-of-care databases** contain evidence summaries, literature reviews, and enhanced content such as pictures, videos, and patient education materials. Evidence summaries are a synopsis of the existing evidence on a topic. It is important to note that the evidence summaries typically only include evidence that exists from the publisher. For example, evidence on fall prevention by one point-of-care database called UpToDate by Wolters Kluwer will only include evidence published by Wolters Kluwer or Lippincott Williams & Wilkins since they own the UpToDate point-of-care database. Examples of point-of-care databases include UpToDate or DynaMed, which are available on hand-held devices including smartphones and tablets. Point-of-care databases are designed to provide quick access to patient care information at the point of care. Though access to point-of-care databases is beneficial, not all of them are transparent on how they search, select, appraise, or describe their information and therefore should be used with caution. Access to point-of-care databases is often funded by hospitals, medical centers, and physician practices, and some can be purchased as an individual subscription by a practitioner.

TABLE 9.3 SELECT POINT-OF-CARE DATABASES

Lippincott's Nursing Advisor, https://tinyurl.com/bdxhxfwm, is a point-of-care tool developed specifically for nursing; it includes drug information, patient education handouts, evidence-based care guidelines, and care plans.	**Essential Evidence Plus**, www.essentialevidenceplus.com, is a point-of care database that uses unique evaluation criteria called POEMS, Patient-Oriented Evidence that Matters, to determine the value of the content.
Mosby's Nursing Consult, www.clinicalkey.com/nursing, is a point-of-care tool developed specifically for nursing; it includes drug information, patient education handouts, evidence-based care guidelines, and care plans.	**UpToDate**, www.uptodate.com, is designed primarily for healthcare practitioners; it is a point-of-care tool containing frequently updated information on hundreds of conditions and treatments and patient education materials.
DynaMed, www.dynamed.com/home, is an evidence-based point-of-care reference database for nurses, nurse practitioners, physicians, residents, and other healthcare professionals.	

BOX 9.1 Select Practice Guideline Tools

Agency for Healthcare Research and Quality, National Guideline Clearinghouse(www.guideline.gov)

Guidelines International Network (www.g-i-n.net)

Registered Nurses' Association of Ontario (www.rnao.ca/bpg)

Select Clinical Practice Guidelines

Clinical practice guidelines (CPG) are summaries of information developed by practitioners, professional organizations, expert groups, and others who critically analyze and synthesize information about a clinical topic, procedure, or scenario and make recommendations for clinical practice. Summaries of guidelines are available for free via the Agency for Healthcare Research and Quality (AHRQ) and the Registered Nurses' Association of Ontario (RNAO). The fulltext of guidelines can often be found on professional organization websites or published within scholarly peer-reviewed journal articles.

LITERATURE SEARCHING WITH KEYWORDS AND SUBJECT HEADINGS

A literature search can be done with keywords and with subject headings. A **keyword** is a search term that uses natural language terminology to search the literature. For example, when searching for evidence on dyspnea, natural language would be considered anything that comes to mind related to dyspnea such as shortness of breath, breathlessness, or problems breathing. A **subject heading** is a search term or phrase that is standardized. Subject headings use consistent terms to represent a concept for data organization and retrieval. Subject headings are part of a larger system of controlled vocabulary, one that is structured as a hierarchy with broad terms and narrow subtopic terms.

Keyword Searching

Keyword searching allows the searcher to enter any keywords or groups of keywords into an electronic database. The electronic database matches the words exactly as entered; it does not evaluate the usefulness or relevancy of the words entered. Different electronic databases use different search screens and processes. In PubMed, for example, each of the keywords are entered into the PubMed search bar. After each search, click on *Advanced*. Then, on the *Results* screen, scroll down to *History* and click *Add* to combine search results together. A search done on October 20, 2020, within PubMed for *type 2 diabetes* retrieved 184,961 articles; then, a search for *diet* retrieved 535,238 articles. When the searcher clicked on *Advanced* on the *Results* screen, scrolled down to *History,* and clicked on *Add* to combine the two search topics together, the combined search identified 25,011 articles that address both of these keywords together. Another technique, called **phrase searching,** is a search for a specific phrase that is enclosed within quotes in the literature search box. For example, searching for type 2 diabetes and searching for "type 2 diabetes" will have a different number of results.

Subject Headings/MeSH Subject Headings

Electronic literature databases usually employ a subject heading system. These systems attach an index term to information using a single controlled vocabulary subject heading, regardless of the keywords or phrases used within the information written by the author. **MeSH,** medical subject headings, are the current controlled vocabulary thesaurus of biomedical terms used to describe the subject(s) of each piece of literature in MEDLINE. MeSH contains approximately 28,000 subject heading descriptors and is updated regularly to reflect changes in medical terminology. MeSH subject headings are arranged hierarchically (see Box 9.2 for example) by subject categories with more specific subject headings arranged beneath broader subject headings. The MeSH hierarchy in its entirety is available at https://meshb.nlm.nih.gov/search.

Anyone who has used hashtags within social media tools such as Twitter or Instagram has used subject headings. Hashtags categorize content within social media just like subject headings categorize content within electronic databases and internet resources. When

BOX 9.2 MeSH Subject Heading Structure

Education
- Education, Nonprofessional
- Health Education
- Consumer Health Information
- Health Education, Dental
- Health Fairs

tagging a tweet with a photo taken while on a vacation, a user might tag it #vacation. The same hashtag, #vacation, is likely to have been used by others to tag their tweets or photographs related to vacations. There may be other similar hashtags like #roadtrip or #springbreak which further categorize the same tweet or photo. When a person searches for vacation tweets or photographs, a search for the #vacation hashtag will retrieve other items tagged with the same hashtag. Like hashtags, using subject headings makes searching more efficient and precise because it groups similar information together. Because of the efficiency and precision in which subject headings search for similar information, it is important to learn how to search the literature using them.

MeSH headings are commonly used within nursing and medical databases such as MEDLINE, the Cochrane Library, and many other electronic databases and internet resources. Other databases use a slightly different set of subject headings. CINAHL's subject heading structure, called CINAHL Headings, is a system of controlled vocabulary similar to MeSH. PsycINFO's information is indexed by a thesaurus developed by the American Psychological Association, which operates similarly as MeSH.

Because of the controlled vocabulary and structure, a literature searcher wishing to find articles on weight loss surgery in an electronic database using a controlled subject heading vocabulary will not need to search with the keywords "weight loss surgery", "weight loss surgeries" "gastric bypass," and so on. Instead, the literature searcher can identify and search using the relevant subject heading in that database. In PubMed, the MeSH subject heading for weight loss surgery would be bariatric surgery. Specific categories within bariatric surgery include gastric bypass, gastroplasty, and lipectomy. Subheadings within bariatric surgery include complications, economics, epidemiology, mortality, nursing, pharmacology, and therapy. If the complications subheading is selected, literature that does not discuss complications will be eliminated from the search results. Subject heading searches result in relevant and focused results while keyword search results tend to be broader and include less-relevant results.

CASE STUDY

A nurse, a nutritionist, and a physical therapist have been caring for an overweight young adult patient with type 2 diabetes. They all are aware that type 2 diabetes is a widespread disease and traditional treatments often fail to provide adequate control. The patient has heard discussions on television about weight loss surgery providing better outcomes than traditional management with pharmaceuticals, diet, and exercise. The interprofessional team decides to conduct a literature search to find information related to the intervention options.

1. *How will exploring the evidence be useful to the patient? To the interprofessional team?*
2. *What keywords or MeSH subject headings could be used in the literature search?*
3. *How will literature results be shared with the patient?*

Search Techniques

Almost all electronic databases make use of Boolean logic to define relationships between relevant terms in literature searches. **Boolean operators** are terms such as "AND," "OR," or "NOT" that are used to expand or limit literature search results. A literature search in an electronic database using the phrases "weight loss surgery" *AND* "type 2 diabetes" makes use of the Boolean operator *AND* (see Figure 9.2). The specific attributes of the *AND* and *OR* Boolean operators are frequently confused. The *AND* Boolean operator means that all terms linked by the *AND* operator must be present in the literature to be included in the search results. If conducting a literature search for "myocardial infarction" *AND* aspirin, both terms must be present within the text for the information to be included in the search results.

When the *OR* Boolean operator is used to connect a list of terms, literature search results will be returned if either term is present, for example, aspirin *OR* ibuprofen (see Figure 9.3). All literature containing the keyword "aspirin" or "ibuprofen" will be returned. The *NOT* Boolean operator will eliminate the term that follows the *NOT* operator from your literature search results; for example, aspirin *OR* ibuprofen *NOT* acetaminophen. Literature with the terms "aspirin" or "ibuprofen", but not literature with the term "acetaminophen" present, will be returned. Literature searchers should be cautious when using the *NOT* operator because it eliminates all literature which contains the keyword regardless of the context in which the keyword is being used. Inappropriate use of the *NOT* operator can eliminate relevant and useful literature.

Search Limits

Employing **search limits** can help refine the results. For example, most students are asked to write a paper using evidence that is less than 5 years old. The date range limiter helps

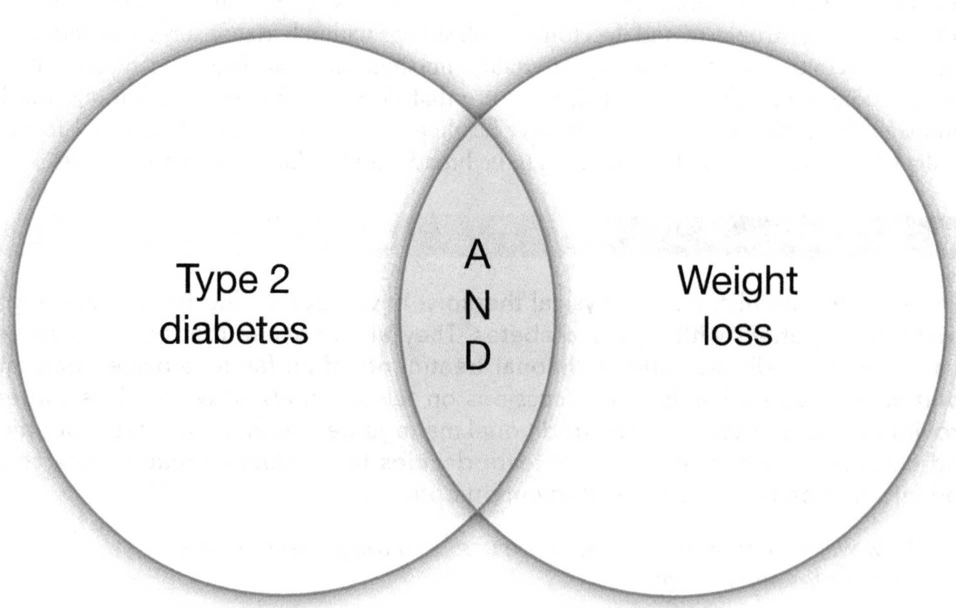

FIGURE 9.2 Using the *AND* Boolean Operator.

Search results will include only literature that includes both phrases.

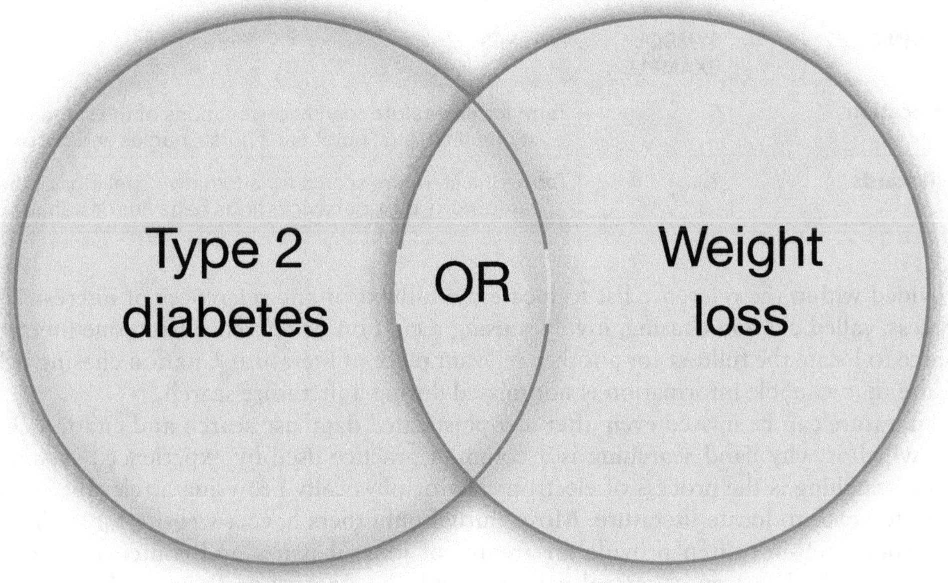

FIGURE 9.3 Using the *OR* Boolean Operator.

Search results will include all literature that includes either phrase.

to reduce the likelihood of retrieving outdated literature in the results. Every database has slightly different search limits, but common search limits include the following:

- Limit results to English language publications. Note that larger electronic databases often index and provide full-text results in many languages.
- Limit results to scholarly peer-reviewed sources. Note that larger electronic databases often include scholarly and non-scholarly sources including newspaper articles and trade publications.
- Limit results by the date of publication, for example, current year, past 5 years, and so on.
- Limit results to the type of publication, for example, randomized controlled trials (RCTs), literature reviews, meta-analysis, practice guidelines, and so on.

Even the most basic of literature search limits can lower the number of literature search results considerably. It is often best to start with basic literature search limits, for example, limit to English language and limit by publication date. Literature searchers should add more specific literature search limits as needed within subsequent searches.

Truncation and Wildcards

Other literature search techniques (Table 9.4) can improve the quality of literature search strategies and results. Literature searchers should be cautioned, however, that **truncation** and **wildcard** symbols can vary based on the database used for the search. Inappropriately placed search techniques can result in poor results, so use the techniques wisely.

Citation Chasing and Hand Searching

Reviewing the reference list of those articles retrieved from a search can provide additional evidence that was not accessed through the initial search. Use the citation information

TABLE 9.4 TRUNCATION AND WILDCARDS

TECHNIQUE	SYMBOL EXAMPLE	END RESULT
Truncation	*	Term for a literature search for variations of the same word at one time, e.g., nurs* finds nurse, nurses and nursing
Wildcards	?	Term for a literature search for alternative spellings of the same word, e.g., behavio?r finds behavior or behaviour

provided within the reference list to locate the fulltext of any references of interest. This process, called **citation chasing,** involves using a citation or reference from one literature source to locate the fulltext for another relevant piece of literature. Citation chasing helps ensure that valuable information is not missed during a literature search.

Literature can be missed even after a sophisticated database search and citation chasing, which is why hand searching is a common practice used by experienced searchers. **Hand searching** is the process of electronically or physically browsing a relevant journal cover-to-cover to locate literature. Most journal publishers have a website for each journal. These websites often provide an archive of journal issues and contents. Common headings to look for on a journal website would be *Archive* or *Previous Issues*. Then, click or page through to the table of contents. Skim article titles, abstracts, and any fulltext literature that appears relevant. Researchers conducting systematic reviews and other in-depth analysis regularly conduct a hand search of key journals for a period of years as part of their evidence-gathering process.

CASE STUDY

The nurse is working in a pediatrician's office. Some new patients' parents are concerned about the COVID-19 vaccinations causing harm to their child and are refusing to have their child vaccinated. The physician asks the nurse to help find authoritative and current professional information about vaccinations so she can develop a vaccination policy for the office.

1. *What are two to three authoritative and professional information sources that could be used to search for information?*
2. *What are one to two types of information sources that should not be included in your search?*
3. *How might the nurse share the results with the physician? And with the parents of the patients?*

Search Structure

When searching electronic databases for evidence, it is best to start the search broadly. A broad initial search helps to identify what literature is available on the topic before applying keywords, subject headings, and limiters to the search. For example, if a nurse is interested in finding evidence to indicate whether or not weight loss surgery is a more effective treatment option for type 2 diabetes compared to diet and exercise, it would be best to initially search an electronic database for the keywords "weight loss surgery" *AND* "Type 2 diabetes." If a large enough data set is returned, add the additional term of "ideal body weight" *OR* "normal body weight." If the literature is abundant, add the additional terms of "diet and exercise." If the initial keywords return a small set of literature, adding more keywords, and thus limiting the search further, will not be helpful. Box 9.3 illustrates a narrow PubMed search with limited results.

When searching with subject headings, begin the initial search with a broad subject heading, since more specific subtopics will automatically be included in the literature search. For example, in the MEDLINE electronic database, a literature search using the subject heading *bariatric surgery* will automatically include the subject heading *gastric bypass*, a specific type of bariatric surgery. It is also beneficial to search for information about each individual subject heading separately before combining search results. Adding more subject headings, keywords, and limiters to subsequent searches will refine and focus the results.

BOX 9.3 Searching PubMed With a Narrow Search

QUESTION: For patients with type 2 diabetes with uncontrolled blood glucose, what is the effectiveness of bariatric surgery versus diet and exercise in controlling blood glucose levels?

1. Start by brainstorming possible search terms for this topic, for example,
   - Insulin pump
   - Uncontrolled blood glucose
   - Type 2 diabetes
2. Identify electronic databases available for your literature search. Databases frequently chosen for nursing-related literature searching include:
   - CINAHL
   - MEDLINE
   - PubMed
3. Access the database and begin a preliminary search

   For example, PubMed, www.ncbi.nlm.nih.gov/pubmed

   Within PubMed, click the *Advanced* search link at the top of the database under the search box. Type the first keyword phrase, identified in Step 1. For example, type "insulin pump."

   Note that when a literature search for the phrase "insulin pump" was done in PubMed, 1,730 items were found. Type another keyword exact phrase from Step 1 into the search box. For example, type "uncontrolled blood glucose."

   Note that when a literature search for the phrase "uncontrolled blood glucose" was done in PubMed, 44 items were found.

   Now within the *History* section, *Add to search builder* both searches and click *Search*.

   Note that when the search was combined in PubMed, two items were found.
4. Limit the literature search further, as needed, by choosing filters from the left column of the PubMed search results page, for example, choose:
   - *Free full text* within the *Text availability* section
   - *5 years* within *Publication dates* section

   Note that when these search limits were applied to the previous literature search, one item was returned. This is a very small number of results, so go back to Step 3 and adjust the search terms used. The phrase "uncontrolled blood glucose" might not be the best way to describe the patient scenario. The searcher might need to go back to Step 1 and brainstorm new keywords or phrases such as "blood glucose" and "control" Or "glucose levels" and *control*?

   Note that it often takes multiple adjustments to create an effective search.

Evidence Types

When considering what constitutes evidence, it is important to take a **pluralistic approach** that considers all the literature on the specific topic when searching for evidence (Pearson et al., 2007). A pluralistic approach is based on a philosophical view that there is more than one way to look at something. A pluralistic approach is inclusive of all types of evidence, from the highest level of evidence (i.e., systematic reviews using meta-analysis of high-quality appraised RCTs) to the lowest form of non-research evidence called expert opinion. This is particularly important when there is little research conducted on a novel problem.

Hierarchies of evidence (also known as **levels of evidence**) provide a visual representation of types of evidence, from the least reliable (at the bottom) to the most reliable (at the top). Hierarchies provide a way to understand the strength and reliability of the evidence based on the type of study or type of evidence. An important distinction between strength and reliability of evidence and the quality of evidence must be made. Hierarchies, or levels of evidence, can only tell the type of evidence. It does not tell the searcher anything about the quality of the evidence. The quality of the evidence is determined through appraisal, discussed later in the chapter. There are conflicting representations of what type of evidence is found at what level. For the most part, there is a general consensus on levels of evidence.

Table 9.5 illustrates how the first level includes the strongest type of evidence. Each level decreases in strength and reliability of evidence. While the higher levels (levels I–IV)

TABLE 9.5 SYNTHESIS OF TYPES AND LEVELS OF EVIDENCE RANKED STRONGEST TO WEAKEST

LEVEL OF EVIDENCE	TYPE OF EVIDENCE
I (strongest) Experimental Designs	Systematic reviews (SR) of randomized controlled trials (RCTs) using meta-analysis
	Comprehensive systematic reviews of RCTs and other types of studies
	Clinical practice guidelines based on SRs with meta-analysis
	Randomized controlled trials
II Quasi-Experimental Designs	Systematic review of quasi-experimental designs
	Controlled trial without randomization
III Observational and Analytical Designs	Qualitative systematic reviews of cohort or case studies
	Cohort study
	Case-control study
IV Observational or Descriptive Studies	Qualitative systematic reviews of descriptive studies using meta-aggregation
	Single descriptive or qualitative study
V (weakest) Text and Expert Opinion	Expert opinion, reports from committees, grey literature, literature reviews

Source: Data from Ackley, B. J., Swan, B. A., Ladwig, G., & Tucker, S. (2008). *Evidence-based nursing care guidelines: Medical-surgical interventions.* (p. 7). St. Louis, MO: Mosby Elsevier; Hopp, L., & Rittenmeyer, L. (2020). *Introduction to evidence-based practice: A practical guide for nursing. 2nd Ed.* Philadelphia, PA: F.A. Davis. ISBN 13:978-0-8036-2328-6; Melnyk, B.M. and Fineout-Overholt, E. (2011). *Making the Case for Evidence-Based Practice.* In: Melnyk, B.M. and Fineout-Overholt, E., Eds., *Evidence-Based Practice in Nursing & Healthcare. A Guide to Best Practice. 2nd Edition,* Lippincott Williams & Wilkins, Philadelphia, 3-24; The Joanna Briggs Institute (2021). https://ospguides.ovid.com/OSPguides/jbidb.htm.

describe forms of research evidence, there are other types of evidence that can be used when there is a lack of research articles on a topic. For example, a new idea is tried in practice where a nurse wears a yellow vest to reduce interruptions and signify "do not disturb" while removing medications from an electronic medication dispensing system. While this seems appropriate and does not cause harm, what is not known is if wearing the vest actually decreases interruptions during the medication removal activity. A thorough search of the literature on this topic may only produce one article, written by a nurse, about the experience and perception of reduced interruptions while wearing a yellow vest. This type of evidence is considered expert opinion. While it is one of the lower quality forms of evidence, an argument can be made that it still constitutes evidence and can inform practice but only in the absence of research evidence.

Pre-appraised evidence includes systematic reviews and CPGs. These types of evidence theoretically should include an appraisal of all evidence up to the date the literature was written. For both systematic reviews and CPGs, there should be a section on inclusion and exclusion criteria that details the data range for the literature search. This is important so that the user understands how far the date range is for the search and the studies included. For example, a systematic review on clinical decision support systems in electronic documentation may have a date range of 2000 to 2020. This is appropriate since clinical decision support systems are a relatively new innovation and were not used prior to 2000. If a qualitative systematic review on patient isolation had a date range of 2000 through 2020, one might suspect that some evidence is missing since isolation has been a healthcare practice since the inception of nursing. A date range of 1970 to 2020 would be appropriate as this range captures the beginning of published evidence.

CASE STUDY

The nurse is part of a team working on a project to reduce 30-day hospital readmissions for heart failure. The team consists of a social worker, pharmacist, cardiologist, case manager, dietitian, and yourself. After conducting a review of the literature on best practices to reduce 30-day readmissions for heart failure, the team reassembles to review the findings. Each team member wants to know what the evidence shows for a particular reason. The social worker wants to know what support services are needed to help the patient at home. The pharmacist wants to know which medications are the most effective in maintaining a balance for the patient. The cardiologist wants to know the evidence that influences his decisions about prescribing and ordering care. The nurse wants to know what evidence shows which interventions and education are important for the patient.

1. *What are the ideal types of evidence for each team member's focus?*
2. *What are the implications if each member brought only one piece of evidence rated at a level 4 or level 5? Would this be considered the best available evidence?*

Evidence Appraisal

Once the available evidence from the literature is located, the nurse should appraise the quality of the evidence and the generalizability of the information to the practice setting. A determination should be made whether the evidence is strong enough, or rigorous enough, to support a change in patient care practice and if the evidence is strong enough to inform clinical decisions. The nurse should also determine if the evidence can be applied as is or needs to be adapted to the nurse's clinical setting. The willingness of the nurse's individual institution to adopt change based on their unique situation, availability of resources, and culture of change should also be addressed. These issues drive the appraisal of evidence.

Tools to Appraise Evidence From the Literature

Critical appraisal of evidence is one of the most important steps in EBP to determine if the evidence is truly the "best available." Critically appraising the evidence to determine if it is valid, reliable, and appropriate helps to focus only on high-quality evidence and eliminate evidence that is either not applicable or of low quality. It is important to understand that every piece of evidence should go through a rigorous appraisal process to judge the quality of the evidence. This action is taken to ensure that only the best available evidence is used to inform clinical decision-making and that any proposed changes based on the evidence are defensible. The following are tools to assist both novice and expert nurses and the interprofessional team to appraise different types of evidence.

Appraisal of Guidelines for Research and Evaluation Instrument

The Appraisal of Guidelines for Research and Evaluation (AGREE) II instrument provides a framework to evaluate CPGs (Brouwers et al., 2010). The AGREE II is both valid and reliable and comprises 23 items organized into six quality domains The AGREE Next Steps Consortium (2009):

- scope and purpose
- stakeholder involvement
- rigor of development
- clarity of presentation
- applicability
- editorial independence (Brouwers et al., 2020)

Each of the 23 items in the quality domains target various aspects of practice guideline quality. The AGREE II also includes two final overall assessment items that require the appraiser to make overall judgments of the practice guideline. The AGREE II tool is easy to use for the purposes of the nurse evaluating clinical guidelines for the best available evidence. The tool is free of charge and can be accessed on the world-wide web at www.agreetrust.org. Tutorials are available on the website.

The Critical Appraisal Skills Program

The Critical Appraisal Skills Program (CASP; 2019) is another available free resource that provides the nurse with tools to judge the quality of various types of research evidence. In contrast to the AGREE II tool for appraising CPG, CASP has different appraisal tools for different types of evidence. CASP provides checklists specific to types of research including randomized controlled trials, systematic reviews, cohort studies, case-control studies, and qualitative research studies. See Table 9.6, Research Terminology. The CASP tools can be located on the world-wide web at https://casp-uk.net/casp-tools-checklists. The website also provides tutorials for new users.

TABLE 9.6 RESEARCH TERMINOLOGY

TERM	DEFINITION
Case-control study	A study comparing cases of two study participants in order to identify causes of what makes them different. For example, a case-control study might compare two nursing home patients, one with recurrent urinary tract infections (UTI) and one who never had a UTI, in order to identify elements that might predict the condition in others (e.g., incontinence, immobility).
Clinical practice guidelines (or practice guidelines)	Statements with recommendations to assist healthcare professionals regarding the most appropriate treatment for specific clinical situations. Evidence-based CPGs provide the strongest level of evidence to guide practice, and are based on systematic reviews of RCTs or the best available evidence on a specific clinical circumstance or situation.
Cohort study	A prospective study of two groups conducted over time in order to collect and analyze data in comparison to one another. For example, a cohort study might examine a group of inner-city elementary children from birth through age 18 compared to a similar group in a rural setting.
Integrative review	An analysis of the literature on a specific topic or concept leading to implications for practice. It may or may not include a search strategy or list the databases searched.
Meta-analysis	A comprehensive and systematic approach using statistical methods to pool the results of independent randomized controlled studies on a topic that leads to inferences or conclusions about that topic.
Mixed methods	A study that uses both quantitative and qualitative study designs.
Non-experimental research	A study in which the researcher collects and analyzes data based on what is observed about a phenomenon without using a comparison.
Outcomes research	A study conducted to measure the effectiveness of an intervention. For example, hospitals frequently conduct outcomes research to document the effectiveness of their services by measuring the end results of patient care (e.g., infection rates, rates of readmission).
Prospective study	A non-experimental study that begins with an examination of assumed causes (e.g., high fat diet), which then goes forward in time to the presumed effect (e.g., obesity).
Qualitative research	A study that examines a phenomenon with words and descriptions rather than statistics or numbers in order to determine underlying elements and patterns within relationships.
Quantitative research	A study that examines a phenomenon with numeric data and statistics rather than words or descriptions in order to determine the magnitude and reliability of relationships between variables or concepts.
Randomized controlled trial (RCT)	A study that uses a true experimental design (research that provides an intervention or treatment to research participants who have been randomly chosen to be either in the experimental group receiving a treatment or the control group where they receive no intervention or treatment).
Systematic review (SR)	An exhaustive and transparent systematic approach to searching all the literature on a topic and then critically examining and synthesizing all the evidence on that specific topic.
Text and expert opinion	Opinions from experts or committees. Literature reviews, white papers, and editorials are forms of expert opinions.

CPG, clinical practice guidelines; RCT, randomized controlled trials.

Source: Data from Dicenso, A., Guyatt, G., & Ciliska, D. (2005). *Evidence-based nursing: A guide to clinical practice*. New York. Elsevier. ISBN: 9780323025911; Hopp, L., & Rittenmeyer, L. (2020). *Introduction to evidence-based practice: A practical guide for nursing. 2nd Ed*. Philadelphia, PA: F.A. Davis. ISBN 13:978-0-8036-2328-6; Melnyk, B.M. and Fineout-Overholt, E. (2011). *Making the Case for Evidence-Based Practice*. In: Melnyk, B.M. and Fineout-Overholt, E., Eds., *Evidence-Based Practice in Nursing & Healthcare. A Guide to Best Practice. 2nd Edition*, Lippincott Williams & Wilkins, Philadelphia, 3-24.

Resources for Lifelong Learning

One way to keep up-to-date is through database features that save literature searches and provide email alerts of new information which meet the search criteria. PubMed has a free self-registration feature called My NCBI (National Center for Biotechnology Information). My NCBI allows a literature searcher to save complex search strategies with limits and will automatically run the searches at a later time. The service sends an email with new results to the literature searcher on a predetermined schedule. Literature searches are saved on the National Library of Medicine servers, not on a specific computer, so they can be accessed anywhere with internet access. CINAHL and PsycINFO via the EBSCO platform, MEDLINE via the OVID platform, and most databases on the ProQuest platform also allow literature searchers to create an account and save searches that can be accessed and rerun on demand.

Another way to keep up-to-date is through email alert services offered through professional organizations or information providers. Examples include:

- The American Nurses Association (ANA) offers ANA SmartBrief, a regular news update service offered for free to non-members. Sign up at www.smartbrief.com/ana.
- Medscape offers medical news, journal articles, and expert perspective news updates for free. Register at www.medscape.com/nurses.

Taking advantage of free training resources, features that save a search within electronic databases, and email alert services can make it easy to stay current on topics of interest.

CLINICAL EXPERTISE

In 1984, Benner published a landmark book in which she disseminated the idea that nurses constantly evolve in their practice along a continuum from novice to expert. This evolution occurs with the acquisition of additional education, advanced skills, experience, and an understanding of patients, families, and their unique needs (Benner, 1984). Benner further stated that regardless of how much education a nurse possessed, the nurse could never become an expert without actual clinical experience. In practical terms, what this implies is that based on knowledge and experience, each nurse brings unique perceptions and strengths to the healthcare setting.

There is an expectation in society that nurses will bring theoretical and practical clinical knowledge and expertise to their practice as a credentialed nursing expert. As a professional, there is an assumption that every registered nurse will provide safe and competent care to every patient. **Clinical expertise** develops as the nurse tests and refines both theoretical and practical knowledge in actual clinical situations (Benner, 1984). Hopp and Rittenemeyer (2021) stated that clinical expertise is more than the education, skills, and experience of a nurse; clinical expertise must be explicit, or clearly visible to others, so that it can be subjected to analysis and critique. Nurses demonstrate clinical expertise when they assess their patient and family, consider the setting of the provision of care, make clinical decisions that place the patient's values at the center of care, and coordinate patient care based upon available resources. Analysis and critique of clinical expertise most commonly occurs through performance evaluations, competency assessment, certification from a professional organization, or peer evaluations based on standardized nursing performance criteria.

Real World Interview

Clinical expertise has not been exhaustively defined in the literature. But we have models that help us understand its role in EBP. I think the group that originated the Promoting Action on Research Implementation in Health Services (PARIHS) framework has examined the idea of clinical experience quite thoughtfully. In their original articles, they argued that clinical experience or practical, tacit knowledge can be a source of evidence (Rycroft-Malone et al, 2004). However, like other sources of evidence, it falls along a continuum of low to high. Low clinical experience is anecdotal, lacking critical reflection and testing against external sources, and therefore is limited as a source of knowledge. In contrast, high clinical experience has been tested by others, represents consensus, and others regard it "judiciously" in order to find it credible. That means that the value and validity of the experience and expertise has been reflected upon and weighed as to its relevance and importance. Importantly, legitimate clinical expertise is much more than accumulating experience; it requires critical reflection, externalization, and is critically reviewed (Rycroft-Malone, 2004).

Others may view clinical expertise as the "glue" of EBP. By that I mean the ability of the expert practitioner to seamlessly blend their judgment of the quality and magnitude with the patient's preferences and values, the context of the clinical decision-making, and available resources with their practical knowledge.

In the earliest days of EBP, many clinicians felt that the emphasis only on evidence removed clinical judgment and created a "cookbook" approach to EBP. Some have argued that EBP leads to rule-driven approaches to decision-making and threatens clinical expertise (Day, 2009). But the modern definition of EBP embraces clinical expertise as an important element of accomplishing optimal patient outcomes. Clinical expertise and evidence are not dichotomous but rather partners, bringing together the best available evidence and the clinical tacit knowledge of clinical experts.

Lisa Hopp, PhD, RN, FAAN

Day, L. (2009). Evidence-based practice, rule-following, and nursing expertise. *American Journal of Critical Care, 18*, 479–482. https://doi.org/10.4037/ajcc2009147

Rycroft-Malone, J. (2004). The PARIHS framework—A framework for guiding the implementation of evidence-based practice. *Journal of Nursing Care Quality, 19*, 297–304. https://doi.org/10.1097/00001786-200410000-00002

Rycroft-Malone, J., Seers, K., Titchen, A., Harvey, G., Kitson, A., & McCormack, B. (2004). What counts as evidence in evidence-based practice? *Journal of Advanced Nursing, 47*, 81–90. https://doi.org/pnw.idm.oclc.org/10.1111/j.1365-2648.2004.03068.x

For example, a physically debilitated patient requires assistance transferring from the chair to the bed. The nursing staff used a gait belt to assist with this procedure. Two nurses, with differing experience and background, can approach the care of this patient differently while at the same time they both ensure the safety and well-being of the patient. A novice nurse, with limited practical experience and knowledge related to the patient, decides to ask the physical therapist to assist her by showing her the proper techniques needed for the safe transfer of the patient to the bed. A more experienced nurse, familiar with proper body mechanics, gait belt transfers, and the patient's physical ability chooses to assist the patient with the gait belt by herself. Both nurses achieved the same goal of safely transferring the patient to bed; however they approached the issue differently based on personal experience and knowledge. This example demonstrates how the individual nurses' varying clinical expertise can impact how care is delivered to this patient.

To ensure optimal patient outcomes and patient safety, all nurses need to constantly be aware of their strengths and limitations as they plan and implement care.

CURRENT LITERATURE

CITATION

Gigli, K. H., Davis, B. S., Ervin, J., & Kahn, J. M. (2020). Factors associated with nurse's knowledge of and perceived value in evidence-based practices. *American Journal of Critical Care*, *29*(1), e1–e8. https://doi.org/10.4037/ajcc2020866

DISCUSSION

A cross-sectional survey was conducted with nurses from 12 adult intensive care units. The objective of the research was to examine the relationship between nurses' education level and specialty certification with their perceptions of evidence-based practice on their units. Findings suggest that nurses with specialty certification demonstrate a positive perception, self-efficacy, and role clarity in regards to evidence-based practices whereas educational level was not a factor. Certification was also associated with a greater perceived value in specific daily evidence-based practices of lung-protective ventilation and sedation interruption of ventilated patients.

IMPLICATIONS FOR PRACTICE

This study contributed to the body of knowledge regarding the impact of specialty certification. Supporting specialty certification of nurses can influence the adoption of evidence-based practices as a means to improve patient safety and quality patient care outcomes.

PATIENT PREFERENCES

Patient preferences refer to the involvement of the patient and family with a consideration of their values and beliefs in clinical shareddecisions (Hopp & Rittenmeyer, 2021). Some patients like to leave healthcare decisions up to their provider while others like full disclosure about their health issues. When patients are included in their healthcare decisions there is an improvement in cognitive (e.g., ability to retain education, memory recall) and behavioral (e.g., the ability to adhere to a prescribed regimen) outcomes (Shay & Lafata, 2016). Evaluating the patient's preferences for inclusion in decisions should be part of providing care to each and every patient. Chapter 6 explores tools that help assess the patient's preferences and guides to help patients make healthcare decisions. While considering the patient's preferences seems easy, sometimes patient preferences go against the nurse's own belief system. For example, the patient may continue to smoke after receiving a diagnosis of lung cancer, choose alternative treatments over conventional therapy, refuse life-saving blood transfusions, or decide not to treat a condition altogether. Remaining nonjudgmental, keenly aware, and accepting of a patient's wishes are important elements of evidence-based nursing practice.

Shared decision-making is an approach that involves both clinicians and patients in considering the best available evidence to make healthcare decisions. Patients are empowered, engaged, and supported to make autonomous decisions about healthcare (Truglio-Londrigan et al., 2014). A variety of models exist to guide shared decision-making. One particular model describes the responsibilities required of the healthcare provider and essential skills needed for shared decision-making:

- Involve the patients either implicitly or explicitly in the decision-making process.
- Explore ideas, fears, and expectations of the problem and possible treatments.
- Describe treatment options with consideration for equilibrium and balance.
- Identify the patient's preferred format for education and provide tailor-made information.
- Check the patient's understanding of information and reactions.
- Include the patient to the extent they desire to be involved in the decision-making process.
- Discuss the options and either make or defer the healthcare decision (Elwyn et al., 2012).

NURSES, ROLE IN EVIDENCE-BASED PRACTICE

The ANA made it clear that EBP is a critical component of the nurse's role by embedding it into the guiding standards for nursing practice. The *Scope and Standards of Nursing Practice* (American Nurses Association, 2015) and *The Nursing Social Policy Statement* (American Nurses Association, 2010) both indicate that it is the responsibility of the nurse to provide care that is evidence based. While the Scope and Standards are currently being revised, the draft continues the focus on EBP by nurses. Following suit, the accreditation bodies for nursing programs, the American Association of Colleges of Nursing and the

BOX 9.4 Developing Clinical Judgment

Mr. Armitage is a 56-year-old patient admitted 1 day ago with atrial fibrillation, an abnormal heart rhythm, along with fatigue and dizziness. During an assessment of Mr. Armitage, the nurse notes the presence of rales in his lung bases bilaterally. Upon further assessment, the patient is noted to have 1+ pitting edema in his feet bilaterally. Neither of these findings were relayed at change of shift report. The patient states that he does not want to stay in the hospital and, if possible, he would like to continue care at home. The nurse checks the previous nursing assessment findings in the electronic medical record and finds no mention of rales or edema. Considering the causes of edema and rales, the nurse checks the electronic medical record and finds a report of an echocardiogram completed a day ago that shows an ejection fraction of 35%. The patient's medication list includes Cardizem 30 mg once a day, Lopressor 50 mg twice a day, and aspirin 81 mg once a day. The patient states that his physician ordered a water pill for him to take twice a day but he couldn't afford the medication since he is self-employed with private insurance so he didn't take it.

1. What **CUES** (Assessment) might the nurse consider?
2. What additional information might the nurse need to form a conclusion about the patient's assessment findings?
3. What **HYPOTHESIS (Diagnosis)** can the nurse consider?
4. What **ACTION (Plan and Implement)** plan will be most effective for the nurse to take to ensure the safety of the patient while adhering to the patient's preferences for care?
5. What should the nurse evaluate for the purpose of arriving at a satisfactory clinical **OUTCOME (Evaluation)**?
6. How could the nurse incorporate the patient's preferences into treatment of the patient?

National League for Nursing Accreditation Commission, have increased focus on required competencies for evidence-based nursing practice.

While it may seem that doing the right thing the right way for the right patient at all times should be second nature, many times making a change from "doing it the way it has always been done" to "basing nursing care on evidence" can be difficult. Practices done the way they have always been done are known as "sacred cows" and some workers use these to resist change. They may hold on to old practices believing they are the best approach to patient care. New nurses will be faced with the challenge of basing nursing interventions on the best available evidence. Maintaining a focus on questioning current practice and keeping up-to-date with changes to nursing care in the practice setting is important. Vocalizing evidence-based changes and guiding others to question their nursing practice can help to shift the culture from "sacred cows" to nursing care based on current best available evidence.

The direct care nurse is in the perfect position to identify problems with patient care. During a normal workday, a nurse will care for a team of patients and coordinate care with an assortment of interprofessional healthcare providers. These interactions can highlight problems that are perfect for EBP changes. Communicating patient care problems or issues to a person in a position of influence is critical to initiate change. Such positions of influence can include the unit director or manager, the quality representative on the unit, or the unit practice council. Becoming familiar with appropriate venues for conveying patient care problems is critical as a new nurse.

Nurses can promote a positive attitude regarding innovation and embrace the opportunity to assist with developing EBPs, serving as mentors to others, and encouraging inquisitiveness regarding best practices. Enlightened users of EBP can provide encouragement to others as they incorporate innovative change. Professional nurses who choose to take on the challenge of creating an EBP culture with their colleagues will promote patient safety and improve the quality of healthcare that leads to excellence in patient care. This chapter covered knowledge of basic EBP principles that are essential for the new nurse. New nurses should be able to engage at a beginner level by identifying patient care problems, collaborate with others to identify the best available evidence, and support implementation of evidence in patient care.

END-OF-CHAPTER RESOURCES

KEY CONCEPTS

1. Evidence-based practice (EBP) requires a combination of three elements: the best available evidence, the nurse's clinical expertise, and consideration for the patient's preferences.
2. Developing a good research question using PICO as a framework can help develop a clear, purposeful research direction.
3. Keywords and subject headings are used to search electronic literature databases for evidence.
4. While searching with subject headings is preferable, some literature search topics are better searched with keywords in one's own natural language.
5. Using Boolean operators, synonyms and search techniques like truncation and phrase searching can help identify important content in electronic literature databases.
6. There are several high-quality electronic databases for searching scholarly peer-reviewed professional journals and professionally published information sources.
7. It is often better to first approach a literature search broadly and then narrow the search after the initial literature search results are returned.
8. Examining the type of evidence using a hierarchy of evidence or level of evidence is critical to knowing the strength and reliability of the evidence used to inform a practice change.
9. A standardized appraisal tool, such as AGREE II and CASP tools, provides a valuable, easy to use guide for the nurse to judge the quality of the evidence.
10. Clinical expertise is a combination of knowledge and experience along with externally validated expertise in a given field.
11. Lifelong learning can be facilitated with the use of resources on the internet.

CRITICAL DISCUSSION POINTS

1. The definition of EBP includes three distinct areas: best available evidence, clinical judgment, and patient preferences. How would a nurse prioritize the three areas for a successful EBP project? Which area has the greatest impact? Which area is most likely to be forgotten during EBP projects? How can a nurse make sure that all three areas are considered for an EBP project?
2. What resources are needed for direct care nurses to regularly be able to engage in basic literature search activities?
3. When looking through the literature for information on a topic for an assignment, how is the best available evidence located? What could be done to ensure capture of the best available evidence on a topic?
4. Think about your last clinical experience. How did you demonstrate consideration for the patient's preferences in your care? What changes can you make in the future to include the patient's preferences when providing care?
5. Locate one peer-reviewed article on a nursing topic of your choice. Select the appropriate appraisal tool (CASP or AGREE II) to examine the quality of the evidence. What judgments can you make about the quality of the evidence? Would you use the evidence to inform a change in your clinical practice?

6. What is the importance of using a hierarchy of evidence to determine the types of evidence for an EBP project? Locate one hierarchy online by searching for "nursing evidence hierarchies" or "levels of evidence" using www.google.com and explain why the hierarchy appeals to you.

KEY TERMS

> Best available evidence
> Bibliographic databases
> Boolean operators
> CINAHL (Cumulative Index to Nursing and Allied Health Literature)
> Citation chasing
> Clinical expertise
> Clinical practice guidelines
> Evidence-based practice
> Full-text databases
> Hierarchies of evidence
> Hand searching
> Keyword
> Levels of evidence
> MEDLINE
> MeSH
> Patient preferences
> Phrase searching
> PICO
> Pluralistic approach
> Point-of-care databases
> Practice guidelines
> PubMed
> Search limits
> Shared decision-making
> Subject heading
> Truncation
> Wildcards

REVIEW QUESTIONS

Answers to Review Questions appear in the Instructor's Manual. Qualified instructors should request the Instructor's Manual from textbook@springerpub.com.

1. You are a member of a clinical practice interprofessional team that is looking at the best available evidence to reduce hospital-acquired pressure ulcers on the medical-surgical unit. Which of the following actions by the team demonstrate actions to locate the best available evidence? *Select all that apply.*

   A. Conducting a thorough search of the literature using Google to find evidence
   B. Searching all nursing databases for evidence on the care of hospital-acquired pressure ulcers
   C. Conducting a thorough search of the literature using CINAHL and Medline

D. Using an article based on guidelines from the medical-surgical nursing professional organization.
E. Locating information from Up-To-Date
F. Asking what others have done on the Magnet® listserv

2. The nurse is giving a presentation to coworkers regarding the patient benefits of adopting policies based on evidence-based practice (EBP). Which of the following benefits of EBP should be included in the presentation? *Select all that apply.*
A. Improved quality of care
B. Improved cost savings
C. Decreased patient satisfaction
D. Decreased lengths of stay
E. Improved patient outcomes
F. Decreased cost savings

3. The nurse cares for a patient who has been diagnosed with reoccurring lung cancer. The oncology unit has a nurse-led support group for improving quality of life for cancer patients. The patient declines participation stating that he is a private person and he is not interested in participating in a group. Which of the following is the best response by the nurse?
A. "The grieving process will bring you through many phases. Many patients experience denial initially. If you change your mind at a later date, let me know."
B. "This program is based on research which found that support groups help cancer patients cope with their disease. I suggest that you consider coming to the next meeting anyway."
C. "I will bring over another patient who says the program has been life-changing so you can make an informed decision."
D. "What types of support have you found helpful in dealing with trying situations in the past?"

4. The nurse is gathering evidence on interventions to reduce the risk for falls for patients who are at high risk for falls. The nurse finds a variety of types of evidence. All evidence types are appraised using the appropriate tool and found to be high quality. Which of the following are inappropriate types of evidence to use considering all listed types of evidence are found? *Select all that apply.*
A. Systematic literature review
B. Report from a national committee on fall prevention
C. Clinical practice guidelines
D. Editorial
E. Systematic review using meta-analysis
F. Meta-analyses of randomized controlled trials
G. Case studies
H. Qualitative study

5. The nurse is gathering the best available evidence on interventions to reduce hospital-acquired pressure ulcers. Which of the following would be considered the highest level of evidence?
A. Clinical practice guideline
B. Randomized controlled trial
C. Phenomenological study
D. Meta-analysis systematic review

6. The nurse is involved in a task force to design patient care plans using the best available evidence. Which of the following statements is true regarding EBP? *Select all that apply.*

A. All patients should receive the same care based on evidence.

B. Lower level evidence (levels 4 or 5) should not be used to impact patient care decisions.

C. Patient values are a key component of EBP.

D. All systematic reviews are considered the highest level of evidence.

E. Given the ease of access to scientific data, EBP can be quickly incorporated into care plan design.

F. Evidence from a textbook publisher is considered high quality.

G. Clinical practice guidelines should not be used to develop care plans.

H. If a systematic review is found during the search, the person can stop their literature search.

7. The nurse wants to implement EBP in the care of patients on the unit. Identify the correct order to implement EBP.

A. Measure outcomes from the change.

B. Appraise the evidence.

C. Ask a searchable question.

D. Incorporate the change into practice.

E. Sustain the change.

F. Create a change based on the evidence.

G. Identify a clinical problem.

H. Locate the best available evidence.

I. Determine the level of evidence.

8. A nurse is leading an interprofessional team working on strategies to improve patient satisfaction in the emergency department (ED). A social worker is part of the team and asks the nurse, "Why do we have to appraise all the research articles we found, isn't it good enough to use the findings from the articles since they are all research?" What would be the most appropriate way for the nurse to respond?

A. "We need to know which of the articles have the best evidence."

B. "By appraising the evidence, we will find out the level of each article."

C. "The appraisal will direct us on what evidence supports each intervention."

D. "Appraisal helps us determine the quality of the evidence."

9. The ED nurse reads an article stating that patient morbidity and mortality are increased when patients are given plasma volume expanders in the initial treatment of hypovolemic shock. The nurse is concerned about patient outcomes in the ED as plasma volume expanders are often prescribed. What is the best action by the nurse?

A. Narrow the issue to develop a searchable PICO question and then conduct a search of the literature. Contact a local university to use their library database resources.

B. Contact the chief of emergency medicine and nurse manager to request creating an interprofessional team to investigate the clinical problem.

C. Discuss the article with the unit practice council. Request that the issue be taken to the next nursing quality committee.

D. Post the article in the breakroom. Make copies of the article and place it in conspicuous areas to disseminate the information.

10. Before conducting a literature search in Medline, PubMed or CINAHL, it is important to remember which of the following?

A. In most cases, the best search results will be returned if you search using multiple keywords, exact phrases, subject headings, and limiters all together in your initial search.

B. In most cases, it is preferable to search using the electronic database's system of controlled vocabulary subject headings.

C. In most cases, the best search results will be returned if you search an electronic database with one keyword.

D. In most cases, the best search results will be returned if you search an electronic database with one specific phrase.

REVIEW ACTIVITIES

1. Use information presented in this chapter about the EBP process and required skills to create an interview guide. Use the guide you created to interview a nurse about their experiences with EBP projects. You can ask a nurse you know or one you have contact with during your clinical experiences. Examine your findings against the knowledge and skills required for nurses to participate in EBP.

2. Some literature searches work better with subject headings than with keywords and exact phrases. For example, try to find evidence to support the use of aspirin with patients who have had a heart attack. Try searching this topic using PubMed (www.PubMed.gov). Type "myocardial infarction" *AND* aspirin into the search bar at the top of your computer screen. See how many results you get. Assess the usefulness and relevancy of those results. Then, click the MeSH link found in the drop-down box under PubMed, just left of the main search box. Instead of typing both terms together with the Boolean operator *AND* in between, type one term at a time, search for it, select the best match from the MeSH results on the left side of the screen, click the link *Add to search builder* on the screen, and repeat the process until you are ready to click the *Search PubMed* button to run the search. Assess the usefulness and relevancy of the results returned from the MeSH search. What did you find? Which of the searches yielded more relevant and useful results?

3. Go to the website WhyNotTheBest: www.whynotthebest.org/contents. Review the list of case studies and select one of your choice. Look at the information presented, paying particular attention to how evidence was used to make the change and how nurses were involved as part of the team. Based on what you've learned in the chapter, would you make any changes to the project? What suggestions would you give?

4. Form groups of five to ten students, depending on the number and availability of library databases. Create a PICO question about barriers and facilitators to EBP by new nurses in a hospital setting. Inclusion and exclusion criteria can be set by the students but all articles must be peer-reviewed. Each student should search a different database and all evidence should be appraised using the appropriate tool. As a group, combine all findings from the best available evidence into categories of barriers and facilitators. From each list, the group can come up with strategies to overcome barriers and to enhance facilitators. Share your group's findings with the class. Retain your findings to help you assimilate into nursing practice after graduation.

EXPLORING THE WEB

1. Learning how to search for literature within electronic databases and online tools can be tricky. Online tutorials, videos, and webinars developed by the companies that sell electronic databases can help to improve search skills and strategies. PubMed's *PubMed for Nurses* tutorial can be completed in 30 minutes (www.nihlibrary.nih.gov/training/online-tutorials/pubmed-nurses). EBSCO Information Services has a YouTube channel of database videos and search guides (www.youtube.com/user/ebscopublishing). The National Guideline Clearinghouse has an extensive list of video tutorials, frequently asked questions, and help information available (www.ahrq.gov/gam/index.html). All of these tools and tutorials can keep nurses up-to-date on basic literature search skills, databases, and patient care information tools.

2. The Cochrane Collection (www.cochrane.org) produces systematic reviews and other types of evidence reports. Holdings can be searched by topic or keyword. Review an executive summary from a Cochrane systematic review. The Joanna Briggs Institute (http://joannabriggs.org) produces peer-reviewed highquality systematic reviews, evidence summaries, and best practice series that tend to be nursing focused. Holdings can be searched by topic or keyword. Review best practice information sheets from JBI. How can each of these be used to guide changes in clinical practice?

3. Go to the Indiana Center for Evidence-Based Nursing Practice (ICEBNP) at www.ebnp.org/evidence. Review the tools available to assist nurses with EBP.

4. Go to the following website to further develop your knowledge of evidence-based healthcare: EBM Education Center of Excellence, North Carolina: http://library.ncahec.net.

5. Go to the QSEN website (www.qsen.org) and search for the teaching strategy, Using Evidence to Address Clinical Problems (http://qsen.org/USING-EVIDENCE-TO-ADDRESS-CLINICAL-PROBLEMS. Follow the directions on the teaching strategy page to help students identify how to use evidence during clinical rotations.

6. Locate "Nurse as the leader of the team huddle. An unfolding oncology case study" on the QSEN website (http://qsen.org/nurse-as-the-leader-of-the-team-huddle-an-unfolding-oncology-case-study/) Focus on the identification of evidence-based interventions for the patient in the case study as well as the patient's preferences. PowerPoints and YouTube videos accompany the unfolding case study.

7. As a nurse on the medical-surgical inpatient floor, you have noticed several patients have experienced phlebitis at the site of insertion for intravenous catheters. You start to wonder if there are EBP changes that could be made to decrease the incidence of phlebitis. Locate two articles and use the appropriate CASP or AGREE II tool to appraise the quality of the evidence. Explain why you selected the two articles including the level of evidence from the evidence hierarchy. How would you use the evidence to create guidance for interventions to reduce the incidence of phlebitis?

8. Access a nursing policy from your clinical laboratory experience. Review the evidence that supports the policy. Conduct a literature search on the topic of the policy. Is the evidence currently used to support the policy the best available evidence? Is there better evidence available? What changes would you propose to the policy based on your findings?

A robust set of instructor resources designed to supplement this text is located at **http://connect.springerpub.com/content/book/978-0-8261-6145-1.** Qualifying instructors may request access by emailing **textbook@springerpub.com.**

REFERENCES

The AGREE Next Steps Consortium. (2009). *Appraisal of guidelines for research and evaluation II instrument.* The AGREE Research Trust. https://www.agreetrust.org/wp-content/uploads/2013/10/AGREE-II-Users-Manual-and-23-item-Instrument_2009_UPDATE_2013.pdf

American Nurses Association. (2010). *Nursing's social policy statement: The essence of the profession.* American Nurses Association.

American Nurses Association. (2015). *Scope and standards of nursing practice* (3rd ed.) American Nurses Association.

Benner, P. (1984). From novice to expert, excellence and power in clinical nursing practice. Menlo Park, CA: Addison-Wesley Publishing Company. https://doi.org/10.1002/nur.4770080119

Brouwers, M. C., Kho, M. E., Browman, G. P., Burgers, J. S., Cluzeau, F., Feder, G., Fervers, B., Graham, I. D., Grimshaw, J., Hanna, S., Littlejohns, P., Makarski, J., & Zitzelsberger, L. (2010). AGREE II: Advancing guideline development, reporting and evaluation in healthcare. *Canadian Medical Association Journal, 182*(18), E839–E842. https://doi.org/10.1503/cmaj.090449

Brouwers, M. C., Spithoff, K., Lavis., J., Kho, M. E., Makarski, J., & Flórez, I. D. (2020). What to do with all the AGREEs? The AGREE portfolio of tools to support the guideline enterprise. *Journal of Clinical Epidemiology, 125,* 191–197. https://doi.org/10.1016/j.jclinepi.2020.05.025

Critical Appraisal Skills Program. (2019). *CASP checklists.* https://casp-uk.net/casp-tools-checklists/

Elwyn, G., Frosch, D., Thomson, R., Joseph-Williams, N., Lloyd, A., Kinnersley, P., … & Barry, M. (2012). Shared decision making: A model for clinical practice. *Journal of General Internal Medicine, 27*(10), 1361–1367. http://doi.org/10.1007/s11606-012-2077-6

IOM (Institute of Medicine). (2011). *Clinical Practice Guidelines We Can Trust.* Washington, DC: The National Academies Press. http://www.nationalacademies.org/hmd/Reports/2011/Clinical-Practice-Guidelines-We-Can-Trust.aspx

Pearson, A. (2014). Evidence-based nursing: Synthesizing the best available evidence to translate into action in policy and practice. *Nursing Clinics of North America, 49*(4). Preface. https://doi.org/10.1016/j.cnur.2014.09.001

Pearson, A., Wiechula, R., Court, A., & Lockwood, C. (2007). A Re-consideration of what constitutes "evidence" in the healthcare professions. *Nursing Science Quarterly, 20*(1), 85–88. doi:10.1177/0894318406296306

Quality and Safety Education for Nurses. (2012). *Evidence-based practice.* http://www.qsen.org/definition.php?id=3

Sackett, D. L., Rosenberg, W. M., Gray, J. A., Haynes, R. B., & Richardson, W. S. (1996). Evidence based medicine: what it is and what it isn't. *BMJ: British Medical Journal, 312*(7023), 71–72.

Shay, L. A., & Lafata, J. E. (2015). Where is the evidence? A systematic review of shared decision making and patient outcomes. *Medical Decision Making: An International Journal of the Society for Medical Decision Making, 35*(1), 114–131.

Truglio-Londrigan, M., Slyer, J. T., Singleton, J. K., & Worral, P. S. (2014). A qualitative systematic review of internal and external influences on shared decision-making in all health care settings. *JBI Database of Systematic Reviews & Implementation Reports, 12*(5), 121–194. https://doi.org/10.11124/jbisrir-2014-1414

SUGGESTED READINGS

Baumann, N. (2016). How to use the medical subject headings (MeSH). *International Journal of Clinical Practice, 70*(2), 171–174. https://doi.org/10.1111/ijcp.12767

Brusco, J. M. (2010). Effectively conducting an advanced literature search. *AORN Journal, 92*(3), 264–271. https://doi.org/10.1016/j.aorn.2010.06.008

Chan, E.-Y., Glass, G. F., & Phang, K. N. (2020). Evaluation of a hospital-based nursing research and evidence-based practice mentorship program on improving nurses' knowledge, attitudes, and evidence-based practice. *Journal of Continuing Education in Nursing, 51*(1), 46–52. https://doi.org/10.3928/00220124-20191217-09

Hasanpoor, E., Siraneh Belete, Y., Janati, A., Hajebrahimi, S., & Haghgoshayie, E. (2019). Nursing managers' perspectives on the facilitators and barriers to implementation of evidence-based management. *Worldviews on Evidence-Based Nursing, 16*(4), 255–262. https://doi.org/10.1111/wvn.12372

Malfait, S., Eeckloo, K., Van Biesen, W., & Van Hecke, A. (2019). Barriers and facilitators for the use of NURSING bedside handovers: Implications for evidence-based practice. *Worldviews on Evidence-Based Nursing, 16*(4), 289–298. https://doi.org/10.1111/wvn.12386

Robinson, C. H., Yankey, N. R., Couig, M. P., Duffy, S. A., & Sales, A. E. (2018). The Veterans Health Administration registered nurse transition-to-practice program: A qualitative evaluation of factors affecting implementation. *Journal for Nurses in Professional Development, 34*(6), E8–E22. https://doi.org/10.1097/NND.0000000000000488

Speroni, K. G., McLaughlin, M. K., & Friesen, M. A. (2020). Use of evidence-based practice models and research findings in Magnet-designated hospitals across the United States: National survey results. *Worldviews on Evidence-Based Nursing, 17*(2), 98–107. https://doi.org/10.1111/wvn.12428

CHAPTER **10**

Patient Safety

Christine Rovinski-Wagner and Peter D. Mills

"Maintaining safety reflects a level of compassion and vigilance for patient welfare that is as important as any other aspect of competent health care."

–Stone et al., 2008

Upon completion of this chapter, the reader should be able to:

1. Define safety.
2. Discuss the quality measures of structure, process, and the monitoring of outcomes related to a safe healthcare system.
3. Describe the behaviors necessary for the nurse and interprofessional team to create a just culture of safety in a healthcare environment, that is, leadership, measurement, risk identification and reduction, high reliability, and teamwork.
4. Describe how utilization management (UM) supports a just culture of safety.
5. Differentiate overuse, underuse, and misuse of healthcare services.
6. Distinguish between a person approach and a system approach to patient care safety.
7. Explain strategies that reduce variation in healthcare delivery and standardize the provision of safe patient care.
8. Identify characteristics of organizations that sustain and spread healthcare safety.
9. Discuss current safety initiatives in healthcare.
10. Discuss safety initiatives for healthcare staff.
11. Identify healthcare ranking sources and other information sources for safe, high-quality healthcare.

CROSSWALK

This chapter addresses the following:

QSEN Competency: Safety

The American Association of Colleges of Nursing. (2021). *The essentials: Core competencies for professional nursing education.*

Domain 5: Quality and Safety

OPENING SCENARIO

The nurse decided to help another nurse and ambulate Mr. Smith as he said that he wanted to get out of bed and try to walk. The nurse had heard morning report and knew the patient had his surgery the day before. The nurse had Mr. Smith sit up on the side of the bed, and then began to assist him with ambulation. As Mr. Smith walked down the hallway, he suddenly became weak in the knees and started to fall. The nurse attempted to stop the fall by leaning against Mr. Smith so that he could go down to the floor in a gentle manner, breaking the fall. The nurse immediately yelled for help and started to assess the patient. After another staff member arrived, Mr. Smith's vital signs were taken. His heart rate was 120, respiratory rate 16, temperature 98.6 °F., and his blood pressure 90/60, while lying on the floor. The staff asked Mr. Smith if he could stand long enough to have the staff check orthostatic vital signs, but he stated that he was still dizzy. He felt that he could get up into the wheelchair to go back to his bed with help. The staff successfully moved Mr. Smith to the bed.

Afterwards, the nurse who had been assigned to Mr. Smith initially said the patient had not been out of bed earlier because he felt nauseated each time he tried to sit up and he had refused to walk. His hemoglobin and hematocrit had been low. There were concerns that he might require blood and he had been receiving serial laboratory draws. The physician had just received the laboratory results and was talking to the assigned nurse about initiating a blood transfusion when the fall occurred. The assigned nurse and the physician had been unaware of the other nurse walking the patient.

1. What role did communication play in this scenario?
2. Are there any individual and/or system actions that would have increased the likelihood of a safe patient outcome?
3. Use Table 10.1 and identify a few structures, processes, and outcomes that should be set up and periodically reviewed for this type of patient.

INTRODUCTION

In this chapter, safety is defined and discussed. Quality structures, processes, and outcome monitoring related to safe healthcare systems are aslo discussed. Behaviors necessary for the nurse and interprofessional team to create a just culture of safety are described. The role of utilization management (UM) in supporting patient safety is discussed. The overuse, underuse, and misuse of healthcare services are considered. The difference between a person approach and a system approach to the process of improving patient safety is reviewed. Strategies that reduce variation and standardize the provision of safe patient care are introduced. Characteristics of organizations that sustain and spread healthcare safety are identified, as are healthcare rankings and other measurements and information sources related to patient quality and safety. Current safety initiatives in healthcare for patients and staff such as initiatives in reduction of workplace violence, improvement of healthcare rankings, safe staffing, medication safety, nurses with impairing conditions, hand hygiene, safe patient handling and mobility (SPHM), suicide prevention, environmental safety, and disaster planning are examined. Finally, healthcare ranking sources and other information sources for safe, high-quality healthcare are noted.

HIGH-QUALITY STRUCTURES AND PROCESSES TO ACHIEVE HIGH-QUALITY OUTCOMES AND SAFETY

Safety is the process of minimizing risk of harm to patients and providers through both system effectiveness and individual performance (QSEN Institute, 2020). Patient safety concerns identified by the Emergency Care Research Unit (ECRI) for 2020 include the following:

- diagnostic errors
- maternal health (childbirth-related complications)
- behavioral health needs and inadequate resources
- medical device problems
- device cleaning, disinfection, and sterilization
- standardizing safety policies and education across the healthcare system
- inconsistent use of standard patient identifier conventions, attributes, and formats in all patient encounters and the electronic health record
- overprescribing of antibiotics contributing to antimicrobial resistance
- overrides of automated dispensing cabinets to remove medications
- communication breakdowns across care settings, resulting in patient readmissions, missed diagnoses, medication errors, delayed treatment, duplicative testing and procedures, and patient dissatisfaction (Finnegan, 2020).

Safety does not occur naturally or without effort. Nurses must utilize their leadership and management skills to work with the interprofessional team to build or structure healthcare systems to provide safe outcomes for patients. Nurses also use reviewed activities or processes to achieve safe, high-quality outcomes. Nurses use all these structure and process resources to create, nurture, and sustain safe outcomes. In a safe healthcare system, nurses and the interprofessional team identify and correct quality problems before a patient and/or staff is harmed.

When the nurse accepts a patient care assignment, the nurse develops and/or uses a healthcare system's elements of safe, high-quality structures and processes to ensure safe, high-quality patient outcomes (Table 10.1). First, the nurse develops appropriate patient care using structures and processes to achieve positive outcomes. Then, the nurse learns from positive outcomes, for example, improvements shown in data dashboards and measurements such as those showing decreases in common hospital-acquired infections, such as central line-associated bloodstream infections (CLABSIs), catheter-associated urinary tract infections (CAUTIs), ventilator-associated events (VAEs), surgical site infections (SSIs), methicillin-resistant *Staphylococcus aureus* (MRSA) bloodstream events, *Clostridioides difficile* (*C. difficile*), and others.

The nurse also learns from negative outcomes, for example, close calls and adverse events. A close call, also called a near miss, is an unplanned occurrence that did not result in injury, illness, or damage, but had the potential to do so. One example of a close call is when a nurse double-checks a medication dose and realizes the wrong amount was prepared. An **adverse event** is an incident that occurs during healthcare delivery when the patient suffers injury resulting in prolonged hospitalization, disability, or death, for example, the wrong medication was given to the patient, resulting in difficulty breathing.

When a nurse comes on duty to the emergency department (ED) and is assigned four empty patient rooms, the nurse checks the ED's safety structures, that is, supplies, suction equipment, and monitors in the nurse's four assigned patient rooms. The nurse verifies

TABLE 10.1 NURSING IN A SAFE, HIGH-QUALITY HEALTHCARE ENVIRONMENT

QUALITY MEASURE	EXAMPLE
Structure–The setting where healthcare occurs. Includes physical facility structures, ventilation systems, hospital equipment, human resources, staffing, and so on.	The patient environment, staffing, and access to the interprofessional team and supervisor are set up and structured to ensure patient safety and quality care before beginning patient care. Quality patient standards are put in place by the nurse and interprofessional team to ensure delivery of quality patient care with a high degree of reliability. A just, fair-minded culture of safety is in place. This culture realizes that errors are often organization-wide healthcare system problems, and that errors are often not just a one-time occurrence of an individual problem. When errors in patient care occur in a just culture of safety, the performance of the entire healthcare delivery system is reviewed to identify healthcare system problems, not just the performance of the individual person(s) involved in the error. Patient care assignment sheets are in place to communicate elements of patient care to the interprofessional team.
Process–All actions in healthcare delivery. Includes the process of patient diagnosis and treatment, the technical way patient care is delivered, and the interpersonal way patient care is delivered.	The nurse utilizes hospital policies that reflect the Five Rights of Delegation (National Council of State Boards of Nursing, National Guidelines for Nursing Delegation, 2019). The nurse and interprofessional team follow evidence-based policy and procedures, patient care standards, guidelines, and bundles when giving patient care. The nurse and interprofessional team set priorities when delivering patient care processes to ensure patient safety. Clinical safety precautions, such as chain-of-command reporting guidelines for patient care problems, allergy alerts in the medical records, and nonclinical safety precautions, such as signs alerting people about wet floors, are used.
Outcomes–The effects of healthcare on patients and staff. Includes monitoring changes in patient and staff knowledge, behavior, health status, cost, and patient and staff satisfaction.	The nurse and interprofessional team monitor the following outcomes on an ongoing basis: patient clinical outcomes, patient satisfaction, patient safety, staff safety, staff satisfaction, staff adherence to policy and procedure and evidence-based standards, and other key healthcare structures, processes, and outcomes.

that safe healthcare processes are in place, such as following evidence-based guidelines and checking team assignments and responsibilities with the physician, other nurses, and nursing assistive personnel. Then the nurse is ready for the arrival of a patient needing emergency healthcare, having ensured that the structures and processes are in place to ensure the outcomes of patient safety and quality patient care.

Financial Consequences

Safety has major financial consequences for patients, providers, insurers, family, and/or caregivers. Hospital-acquired infections are associated with increased use of laboratory tests, radiology imaging, antibiotics, and hospital days (Benenson et al., 2020). The cost of a single case of infection can range from just under $1,000 to nearly $50,000, depending upon the type of infection (The Leapfrog Group, 2018). An extended length of hospital stay is also associated with an increase in risk of harm to patients, including health-care-associated infections (HAIs) and death. Additionally, when a patient experiences harm in a hospital, both in-hospital and postdischarge use of health services and costs of care are significantly affected (Tessier et al., 2019). The way to improve safety is to learn about the causes of error and to use this knowledge to design safer systems of patient care to reduce the incidence and harm from errors. A nurse who identifies unsafe conditions and the risks of potential error, who knows what to report, how to communicate with other leaders about risks, and understands the potential organizational consequences of not reporting unsafe conditions, demonstrates leadership.

A JUST CULTURE OF SAFETY

Safety flourishes best when it is part of an organization's just culture of safety. The term "culture" broadly relates to a learned structure where people work together, and which includes the practices of people who lead and people who follow (Schein & Schein, 2019). The term **"just culture of safety"** has four key features:

- acknowledgment of the high-risk nature of an organization's activities and the determination to achieve consistently safe operations.
- a blame-free environment where individuals can report errors or near misses without fear of reprimand or punishment.
- encouragement of collaboration across healthcare positions and disciplines to seek solutions to patient safety problems.
- organizational commitment of resources to address safety concerns (Patient Safety Net, 2019)

A just culture of safety promotes an atmosphere of trust where all nursing, medical, and administrative staff in a healthcare system collaborate and seek solutions to patient safety problems. A just culture of safety ensures balanced accountability and recognizes that an individual may be at fault for an error, but frequently the healthcare system is also at fault. Errors or close calls are reported in a just culture of safety without excessive fear of blame, reprimand, or reprisal. A just culture of safety does not absolve a nurse or others from personal responsibility. Nurses and others remain responsible for at-risk, reckless, or malicious choices and are responsible for the behavioral choices they make.

Note in Figure 10.1, there are two similar looking glass medication vials with yellow tops that contain different medications. One glass vial contains midazolam, used to induce sedation, and the other glass vial contains furosemide, a diuretic. If the nurse does not recognize this similar labeling as high risk and unsafe, and then inadvertently chooses the wrong glass vial of medication to quickly give medication to a patient, the nurse could be blamed for reckless behavior. If a nurse does not call the prescribing physician to clarify an order, a choice has been made by the nurse. The nurse either rationalized the risk, "The doctor will yell at me," or the nurse did not recognize the risk of potential harm to the patient. This choice is classified as at-risk behavior in a just culture of safety. Also, in a just culture of safety, the organization looks beyond just blaming the nurse. It recognizes the high-risk similar appearance of the two glass vials with different medications and encourages collaboration across the healthcare system and healthcare disciplines—for example, nursing, pharmacy, and medicine—to solve this healthcare system's medication safety problem. The organization will commit resources to solve this safety problem. As part of the solution, the pharmacy will probably change the medication labels to assure safety and prevent future medication errors throughout the healthcare system.

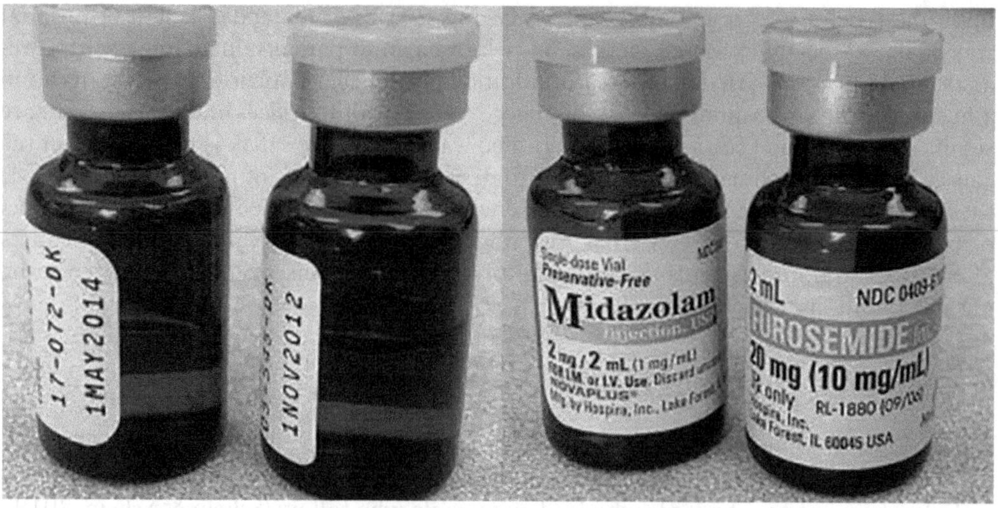

FIGURE 10.1 Similar Medication Vials.

Source: Courtesy of Institute for Safe Medication Practices. Reprinted with permission.

Medication Safety

Improved medication safety outcomes are seen in healthcare facilities that implement prospective and retrospective risk identification and risk reduction activities, such as working with the Institute for Safe Medication Practice (ISMP), to prevent harm to patient or staff. The ISMP (www.ismp.org) is an independent patient safety organization devoted entirely to medication error prevention and safe medication use. The ISMP sponsors, for member healthcare organizations, a confidential, voluntary medication error reporting program, and databank on the same website, which allows data analysis of system causes of medication errors reported by all the member hospitals. This analysis helps member hospitals identify and share some of the best evidence-based practices to improve medication safety. One error reported to the ISMP databank involved an accidental programming by a pediatric nurse of an infusion pump for 10 times the dose ordered. The ISMP issued evidence-based recommendations on its website for improving patient safety during pediatric administration of IV acetaminophen, including using “smart” IV infusion pump technology when giving maximum dosages of medications and requiring pharmacy preparation of medication doses that are different from the usual strength available commercially.

Five Important Behaviors in a Just Culture of Safety

There are five important behaviors in a just culture of safety in healthcare: leadership, measurement, risk identification and reduction, high reliability, and teamwork (Table 10.2).

A healthcare organization that wants to strengthen its just culture of safety may also incorporate the components of **high-reliability organizations** (HROs), which have a preoccupation with failure, reluctance to simplify, sensitivity to operations, commitment to resilience, and deference to expertise. HROs achieve a just culture of safety in dangerous environments, such as aviation, nuclear energy, and healthcare. In healthcare organizations that strive to be HROs, the goal is to deliver exceptionally safe, consistently high-quality reliable care (Table 10.3).

Nurses who role-model behaviors that support a just culture of safety and recognize and honor when others do the same are demonstrating nursing leadership, regardless of their positions. For example, during a unit meeting, a nurse builds teamwork by acknowledging

TABLE 10.2 BEHAVIORS SEEN IN A JUST CULTURE OF SAFETY IN HEALTHCARE

JUST CULTURE OF SAFETY IN HEALTHCARE	BEHAVIORS
Leadership	Encouraging nurses and all staff to assume leadership and report any unsafe conditions that could lead to patient falls Responding with a system approach to safety disruptions, such as when a nurse exhibits reckless behavior by not using correct personal protective equipment (PPE) when caring for a patient with COVID-19, considering the availability of PPE supplies, gloves, staffing ratios, and so on, as well as the need for nursing re-education and competency testing, as needed Being sensitive to reports of any deviations from standard safety protocols even if this slows down work, for example, encouraging staff to complete incident reports about safety close calls
Measurement	Designing the healthcare system to encourage development of evidence-based practices and measuring the outcomes of evidence-based practices as they are developed and implemented Ensuring that removing steps from a healthcare process will not cause adverse events and tracking the number of adverse events after the steps are removed
Risk Identification and Reduction	Identifying risks and reducing the possibility that an adverse event can happen, such as adding safe patient handling instructions to a care plan for a patient with right-sided weakness Designing healthcare systems to avoid errors before they cause harm or result in an adverse event; for example, developing and using a checklist to guide nurses in the timely use of preoperative antibacterial cloths
Teamwork	Building relationships with nurses, physicians, and all other members of the interprofessional team to facilitate ongoing working together toward the goal of a just culture of safety Avoiding a silo mentality where staff from one group in the hospital, for example, nurses, doctors, administrators, and so on, do not communicate with, share information with, understand, or work well with another group in the hospital (e.g., nurses, doctors, administrators, and others working in healthcare. A silo mentality reduces communication and efficiency in the overall operation, reduces morale, and often contributes to a nonproductive company culture Cross-monitoring, watching each other's back, and working together to ensure patient safety Engaging patients in health promotion/disease prevention through interprofessional and patient-centered strategies Empowering the people with the greatest expertise in a specific area to help resolve a potential safety concern rather than always deferring to the person with the highest rank, for example, on a safety QI team, including staff who have expertise and regularly use the healthcare processes being examined Demonstrating behaviors of an effective leader and follower, such as being active in decision-making, taking ownership of team decisions, taking other actions when necessary, and providing honest feedback

TABLE 10.3 HIGH-RELIABILITY ORGANIZATION CHARACTERISTICS

CHARACTERISTIC	ELEMENTS
Preoccupation with Failure	Be alert to near-miss events. Recognize any weaknesses in the healthcare system early.
Reluctance to Simplify	Recognize the complexity of work. Do not focus on superficial causes of failure.
Sensitivity to Operations	Acknowledge the complexity of healthcare processes. Have situational awareness of the environment, distractions, and the availability of resources and supplies. Be aware of nursing, medical, administrative, and other staff relationships.
Commitment to Resilience	Anticipate and mitigate or reduce the disruptive impact of any failure. Determine how to diminish risk of harm to patients. Identify nursing, medical, and administrative and other staff strengths to recover when an adverse event occurs.
Deference to Expertise	Use teamwork that recognizes each member's knowledge, skill, and expertise. Facilitate active participation from all healthcare professionals. Be comfortable in sharing information. De-emphasize the hierarchy among nursing, medical, administrative, and other staff.

Source: Adapted from Weick, K. E., & Sutcliff, K. M. (2015). *Managing the unexpected: Sustained performance in a complex world* (3rd ed.). John Wiley & Sons.

a colleague's good work stating, "Joe did a good job calming an upset patient yesterday." This building of teamwork in a just culture of safety, along with using the other elements of a just culture of safety (Table 10.2) in a healthcare organization, allows for the greatest reduction in accidental harm to patients. A just culture of safety allows for healthcare delivery that is replicable and can be reproduced in another healthcare organization; it is reliable, regardless of the day of the week, area of patient care, patient transfers, or patient background. A healthcare organization with a just culture of safety can be relied upon to deliver the right care to the right patient at the right time in the right setting.

Leadership

Nursing leadership in a just culture of safety acknowledges the high-risk nature of the organization's activities and empowers all nurses and employees to assume leadership and report all safety hazards. Nursing leaders create and sustain a just culture of safety. Employees feel confident that there will be no negative consequences in productively communicating safety problems to supervisors. All nurses are oriented to the chain-of-command and all nurse leaders support the idea that every nurse is a leader and manager responsible for safe, high-quality care. If a patient's safety is threatened, all nurses speak up and work with the interprofessional team and administration to manage the environment for patient safety. At the bedside, nurses demonstrate a just culture of safety leadership with simple yet essential actions. Each shift, nurses consistently maintain a just culture of safety and raise bedside rails, position bedside tables within easy reach for each patient, and create a plan with their team members for regular rounding and prompt responses to call lights. Nurses are personally involved in seeking and understanding gaps in patient safety, making safety a priority, and committing organizational resources needed to close any performance gaps in providing safe, high-quality patient care in a just culture of safety consistently.

Real World Interview

Nurses demonstrate safety leadership through initiating gentle education, collaborative inquiry, and modeling clear, direct, and professional communication with their interprofessional colleagues. These behaviors create trusting relationships and position nurses as trusted organizational leaders, even if they are not in formal leadership roles. When working with a new physician, nurses introduce themselves by name and role. The nurse identifies which patients are the nurse's responsibility and provide direction about how the physician can reach the nurse for any questions or concerns. If the physician does not reciprocate with similar information, for instance, "I am Dr. Smith, the new chief resident. I am covering Dr. David's patients today. My contact information is at the desk," the nurse can step up as a leader. The nurse can ask the physician directly for this information. This establishes the structure and processes for clear communication between the nurse and the physician which supports the outcome of safe patient care. When nurses lead in building relationships across silos they make a significant difference in improving patient safety processes.

Lisa Harmon, PhD
Patient Safety Manager
White River Junction Medical Center, Vermont

In a just culture of safety, successful hospital boards and staff, including nurses, physicians, and the other members of the interprofessional team, use specific measures of safe performance to monitor quality improvement (QI). They hold all staff accountable for high levels of quality and safety, they learn from best practices in the healthcare field, and they implement new knowledge within their organizations. Healthcare and nursing leaders are sensitive to the daily operations of their organizations and they encourage nursing leadership activities and collaboration across the organization's hierarchies, reporting structures, and interprofessional roles that support a just culture of safety (Table 10.4).

Measurement

The second component of a just culture of safety is measurement. Measurement provides information and feedback to leadership and clinicians about a just culture of safety and its clinical outcomes. Nurses promote a just culture of safety by posting outcome graphs and safety dashboards (Figure 10.2) on their units that demonstrate safety gains and losses so that adjustments can be made.

When nurses look at this dashboard, they can see a trend toward a decrease in the fall rate from January through September aligned with an increase in three safety elements:

- use of a nurse-driven fall reduction protocol,
- improved teamwork as measured by using safety huddles, and
- inclusion of "risk for fall" information on the patient assignment sheet.

This trend toward a decrease in the fall rate tells the staff that the activities undertaken to decrease the number of falls has been effective, but that further work is needed to continue to decrease falls. A data display or dashboard is designed to help facilities identify and target areas for QI and promote safe practices.

Clinical outcomes associated with patient safety such as patient falls and risk-adjusted mortality and morbidity are measured, tracked, and analyzed in a just culture of safety. **Risk adjustment** is a statistical process that identifies and adjusts for variation in patient outcome data due to differences in patient characteristics (or risk factors) across healthcare organizations (The Joint Commission [TJC], 2020). To illustrate, a reliable comparison of

TABLE 10.4 LEADERSHIP ACTIVITIES THAT SUPPORT A JUST CULTURE OF SAFETY

LEADERSHIP GROUP	ACTIVITIES SUPPORTING A JUST CULTURE OF SAFETY
Hospital Boards	Include safety as a standing item on board agenda. Establish an organizational baseline measure of safety culture performance. Include representatives with clinical expertise, including nurses, physicians, and other members of the interprofessional team on the hospital board.
Hospital Administration and Nurse Leaders and Managers	Integrate patient safety and evidence-based practice into every activity in the organization. Create an annual patient safety award to recognize outstanding leadership and teamwork in making patient care safer. Listen to the bedside nurse to identify obstacles that are encountered in daily work and continue to enhance patient safety and staff competencies. Implement policies that ensure that nurses and all staff are safe and have adequate resources at work. Provide clinical nursing supervision. Establish clear chain-of-command reporting guidelines. Include nurses in decisions that affect their work environments.
Peer review committees	Focus on clinical practice measured against evidence-based professional standards. Review and evaluate patient records for quality and appropriateness of services ordered or performed by their professional peers. Identify practice patterns that indicate a need for more knowledge.
Staff nurse leaders	Motivate and encourage staff nurse leaders to deliver safe, high-quality patient care with timely and meaningful feedback. Maintain competency in evidence-based practice. Utilize opportunities for professional development. Join nursing and community committees to improve patient care quality.

the in-hospital deaths of healthy patients who were not expected to die based on the condition of the patients upon admission requires a statistical adjustment of the figures for patient risk factor differences, such as tobacco and alcohol use, weight, and level of physical activity.

Measurement and analysis of how and what clinicians feel about their work environment are also reviewed and can predict whether nurse and patient safety outcomes will be

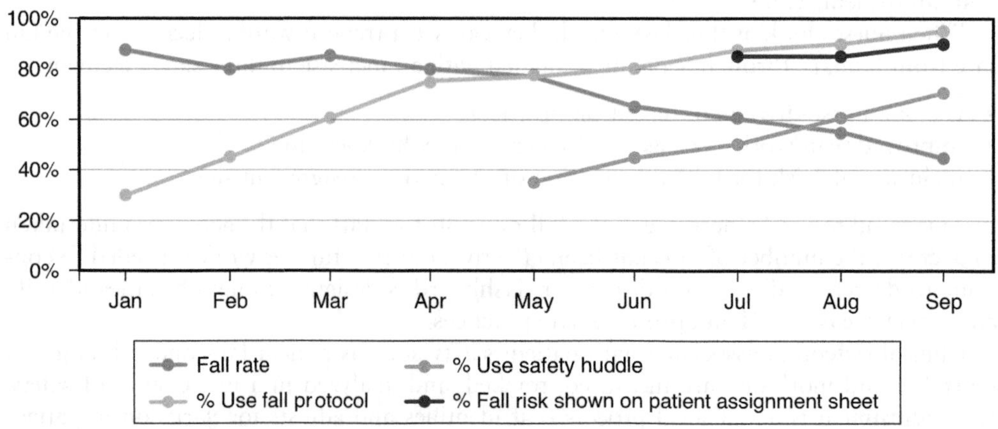

FIGURE 10.2 Example of Dashboard Displaying the Safety Outcome of Patient Fall Reduction.

BOX 10.1 SOPS Hospital Survey Items and Composite Measures, Version 2.0

Teamwork
Staffing and work pace
Response to error
Communication about error
Communication openness
Reporting patient safety events
Handoffs and information exchange
Hospital management support for patient safety
Organizational learning-continuous improvement
Supervisor or clinical leader support patient safety

SOPS, Surveys on Patient Safety Culture

Source: Data from Agency for Healthcare Research and Quality. (2019). SOPS® *hospital survey*. https://www.ahrq.gov/sites/default/files/wysiwyg/sops/surveys/hospital/SOPS-Hospital-Survey-2.0-5-26-2021.pdf

positive or negative. The Agency for Healthcare Research and Quality (AHRQ) Surveys on Patient Safety Culture (SOPS; AHRQ, n.d.) can be administered throughout an organization to collect data to understand how staff perceive various aspects of the patient safety culture (Box 10.1). The SOPS surveys are not mandatory and there are no penalties for poor safety scores. SOPS surveys are done by healthcare organizations to assess a patient safety culture at a level of detail that helps organizations identify specific areas of strength and areas for improvement. Healthcare organizations can upload their SOPS™ survey data and compare it with AHRQ's national database of SOPS. A positive just culture of safety is associated with fewer adverse events (Sammer et al., 2020).

Measurement in a just culture of safety often includes use of the Institute for Healthcare Improvement (IHI) Global Trigger Tool for Measuring Adverse Events, available at www.ihi.org/resources/Pages/IHIWhitePapers/IHIGlobalTriggerToolWhitePaper.aspx. The IHI Global Trigger Tool methodology includes a retrospective review of a random sample of patient records using "triggers" (or clues) to identify possible adverse events. The IHI Global Trigger Tool includes a specific list of triggers and their definitions; detailed information on using the methodology; and step-by-step instructions for establishing a review team and using the tool to accurately identify adverse events (harm) and measure the rate of adverse events over time.

Triggers (Table 10.5) can identify the need to examine a patient care record more carefully to determine if there were any problems in care delivery. As an example, if there is evidence in a patient care record that the patient received a blood transfusion, this may indicate there was a problem in patient care delivery, that is, an unexpected episode of patient bleeding during surgery.

Risk Identification and Reduction

Risk identification and reduction, the third component of a just culture of safety, studies human error and reduces factors that contribute to human error. Risks are identified both prospectively (looking forward) and retrospectively (looking backward). The identification of any human error associated with safety risks will trigger the review of the different factors contributing to the ways that humans make mistakes. Human factors engineering uses what we know about the way humans think, how human minds and bodies work, and how humans interact with the environment to make products and processes that are safer to use. Unconscious human safety errors, such as forgetting to give a medication to a patient or picking up the wrong medication syringe, may derive from a breakdown in an automatic human behavior or a temporary lapse in memory. These human behavior breakdowns and memory lapses leading to unconscious human errors can be influenced by both environmental external factors such as distractions, noise, and time pressure, and by internal factors such as fatigue, expectations about the future, and anxiety. Conscious human safety errors involve a breakdown in a human's decision-making process, for instance, using a work-around. **Work-arounds** occur when one does not follow the rules and/or works around the rules or correct actions of a patient care process or a work process to save time or solve a problem (Table 10.6).

TABLE 10.5 INSTITUTE FOR HEALTHCARE IMPROVEMENT GLOBAL TRIGGER TOOL

General Triggers	Transfusion of blood or use of blood products Code, cardiac or pulmonary arrest, or rapid response team activation Acute dialysis Positive blood culture X-ray or doppler studies for emboli or venous thromboembolism Decrease in hemoglobin or hematocrit of 25% or greater Patient fall Pressure injuries Readmission within 30 days Restraint use Healthcare-associated infections In-hospital stroke Transfer to higher level of care Any procedure complication
Medication Triggers	*Clostridium difficile* positive stool, if history of antibiotic use Partial thromboplastin time (PTT) >100 seconds if on heparin International normalized ratio (INR) >6 if on anticoagulants Glucose <50 mg/dL if on insulin or oral hypoglycemics Rising blood urea nitrogen (BUN) or serum creatinine two times (2×) over baseline if on meds known to cause renal toxicity Vitamin K administration if evidence of bruising, gastrointestinal (GI) bleed, hemorrhagic stroke, or large hematomas Diphenhydramine (benadryl) administration Romazicon (flumazenil) administration Naloxone (narcan) administration Antiemetic administration for nausea and vomiting that interferes with feeding, postoperative recovery, or delayed discharge Oversedation/hypotension Abrupt medication stop
Surgical Triggers	Return to surgery Change in surgical procedure Admission to intensive care postoperatively Intubation or reintubation or use of bilevel positive airway pressure (BiPap) in post-anesthesia care unit (PACU) X-ray intraoperatively or in PACU Intraoperative or postoperative death Mechanical ventilation >24 hours postoperatively Intraoperative administration of epinephrine, norepinephrine, naloxone, or romazicon Postoperative increase in troponin levels >1.5 ng/mL Occurrence of any operative complication
Intensive Care Triggers	Pneumonia onset Readmission to the intensive care unit (ICU) All bedside procedures and other procedures done while patient in intensive care unit Intubation or reintubation or use of BiPap in post-anesthesia care

(continued)

TABLE 10.5 INSTITUTE FOR HEALTHCARE IMPROVEMENT GLOBAL TRIGGER TOOL (*continued*)

Perinatal Maternal Triggers	Terbutaline use Third- or fourth-degree lacerations Platelet count <50,000 Estimated blood loss >500 mL for vaginal delivery or >1,000 mL for cesarean delivery Specialty consult Administration of oxytocic agents, such as oxytocin, methylergonovine, or 15-methyl-prostaglandin postpartum Instrument delivery in the prenatal delivery, postpartum, and neonatal and infant healthcare areas of the hospital Administration of general anesthesia
Emergency Department (ED) Triggers	Readmission to the ED within 48 hours Time in ED >6 hours

Source: From Griffin, F. A., & Resar, R. K. (2009). *IHI global trigger tool for measuring adverse events*. (IHI innovation series white paper, 2nd ed.). Institute for Healthcare Improvement. http://app.ihi.org/webex/gtt/ihiglobaltriggertoolwhitepaper2009.pdf

Human beings are prone to making safety errors because humans have limited capacity in their short-term memory. Safety improves when healthcare providers use strategies to reduce their reliance on memory. A patient with chronic heart failure (CHF) will be at risk if intake and output amounts are not documented at the time they are measured. It is very possible that the undocumented intake and output amounts will not be accurately remembered at the end of a busy shift as human beings have a limited capacity to recall facts and are susceptible to a bias in thinking that can distort remembrance of past events. Unfortunately, this bias in thinking sometimes trips humans up, distorts our thinking, influences our beliefs, and leads to poor decisions and bad judgments.

Another bias in thinking that can lead to a potential safety error may occur when all patient care units have similar infusion pump units without easily readable directions posted right on the infusion pumps. If the nurse has been using a specific type of infusion pump on one unit and then is floated to another unit, the nurse may assume that the new unit has a similar type of infusion pump. The nurse might use this bias in thinking and make a programming

TABLE 10.6 WORK-AROUND EXAMPLES

CORRECT ACTION	WORK-AROUND
Manually enter the information from a medication package into the electronic health record (EHR) when the barcode is wet or unreadable.	Scan an intact package of the medication from the medication drawer but give the patient the medication from the medication package with the unreadable barcode.
Clarify a written order with the physician who wrote the order.	Ask other staff what they think the written order means without contacting the physician.
Use personal protective equipment (PPE) as indicated by the patient's condition.	Enter a patient's room without required PPE for only a minute, not intending to touch anything.
Observe the patient consuming their medications.	Leave medications on the patient's bedside table because the patient is on the telephone.
Use abbreviations sparingly and consistent with the healthcare organization's approved abbreviations list.	Use personally preferred abbreviations when documenting to save time.

error on the unit's different infusion pump. Then, the wrong dose of medication would be delivered to the patient. It is probably impossible to eliminate all human errors in healthcare. However, it is possible and especially important to work to design a just culture of safety that can prevent as many errors as possible before any potential harm caused by errors reaches the patient. Note that some hospitals now purchase the same infusion pumps to be used on all units throughout the hospital to prevent errors when nurses are assigned to work on units other than their own. This is an example of a system-based safety strategy.

Another example of error prevention in a just culture of safety is using white boards to communicate patient information. White boards are communication tools used to display patient assignments, contact information, and critical clinical information. They are placed in patient rooms and include specific patient information that can reduce the risk of errors that occur through misinterpreted or unclear communication between patients, nurses, and physicians.

CASE STUDY

The nurse is administering morning medications. The unit is noisy and busy. Physicians are making rounds with the resident teams, breakfast trays are being delivered, and patients are ringing their call bells. Several physicians walk past the nurse saying medication orders have changed for their patients. The supervisor walks past and reminds the nurse about the mandatory staff training at 10 a.m. The nurse is feeling distracted and rushed.

1. *What can the nurse do now to maintain patient safety during medication administration?*
2. *What actions can the nurse take later to improve the structure of medication administration to ensure an outcome of safe patient medication administration?*
3. *What actions can the nurse take now to improve the process of medication administration to ensure an outcome of safe patient medication administration?*

High Reliability

No matter how careful people are, they may still misperceive, misjudge, or just not recognize errors in judgment and action. To counter this normal human behavior, the nurse and interprofessional team use standardized structures and processes to deliver, with a high degree of reliability, the outcomes of quality patient care. Highly reliable healthcare organizations use standardized evidence-based routines, for example, guidelines, practices, protocols, and tools in areas where patient care variation would be unacceptable, such as in hand hygiene, infection control, and blood transfusions. As a result, safety is promoted, and patient care variation is reduced. Efficiency is increased since evidence-based routines support coordination of the actions needed to be done by each member of the interprofessional team. A highly reliable healthcare organization strives to radically reduce the frequency of negative clinical and nonclinical quality and safety outcomes., for example, hospital-acquired infections, patient and visitors falls, and so on. Situational awareness is required to reduce these negative outcomes and develop complex, dynamic, safety sensitive, and highly reliable healthcare environments. **Situational awareness** occurs when a nurse knows what is happening in the work environment and is ready to help quickly as the nurse is aware of situations that threaten safety. The nurse who practices situational awareness demonstrates high reliability. As a highly reliable healthcare organization matures, the interprofessional healthcare team has more opportunities to participate in robust and innovative process improvements. These process improvements involve more complex issues and use systematic QI initiatives to achieve a fully functioning just culture of safety.

Teamwork

Teamwork, the fourth component of a just culture of safety, must be valued and be evident in healthcare. For safe care to be delivered in today's extraordinarily complex healthcare systems, it is critical for clinicians to collaborate in interprofessional teams of nurses, physicians, pharmacists, dietitians, and others. It is often impossible to safely deliver care, monitor patients, document treatments, and manage changes in the health status of multiple patients while working alone. Interprofessional teams can support each other, identify potential safety hazards, find solutions to patient safety problems, and provide patient care effectively. For good working teams to exist there must be mutual respect, understanding of respective roles, and trust. An attending physician who asks a student nurse to accompany the medical resident team on morning rounds and provide the nursing assessment about the patient is showing respect to the student as part of the healthcare team.

Psychological safety is another aspect of teamwork. Psychological safety means one can speak up about mistakes or ask questions without being afraid of being criticized, ostracized, or punished. Staff members are more likely to report a mistake when they believe they work in a psychologically safe healthcare organization because there is less fear of reprisal for reporting the mistake. Patients are part of the healthcare team and are encouraged to speak up when they have a question about their care. Psychological safety is created for patients when they know who is taking care of them, such as when nurses introduce themselves during change of shift bedside rounds. These shift bedside rounds are an opportunity for patients to know their healthcare teammates by name and face. During the COVID-19 pandemic, infection control safety requirements mandated expanded use of personal protective equipment (PPE) for employees. As a result, faces were not fully visible. One healthcare organization created photograph buttons for all staff, as seen in Figure 10.3, an action which supported psychological safety among patients and staff.

Teamwork requires good communication. A study about perioperative medication errors found that more than three-fourths of the errors were attributable to communication breakdowns in transitions of care, handoffs, medication ordering processes, and lack

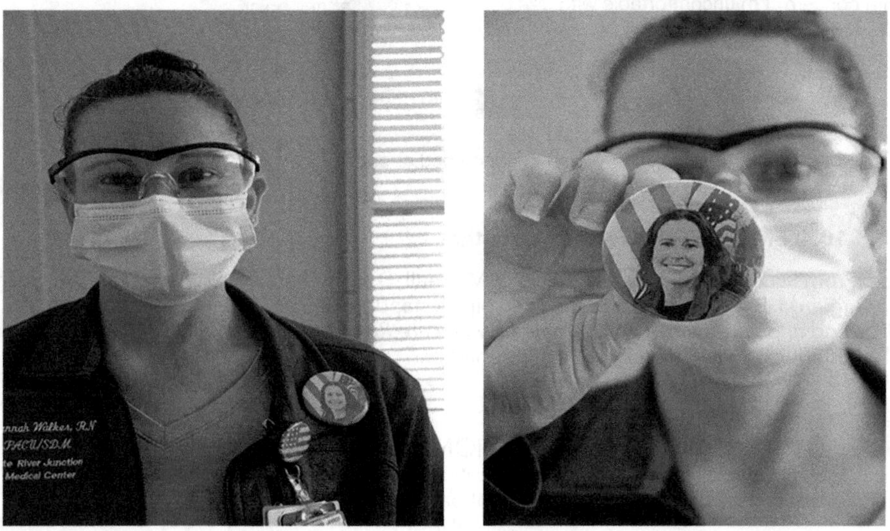

FIGURE 10.3 Wearing a Full-Face Button Supports Psychological Safety of Patients and Nurses.

Source: Photo by Katherine Tang, Public Affairs Officer, White River Junction VA Medical Center, Vermont. Used with permission.

of adequate documentation (Cierniak et al., 2018). Effective team communication quickly resolves clinical concerns and conflicts.

The Effective Followership Algorithm

The Effective Followership Algorithm (Figure 10.4) is a communication tool that directly addresses the ability to immediately challenge authority at a moment in time (Sculli et al., 2015) and can help the nurse act anywhere, at any point, avoiding unclear nursing communication that only "hints" at problems and "hopes" another will understand. Instead, nurses can use specific, direct, clear, and concise communication tools such as the 4-Step Tool in the Effective Followership Algorithm to get attention, state the concern by saying "I'm uncomfortable with . . .," offer a solution, and pose a question.

The 3Ws Method of Communication (Table 10.7) in the Effective Followership Algorithm also clarifies communication. Using the 3Ws Method of Communication, the nurse demonstrates professional and effective **followership** through critical thinking; assertive, respectful communication; and by raising concerns to supervisors. Communications with supervisors, physicians, and others are then more productive.

When professional communication is used, such as with the 3Ws, there is little doubt on the part of any member of the team and the physician what the nurse's concerns are and what the nurse wants to happen to keep the patient safe. If any member of the team chooses to not respond appropriately, the nurse can take action, anywhere, at any step of

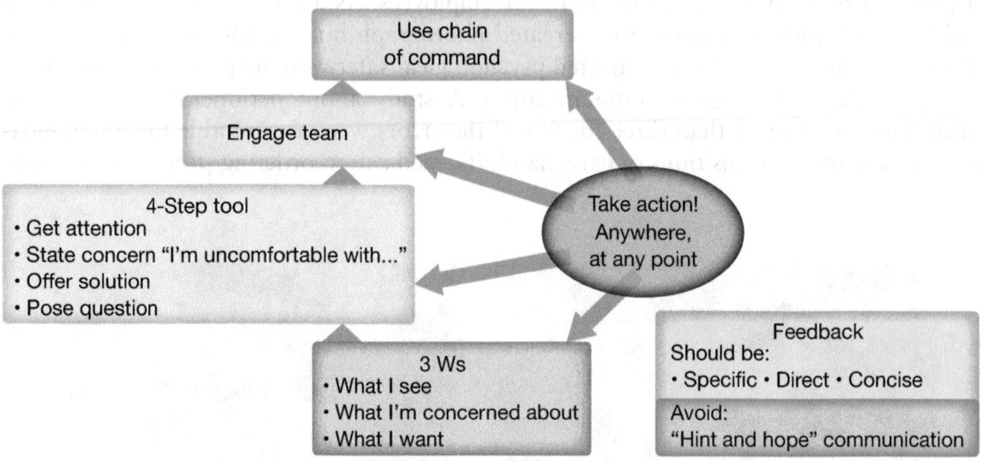

FIGURE 10.4 Effective Followership Algorithm.

Source: From Sculli, G. L., Fore, A. M., Sine, D. M., Paull, D. E., Tschannen, D., Aebersold, M., Seagull, F. J., & Bagian, J. P. (2015). Effective followership: A standardized algorithm to resolve clinical conflicts and improve teamwork. *Journal of Healthcare Risk Management, 35*(1), 21–30. https://doi.org/10.1002/jhrm.21174. Reprinted with permission.

TABLE 10.7 THE 3Ws COMMUNICATION

The nurse contacts a surgeon about a surgical patient and says:	
What I see.	"The patient's blood pressure is 90/50."
What I am concerned about.	"I am concerned that the patient is bleeding internally."
What I want to happen.	"Please come evaluate the patient."

Source: Data from U.S. Department of Veterans Affairs. (n.d.). *Quality, safety & value: Stop the Line for Patient Safety Initiative.* https://www.qualityandsafety.va.gov/stoptheline/stoptheline.asp

the Effective Followership Algorithm (Figure 10.4) to get attention and state the nurse's concern, for example, "I am uncomfortable with." Then the nurse can offer a solution and pose questions. Other steps of the Effective Followship Algorithm engage the rest of the patient's healthcare team, usually by calling for a team conference. The nurse can also use the chainofcommand and elevate any concerns to supervisors. This requires clinical judgment. For example, if the physician is not responding to the nurse's initial communications of concern and the nurse feels the patient's safety is in danger, the nurse can then use the chain of command and contact the supervisor for help in protecting the patient's safety.

Teamwork and improved patient safety can also be fostered through programs such as Team*STEPPS*. See Chapter 7 for more information about Team*STEPPS*.

CURRENT LITERATURE

CITATION

Umberfield, E., Ghaferi, A. A., Krein, S. L., & Manojlovich, M. (2019). Using incident reports to assess communication failures and patient outcomes. *Joint Commission Journal on Quality and Patient Safety, 45*(6),406–413. https://doi.org/10.1016/j.jcjq.2019.02.006

DISCUSSION

Incident reports were examined to identify and describe types of communication failures involving nurses and physicians to determine how these might affect patient outcomes. Breakdowns in the communication process included the absence of necessary communications, poor or unsuccessful information exchanges, misunderstanding about the goal of the communication, not including the right people in the information exchange, and lack of shared understanding about the contents of the communication. Patient outcomes included delays in care, physical harm, and patient dissatisfaction.

IMPLICATIONS FOR PRACTICE

Communication, oral and written, between nurses and physicians is more than an exchange of information. Their communications must be clear, open to questions, and use content that means the same to both nurses and physicians to ensure a safe healthcare environment.

THE ROLE OF UTILIZATION MANAGEMENT IN SUPPORTING A JUST CULTURE OF SAFETY

Utilization management (UM) is a process of hospitalized patient case management using evidence-based and standardized criteria such as InterQual to evaluate a patient's level of care from hospital admission to discharge and determine the safest and most efficient care level based on severity of illness, comorbidities, complications, and the intensity of services being delivered (Change Healthcare, 2020). UM supports a culture of patient safety by promoting shorter patient lengths of stay and reduced patient readmissions to the hospital using evidence-based decisions about patient care delivery. One hospital changed its patient care processes to include UM in daily huddles which helped improve communication between nurses and physicians about patient transfers and discharges. These changes resulted in an overall shortening of patient length of stay in the hospital without increasing the hospital readmission rate (Health Catalyst, 2018). Prolonged hospital stays are associated with a higher frequency of complications and increased risk of hospital-acquired conditions including infections and skin breakdown. When hospitals use UM, the patient receives the healthcare services and supplies that are no more or less than the patient needs at that point in time. Evidence-based criteria are used along with interprofessional team judgment to measure the appropriateness of the patient's level of care. Documentation in the medical records should support why a patient needs to be in the hospital receiving a particular level of care. Documentation of the stability of the patient's vital signs, diagnosis, treatment plan, and interventions help determine if the patient is in the right place receiving the right care to address the patient's care needs.

UM facilitates cooperative teamwork and clear and effective communication among the patient's healthcare providers. For example, an interprofessional UM team caring for a group of medical-surgical patients meets daily to discuss each patient's readiness for discharge or transfer from the hospital. The team reviews and, as necessary, revises each patient's care plan to support each patient's progress toward a timely and appropriate discharge. The nurse caring for the patient contributes information about the patient's pain and symptom management and learning needs. UM reviews standardized diagnosis-specific InterQual UM criteria, such as objective patient and clinical data, imaging studies, and laboratory findings. UM provides the information needed to know if, given a patient's status, the patient could receive healthcare services in a different level of care, such as on a step-down unit or at home.

The UM review helps evaluate whether the service intensity, which is the amount and type of hospital care services provided to the patient, is appropriate for the patient and follows the UM standards. A patient with pneumonia is transferred from an ICU to a medical patient care unit as the patient's breathing improves and the need for hourly respiratory therapy interventions and one-to-one nursing care decreases. This follows physician agreement with evidence-based recommendations made by UM to the patient's healthcare team (Figure 10.5).

The findings from UM reviews are tracked, measured, and shared on a regular, often monthly basis, at executive level QI meetings to help leadership determine if patients are consistently admitted to the most appropriate level of care, transitioned to the most appropriate level of care, and discharged in a timely manner to help prevent patient readmission

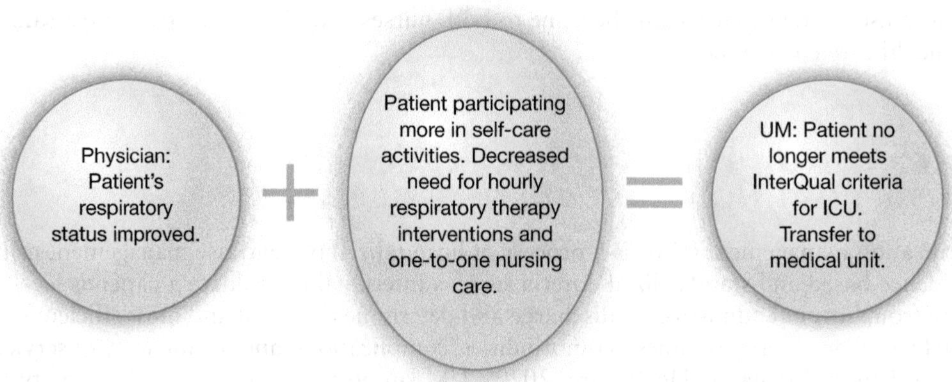

FIGURE 10.5 Utilization Management (UM) Process.

Source: Data from Change Healthcare. (2020). *Interqual®*. https://www.changehealthcare.com/solutions/clinical-decision-support/interqual

TABLE 10.8 EXAMPLES OF NURSING OVERUSE, UNDERUSE, AND MISUSE OF HEALTHCARE SERVICES

	NURSING EXAMPLE	POTENTIAL HARM TO PATIENT
Overuse	Giving a patient frequent PRN medication for pain without evaluating the need for the medication.	Patient is overly sedated.
Underuse	Not using culturally sensitive patient education materials to teach patient about the effects of smoking.	Cardiopulmonary damage continues when patients do not understand the impact of smoking on their bodies.
Misuse	Putting a sphygmomanometer over a patient's clothing rather than on patient's bare skin to take a blood pressure (Ozone et al., 2016).	Inappropriate assessment and treatment for hypertension based on inaccurate blood pressure readings.

to the hospital. UM review data can also help identify overuse, underuse, and misuse of healthcare services. For example, hospital leadership at an acute care hospital approves creation of a substance abuse residential rehabilitation unit after analysis of utilization review data showing that many patients admitted to the medical unit for detoxification are readmitted for another detoxification within 30 days of discharge. This finding is presented to the hospital leadership during an executive leadership QI meeting. Further examination of the UM review data reveals a lack of available residential substance abuse rehabilitation facilities. Leadership also notes the need for more teaching and follow-up pre- and postdischarge of these patients. The UM review data reveals an overuse of hospital admissions for detoxification and helps hospital leadership document the need to improve the provision of the community's healthcare services to people with substance abuse problems.

OVERUSE, UNDERUSE, AND MISUSE OF HEALTHCARE SERVICES

Overuse, underuse, and misuse of healthcare services undermines efficiency and patient safety. **Overuse of healthcare services** occurs when a healthcare service is provided even though it is not justified by the patient's healthcare needs. **Underuse of healthcare services** occurs when a healthcare service is not provided even though it would have benefited the patient. **Misuse of healthcare services** occurs when incorrect diagnoses, medical errors, and avoidable healthcare complications occur. Overuse, underuse, and misuse of healthcare services all have the potential to cause harm or an adverse event to a patient (Table 10.8).

A PERSON APPROACH VERSUS A SYSTEM APPROACH TO PATIENT CARE SAFETY

When an adverse patient care event occurs, it is possible to analyze what happened in different ways, that is, with a person approach to safety and/or with a system approach to safety. Too often in healthcare, we have taken only a **person approach to safety,** in which we blame the person at the end of a long chain of actions for making an error that caused an adverse event from overuse, underuse, or misuse of healthcare services. A **system approach to safety** takes a broader look at an adverse event, reviews the total healthcare system in which the adverse event took place, and considers how to prevent future occurrences through QI of the total healthcare system and not just the person.

In a just culture of safety that uses a system approach to safety, when a nurse gives a wrong dose of a medication to a patient on a specialty unit, a fishbone diagram may be used to do a root cause analysis of the total system of medication administration. The fishbone diagram in Figure 10.6 encourages the healthcare team to consider nurse characteristics, patient characteristics, practice breakdown categories, and system factors as causes of actual or potential harm to a patient in a healthcare system. Nurse characteristics may include how many years one has worked as a nurse, level of education, and years of experience on the unit or in the specialty. Patient characteristics may include patient age, level of cognition and mental status, and patient's willingness to participate in self-care. Practice breakdown categories may include safe medication administration, documentation, attentiveness/surveillance, clinical reasoning, prevention, intervention, interpretation of authorized provider's orders, and professional responsibility/patient advocacy. System factors may include communication, leadership/management, backup and support, environment, other health team members, staffing issues, and the healthcare team.

In a just culture of safety, healthcare leadership fosters both a person approach and a system approach to safety. Sometimes leadership will examine trends from a large group of similar adverse events, such as falls. Data from fall events for a 3- to 6-month period can be combined and reviewed. The fall events are then separated into subsets of patient injury levels, such as falls causing serious injury and falls causing less serious injury. This separation into injury subsets allows differentiation of the causes of each subset of falls, such as time, location, medications, and environmental conditions during the aggregate review of the falls. An aggregate review is a multistep review process in which critical factors from a group of similar adverse events—for example, all falls occurring in a specific period—are analyzed together. Based on this aggregate review, common root causes of the falls are identified, and actions are developed to reduce the causes. The advantage of this aggregate review of falls is that the actions taken to improve care are based on data from

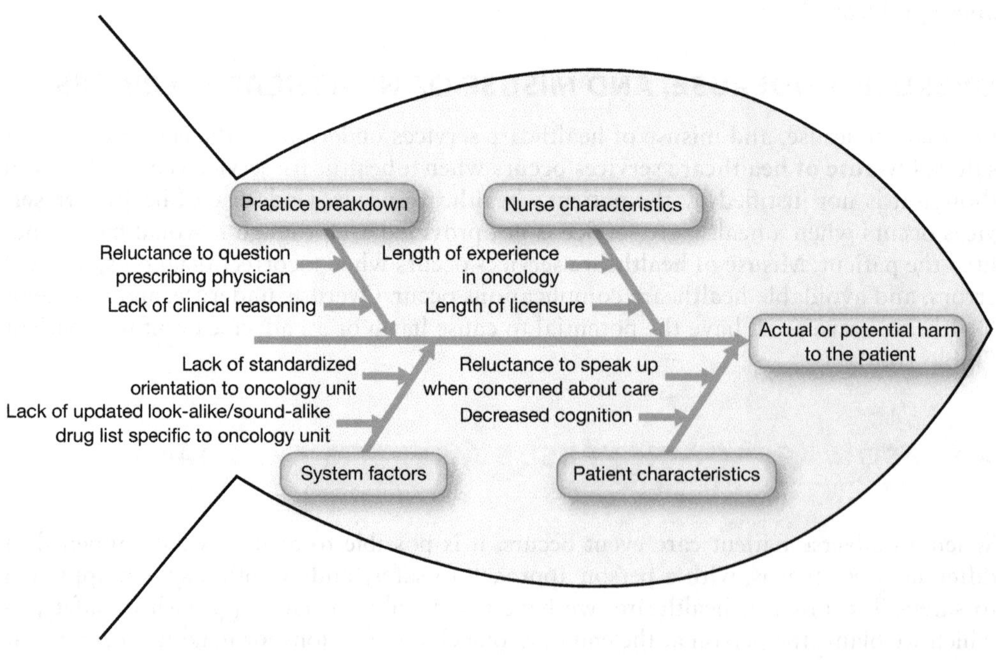

FIGURE 10.6 Use of a Fishbone Diagram to do a Root Cause Analysis of a Medication Administration Error.

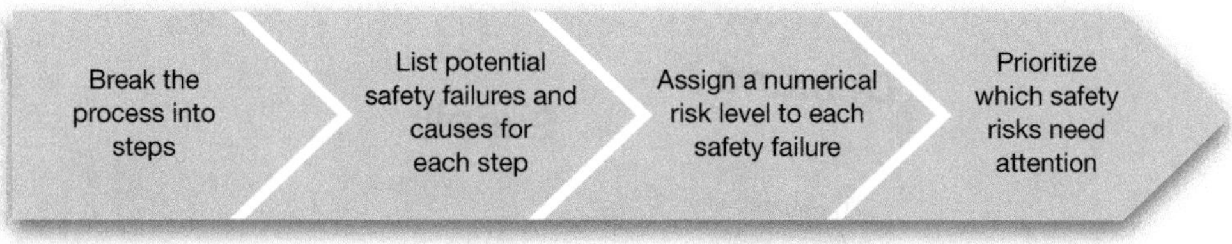

FIGURE 10.7 Healthcare Failure Mode and Effect Assessment (HFMEA) Process.

multiple adverse events and so are more likely to address problems common to many of them to prevent future falls.

Healthcare leadership often partners with risk management to review adverse events through root cause analysis and to use the aggregated data to decrease safety risk by improving performance. **Risk management** is a program that protects the assets of the organization by identifying potential threats or actual harm and seeking to prevent and reduce injury to the organization, patients, and employees. Leadership and risk management also come together to discuss the results and suggested actions from **Healthcare Failure Mode and Effect Assessment (HFMEA)** Figure 10.7. An HFMEA is a proactive step-by-step process that examines activities having a high possibility of a negative outcome, such as infrequent administration of an intravenous (IV) chemotherapeutic medication that can cause extravasation. Using the HFMEA process, leadership, including nurse leaders, and risk management break the IV administration process into steps. Then they list potential causes for the potential failure of each step of the process, assign a numerical risk level to each safety failure, and prioritize which safety risks need attention. Then, leadership, including nurse leaders, and risk management make recommendations about what steps could be taken to improve patient and staff safety.

STRATEGIES THAT REDUCE VARIATION AND STANDARDIZE SAFE PATIENT CARE DELIVERY

Reducing variation or differences in care and standardizing safe patient care delivery contribute to creating a just culture of safety. One way to reduce variation in patient care delivery is to examine differences in healthcare delivery that cannot be explained by illness, medical needs, or evidence-based healthcare. If a nurse's actions do not follow the hospital's evidence-based procedure for urinary catheter care. there is variation in the care provided to the patient. The patient is at risk for a urinary tract infection (UTI) due to the variation in care delivery by the nurse. Another example of variation in care delivery that negatively affects patient safety is when a nurse caring for a patient with reduced mobility feels time is short in the nurse's workday and decides to use a work-around or short cut and vary the evidence-based standards for patient skin care. By choosing a skin care work-around shortcut, the nurse is not providing quality skin care for this patient. This patient is now at increased risk for decubitus ulcer formation.

A nurse who applies restraints to a patient with dementia before using a behavioral intervention is varying patient care from the restraints standard and negatively affecting patient safety as the patient can experience self-harm if the patient tries to get out of the restraints. This is also called preference-sensitive care, that is, the nurse prefers to apply restraints rather than using nonphysical interventions first. Nurses who are culturally competent reduce variation in care. Race, ethnicity, and primary language affect safety outcomes (Chauhan et al., 2020). The nurse at the bedside can reduce disparities in patient safety by effectively delivering healthcare services that meet the social, cultural,

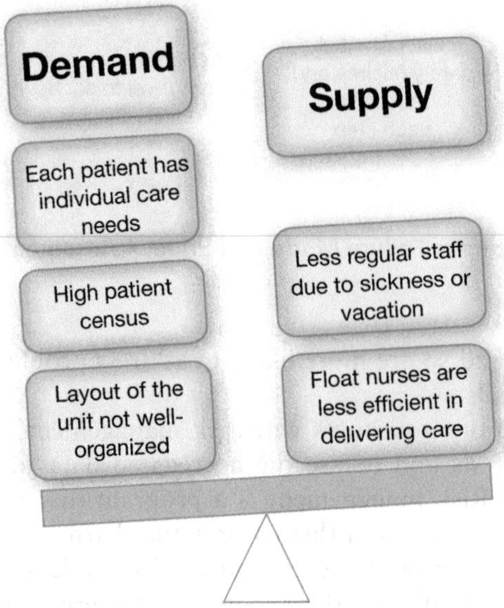

FIGURE 10.8 Increased Demand and Decreased Supply Affecting Delivery of Safe Patient Care.

and linguistic needs of a patient. Lastly, variation in healthcare delivery can be reviewed by examining supply and demand concerns (Figure 10.8). The demand for services is higher when each patient has individual care needs that must be met, there are many patients on the unit, and the unit layout is not organized for efficiency. The supply of skilled staff on the unit is lower when there is sickness or vacation of regular staff and there is increased use of float nurses who are unfamiliar with the unit and who may be less efficient in delivering patient care. Safe patient care delivery is at risk when the demand for patient care is higher than the supply of competent nurses.

When patterns of patient care delivery vary widely, safety is compromised, and patient clinical outcomes suffer. UM, discussed earlier, is one process in a just culture of safety that reduces variation in healthcare delivery by using evidence-based criteria to support appropriate hospital length of stay and minimize HAIs by shortening a patient's exposure to the many microorganisms found in hospitals.

Two other effective ways to reduce variation in patient care delivery are simplification of work processes and standardization of simplified work processes. **Simplification of work processes** is the act of reducing a work process to its basic components and, in so doing, making it easier to complete the work and to understand it. Simplification of work processes requires that only the essential elements of a work process are retained. For example, when the nurse takes a patient's vital signs, the patient's temperature, pulse, and respirations are taken and documented. The nurse then checks the patient's blood pressure reading and asks what level of pain the patient is experiencing on a scale of 1 to 10. Collecting this vital sign data in this format simplifies the work process, decreases the likelihood of variation in the data set of vital signs, and improves the understanding of vital signs among health team members.

Standardization of simplified work processes in an organization facilitates safety, QI, and accurate communication by using a single set of standardized terms, definitions, practices, and/or clinical tools. Clinical tools include bundles, routines, checklists, pathways, protocols, and guidelines to reduce variation in patient care delivery (Table 10.9). Standardization of simplified work processes makes it easier to do the right thing to improve healthcare quality and reduce complications.

TABLE 10.9 STANDARDIZED AND SIMPLIFIED WORK PROCESSES USED IN PATIENT CARE

CLINICAL TOOL	DESCRIPTION	EXAMPLE
Bundle	A small set of simple evidence-based interventions that have been proven to improve patient outcomes	The Hour-1 Bundle reduces the time to treatment and acknowledges the urgency that exists for patients with sepsis and septic shock. Available at www.sccm.org/SurvivingSepsisCampaign/Guidelines/Adult-Patients
Checklist	List of reminders that help reduce healthcare variation by compensating for errors in human memory.	"CHIEF O" is a nurse-driven checklist used to improve the quality, safety, and discharge planning of patients at risk for a catheter-associated urinary tract infection (CAUTI) and/or a central line-associated bloodstream infection (CLABSI). Available at www.myamericannurse.com/wp-content/uploads/2018/11/ant11-Focus-On-PATIENT-SAFETY-1015.pdf
Guideline	Interprofessional evidence-based recommendations for the diagnosis, management, or prevention of specific diseases or conditions that meet the needs of most patients in most circumstances. A guideline is individualized to the patient.	To improve outcomes and reduce the need for renal replacement therapy, use a guideline to prevent, detect and manage acute kidney injury in adults in the hospital with known or suspected COVID-19. Available at www.nice.org.uk/guidance/ng175
Pathway	Evidence-based algorithm or map that recommends clinical management and decision-making based on the patient's status and needs.	Use of National Comprehensive Cancer Network Value Pathways allows collaborating healthcare organizations to quickly adopt the latest drugs and therapies backed by clinical evidence to achieve optimal outcomes for oncology patients. Available at www.ajmc.com/view/clinical-pathways-reducing-costs-and-improving-quality-across-a-network
Protocol	Predetermined steps of care management for a single clinical condition. It can be individualized to a patient's needs.	Use of a nurse-initiated pain protocol in an emergency department reduced patient's pain intensity and increased patient satisfaction while maintaining the safety of patients with musculoskeletal trauma. Available at www.painmanagementnursing.org/article/S1524-9042(18)30515-0/fulltext
Routine	A series of actions that ordinarily is followed in each situation.	Use of mobile devices and virtual technology for routine rounding enables healthcare teams to reduce the need for personal protective equipment during a pandemic and decreases the patient's feelings of isolation. Available at https://healthtechmagazine.net/article/2020/07/virtual-rounding-supports-communication-during-pandemic

ORGANIZATIONS THAT SUSTAIN AND SPREAD HEALTHCARE SAFETY

There are many national and international organizations that sustain and spread safe healthcare outcomes by reducing variation in healthcare practices (Table 10.10). They collect, analyze, disseminate, and share evidence-based best practices. These organizations welcome organizational membership and participation by nurses involved in the development and use of standardized clinical practice tools and strategies.

SAFETY INITIATIVES IN HEALTHCARE

Safety initiatives are programs that use standardized clinical practice tools and strategies and focus on reducing healthcare errors and improving patient safety in selected areas of healthcare (Table 10.11). One area of focus is on high-alert medications which are drugs with a heightened risk of causing devastating patient harm when used in error. The ISMP has lists of high-alert medications for acute care, ambulatory care, and long-term care settings. These high-alert lists identify medications requiring special safeguards, such as standardizing the ordering, storage, preparation, and administration of these medications and using independent double-checks when necessary to reduce the risk of error. An independent double-check requires two nurses to separately check a medication without knowing the results of the other nurse. This independent double-check reduces the risk of confirmation bias that may occur if the same person prepares and checks a medication, as they likely will see only what they expect to see, even if an error has occurred. So, holding up a syringe and a vial and saying, "This is 5 units of insulin, can you check it?" is not effective because the person asking for the double-check is influencing the person checking the product.

Note that manual independent double-checks are not always an optimal error-reduction strategy and may not be practical for all the medications on the list (ISMP, 2019). A few of the medications included on the high-alert list for acute care settings are potassium chloride, insulin, heparin, methotrexate, and magnesium sulfate (ISMP, 2018). Complete lists of high-alert medications are available at https://www.ismp.org/sites/default/files/attachments/2018-08/highAlert2018-Acute-Final.pdf.

TABLE 10.10 ORGANIZATIONS THAT SUSTAIN AND SPREAD HEALTHCARE SAFETY

ORGANIZATION	UNIQUE SAFETY FEATURES
Emergency Care Research Institute (ECRI), www.ecri.org	Shares best practices, guidance, benchmarking, and recommendations about patient safety, evidence-based medicine, and technology decision support.
Guidelines International Network (G-I-N), www.g-i-n.net	Provides the world's largest international guidelines library website.
Joanna Briggs Institute, https://joannabriggs.org	Shares evidence-based information, software, education, and training designed to improve healthcare practice and health outcomes for nursing, healthcare providers, and consumers.
U.S. Department of Veterans Affairs (VA) Department of Defense (DoD) VA/DOD Clinical Practice Guidelines, www.healthquality.va.gov	Shares evidence-based clinical practice guidelines for patient populations, to reduce errors, and provide consistent quality of care and utilization of resources.

TABLE 10.11 A SAMPLING OF HEALTHCARE SAFETY INITIATIVES

INITIATIVE	EXAMPLE AND SPONSORING ORGANIZATION
Medication safety	Read medication labels carefully Institute for Safe Medication Practices (ISMP) www.ismp.org/recommendations/high-alert-medications-acute-list
Safe patient handling	Implement an effective safe patient handling and mobility (SPHM) program and control patient handling of ergonomic risk to reduce harm to patients and staff. American Industrial Hygiene Association (AIHA) Position Statement: Ergonomics https://aiha-assets.sfo2.digitaloceanspaces.com/AIHA/resources/Occupational-Ergonomics-Position-Statement.pdf
Comprehensive Unit-Based Safety Program (CUSP)	Identify recurring negative events in the healthcare system, such as missing equipment on carts, and reduce the risk of future harm to patients using an evidence-based set of tools and strategies for change. Agency for Healthcare and Research and Quality CUSP. Available at www.ahrq.gov/hai/cusp/modules/identify/index.html
Alarm safety	Collect data about baseline Saturation of Peripheral Oxygenation (SpO2) alarm conditions in the unit-care environment to determine which SpO2 alarms (technical versus patient related), in relation to specific patient populations and hospital units, are causing the falsest or nonaction-able alarms. This knowledge helps identify which SpO2 alarm management strategies will work best in a unit. Association for the Advancement of Medical Instrumentation (AAMI). Available at https://www.aami.org/docs/default-source/foundation/alarms/aamifdn_2017_spo2_toolkit.pdf

TJC gathers information yearly about emerging patient safety issues and develops the National Patient Safety Goals (NPSG, 2021). The NPSG includes using at least two patient identifiers when providing care, treatment, or services to improve accurate patient identification, maintaining and communicating accurate patient medication information to improve patient outcomes associated with medications, and using approved protocols and evidence-based practice guidelines for the initiation and maintenance of anticoagulant therapy to reduce patient harm associated with anticoagulants (TJC, 2021).

Safety initiatives are often started by hospital leadership in a just culture of safety. Employees are encouraged to communicate perceived safety issues up and down the power hierarchy of the hospital. This communication can happen with the use of incident reports and during staff meetings with nursing leaders or hospital administration. Using safety stories which focus on avoidance of a negative safety outcome or a change in a healthcare process due to a negative occurrence is another way to raise the awareness of all healthcare staff about safety and encourage a safety initiative. Effective communication among healthcare professionals in the work setting is essential to patient safety.

Avoidance of Workplace Violence

One of the most lethal barriers to effective communication is workplace violence. Workplace violence in healthcare is an important public health issue. Workers in healthcare and social service industries experience the highest rates of injuries caused by workplace violence and are 5 times as likely to suffer a workplace violence injury than workers overall (U.S. Bureau of Labor Statistics, 2020). The terms "workplace violence," "disruptive behavior," and "workplace bullying" are often used interchangeably but they are different (Table 10.12). Workplace violence and disruptive behavior erodes professional behavior and is an obstacle to creating a just culture of safety.

TABLE 10.12 EXAMPLES OF DIFFERENT TYPES OF WORKPLACE VIOLENCE

Workplace violence	Violent acts, such as verbal or physical abuse, sexual assault, and active shooter situations, directed toward persons at work or on duty.
Disruptive behavior	Insults, intimidation, verbal threats, humiliation, sabotage, sexual harassment, unresponsiveness, shouting, sarcasm, exclusion, and intentionally distancing the targeted individual(s).
Workplace bullying	Unwelcome behavior in the workplace meant to harm someone who feels powerless to respond, for example, a staff person or physician purposefully intimidates a newly hired nurse.

Source: Data from American Association of Nurse Anesthetists. (2018). *Promoting a culture of safety and healthy work environment.* https://www.aana.com/docs/default-source/practice-aana-com-web-documents-(all)/promoting-a-culture-of-safety-and-health-work-environment.pdf?sfvrsn=e4fa54b1_2

BOX 10.2 Developing Clinical Judgment

The oncoming nurse is doing bedside rounds with the offgoing nurse. One of the patients is a 57-year-old male admitted for a poorly healing lower extremity wound. The offgoing nurse stops outside the patient's room saying, "He has been nasty all day. Nothing anyone does is right. He smells but refuses to be washed. I just go in, do what I have to do, and get out as fast as I can. I'm glad I'm going home." The oncoming nurse checks the patient's care plan where the only reference to behavior is that the patient is difficult.

1. What **CUES (Assessment)** can the nurse assess?
2. What **HYPOTHESIS (Diagnosis)** will the nurse consider?
3. What **ACTION (Plan and Implement)** will be most effective for the nurse to take to ensure the patient's safety in this situation?
4. How will the nurse evaluate the patient's **OUTCOME (Evaluation)** for the purpose of arriving at a satisfactory clinical outcome?

Workforce bullying refers to both negative behaviors and to the verbal and nonverbal communications that nurses and other interprofessional team members may inflict on each other, such as rolling their eyes, sighing deeply, or turning away every time a team member speaks, not returning phone calls, being reluctant to answer questions, and using a condescending tone of voice. Workforce bullying can go from peer to peer or from supervisor to employee. A new nurse or team member is particularly susceptible to workplace bullying. The new nurse may avoid staff interactions necessary for patient care as a means of avoiding workforce bullying. Sometimes nurses will adopt the behaviors of workforce bullying, seeing it as the "norm" or to survive in the workplace. Many nurses prefer to quit rather than work in a healthcare system tolerant of workforce bullying. Patient safety is in jeopardy when workforce bullying occurs and is allowed to continue. For instance, staffing patterns may be negatively impacted when the number of nurse aides or healthcare technicians is increased because of workplace bullying of nurses and there are fewer nurses available to assign to a unit. Recruitment of new staff may be hard for an organization when team members share their stories about workforce bullying experiences with the healthcare community. Confronting workforce bullying in an organization is difficult, but necessary. Strategies for helping nurses deal with workplace violence are discussed in Chapter 7. The Centers for Disease Control and Prevention's (CDC) free course, Workplace Violence Prevention for Nurses, available at www.cdc.gov/niosh/topics/violence/training_nurses.html, also contains suggestions for creating a healthy and safe work environment.

CASE STUDY

The experienced nurse is working on a medical unit with a new graduate nurse who has a reputation of being forgetful. When approaching the unit station, the experienced nurse overhears a physician and a physical therapist making jokes about the new graduate. The nurse laughs and keeps walking. As the nurse turns a nearby corner, the new graduate is found standing in the corridor, listening.

1. *Is the experienced nurse's behavior consistent with workforce bullying?*
2. *Should the experienced nurse interact with the new graduate right then? If yes, how? If no, why not?*
3. *What can the experienced nurse do to support the new graduate and other colleagues with the same habit of forgetfulness?*

Healthcare Ranking and Information Sources

Healthcare rankings and other information sources for safe, high-quality healthcare are developed by many organizations (Table 10.13).

The healthcare rankings use patient outcome data to measure and compare the safety of different healthcare facilities and organizations, nationally and worldwide. Healthcare rankings provide information on national and international benchmark data. Staff can use the data to focus their efforts and resources and improve safety by reducing risks to

TABLE 10.13 HEALTHCARE RANKINGS AND INFORMATION SOURCES FOR SAFE, HIGH-QUALITY HEALTHCARE

Leap Frog Hospital Safety Grade www.hospitalsafetygrade.org	Types of infections and infection rates
U.S. Centers for Medicare & Medicaid Services www.medicare.gov/hospitalcompare/search.html	Timely and effective care
U.S. News and World Report https://health.usnews.com/best-hospitals/rankings	Performance in clinical specialties such as cancer care
United Health Foundation www.americashealthrankings.org	Reviews outcomes in healthcare for seniors
The Commonwealth Fund www.commonwealthfund.org/publications/issue-briefs/2020/jan/us-health-care-global-perspective-2019	Health outcomes of vulnerable populations
World Health Organization World Health Statistics (who.int)	Reports current health statistics for the WHO member countries
Healthgrades www.healthgrades.com/quality/americas-best-hospitals?filter=top250&year=2021	Identifies America's best hospitals
IBM Watson Health www.ibm.com/watson-health/services/100-top-hospitals	Measures performance of top hospitals.
Health.gov https://health.gov/our-work/health-literacy	Offers evidence-based health literacy and communication tools, practices, and research for health professionals.

patients. For example, if the Leapfrog ranking for Hospital A shows a higher occurrence of HAIs than other similar hospitals, nurses and the interprofessional team can investigate and note that the increase in HAIs is associated with large turnover in staff. They can implement an immediate and aggressive hospital-wide education program about how to reduce HAIs and prevent the transmission of communicable diseases between patients and healthcare workers.

Disparity in Safety Outcomes

Comparisons of healthcare outcomes take on different meanings when reviewed with regional, ethnic, and racial variations. It is important to recognize how the comparison information applies to the nurse's practice setting and patient population. The nurse learns the details that describe the particular patient population and healthcare work setting. This information can be obtained from websites such as the American Hospital Directory, (www.ahd.com) and Kaiser Family Foundation (www.kff.org/statedata). These websites provide information on the demographics of patient populations and whether these demographics are like other healthcare settings in the region.

Race, ethnicity, and primary language affect safety outcomes (Chauhan et al., 2020). The nurse at the bedside can reduce disparities in patient safety through culture proficiency. **Culture proficiency** is the ability to effectively deliver healthcare services that meet the social, cultural, and linguistic needs of a patient. This is accomplished through showing respect for the patient's cultural beliefs and values, and then responding to the whole individual's health requirements and preferences. The nurse can ask questions such as how to pronounce someone's name or how the patient would prefer to receive information, perhaps in their own language. Nurses who are culturally proficient reduce variation in care and increase patient safety. The U.S. Department of Health and Human Services has published the National Standards for Culturally and Linguistically Appropriate Services in Health and Health Care, accessible at https://thinkculturalhealth.hhs.gov/assets/pdfs/EnhancedNationalCLASStandards.pdf to provide safe, effective, equitable, understandable, and respectful quality care and services that are responsive to diverse cultural health beliefs and practices, preferred languages, health literacy, and other communication needs.

Safe Nurse Staffing

Safe nurse staffing is significantly associated with better patient care and lower mortality (Aiken et al., 2018). Nurse staffing plans are guidelines that identify the number of nurses needed to provide safe and adequate care in each healthcare setting. Fourteen states have enacted legislation or adopted regulations about nurse-to-patient ratios as of September 2015, and 16 states have enacted legislation to restrict mandatory overtime for nurses (AHRQ, 2021, https://psnet.ahrq.gov/primer/nursing-and-patient-safety). The only state to enact specific patient-to-nurse staffing ratios is California (Table 10.14). Federal legislation, H.R.2581—Nurse Staffing Standards for Hospital Patient Safety and Quality Care Act of 2019, accessible at www.congress.gov/bill/116th-congress/house-bill/2581/text, was introduced during the 2019–2020 U.S. congressional session but was not acted upon.

Nurse staffing plans are associated with patient acuity measurements. **Patient acuity** refers to the degree of healthcare service complexity needed by a patient related to their physical or mental status.

Note that patient acuity is higher for a patient who has a central line infusion than for a patient who is receiving oral medications, as the higher acuity patient with a central line infusion will need more nursing resources to provide safe care. Likewise, patients in an ICU with higher acuity need more clinical attention than patients on a telemetry unit due to the instability of their conditions. Thus, a patient care unit with high patient acuity

TABLE 10.14 PATIENT ACUITY AND NURSE STAFFING RATIOS

UNIT TYPE	TYPE OF PATIENTS	NURSE-TO-PATIENT STAFFING RATIO
Medical-surgical unit	Patients who require less care than that available in intensive care units (ICUs), step-down units, or telemetry units and receive 24-hour inpatient general medical services, postsurgical services, or both general medical and postsurgical services.	1:5 or fewer
Telemetry unit	Patients who require more care than patients in medical-surgical units and have, or are suspected of having, a cardiac condition or a disease requiring the electronic monitoring, recording, retrieval, and display of cardiac electrical signals.	1:4 or fewer
ICU	Patients who require intensive care and need medical technology to aid, support, or replace a vital function of the body that has been seriously damaged and needs specialized equipment and/or personnel providing for invasive monitoring, telemetry, or mechanical ventilation for the immediate repair or cure of a patient's severe pathology.	1:2 or fewer

Source: Data from California Code of Regulations (22CCR, 70217). (2020). https://govt.westlaw.com/calregs/Document/I8612C410941F11E29091E6B951DDF6CE?contextData=%28sc.Default%29&transitionType=Default#:~:text=(11)%20The%20licensed%20nurse%2D,or%20fewer%20at%20all%20times

such as in an ICU will require more nursing staff to provide safe care. The lower acuity telemetry patient care unit requires less staffing.

The Nursing Hours Per Patient Day (NHPPD) calculation, used worldwide, is one of the National Database of Nursing Quality Indicators (NDNQI). The NDNQI computes nurse staffing, that is, RN and/or licensed practical nurse (LPN) staffing. The NHPPD calculation provides a measurement to compare to the desired patient acuity guidelines in the nurse staffing plan. NHPPD indicates the minimum number of nurses required for safe staffing based on patient need rather than patient volume. To calculate the NHPPD, multiply the hours worked by each nurse by the number of nurses to equal total nursing hours. Divide the total nursing hours by the number of patients. The result is the nursing hours needed to care for each patient each day on the unit. For instance, 14 nurses worked on Friday on a same-day procedure unit. All nurses worked an 8-hour shift to staff the 35-bed unit that is open 12 hours daily. The unit cared for 40 patients on Friday. The number of NHPPD is 2.8 hours. To calculate the NHPPD, multiply the hours worked by each nurse by the number of nurses (8 multiplied by 14 equals 112 total nursing hours). Divide the total nursing hours by the number of patients cared for (112 divided by 40 equals 2.8 NHPPD). Neither the number of beds on the unit nor the 12 hours that the same-day unit is open are used in the calculation.

NHPPD staffing calculation can provide retrospective information for an aggregate analysis of adverse events, for example, to determine if a relationship exists between the number of patient falls during a shift and the NHPPD. If the number of patient falls increases when nursing staffing is low, this is an unsafe situation. Nurses need to take action to provide safe care for patients. Nurses can bring concerns about unsafe nurse–patient ratios to nursing and hospital leadership. Another importance of NHPPD is that it allows for comparison across hospitals. A larger comparison of data encourages collaboration between healthcare facilities and helps to justify the safety benefits of appropriate nurse staffing more strongly.

Having more nurses does not guarantee better outcomes. However, higher proportions of nurses with baccalaureate degrees in acute care hospitals are associated with lower rates of mortality and failure to rescue (Audet et al., 2018). **Failure to rescue** occurs when clinicians fail to notice patient symptoms, or they fail to respond adequately or quickly enough to clinical signs that may indicate that a patient is dying of preventable complications in a hospital. Leadership commitment to safe nurse staffing levels and effective nurse retention strategies such as zero tolerance for workforce violence may also influence the achievement of better and safer patient outcomes due to the stability of clinical staff.

CASE STUDY

The nurse is assigned a 79-year-old female patient who was admitted to the unit after experiencing a cerebrovascular accident. The patient has limited mobility in bed and prefers a supine position. Previously assigned nurses had done skin assessments every shift and documented that the patient's skin was intact, warm, and dry. One nurse documented that the sacral skin was slightly darker and harder than the surrounding skin but did not address this in the care plan.

1. *What safety precautions should the nurse take to prevent the patient from developing skin breakdown?*
2. *What other actions by the interprofessional team will keep the patient safe?*
3. *Align the answers from the previous questions with the behaviors seen in a just culture of safety in healthcare (refer to Table 10.2).*

Nurses With Impairing Conditions

Nurses with impairing conditions are unable to meet the requirements of the Code of Ethics (American Nurses Association, 2015a) and Scope and Standards of Practice (American Nurses Association, 2015b) of the profession. **Impairing conditions** are substance use disorders, psychiatric conditions, and physical conditions that can impact a nurse's ability to practice safely. Employers refer nurses with impairing conditions to state boards of nursing when they have a concern about a nurse's ability to practice safely. Most state boards of nursing have alternatives-to-discipline programs, such as Florida's Intervention Project for Nurses, available at www.ipnfl.org. An alternatives-to-discipline program ensures patient safety by promoting early identification of nurses with impairing conditions and requiring evidence-based interventions such as comprehensive monitoring and support services. The benefits to the nurse include the opportunity to demonstrate to the board of nursing in a nondisciplinary and nonpublic manner that the nurse can become safe and remain safe while retaining their nursing license.

Hand Hygiene

Another risk reduction strategy in a just culture of safety is a focus on hand hygiene. Hand hygiene is the single most effective way to prevent the spread of HAIs. Hand hygiene is well suited for prospective quality reviews of available hand sanitizer resources and retrospective quality reviews, such as looking at data about HAI rates. Although the CDC (2019) and the World Health Organization (WHO, 2009) issued guidelines for

BOX 10.3 Developing Clinical Judgment

The nurse is working a weekend evening shift on a medical unit. While the nurse is passing medications, one of the patients, an obese patient who is unsteady on his feet, wants to get out of bed and sit in the bedside chair. The patient has been instructed to ask for help when transferring and there is a bed alarm on the bed. The chair is right next to the bed. The nurse assists the patient into a sitting position on the edge of the bed. The nurse's cell phone starts to vibrate, indicating a call. The nurse turns away to answer the cell phone, telling the patient to stay right where he is. The patient does not respond. He stands suddenly, reaching for the arm of the chair. The bed alarm sounds. The nurse looks over, moves quickly, and tries to stop the patient. The patient falls to the floor, and so does the nurse. The fall results in a broken hip for the patient and a broken wrist for the nurse.

1. What **CUES (Assessment)** should the nurse have assessed to support the patient's safety?
2. What **HYPOTHESIS (Diagnosis)** should the nurse have considered to support the patient's safety?
3. What **ACTION (Plan and Implement)** would have been most effective for the nurse to take to assure the patient's safety in this situation?
4. How could the nurse have evaluated the patient's **OUTCOME (Evaluation)** to support this patient's safety?

hand hygiene that include having the patient remind all healthcare providers to wash their hands, the compliance of healthcare providers with hand hygiene protocols is frequently low. Healthcare staff may sometimes think that a certain type of physical contact with patients is less likely to require handwashing, such as checking blood pressure or straightening bed linens. Staff members are often reluctant to correct or remind coworkers to wash their hands. Reminders to a coworker about handwashing include saying, "Do you want to use the sink before I do to wash your hands?" or "Do you need hand sanitizer? I have a bottle right here." When done with tact and a professional demeanor, communication from one healthcare provider to another about hand hygiene is not only appropriate but can also be effective in improving hand hygiene compliance.

Suicide Prevention

Suicide remains the 10th-leading cause of death for all age groups in the United States (Heron, 2019). Suicide rates increased by more than 30% in 25 states from 1999 to 2016. Nearly 90% of counties in the United States had an increase greater than 20% from 2005 to 2015 (Steelesmith et al., 2019). In response, TJC re-evaluated the National Patient Safety Goals for suicide prevention and implemented new and revised goals considering current evidence-based practices relative to suicide prevention (TJC, 2019). Suicide prevention involves prospective and retrospective risk identification and risk reduction for individual patients and high-risk populations (Box 10.4).

It is likely that nurses in all areas of the hospital will encounter suicidal patients. Nurses need to understand how to care for these patients and how to avoid an inpatient suicide. Recommendations for treating people with suicide risk in primary care, inpatient units, EDs, outpatient behavioral health clinics, and mental health units include patient screening; safety planning; means-to-harm reduction, such as removing belts and ensuring that patients are swallowing administered medications; and follow-up mental healthcare (National Action Alliance for Suicide, 2018).

BOX 10.4 Risk Factors and Risk Reduction for Suicide

Poor prognosis
Social stressors
Suicidal thoughts
Mental health diagnosis
Physical health problems
Previous suicide attempts
Veterans and military personnel
Experience of violence including child abuse, bullying, or sexual violence
Non-Hispanic American Indian/Alaska Native and Non-Hispanic White populations
Sexual minority youth (youth who identify as lesbian, gay, or bisexual (LGB), who are not sure of their sexual identity, or who have any same-sex partners

Source: Data from Centers for Disease Control and Prevention. (2018). *Preventing suicide fact sheet.* https://www.cdc.gov/violenceprevention/pdf/suicide-factsheet.pdf; Centers for Disease Control and Prevention. (n.d.). Hand hygiene in healthcare settings. https://www.cdc.gov/handhygiene; Centers for Disease Control and Prevention. (n.d.). *Health disparities among LGBTQ youth.* https://www.cdc.gov/healthyyouth/disparities/health-disparities-among-lgbtq-youth.htm

When working with a patient whom the nurse thinks is suicidal, the nurse should ask if the patient is thinking about hurting themself or committing suicide. The nurse's priority with this patient is to assure that the patient does not have access to sharps, ropes, medications, or other means of self-harm and that the patient is under continuous observation until the patient can be moved to a safe environment. Suicide prevention includes removing clothes hooks and unnecessary doors from a psychiatric unit and patient rooms since these could be used for a suicide by hanging. In the meantime, the nurse should notify the patient's provider or the psychiatry department per the facility's protocol so that a more thorough patient evaluation can be done. Most often, suicidal patients are only feeling suicidal for a short period of time. It may be a moment of desperation when they are feeling hopeless about the future or devastated by recent losses or overwhelming social stressors. The job for nurses is to get these patients through this time without allowing the patients to hurt or kill themselves.

Environmental Safety

A safe healthcare environment minimizes potential errors and maximizes safe healthcare practice. Nursing care units must be accommodating to patient needs. Door alarms alert staff when a patient goes through a door on a healthcare unit that has cognitively impaired inpatients. Pressure-sensitive bed and chair alarms alert staff to patient movement and facilitate interventions to prevent falls when a patient does not call for transfer assistance. A safe healthcare environment controls noise and keeps distractions to a minimum so that staff can focus on patient care. Nurses must be aware of "accidents waiting to happen." If there is an uneven surface in the floor, nurses can report that problem, so a patient does not trip and fall. The nurse must speak up. The nurse's perspective is important. Reporting unsafe situations can help change a healthcare system and prevent future adverse events.

SAFETY FOR HEALTHCARE STAFF

Safety is an important concern for healthcare staff as well as patients. Healthcare staff face serious safety threats, including blood-borne pathogens and biological hazards, potential chemical and drug exposures, respiratory hazards, ergonomic hazards from lifting and

BOX 10.5 Developing Clinical Judgment

During change of shift bedside assessment, the oncoming nurse sees that the trachea of a patient, who is postop carotid endarterectomy, is not midline, and the patient is drooling. The offgoing nurse states the dressing was not removed to evaluate the site as, "We are not supposed to." The oncoming nurse removes the dressing and sees a hematoma along with a shift of the patient's trachea.

1. What **CUES (Assessment)** can the nurse assess?
2. What **HYPOTHESIS (Diagnosis)** will the nurse consider?
3. What **ACTION (Plan and Implement)** will be most effective for the nurse to take to assure the patient's safety in this situation?
4. How will the nurse evaluate the patient's **OUTCOME (Evaluation)** for the purpose of arriving at a satisfactory clinical outcome?

repetitive tasks, laser hazards, and workplace violence. Other hazards are associated with laboratories, radioactive material, and exposure to anesthetic gases. The total number of work-related injuries and illness reported by hospitals in 2018 was 39% of the total number reported by all industries including private, state, and local government (United States Bureau of Labor Statistics, 2018).

Safety Risks for Nurses

Historically, nurses experience some of the highest injury and illness rates in the healthcare and social assistance employment sector. Nurses spend time walking, bending, stretching, and standing; lifting and moving patients; and encountering potentially harmful and hazardous substances, including drugs, diseases, radiation, accidental needlesticks, and chemicals used for cleaning (Table 10.15). In 2016, 74.1% of all reported injuries and illnesses experienced by RNs occurred in a hospital setting (United States Bureau of Labor Statistics, 2018). Nearly half of the cases were due to overexertion and bodily reaction to motions like lifting, bending, or reaching related to moving or transferring patients who have limited mobility.

Safe Patient Handling

Safe patient handling requires that healthcare facilities and nurses use principles of ergonomics as many patient care activities put nurses at high risk for physical injury and involve lifting, moving, or positioning patients and equipment. Unsafe patient handling and mobility activity is one of the most frequent causes of injuries to nurses and healthcare staff (Dressner & Kissinger, 2018). Ergonomics is the scientific study of the relationship between work being performed (occupation/job), the physical environment where the work is performed (workplace), and the tools (equipment) used to help perform the work (Cohen et al., 2010). Areas that should be addressed in a facility's safety and health program (to address ergonomic needs) include leadership by management, employee participation, analysis of the workplace through hazard identification, assessment, prevention and control, performance improvement, and training.

The consequences of work-related nursing musculoskeletal injuries, that is, chronic pain, functional disability, absenteeism, and high turnover, are substantial. Costs associated with back injuries in the healthcare industry are estimated to be $20 billion annually (Occupational Safety and Health Administration [OSHA], 2020). As many as 20% of nurses who leave direct patient care positions do so because of risks associated with the work (OSHA, 2020). Nurses and other healthcare employees who experience pain and

TABLE 10.15 INCIDENCE RATES OF OCCUPATIONAL HAZARDS IN NURSING

OCCUPATIONAL HAZARDS	INCIDENT RATES BASED ON REPORTED CASES	PREVENTION STRATEGIES
Blood and Body Fluid Exposure (includes exposure via respirations, vomit, peritoneal, urine, etc.)	Nurses account for 55% of all hospital workers exposed. The International Council of Nurses confirms that as of October 28, 2020, 1,500 nurses have died from COVID-19 in 44 countries and estimates that healthcare worker COVID-19 fatalities worldwide could be more than 20,000, as of October 28, 2020.	Wear all appropriate personal protective equipment (PPE), that is, gown, gloves, eye protection, and respirator, including goggles or face shields, while performing procedures. Participate in annual TB test assessment. Accept hepatitis B vaccine and COVID-19 vaccine. Volunteer to serve as nursing representative on hospital PPE supply committee.
Musculoskeletal disorders (MSD) and back injuries	Accounts for 44.1% of all RN injury cases reported; back injuries account for 51.8% of all musculoskeletal disorder cases reported.	Use appropriate body mechanics and the correct equipment and help when lifting, transferring, repositioning, and ambulating patients.
Needlestick	Nurses account for 27% of all hospital workers who experience needlestick.	Do not put used needles in an overfilled collection container. Do not recap needles after use.
Workplace violence	Workplace violence caused 12% of all injuries to nurses.	Use conflict management techniques, such as confronting the issue and problem-solving with supervisors and others to deal with inappropriate communications and behavior.
Substance misuse, abuse, and addiction	10% of nurses misuse drugs or alcohol during the course of their career.	Maintain a healthy lifestyle, use stress-reducing strategies, and ask for help.

*Nursing occurrence percentages do not add up to 100% as chart is a sampling of reported occupational hazards from multiple sources.

fatigue may be less productive, less attentive, more susceptible to further injury, and may be more likely to affect the safety of others (OSHA, 2020).

A safe healthcare environment reduces the risk of harm to patients and staff by using assistive patient handling equipment that helps lift, transfer, and reposition patients to reduce the potential for musculoskeletal injuries. Leadership support and staff participation in ergonomic training in using the correct patient handling equipment, such as ceiling-mounted patient lifts, along with patient assessment protocols, have been identified as being effective in reducing harm to patients and staff.

A safe healthcare environment encourages the use of good body mechanics and does handling and mobility patient assessments to determine the safest way to lift and move each individual patient. OSHA has identified some facts about safe patient handling (Box 10.6).

Safety Leadership by Nurses in a Pandemic

Nurses are often found on the frontline in disaster preparedness and management. Many nurses demonstrated safety leadership as they delivered nursing care during the COVID-19 pandemic despite the risk of potential infection and the emotional impact of fearing for themselves and their families (Table 10.16). Healthcare organizations, government agencies, and nursing organizations support safety during pandemics by ensuring adequate staffing, availability of appropriate and sufficient resources such as PPE, providing timely

BOX 10.6 Safe Patient Handling

There is no such thing as safe manual lifting of a patient. Do not rely on only "proper" body mechanics (including use of back belts) to reduce injuries.

Mechanical lifts are safer for both patients and healthcare workers and they reduce injuries to workers and lower costs.

Manual lifting can cause micro-injuries to the spine. and should be limited to 35 pounds or less.

Cumulative micro-injuries to the spine can result in a debilitating spine injury.

If patient handling equipment is located conveniently, accessing it will not take a long time.

It is often more time-consuming to round up a team of workers to manually lift a patient than to get safe patient handling equipment.

Good health and strength may put workers at increased risk because their peers are much more likely to seek their assistance when manually lifting patients.

Source: Data from Occupational Safety and Health Administration (2020).

TABLE 10.16 SAFETY LEADERSHIP BY NURSES IN A PANDEMIC

Caregiving	Providing safe, timely, effective, efficient, equitable, and patient-centered care despite rapidly changing information Redesigning care and staffing models to care for large groups of patients Providing accurate screening information, confinement guidelines, and triage protocols to patients and staff based on the latest guidance
Creativity and Adaptability	Collaboration with interprofessional colleagues to develop alternatives when ICU beds and personal protective equipment (PPE) supplies are low. Working with hospital/nursing/community leadership to assure access to adequate PPE supplies and maintain personal safety and safety for patients, staff, family, friends, and the community. Developing crash courses on critical care COVID nursing for appropriately trained staff to care for the large numbers of critically ill patients
Leadership	Adapting quickly to changes due to high patient turnover and limited isolation rooms Developing policies for quick recognition of diseases in community Providing accurate information to patients and staff regarding the pandemic and dispelling myths Offering screening information, confinement guidelines, and triage protocols based on the latest guidance Serving as hospital board member and member of various hospital and community committees to assure adequate PPE supplies Supporting nurses, right to reimbursement, psychological counseling, and therapeutic care if they are diagnosed with illness through contact at work Encouraging the International Council of Nursing (ICN), World Health Organization (WHO) Dept. of Pandemic and Epidemic Diseases, the U.S. Department of Health and Human Services Office of Pandemic and Emerging Threats, the U.S. Centers for Disease Control and Prevention (CDC), and national nurse leaders to build an in-country community health worker-to-clinic nurse-to-physician/lab technologist network (Corless et al., 2018).
Collegiality	Encouraging a team spirit and willingly working together

TABLE 10.17 SAFETY AND RISK REDUCTION FOR HEALTHCARE STAFF AND PATIENTS

RISK CATEGORY	RISK EXAMPLES	RISK REDUCTION EXAMPLE
Biological	Drug-resistant pathogens	Change gloves and wash hands, especially after contact with body fluids, and even between procedures on the same patient to prevent cross contamination to different body sites.
	COVID-19 pathogen	Get vaccine. Follow all safety precautions.
Chemical	Powdered latex gloves	Use nonpowdered alternative gloves that do not carry any of the risks associated with glove powder, such as skin irritation, called irritant contact dermatitis.
Physical	Slips, trips, and falls	Clean spills promptly.
Ergonomic	Computer usage and prolonged sitting	Request ergonomic evaluation and workplace accommodation.
Psychological	Shift work and circadian rhythms	Allow sufficient time off to catch up on sleep deficit after working night shift.

and clear information about nursing care, and responding quickly to provide services to support the physical and emotional needs of healthcare workers (Fernandez et al., 2020).

Developing a just culture of safety and risk reduction for healthcare staff as well as for patients is an important consideration in healthcare organizations today (Table 10.17).

CURRENT LITERATURE

CITATION

Hughes, M. M., Groenewold, M. R., Lessem, S. E., Xu, K., Ussery, E. N., Wiegand, R. E., Qin, X., Do, T., Thomas, D., Stella Tsai, S., Davidson, A., Latash, J., Eckel, S., Collins, J., Mojisola Ojo, M., McHugh, L., Li, W., Chen, J., Chan, J., . . . Stuckey, M. J. (2020). Update: Characteristics of health care personnel with COVID-19—United States, February 12–July 16 2020. *Morbidity and Mortality Weekly Report, 69*, 1364–1368. https://doi.org/10.15585/mmwr.mm6938a3

DISCUSSION

As of July 16, 2020, over ten thousand cases of COVID-19 in healthcare personnel (HCP) and 641 deaths among HCP have been reported to the CDC. HCP are essential workers at risk for exposure to patients or infectious materials. Risk to HCP can also occur through exposure to coworkers, household members, or persons in the community. Nurses are the most frequently identified single occupation type, and nursing home/assisted living and residential care facilities are the most common job setting.

IMPLICATIONS FOR PRACTICE

Safety practices such as assuring training and access to PPE and practices such as screening healthcare providers for illness before workplace entry, good hand hygiene, universal use of face masks at work and in the community, observing social distancing, and providing nonpunitive sick leave options are important to protect HCPs and patients.

END-OF-CHAPTER RESOURCES

KEY CONCEPTS

- Safety minimizes the risk of harm to patients through system effectiveness and individual performance.
- Quality structures, processes, and the monitoring of outcomes contribute to a safe healthcare environment.
- A just culture of safety has five necessary components: leadership, measurement, risk identification and reduction, high reliability, and teamwork.
- Utilization management facilitates patient safety and teamwork.
- Overuse, underuse, and misuse of healthcare services increases the incidence of patient harm.
- A just culture of safety is strengthened by a system approach to analysis of adverse events and work processes.
- A just culture of safety reduces variation and standardizes the provision of safe patient care.
- Several national and international organizations sustain and spread healthcare safety by sharing evidence-based best practices.
- A just culture of safety improves patient care by implementing safety initiatives and programs, such as prevention of workforce violence, safe staffing, medication safety, programs for nurses with impairing conditions, use of hand hygiene, safe patient handling and mobility (SPHM), suicide prevention, and environmental safety.
- Developing a just culture of safety for staff as well as for patients is an important consideration in healthcare organizations today.
- Healthcare ranking sources help identify safe, high-quality healthcare agencies

CRITICAL DISCUSSION POINTS

1. During a prior clinical rotation, what safety precautions for patients, staff, and others were visible? What were the clinical safety precautions in the medical records, or near patient beds? What nonclinical safety alerts were evident?
2. Think about prior clinical rotations. Which location felt the most comfortable? What aspects of structure, process and outcomes related to patient and staff safety influenced that feeling of comfort?
3. How can a nurse at the bedside develop the ability to have productive conversations with supervisors and physicians about safety concerns?
4. When would the nurse change a standardized clinical process to meet a patient's individual healthcare needs and support safe outcomes? How would the nurse justify the change? Would the nurse need permission to do this? If so, from who? How would the nurse communicate the change to the interprofessional team?
5. During prior clinical rotations, what indicated that nursing behaviors were safe patient care practices rather than work-arounds that had become the healthcare organization's "cultural norm"?

KEY TERMS

> Adverse event
> Culture proficiency
> Failure to rescue
> Followership
> Healthcare Failure Mode and Effect Analysis (HFMEA)
> High-reliability organizations
> Impairing conditions
> Just culture of safety
> Misuse of healthcare services
> Overuse of healthcare services
> Patient acuity
> Person approach to safety
> Psychological safety
> Risk adjustment
> Risk management
> Safety
> Safety initiatives
> Simplification of work processes
> Situational awareness
> Standardization of simplified work processes
> System approach to safety
> Underuse of healthcare services
> Utilization management
> Work-arounds
> Workforce bullying

REVIEW QUESTIONS

Answers to Review Questions appear in the Instructor's Manual. Qualified instructors should request the Instructor's Manual from textbook@springerpub.com.

1. During a staff meeting, the nurse manager says the rate of patient falls has increased. Which of the following would help identify potential reasons for the increase? *Select all that apply.*
   A. Fishbone diagram
   B. Healthcare mode failure and effect assessment
   C. Aggregate root cause analysis
   D. Comparison and analysis of staffing and falls
   E. Staff re-education for nurses on all shifts
2. A patient is being treated for a late-stage lung cancer. The patient says to the nurse, "I don't think I would do it but sometimes, like now, I think about ways to kill myself." Of the following, which should be the nurse's priority safety action?
   A. Contact the hospital's psychiatry service.
   B. Remove the patient's access to means of self-harm.
   C. Keep the patient under continuous observation.
   D. Alert other staff members about the patient's statement.

3. The nurse overrode the hospital's electronic prescribing cabinets, which allowed a search for medicines by name through a computer system. Instead of selecting the prescribed medication, the nurse selected and administered the first medication having the prescribed medication's first two letters. The patient died. This is classified as which of the following?
   A. Deliberate error
   B. Close call
   C. Adverse event
   D. Biased action
4. A nurse makes a serious medication error and realizes it when the patient experiences an adverse reaction. The hospital has a just culture. Which of the following would be the nurse's first most appropriate safety action?
   A. Deny any knowledge of change in the patient's condition.
   B. Create a fishbone diagram about the reasons for the error.
   C. Report the error to the supervisor and the patient's physician.
   D. Report the error to the healthcare organization's risk manager.
5. During the medication administration process, a nurse notices an alert about a potentially dangerous drug interaction for a patient who has been hospitalized and taking the medication for a week. What is the nurse's safest action?
   A. Override the alert on the electronic medication administration system.
   B. Check with the pharmacy about the alert before giving the medication.
   C. Call the physician and ask for a clarification of the medication order.
   D. Administer the medication since the patient has probably been receiving it for a week.
6. The nurse assesses a patient who had abdominal surgery 2 days ago. The patient's pulse is elevated, and the blood pressure is lower. The patient is pale. Which action should the nurse take first to ensure the patient's safety?
   A. Call the rapid response team.
   B. Ask another nurse to assess the patient.
   C. Bring the code cart into the patient's room.
   D. Continue to assess the patient.
7. The nurse is caring for a mobile patient who is recovering from injuries sustained in a car accident. The patient also has hypotension. Which of the following would create a safe environment for this patient? *Select all that apply.*
   A. Skid-resistant floor mat
   B. Ceiling-mounted transfer equipment
   C. Bed and chair alarms
   D. Raised side rails
   E. Bright lighting in the patient's room

8. The nurse is starting a shift on the medical-surgery unit. The nurse sees Mr. Jones wrapping the call light cord around his neck and attempting to hang on it. The nurse intervenes and unwraps the cord. Mr. Jones says: "I don't want to live anymore with this cancer." Which one of the following is the nurse's most appropriate next step?
   A. Leave the room remembering to make a note of the incident.
   B. Reassure Mr. Jones that his cancer is not yet terminal.
   C. Find the doctor to increase Mr. Jones's medications.
   D. Stay with Mr. Jones and call for help while continuing to monitor him.
   E. Leave to call the psychiatric liaison team to come and assess Mr. Jones.
9. The nurse is writing a care plan for a patient who was admitted with a diagnosis of heart failure. Which of the following includes standardized clinical patient care and might be useful? *Select all that apply*.
   A. Routine
   B. Bundle
   C. Protocol
   D. Checklist
   E. Pathway
10. The nurse is reviewing assignments with the only nursing assistant on the shift. One of the patients requires the use of ceiling-mounted transfer equipment. The nursing assistant tells the nurse it would be better to reassign the patient because, "I haven't worked with that kind of equipment before. I've only used the regular Hoyer lift." What actions should the nurse take to support this patient's safety? *Select all that apply*.
   A. Contact the nursing supervisor for another nursing assistant.
   B. Demonstrate use of the ceiling lift to the nursing assistant.
   C. Plan care so the patient does not need to be moved much.
   D. Assist the nursing assistant with moving the patient.
   E. Tell the nursing assistant to use the regular Hoyer lift.

REVIEW ACTIVITIES

1. Discuss the structure, process and outcomes that reflect safe medication administration with a staff nurse. Ask the nurse how medication administration safety is monitored.
2. Ask members of the interprofessional team in the clinical area which safety initiatives are most important and why. Is there a difference between the team members, that is, between nurses, physicians, therapists, and others?
3. Find dashboards or graphs related to patient safety posted in the clinical area. Ask a staff member how to read and interpret the dashboard or graph.

EXPLORING THE WEB

1. Go to the Quality and Safety Education for Nurses (QSEN) website (www.qsen.org) and search for *Safety*. Click on *Safety* and then the *Patient Safety America Newsletter*. Read the review of a patient-oriented book on protection against medical errors in the January 2019 issue. Discuss whether a communication error is a type of patient harm or whether it is a process that leads to patient harm.

2. Go to the QSEN website (www.qsen.org) and search for *Safety*. Select *Safety One Minute Checklist*. Review the material, including the checklist. Consider how the nurse can achieve the integration of the "all at once" ability to talk with the patient, deliver quality care, and observe for safety issues in the environment.
3. Search the Cochrane Collaboration site for the abstract "Do education and training programs reduce aggressive behavior toward healthcare workers?" (www.cochrane.org/CD011860/OCCHEALTH_do-education-and-training-programs-reduce-aggressive-behavior-toward-healthcare-workers). Discuss what other structures and processes besides education might lead to increased reports of workplace violence.
4. Register on the Institute for Safe Medication Practice (ISMP) website. Read the article "During the Pandemic, Aspire to Identify and Prevent Medication Errors and to Avoid Blaming Attitudes" (www.ismp.org/resources/during-pandemic-aspire-identify-and-prevent-medication-errors-and-avoid-blaming-attitudes). Discuss how a nurse is a leader in medication safety during "pandemic nursing."

SPRINGER PUBLISHING CONNECT™

A robust set of instructor resources designed to supplement this text is located at **http://connect.springerpub.com/content/book/978-0-8261-6145-1.** Qualifying instructors may request access by emailing **textbook@springerpub.com.**

REFERENCES

Agency for Healthcare Research and Quality. (2021). Nursing and patient safety. Patient Safety Network. psnet.ahrq.gov/primer/nursing-and-patient-safety.

Agency for Healthcare Research and Quality. (n.d.). *Surveys on patient safety culture™ (SOPS®)*. https://www.ahrq.gov/sops/index.html

Aiken, L., Ceron, C., Simonetti, M., Lake, E. T., Galiano, A., Garbarini, A., Soto, P., Bravo, D., & Smith, H. (2018). Hospital nurse staffing and patient outcomes. *Revista Medica Clinica Las Condes, 29*(3), 322–327.

American Association of Colleges of Nursing. (2021). *The essentials: Core competencies for professional nursing education*. https://www.aacnnursing.org/Portals/42/AcademicNursing/pdf/Essentials-2021.pdf

American Association of Nurse Anesthetists. (2018). *Promoting a culture of safety and healthy work environment*. https://www.aana.com/docs/default-source/practice-aana-com-web-documents-(all)/promoting-a-culture-of-safety-and-health-work-environment.pdf?sfvrsn=e4fa54b1_2

American Nurses Association. (2015a). *Code of ethics for nurses with interpretive statements*. https://www.nursingworld.org/practice-policy/nursing-excellence/ethics/code-of-ethics-for-nurses/coe-view-only

American Nurses Association. (2015b). *Nursing: Scope and standards of practice* (3rd ed.). Author.

Audet, A., Bourgault, P., & Rochefort, C. M. (2018). Associations between nurse education and experience and the risk of mortality and adverse events in acute care hospitals: A systematic review of observational studies. *International Journal of Nursing Studies, 80*(4), 128–146. https://doi.org/10.1016/j.ijnurstu.2018.01.007

Benenson, S., Cohen, M. J., Schwartz, C., Moses, A. E., & Levin, P. D. (2020). Is it financially beneficial for hospitals to prevent nosocomial infections? *BMC Health Services Research, 20*(1), Article 653. https://doi.org/10.1186/s12913-020-05428-7

Centers for Disease Control and Prevention. (2019). *Hand hygiene in healthcare settings*. https://www.cdc.gov/handhygiene

Change Healthcare. (2020). *Interqual®*. https://www.changehealthcare.com/solutions/clinical-decision-support/interqual

Chauhan, A., Walton, M., Manias, E., Walpola, R. L., Seale, H., Latanik, M., Leone, D., Mears, S., & Harrison, R. (2020). The safety of health care for ethnic minority patients: A systematic review. *International Journal for Equity in Health, 19*(1), Article 118. https://doi.org/10.1186/s12939-020-01223-2

Cierniak, K. H., Gaunt, M. J., & Grissinger, M. (2018). Perioperative medication errors: Uncovering risk from behind the drapes. *Pennsylvania Patient Safety Advisory, 15*(4). http://patientsafety.pa.gov/ADVISORIES/Pages/201812_Perioperative.aspx

Cohen, M., Nelson, G., & Green, D. (2010). *Patient handling & movement assessments: A white paper*. The Facility Guidelines Institute. mnhospitals.org/Portals/0/Documents/ptsafety/lift/FGI_PHAMAwhitepaper_042710.pdf

Corless, I. B., Nardi, D., Milstead, J. A., Kurth, A. E., Kirksey, K. M., & Worth, W. (2018). Expanding nursing's role in responding to global pandemics. *Nursing Outlook, 66*(4), 412–415. https://doi.org/10.1016/j.outlook.2018.06.003

Dressner, M. A., & Kissinger, S. P. (2018). *Occupational injuries and illnesses among registered nurses*. Monthly Labor Review, U.S. Bureau of Labor Statistics. https://doi.org/10.21916/mlr.2018.27

Fernandez, R., Lord, H., Halcomb, E., Moxham, L., Middleton, R., Alananzeh, I., & Ellwood, L. (2020). Implications for COVID-19: A systematic review of nurses' experiences of working in acute care hospital settings during a respiratory pandemic. *International Journal of Nursing Studies, 111*, 103637. https://doi.org/10.1016/j.ijnurstu.2020.103637

Finnegan, J. (2020). *ECRI releases its top 10 patient safety concerns in 2020 list. What's No. 1?* https://www.fiercehealthcare.com/practices/top-10-patient-safety-concerns-ecri-s-2020-list-what-s-number-one

Health Catalyst. (2018). *Systematic, data-driven approach lowers length of stay and improves care coordination*. https://www.healthcatalyst.com/success_stories/reducing-length-of-stay-memorial-hospital-at-gulfport

Heron, M. (2019). Deaths: Leading causes for 2017. *National Vital Statistics Reports, 68*(6), 1–76. https://www.cdc.gov/nchs/data/nvsr/nvsr68/nvsr68_06-508.pdf

Institute for Safe Medication Practice. (2018). *ISMP list of high-alert medications in acute care settings*. https://www.ismp.org/sites/default/files/attachments/2018-10/highAlert2018new-Oct2018-v1.pdf

Institute for Safe Medication Practice. (2019). *Independent double checks: Worth the effort if used judiciously and properly*. https://www.ismp.org/resources/independent-double-checks-worth-effort-if-used-judiciously-and-properly

International Safety Center. n.d. *EPINet sharps injury and blood and body fluid data reports*. https://internationalsafetycenter.org/exposure-reports

The Joint Commission. (2019). *R^3 report: Requirement, rationale, reference: National Patient Safety Goal for suicide prevention. Issue 18*. https://www.jointcommission.org/-/media/tjc/documents/standards/r3-reports/r3_18_suicide_prevention_hap_bhc_cah_11_4_19_final1.pdf

The Joint Commission. (2021). *National Patient Safety Goals*. https://www.jointcommission.org/standards/national-patient-safety-goals

The Joint Commission. (2020). *Specifications manual for Joint Commission national quality measures*. https://manual.jointcommission.org/releases/TJC2020B2/AppendixDTJC.html

The Leapfrog Group. (2018). *Healthcare associated infections*. https://www.leapfroggroup.org/sites/default/files/Files/Leapfrog-Castlight%202018%20HAI%20Report.pdf

National Action Alliance for Suicide Prevention: Transforming Health Systems Initiative Work Group. (2018). *Recommended standard care for people with suicide risk: Making health care suicide safe*. Education Development Center, Inc. https://theactionalliance.org/sites/default/files/action_alliance_recommended_standard_care_final.pdf

National Council of State Boards of Nursing. (2016). National guidelines for nursing delegation. *Journal of Nursing Regulation* 7(1), 5–14. https://www.ncsbn.org/NCSBN_Delegation_Guidelines.pdf

Occupational Safety and Health Administration. (2020). *Safe patient handling*. https://www.osha.gov/healthcare/safe-patient-handling

Ozone, S., Shaku, F., Sato, M., Takayashiki, A., Tsutsumi, M., & Maeno, T. (2016). Comparison of blood pressure measurements on the bare arm, over a sleeve and over a rolled-up sleeve in the elderly. *Family Practice, 33*(5), 517–522. https://doi.org/10.1093/fampra/cmw053

Patient Safety Net. (2019). *Culture of safety*. https://psnet.ahrq.gov/primer/culture-safety

QSEN Institute. (2020). *Pre-licensure KSAs: Safety*. https://qsen.org/competencies/pre-licensure-ksas/#safety

Sammer, C., Hauck, L., Jones, C., Zaiback-Aldinger, J., Li, M., & Classen, D. (2020). Examining the relationship of an all-cause harm patient safety measure and critical performance measures at the frontline of care. *Journal of Patient Safety, 16*(1), 110–116. https://doi.org/10.1097/PTS.0000000000000468

Schein, E. H., & Schein, P. A. (2019). *The corporate culture survival guide*. John Wiley & Sons.

Sculli, G. L., Fore, A. M., Sine, D. M., Paull D. E., Tschannen, D., Aebersold, M., Seagull, F. J., & Bagian, J. P. (2015). Effective followership: A standardized algorithm to resolve clinical conflicts and improve teamwork. *Journal of Healthcare Risk Management, 35*(1), 21–30. https://doi.org/10.1002/jhrm.21174

Steelesmith, D. L., Fontanella, C. A., Campo, J. V., Bridge, J. A., Warren, K. L., & Root, E. D. (2019). Contextual factors associated with county-level suicide rates in the United States, 1999 to 2016. *JAMA Network Open, 2*(9), e1910936. https://doi.org/10.1001/jamanetworkopen.2019.10936 https://jamanetwork.com/journals/jamanetworkopen/fullarticle/2749451

Stone, P. W., Hughes, R. G., & Dailey, M. (2008). Creating a safe and high-quality healthcare environment. In R. G. Hughes (Ed.), *Patient safety and quality: An evidence-based handbook for nurses* (pp. 594–603). Agency for Healthcare Research and Quality.

Tessier, L., Guilcher, S. J. T., Bai, Y. Q., Ng, R., & Wodchis, W. P. (2019). The impact of hospital harm on length of stay, costs of care and length of person-centred episodes of care: A retrospective cohort study. *Canadian Medical Association Journal, 191*(32), E879–E885. https://doi.org/10.1503/cmaj.181621

United States Bureau of Labor Statistics. (2018). *Numbers of nonfatal occupational injuries and illnesses by industry and case types, 2018*. https://www.bls.gov/iif/oshwc/osh/os/summ2_00_2018.htm

U.S. Bureau of Labor Statistics. (2018). *Fact sheet: Workplace violence in healthcare, 2018*. https://www.bls.gov/iif/oshwc/cfoi/workplace-violence-healthcare-2018.htm

World Health Organization. (2009). *The WHO guidelines on hand hygiene in health care*. https://www.who.int/publications/i/item/9789241597906

SUGGESTED READINGS

Agency for Healthcare Research and Quality. (2020). *Making healthcare safer III*. https://www.ahrq.gov/research/findings/making-healthcare-safer/mhs3/index.html

Barto, D. (2019). Nurse-driven protocols. *Nursing Critical Care, 14*(4), 18–24. https://doi.org/10.1097/01.CCN.0000560104.63793.d9

Carbuto, A., Gruden, M., Pionk, C., & Smirl, S. (2020). *Beyond getting started a resource guide: Implementing a safe patient handling and mobility program in the acute care setting* (4th ed.). AOHP Association of Occupational Health Professionals in Healthcare. https://www.aohp.org/aohp/Portals/0/Documents/ToolsForYourWork/BGSpublication/20-06%20BGS%20Safe%20Patient%20Handling.pdf

Hall, K. K., Lim, A., & Gale, B. (2020). The use of rapid response teams to reduce failure to rescue events: A systematic review. *Journal of Patient Safety 16*(3), 3–7. https://doi.org/10.1097/PTS.0000000000000748

Jones, M. M., & Saines, M. (2019). The eighteen of 1918–1919: Black nurses and the Great Flu Pandemic in the United States. *American Journal of Public Health, 109*(6), 877–884. https://doi.org/10.2105/AJPH.2019.305003

Page, A. (Ed.). (2004). *Keeping patients safe: Transforming the work environment of nurses*. The National Academies Press. https://doi.org/10.17226/10851

Prestia, A. S. (2019). Leading with the soul of a warrior. *Nurse Leader, 18*(2), 63–166. https://doi.org/10.1016/J.MNL.2019.09.015

Robert Wood Johnson Foundation. (2011). *Nurses are key to improving patient safety*. http://www.rwjf.org/en/library/articles-and-news/2011/04/nurses-are-key-to-improving-patient-safety.html

Skloot, R. (2011). *The immortal life of Henrietta Lacks*. Broadway Paperbacks/Random House.

Sloane, D. M., Smith, H. L., McHugh, M. D., & Aiken, L. H. (2018). Effect of changes in hospital nursing resources on improvements in patient safety and quality of care: A panel study. *Medical Care, 56*(12), 1001–1008. https://doi.org/10.1097/MLR.0000000000001002

CHAPTER 11

Quality Improvement Essentials

Anthony L. D'Eramo

"Undoubtedly, the most important single requisite is a commitment to quality: an unequivocal desire and determination to dedicate oneself to the best one is capable of, despite every obstacle."

–Donabedian, 2003, p. xxix

Upon completion of this chapter, the reader should be able to:

1. Define quality improvement (QI).
2. Describe the historical evolution of QI.
3. Explain QI in nursing practice
4. Compare and contrast QI, evidence-based practice, and research.
5. Differentiate between QI models and methodologies, including Plan-Do-Study-Act (PDSA), Lean, and Six Sigma.
6. Describe reactive and proactive approaches to QI problems.
7. Explore the role of the nurse in QI projects.
8. Discuss the impact organizational leadership has on QI activities.

CROSSWALK

This chapter addresses the following:

QSEN Competency: Quality Improvement

The American Association of Colleges of Nursing. (2021). *The essentials: Core competencies for professional nursing education.*

Domain 5: Quality and Safety

OPENING SCENARIO

A home care nurse is admitting a new patient. While conducting the medication reconciliation based on the nursing admission policy, the patient hands the nurse a bottle of erythromycin he has been taking for 3 days. However, there is no electronic medical record (EMR) indication that this patient was prescribed erythromycin or any medical history or recent provider notation prescribing erythromycin. The nurse is clearly performing an important assessment and has several questions about the medication. The first question the nurse asks is, "Who prescribed erythromycin for you?" The patient responds that he had a cold and decided to go to urgent care rather than try to see his provider. The provider at urgent care prescribed erythromycin for bronchitis. As the patient explains the situation, the nurse recognizes that the EMR cannot reflect any out of network information.

1. From an interprofessional perspective, who would the nurse initially contact based on this observation?
2. What regulation(s) is the nursing admission assessment policy that stipulates medication reconciliation be conducted on every home visit based on?
3. Is there opportunity to consider a quality improvement activity based on this scenario?

INTRODUCTION

Staff nurses who provide direct patient care are best positioned to participate and lead quality improvement (QI) activities, thus affecting the quality of care patients receive. In such manner, it is important that nurses become familiar with the essentials of QI. The purpose of this chapter is to explore QI processes as they promote patient safety and the achievement of the best patient outcomes. QI will be defined and key concepts pertaining to the history of QI will be presented to showcase its interdisciplinary nature. Research and evidence-based practice (EBP) will be differentiated from the process of QI. The Donabedian model for change and Deming's Plan-Do-Study-Act (PDSA) process will be introduced as models commonly used in QI activities. Improvement methodologies such as Six Sigma and Lean will be explored. A proactive tool, namely the Healthcare Failure Mode and Effect Analysis (HFMEA), is presented. Reactive tools such as the root cause analysis (RCA) process are discussed as evaluation tools used to determine the root cause of a significant near miss, an error, or sentinel event. Implementing and sustaining a culture of safety through the delivery of evidence-based high-quality healthcare using an interdisciplinary approach supported by leadership are key to continuous QI.

DEFINING QUALITY IMPROVEMENT

Quality improvement (QI) is defined the same for both prelicensure and graduate nursing education by the Quality and Safety Education for Nurses (QSEN) competency as "Use data to monitor the outcomes of care processes and use improvement methods to design and test changes to continuously improve the quality and safety of healthcare systems" (QSEN Institute, n.d.-a, n.d.-b). The knowledge, skills, and attitudes (KSAs) differ, however, in that the prelicensure expectations focus on preparing the new nurse to participate in or lead small-scale QI activities while graduate students are expected to take a greater role and facilitate QI activities across the organization. QI is the process of collecting and analyzing data to determine the extent to which quality healthcare is being delivered according to established standards. Standards may be internal, such as those created by the organization, or external, such as those created by regulatory bodies. QI can be considered as both an art and a science (McLaughlin et al., 2012). Indeed, the art of QI involves asking questions and coming up with creative ideas and visionary innovations of how to approach and consider improvement interventions. The science of QI, presented in Chapter 12, involves the ongoing process of testing improvement interventions, to measure if improvements lead to the intended outcomes, and to sustain intended outcomes.

Triggers that may initiate a QI activity may include inconsistent patient outcomes, poor patient outcomes, patient outcomes that do not meet expectations related to evidence-based practice (EBP) or to standards, or patient/family complaints. Such outcomes may be specific to a patient (e.g., a medication error), groups of patients (e.g., hospital-acquired pressure injury rates), or may identify a process that needs improving (e.g., transition from acute care to home care). QI is a continuous process that includes elements of prevention (risk reduction), recognition, and alleviation of harm as well as the ongoing search for performance excellence.

QI is a structured series of events that involves planning, implementing, and evaluating healthcare outcomes (Hughes, 2008b). In addition, the National Academy of Medicine, formerly the Institute of Medicine (IOM, 2001), identified six aims for care delivery: that care delivery is safe, effective, patient-centered, efficient, equitable, and timely. Each aim provides an avenue for data collection and analysis that may trigger evidence that improvement is required or desired.

There are several key steps to formal QI projects, including assembling a team, understanding the organization as a complex system, accessing and interpreting data, implementing interventions to improve outcomes, and sustaining actions when improvement goals are met. Certainly, it is safe to say QI focuses on improving processes and outcomes, including those that result from practice decisions, and measuring or evaluating such outcomes compared to an established, evidence-based standard, goal, or industry benchmark. Many organizations exist to provide QI resources and expertise to individuals, teams, and organizations working to improve. Examples of such organizations are listed in Box 11.1. It is also well recognized that there are cultural factors of the organization that influence

BOX 11.1 Examples of Organizations Associated With Healthcare Quality

Organization and Web Address

Agency for Healthcare Research and Quality (AHRQ) http://ahrq.gov

American Society for Quality (ASQ) http://asq.org

Centers for Medicare and Medicaid Services (CMS) http://cms.hhs.gov

Hospital Compare http://medicare.gov/hospitalcompare/search.html

Institute for Healthcare Improvement (IHI) http://ihi.org/Pages/default.aspx

Institute for Safe Medication Practice (ISMP) www.ismp.org

The Joint Commission (TJC) http://jointcommission.org

The Leapfrog Group www.leapfroggroup.org

National Database of Nursing Quality Indicators http://public.qualityforum.org/actionregistry/Lists/List%20of%20Actions/Attachments/141/NDNQIBrochure.pdf

National Association for Healthcare Quality (NAHQ) www.nahq.org

National Quality Forum www.qualityforum.org/Home.aspx

Quality and Safety Education for Nurses (QSEN) http://qsen.org

improvement activities such as engaged and supportive senior leadership, interdisciplinary teams, staff buy-in, technology support, and direct supervisory commitment for time to work on improvements (Mitchell et al., 2015). The existence of a just culture, or a culture where reporting errors or risks is welcome because such reporting leads to improvements, is another cultural factor that distinguishes organizations that strive and meet performance excellence.

As nurses care for patients or communities, it is their professional responsibility to obtain and apply the KSAs of QI to daily practice. The American Nurses Association (ANA) Code of Ethics, specifically Provision 3, speaks to nurses as patient advocates, protecting patient rights and safety (ANA, 2015). This provides an ethical basis for nurses taking part in QI activities. Organizations do not only hold nurses accountable to recognize and mitigate risk, but also to analyze patient outcomes to determine if improvement is warranted. In addition, nurses must have skills to evaluate organizational processes and report those processes that impede care delivery. Analyzing patient outcomes and evaluating complex processes requires the QI KSAs outlined by QSEN. These QI actions should sound familiar as they mimic the nursing process. It is truly an exciting time to be a nurse! Nurses are not only responsible for impacting the well-being of patients, groups, and communities, but are charged with ethical accountability to pursue continual improvement toward zero harm. It is no wonder why the public consistently ranks nurses as the most trusted, ethical, and honest profession 18 out of the last 19 Gallup polls (Gaines, 2021). Sometimes, the most challenging aspect of QI activities is getting started. The Real World Interview on page 365 describes a newly graduated nurse's experience with her first QI project.

Getting started also includes establishing a project team, gathering support or buy-in for a project, and setting aside time to complete the project. Buy-in and team success can be challenging, as seen in the Developing Clinical Judgment (Box 11.2) scenario.

BOX 11.2 Developing Clinical Judgment

You are the nurse representative on a QI project team that plans to reduce the use of mental health restraints. The project has been going on for 3 months, yet the expectation was it would be completed within weeks. The project meetings are typically attended by half of the participants. The leadership project sponsor, who was away when the project started, has assigned the project lead to a psychiatrist who has delegated the lead role to one of the mental health administrative support staff and does not attend the scheduled meetings. Although the organization's patient safety officer has created a project charter, the psychiatrist also does not think there is a problem that needs improvement. As a project team member, you are frustrated and think the team needs motivation.

1. What CUES for the causes of the project delay could you provide to the leadership project sponsor?
2. What HYPOTHESIS can you consider?
3. What ACTION (plan and implement) would be the most effective in this situation?
4. What OUTCOMES would you consider evaluating?

Real World Interview

When I graduated, I attended a year-long Transition to Practice Residency that included numerous classes and clinical experiences as well as the requirement to complete a QI project. My goal was to do a project where I would eventually practice, the optometry and ophthalmology services, or eye clinic. As a novice nurse, my initial project ideas tended to be grandiose. I wanted to make a significant impact on the patient experience. However, I knew I had to scale back my idea and focus on one part of patient care. As I considered my project idea, two separate events with suboptimal patient outcomes occurred within 1 week.

The first event happened when a veteran called their primary provider complaining of "change in vision." A referral was placed for a "routine" eye examination, typically scheduled within 30 days. The veteran was scheduled nearly 30 days from his complaint. His symptoms persisted, so he contacted the eye clinic directly. He was seen quickly and diagnosed with a retinal detachment requiring surgery. Unfortunately, some permanent visual impairment resulted.

As that was unfolding, a veteran called the Telephone Assistance Program (TAP) complaining of a headache and blurry vision. The TAP operator encouraged the veteran to go to the emergency department. The veteran, however, declined as he was concerned about long wait times. A note was entered into his chart for the primary care staff. Because this occurred during the weekend, the primary care staff did not read the note for 2 days. Sadly, we later learned that this veteran suffered a stroke. Although everyone involved followed procedures, we understood an eye examination may have detected an impending stroke.

These two events highlighted an opportunity for improvement. Could a nurse-led initiative to ensure timely assessment with the goal to minimize these types of outcomes work?

For eye or vision complaints, primary care (or other services) and electronic or telephone referral to the eye clinic occurred, where a nonclinical staff member scheduled the appointment. Because the staff are nonclinical, no triage occurred to determine urgency. Knowing this, I wondered if I could create a way for a healthcare provider to refer a patient to the eye clinic as a way to determine urgency of needed care. Could this be my project?! There's a clear problem, a goal, and potential intervention.

The goal, to improve consultations for appropriate and timely triage of veterans needing eye clinic expertise, was agreed on by leadership. With access being key, the logical intervention was to collaborate with telecommunications to develop a '"triage line." This direct triage line would include both clinic nurse phones and the attending/technician workstations ensuring <u>only</u> clinical staff would be responding. In addition, to ensure timely access, the intervention included <u>no</u> voice mailbox. Telecommunications installed the line and we were set to study the outcome. To support the intervention, I developed a flyer about the new resource, including instructions. This informative flyer was sent to all healthcare providers in the organization, emphasizing the use of this line.

By the end of the first month we had 15 calls, all of which resulted in same day appointments. Three of those patients (20%) required close follow-up. Within 2 months, two veterans with retinal tears were triaged, received immediate intervention, and had outcomes of preserved vision. One veteran already had longstanding visual impairment in one eye; thus, preservation of the vision in the other eye was especially critical. It was clear that this new process improved care outcomes for patients.

Financial costs for this project were minimal: only activation of a new direct line and the paper/time to develop and distribute the informational flyers. It is clear this new process has improved care outcomes for veterans while increasing efficiencies for healthcare providers. The improvement skills I gained from the residency project have professional impact because as nurses, we need to not only have improvement skills, we need to employ them throughout our professional careers.

Christine Dyer, RN, BSN
Staff Nurse
Eye Clinic, Providence VA Medical Center, Providence, Rhode Island

HISTORY AND EVOLUTION OF QUALITY IMPROVEMENT IN HEALTHCARE

Prior to the 20th century, there was no such thing as a standard of care for physicians or hospitals, let alone nursing care standards of practice. Patient outcomes were not tracked or reported. With little to no emphasis on measuring patient care outcomes, it is not surprising that improvement or quality was not a consideration.

The establishment of the American Medical Association (AMA) started in the early 20th century from the efforts of Dr. Ernest Codman. The AMA set out to create standards of care and expectations for physicians, improve medical education, and improve public health. Dr. Codman began encouraging patient case review and the tracking of patients posthospitalization to ensure the care they received was effective. It was through Codman's efforts to track patient outcomes, morbidity, and mortality following hospital stays and surgical procedures that the American College of Surgeons (ACS) was born. The primary responsibility of the ACS was to act as an oversight organization to physicians and hospitals. In the early 20th century, the ACS developed five minimum standards for hospital care. To be certified by the ACS, a hospital had to:

1. Organize the physicians practicing at the hospital into a medical staff.
2. Limit staff membership to well-educated, competent, licensed physicians and surgeons.
3. Have rules and regulations governing regular staff meetings and clinical review.
4. Keep medical records that included the history, physical examination, and results of diagnostic testing.
5. Supervise diagnostic and treatment facilities such as laboratory and radiology departments (Luce et al., 1994).

For the next 40 years, meeting minimum standards for hospital care was considered a satisfactory means to demonstrate quality care. By the 1960s there was a shift from meeting the minimum standards to identifying outcomes outside those that were expected, often referred to as outliers. Identifying and improving physician outliers became the impetus to achieving quality care. To identify physician outliers, a peer review of patient charts was instituted. Individual physician care data were collected from patient charts and analyzed. Patient care characteristics such as readmission rates, transfers to the ICU, needs for transfusion, and antibiotic use were reviewed to identify poorly performing physicians. Efforts could then be made to educate and support QI in physician practice through mentoring. The results of this peer-review process were eventually used by hospitals in credentialing physicians. Physicians not performing up to standards or failing to correct practice deficiencies could potentially lose their privileges to practice at that institution.

As physicians were being peer reviewed, there remained little to no attention to the quality of nursing care. However, that was not the case in the manufacturing sector. The work of many experts including Deming and the Plan-Do-Study-Act (PDSA) model became intriguing to businesses that could demonstrate improved production by employing principles of continuous improvement. As part of this revolution, industrial leaders began welcoming frontline staff participation and evaluation of processes since they were involved with the day-to-day operations. Frontline staff welcomed the opportunity and could easily and often quickly identify opportunities for improvement that could impact production. This belief and even the PDSA, described later in this chapter, eventually influenced healthcare quality methodologies.

There were numerous historical events that have brought light to healthcare quality. For the purpose of this chapter, several will be highlighted including Title XVIII of the Social Security Act that signed Medicare into law; regulatory oversight of healthcare, such as TJC; and several IOM publications.

In 1966, Medicare was signed into law providing healthcare for Americans 65 years and older, followed by Medicaid that provided healthcare resources to low-income Americans. Today, both programs are combined into the Centers for Medicare and Medicaid Services (CMS). These programs have gone through revisions over the years including identifying quality indicators. For example, the Experimental Medical Care Review Organizations were established in 1972 to review quality and appropriateness of care delivered (Owens & Koch, 2015). In 2001, CMS instituted the Hospital Quality Initiative, making aggregated healthcare quality data publicly accessible. The National Quality Foundation identified "never events" in 2001 as sentinel events or preventable errors that should never occur. In 2007, the CMS restructured reimbursement of never events, holding organizations more financially accountable for the cost associated with never events. The **Hospital Value-Based Purchasing** (HVBP) Program introduced by CMS in 2011 is a payment model with roots in the Affordable Care Act (ACA). Traditionally, reimbursement for healthcare has mainly been and remains a fee-for-service model where the patient or the patient's insurer, if an insurer exists, is billed directly. The HVBP model shifts payment from fee-for-service to value based. This shift equates to insurers such as Medicare to reward or penalize hospitals based on patient care and process outcomes. The HVBP recognizes providers who deliver better outcomes at lower costs (Aroh et al., 2015; Figueroa et al., 2016; Haley et al., 2017). With HVBP, hospital performance is based on four quality domains: Person and Community Engagement (25%), Clinical Care (25%), Safety (25%), and Efficiency and Cost Reduction (25%; CMS, 2018a). Because reimbursement is tied to meeting established outcomes, the belief is that HVBP would result in cost containment. There are organizations who maintain high performance, those who improve performance, and others who decline in performance, which impact their reimbursement (Carroll & Clement, 2020).

The Joint Commission on Accreditation of Healthcare Organizations (JCAHO) was founded in 1951 through the collaborative efforts of the American College of Physicians, the American Hospital Association, the AMA, and the Canadian Medical Association. JCAHO was initially charged with regulatory oversight of hospital quality (TJC, n.d.-b). JCAHO, currently called TJC, also assumed regulatory oversight of nursing homes and laboratory facilities, among other duties. TJC sets forth a set of widely recognized standards of performance and quality measure sets that healthcare organizations must achieve for accreditation. One example of a TJC requirement, specifically one of the TJC National Patient Safety Goals (NPSG), is to maintain and communicate accurate patient medication information (TJC, n.d.-c) that was discussed in the chapter opening scenario.

In the 1970s and 1980s, the focus on quality care transitioned from a peer review of patient charts to identify "problem physicians" to improving the performance of a group of physicians and hospitals through implementing practice guidelines. The goal of practice guidelines was to standardize care decision-making. Practice guidelines would apply up-to-date evidence that would inform clinical decision-making, resulting in improved patient outcomes and a reduction in morbidity and mortality.

As TJC matured, the focus moved from quality of care being a physician responsibility to an interprofessional responsibility. All healthcare workers were now responsible and accountable to ensure quality and safety within their practice. The scope of responsibility not only included patients, but staff and visitors who were also in the healthcare environment and could be subject to safety risks. The environment of care, for example, has many TJC requirements to protect patients, visitors, and employees. A simple spill of ice chips on a floor can lead to falls for anyone in that area, not just patients.

In 2002, TJC initiated the requirement that all hospitals seeking their accreditation begin reporting their performance on core patient quality measures. These core patient quality measures are a listing of standardized evidence-based care that should be delivered to certain patient groups, for example, all patients with pneumonia should receive an antibiotic before they leave the emergency department (ED) or all patients with a myocardial infarction should be prescribed a beta-blocker. Since hospital payers (e.g., insurance companies, CMS) often require proof of accreditation before they will reimburse health services, hospitals became motivated to participate in improving their performance given the financial implications. TJC patient quality measures change based on evidence or outcome trends. To learn more about TJC quality measures, visit www.jointcommission.org/measurement/measures.

TJC also changed its approach to how it assessed an organization's compliance to their published standards by shifting from a scheduled to an unannounced site visit. In addition, TJC implemented the **tracer methodology** that traces an individual patient through their transitions of care across the organization, and included "system tracers," such as medication management and infection control, tracing those complex processes across the entire organization. Consider a patient with congestive heart failure (CHF) on an acute care medical unit who has had multiple admissions for CHF. This patient is improving but, on arrival to the ED, was intubated and admitted to the medical ICU (MICU).

When TJC surveyor is ready to conduct a tracer activity, the surveyor will request a complex patient, such as the patient with CHF, who has been admitted across several care settings during one hospital stay. The surveyor will request to meet with the interprofessional team starting with the current team on the medical unit, and then traces the care delivery backward to previous settings, including meeting with those team members. All staff involved in the care of the selected patient, including the nurse caring for the patient while on that unit, are asked to meet with the surveyor. The surveyor asks the team about their care delivery to determine if the team is following their policies and procedures, which are often created based on TJC regulatory requirements. The surveyor may also request to speak to the patient and the family to assess if patient education occurred and if they are satisfied with the care and services they have received. Once the surveyor has completed the discussions, which may take hours, the surveyor traces care and services backwards to meet with the previous care team(s). In this example, the surveyor begins in the MICU followed by the ED team. The surveyor interviews the staff regarding the specific care and services the patient received while under their care. The patient's electronic medical record (EMR) is reviewed, and team documentation and any other aspects of care and services that the surveyor chooses are evaluated. Because the patient experienced multiple levels of care, the surveyor asks about communication that occurred during transfer between transitions as communication failures may result in risks or errors that can impact patient outcomes.

During the team discussions, the surveyor takes notes, such as policy questions to look up after the discussion, and visits other departments involved in the care delivery for this patient. Since the patient was previously intubated, respiratory care services and the radiology department both receive visits from this surveyor. The intent of tracers is to determine if staff followed their policies and procedures based on TJC requirements for accreditation. This level of review adds value to the accreditation and ultimately to patient care because it goes beyond compliance (yes–no type questions) to a process approach ("talk to me about your admission assessment"). For nurses, a tracer is nothing more than explaining what was done for the patient and/or family based on the scope of nursing practice.

The surveyor asks questions about nursing care processes related to medication administration, assessment/reassessment, documentation, patient education, discharge planning, and care coordination across settings. Also appreciate that TJC surveyors are well versed in all TJC requirements. Although they may be on the unit conducting a tracer, they will be assessing the environment, looking in storage areas, and watching staff in action, for example, regarding hand hygiene (HH) compliance. To learn more about tracers, TJC

Real World Interview

Despite my high level of experience and confidence as a homecare nurse, I always feel anxious if I am the nurse involved with a TJC tracer. I think no matter how well prepared, there is always the worry that they will find something, and it will be your fault. I do feel the best way to prepare is to try and do the right thing every day and then you are always ready. During my visit, the patient had a free-standing oxygen tank for supplemental oxygen. Because I immediately saw it and knowing home oxygen is a safety risk, I quickly placed the tank into a storage cylinder where it belonged and re-educated the patient that oxygen tanks cannot be left freestanding, which pleased the surveyor. The patient also had an over-the-counter medication that was not on his medication list. I was able to address that as part of the routine medication reconciliation and ensured it was documented. Home care nurses are well informed that handwashing will be closely watched by the surveyor and should not cause anxiety. Because we know errors can happen, especially when being watched, we make sure our techniques are correct. The process of preparing for a survey or tracer is challenging because one never really knows what they will ask. As a new nurse I was anxious. Experience helps me ***do my job to the best of my ability, to adjust along the way, and*** *to follow the procedures. This makes talking with a surveyor less stressful. I also have found if I do not know an answer, the surveyor helps to coach me and will share best practices the surveyor may have seen at other organizations that can help. All in all, it can be stressful but also educational.*

Carol A. Mello, MSN, RN

offers a brief video overview of the tracer process at www.jointcommission.org/resources/news-and-multimedia/video-resources/mock-tracer-therapeutic-school.

A greater emphasis on risk reduction can be seen in TJC standards and process. In 2017, TJC changed their approach to how deficiencies are identified and scored during surveys. Deficiencies are reported based on risk of harm and scope of the deficiency. This change allows the organization to mitigate or take corrective action on the highest risk deficiencies first by prioritizing them for immediate action (TJC 2016). With TJC's scoring methodology called Survey Analysis For Evaluating Risk (SAFER) Matrix, deficiencies are categorized by the likelihood of harm and the scope of the deficiency. This approach allows the surveyor who identified the deficiency to analyze the deficiency based on the likelihood of harm (high, moderate, and low) as well as the scope of the deficiency (widespread, pattern, and limited). The deficiency is evaluated and inserted into the matrix based on the surveyor's analysis. This provides the organization with a comprehensive visual, risk-based prioritized list of deficiencies to correct. Regardless of risk (except for identification of immediate risk to life or safety), the organization will have 60 days for corrective action. However, for those high-risk deficiencies, TJC will request additional information and evidence of corrective actions and sustainment (TJC, n.d.-a). Visit www.jointcommission.org/accreditation-and-certification/become-accredited/what-is-accreditation/safer-matrix-resources to learn more about and to visualize the SAFER Matrix.

Several publications by the IOM highlighted the continued quality challenges facing the healthcare system. *To Err Is Human: Building a Safer Health System* (2000) recognized the grim reality of patient deaths associated with medical errors. The publication *Crossing the Quality Chasm: A New Health System for the 21st Century* (2001) focused on healthcare system failures, emphasizing it was not the fault of the employees but poor care delivery processes, or systems, that needed improvement. In response, many organizations have taken improvement actions to address these issues utilizing the QI tools discussed later in this chapter.

As the public became better informed about the mounting problems within the healthcare industry, the staggering cost of healthcare continued and continues to rise today at alarming rates. In fact, the U.S. health expenditure is expected to increase by 5.5% annually between 2018 and 2027, with growth of spending expected to be faster than that expected in Gross Domestic Product (GDP) by 0.8% (CMS, 2018b). These predictions indicate the health share of GDP will increase from 17.9% (2017) to 19.4% by 2026 (CMS, 2018b). Despite significant funding, continued evidence of less than optimal healthcare outcomes are realized. Patients complain of long wait times for appointments and access to care challenges. Care coordination and communication gaps exist as do healthcare disparities with the focus on episodic care rather than preventive care (Salmond & Echevarria, 2017). There are many examples that contribute to increased healthcare costs, such as the demand for greater, sophisticated technology, prescription medications (Squires & Anderson, 2015), waste, excessive administrative costs, unnecessary services, and preventive failures (Berwick & Hackbarth, 2012).

With increased healthcare costs, many Americans find healthcare unaffordable. For years, consumers of healthcare have asked for healthcare reform to include affordable healthcare coverage. In response, the ACA was passed by Congress in 2010. At that time, approximately 46.5 million Americans were uninsured (Tolbert et al., 2019). That number decreased because of the ACA to 27.9 in 2018. However, there has been a steady increase in uninsured Americans since 2016 (Tolbert et al., 2019). These authors noted in 2018, 45% of the uninsured Americans reported the cost of insurance being prohibitive to purchase (Tolbert et al., 2019). The ACA went beyond healthcare coverage; it supported many programs and reimbursement models aimed at "fixing" the healthcare system. An example is the Patient-Centered Medical Home program to provide a team-based approach to primary care in the patient's home. Patients with chronic disease are prime candidates for the Medical Home program because the focus is to improve the patient's self-management of their chronic conditions while providing care coordination and evidence-based care.

QUALITY IMPROVEMENT IN NURSING

Traditionally, the practice of nursing has been perceived as a valued, trusted contribution to patient care. Because nurses are members of teams and often carry out interventions identified by other team members, consider the complexity of identifying unique indicators of nursing practice that are specific to nursing. There are many questions as to how the unique practice of nursing equates to quality care outcome measures. How does nursing judgment impact patient outcomes? How is efficiency of nursing practice measured? As these and many other questions have been raised regarding nursing and patient outcomes, the IOM, QSEN, ANA, and others have acted. The IOM has called for a stronger body of EBP for all healthcare disciplines to create a greater empirical evidence-based care delivery by each discipline. Through the KSAs of the QSEN competencies, nurses are being better prepared to question practice, evaluate the literature, and take active roles in QI.

The ANA funded the development of nurse-sensitive quality indicators in 1998 to provide data on specific acute-care outcomes that could directly indicate the quality of nursing care delivery. Participating organizations could submit their outcomes for trending and comparison purposes. Results could be useful to compare nursing care outcomes with like-sized organizations with either evidence that expectations are being met or indications that improvement is warranted. These data in the National Database of Nursing Quality Indicators (NDNQI), now managed by Press Ganey (accessible at www.pressganey.com/resources/program-summary/ndnqi-solution-summary), continue to evolve and are likely to change as new empirical evidence substantiates new, specific, nurse-sensitive indicators. Other organizations have created nurse-sensitive indicators, such as the National Quality Forum (NQF), that include many of the NDNQI indicators (accessible at www.qualityforum.org/Publications/2004/10/National_Voluntary_Consensus_Standards_for_Nursing-Sensitive_Care__An_Initial_Performance_Measure_Set.aspx). In reality, capturing nurse-sensitive indicators that effectively and accurately capture nursing care is challenging. Other sources have identified indicators that are used and are useful but further research is needed that demonstrates unique, empirical relationships between such indicators to specific patient outcomes. In addition, indicators for all practice settings are needed as most of the current nurse-sensitive measures focus on acute care settings.

Today's healthcare organizations are highly complex systems that are often multi-site and provide various levels of care. Perhaps one of the most important aspects of QI is the organization's culture and expectations regarding quality care delivery and outcomes. To create and sustain a culture of continual improvement, leadership must foster innovative systems thinking of all staff and serve as role models by participating with staff in QI activities. Leadership support includes educating employees on QI methods, providing time for QI activities, recognizing staff for identifying opportunities for improvement, ensuring that patients' and families' feedback is used toward improvement, and sustaining those QI outcomes that have met the improvement aim(s).

IS QUALITY IMPROVEMENT EVIDENCE-BASED PRACTICE OR RESEARCH?

It is important to be able to differentiate QI from EBP and research. QI incorporates a data-driven systematic process in which individuals collaborate to improve specific internal processes within a care delivery area or an organization. One key aim of QI is the analysis of data into decision-making information to determine if improvement is warranted. The aim is different from EBP and research.

EBP does not analyze information, data, or seek to problem-solve, but rather it critically appraises all relevant evidence to answer a clinical, educational, or administrative question. The aim of EBP is to determine if evidence supports clinical, educational, or administrative practice. If evidence exists, it validates practice. If evidence does not exist, the need for research to provide new evidence may be supported. One similarity between QI and EBP involves a review of literature. Reviewing the literature is a basic aspect of EBP but there is merit in assessing the literature when conducting QI. The literature may provide relevant interventions that a team may wish to employ. As nurses, QI and EBP are both fundamental expectations of practice. It is important to apply basic QI principles for continued improvement and question practice to determine if practice is based on sound evidence.

Research is a scientific process of generating new knowledge. The aim of research is to test hypotheses that may be generalizable beyond the research setting. Reducing bias is crucial to generalize research outcomes. Quantitative research often includes an intervention group (those who received the study intervention) and a control group (those not receiving the intervention), allowing to test for statistical differences between groups. Conducting research is neither a basic skill nor an expectation of nursing practice. Advanced degrees are necessary for nurses who may wish to become researchers. When conducting research, ethical consideration for approval and oversight by an institutional review board (IRB) is required to ensure the safety of human subjects who will be participating in the research study. Although the aims of research and QI are different, these differences can be vague, especially if patients are included in a QI project.

The scope of QI activities can be a simple, individual act such as reorganizing a utility room, making it easier and quicker to find supplies, to a unit-based team working to improve unit outcomes, to a system-wide initiative that includes professionals from different disciplines, all involved in the process that needs improvement. With QI, there are two distinct types of data. There are **baseline data**, or the data that support the need for improvement, and **postintervention data**, or the data generated after the QI intervention was implemented. Comparing baseline to postintervention data allows for the determination if the QI goal(s) were accomplished. **Outcome data**, often referred to as accountability data or performance measure outcomes, represent the outcomes of healthcare delivery processes. These outcomes are inherent to practice and systems. For example, patient falls can be measured as one outcome indicator of nursing care. The total time it takes from a CT scan order, to scan, to read, and to communicate results, is a process that can be measured. Patient or process outcomes relate to accountability of employees and the organization. These outcomes are frequently public and reported to regulatory bodies as an indication of organizational performance. Analysis of outcome data can be used as baseline data for decision-making, regarding whether improvement is warranted or not. For example, if an indicator such as hand hygiene was measured on a nursing unit for 1 month and was found to be 70% compliant with the Centers for Disease Control and Prevention (CDC) requirements, 70% represents an outcome measure and would serve as the baseline if a project was planned to improve hand hygiene compliance. Analysis of this outcome, including unit trends of hand hygiene compliance over time, is necessary to determine if improvement is warranted. If improvement of hand hygiene compliance is deemed necessary, a QI activity could occur. The QI activity would involve implementing an intervention to improve the baseline outcome measure of 70%. The measurement obtained to evaluate the effect of the intervention is the postintervention measure. In this example, if an intervention was introduced resulting in 88% hand hygiene compliance, the 88% represents the postintervention measure, which is an improvement from the baseline measure of 70%. If an intervention to improve hand hygiene was introduced but the goal was not obtained, an additional intervention may be needed. If the intervention had no effect, the team would need to identify a new intervention or consider reevaluating how the original intervention was implemented, which may be the contributing factor to not meeting the goal.

So far, EBP, research, and QI seem to be very distinct approaches to measurement. As patient care and process outcomes have greater influence on reimbursement, the need for measurement and sophisticated QI interventions will become more important. In addition, the study of QI interventions has become a relevant area of research. In fact, the literature has numerous examples of QI research where the focus of the research hypothesis is on the intervention itself and how the intervention was deployed. Confusing, right? But consider a QI project with the aim to reduce falls on a nursing unit. The intervention consists of one group of patients assessed with Fall Risk Scale A, another group with Fall Risk Scale B, and a third group who did not have a risk assessment performed. Although there would be unit-level baseline outcome data on falls and the scope of the project is within one unit with no intent to generalize outcomes, the fact is patients are being randomized. Randomization is a research methodology; thus, this QI project is now moving into a QI research realm. As described in the example, the QI activity is now QI research because patients were randomized with a control group. If the project aim had been to reduce falls by trialing one fall risk assessment that all patients received, without randomizing patients, there would be no research methodologies underway. Casarett et al. (2000) propose differentiating QI from research can be challenging in that rigorous research guidelines exist while such rigor is currently absent with QI.

Traditionally, there was confidence employees could easily differentiate between "QI," "research," and "data." That confidence may be risky. Understanding the difference among QI Nonresearch, QI Research, and Accountability data that represent patient/ process outcome can increase confidence that staff nurses can take improvement actions appropriately and safely and are not including research methodologies as a member of a QI team. The distinction among QI Nonresearch, QI Research, and Accountability data, as they relate to performance measurement, is important because each has a different value, aim, and specific processes associated with it. O'Rourke and Fraser (2016) differentiate QI as both a research and practice activity. Lloyd (2010) identified three faces of performance measurements. Table 11.1 is useful in differentiating the characteristics of all three measurement approaches. Notice the aim statements clearly provide key differences as they relate

TABLE 11.1 THREE APPROACHES TO PERFORMANCE MEASUREMENT

PERFORMANCE MEASUREMENT APPROACH			
ELEMENTS OF EACH APPROACH	QI - NONRESEARCH	QI - RESEARCH	ACCOUNTABILITY-PATIENT/PROCESS OUTCOME DATA
Aim	Improve patient care within a local context	New knowledge as to why and how QI interventions work in different contexts	Benchmark Evidence of meeting or not meeting a measurable expectation Provides opportunities for improvement
Intervention	Identified, applied, revised based on local context	Tested, explored, often a control group to compare impact of intervention(s)	No intervention, evaluate current performance
Project Lead	Expert in local context	Expert in research methods	No project
Bias	Accept bias	Designed to eliminate bias for greater generalizability	Measure and adjust to reduce bias
Sample Size	Small sample is usually adequate	Statistically calculated	Utilize 100% of available data
Flexibility of Hypothesis	Hypothesis is flexible to allow for changes during intervention	Fixed, unchangeable	No hypothesis
Testing & Time Frame	Sequential tests with goal to complete quickly; rapid cycles	One large test that is time intensive	No testing, technological systems are frequently instituted for review of aggregate data analysis and decision-making
Project Approval	IRB not required	IRB required	Not a project
Determining if Outcome Is an Improvement	Commonly run or control charts	Hypothesis statistical testing	No testing
Confidentiality of Data	Data used only by QI intervention team	Participant data is protected	Data available to stakeholders and usually public

IRB, institutional review board; QI, quality improvement.

Source: Adapted from Lloyd, R. C. (2010). Navigating in the turbulent sea of data: The quality measurement journey. *Clinics in Perinatology, 37*, 101–122. https://doi.org/10.1016/j.clp.2010.01.006; O'Rourke, H. M., & Fraser, K. D. (2016). How quality improvement practice evidence can advance the knowledge base. *Journal for Healthcare Quality, 38*(5), 264–274. https://doi.org/10.1097/JHQ.0000000000000067

to context. In summary, the aim of a QI research project is to understand why and how improvement interventions work in different contexts to determine if they are generalizable. The focus of QI Research is therefore to study and understand the intervention itself. The aim of QI-Nonresearch is to improve processes and outcomes within a local context, not to imply the outcome has implications across settings, although that may well be the case when sharing/standardizing successful projects. Patient and process outcomes are not a project at all, but the measures from care and service delivery that can serve as baseline data for QI decision-making.

QUALITY IMPROVEMENT MODELS AND METHODOLOGIES

There are various QI models that provide a comprehensive framework for evaluating healthcare quality. Some of the most common are Donabedian's Structure, Process, Outcomes Model, and methodologies such as Deming's PDSA, Six Sigma, and Lean. It is important for nurses to familiarize themselves with the types and workings of the models. Regardless of the QI method applied, ultimately QI should improve outcomes. Improved outcomes, however, does not guarantee staff will adopt new practice changes. One factor that influences adaptation, that may be minimized by QI teams, is applying principles of change theory throughout their project. There are a variety of change theories to consider that are beyond the scope of this chapter. Small et al. (2016) described their QI journey in adopting a handoff process that failed until the team applied principles of change theory to the project. After studying various change theories, the team selected a simple but effective theory commonly used in business, Kotter's Change Model, that incorporates eight steps:

1. Create a sense of urgency.
2. Form a guiding coalition.
3. Create a vision.
4. Communicate the vision.
5. Empower others to act.
6. Create quick wins.
7. Build on the change.
8. Institutionalize the change.

Staff's willingness to change practice based on QI outcomes is influenced by how well the QI team applies principles of change theory.

DONABEDIAN'S MODEL

Over 50 years ago, Avedis Donabedian proposed a model of quality assurance that is still used today: structure, process, and outcomes of care (Donabedian, 2003). **Structure** refers to "the conditions under which care is provided" such as nursing staff ratios or supplies available to provide patient care (Donabedian, 2003, p. 46). **Process** refers to "the activities that constitute healthcare" such as healthcare policies and standards of care (Donabedian, 2003, p. 46). **Outcomes** refer to the "changes (desirable or undesirable) in individuals and populations that can be attributed to healthcare" (Donabedian, 2003, p. 46). Outcomes may be clinical (urinary tract infections), functional (mobility), patient safety (medication errors), or patient/family satisfaction measures. It is important to understand that structure, process, and outcomes are not isolated. In fact, structures, processes, and outcomes are interdependent, meaning "specific attributes of one influence another according to the strength of the relationship" (Hughes, 2008a, p. 5). When evaluating outcomes, it is important to consider both the structural and process impacts on the

TABLE 11.2 EXAMPLES OF STRUCTURES, PROCESSES, AND OUTCOMES

STRUCTURE	PROCESS	OUTCOMES
Staffing (nurses, physicians, nursing assistants, advanced practice nurses) Infection control Skill mix Education level of staff Resources (e.g., computers, library databases, etc.) Supplies Technology Budget Leadership commitment/ engagement	Evidence-based guidelines Nursing process Standards of care Pathways Policies Motivated, engaged Staff Core measures Care routines (e.g., hourly rounding)	Hospital-acquired infections (e.g., Catheter-associated urinary tract infections, Central line associated blood stream infections, ventilator-associated pneumonia) Hospital-acquired pressure ulcers Fall rates Patient satisfaction Medication errors Infection rates Sentinel events/Never events

outcomes. Chapter 12's content explains that outcome data are used to determine if outcomes meet, exceed, or fail to meet expectations. When outcome data do not meet expectations, improvement interventions may be warranted. The structural and process elements associated with the outcome provide ideal opportunities for improvement interventions.

Donabedian's model was applied by the ANA's development of the NDNQI. The ANA's aim was to identify nurse-sensitive measures that could demonstrate the impact of nursing care on patient outcomes (Jones, 2016). Table 11.2 provides structure, process, and

CASE STUDY

QI teams often use Dr. W. Edwards Deming's **Plan-Do-Study-Act (PDSA)** model to implement QI projects. Deming incorporated knowledge of engineering, operations, and management with the goal of improving accuracy, reducing costs, and increasing efficiency and safety, all leading to satisfied customers. Deming described his philosophy as "a system of profound knowledge" composed of four parts: (a) appreciation for a system, (b) understanding process variation, (c) applying theory of knowledge, and (d) using psychology (Evans, 2008). The PDSA model and the actions within each step can be seen in Figure 11.1. Although some refer to the cycle as Plan-Do-Check-Act (PDCA), as originally developed by Walter Shewhart, Deming had strong beliefs that the terminology, PDCA, and PDSA, were very different and he only used the "PDSA cycle" to describe process improvement (Moen & Norman, 2009). Deming argued that "study" implied more of a rigorous scientific approach to QI measurement and outcomes analysis where "check" did not have the same connotation.

The advantage of using the PDSA cycle is that it is easy to understand, can be used cyclically on a smaller scale to perform small tests of change, or can be used when implementing large, system-wide improvements. The following questions can be used during the PDSA process (Langley et al., 2009):

1. *What is the goal of the project?*
2. *How can it be determined that the goal of the project was reached?*
3. *What needs to be done in order to reach the goal?*

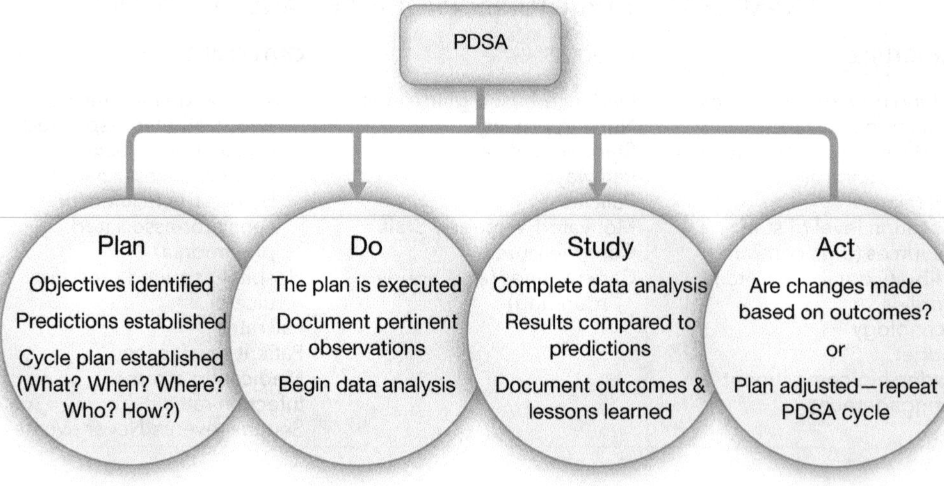

FIGURE 11.1 Plan-Do-Study-Act Model.

outcomes examples that support the delivery of patient care. This table will serve as a resource to use while working through the corresponding Case Study.

In the "Plan" stage, a plan to improve quality is developed. In this beginning project stage, planning includes a problem statement, evidence of the problem (baseline data), and a clear aim or specified goal used to evaluate the outcomes of the QI project. In addition, the Plan will include what the intervention will consist of and how it will be introduced. The "Do" stage is the actual implementation of the improvement intervention. No change can occur without taking some action. It is important to understand that one intervention is to be introduced within the PDSA cycle. The outcome of one intervention allows for the testing of that single intervention's ability to meet the goal. If multiple interventions are introduced simultaneously, it will be unclear which intervention is making the impact, or which one did not impact. After the intervention has been introduced over a period of time, evaluation of the impact the intervention had toward meeting the QI goal can now be determined or studied. The "Study" stage focuses on measurement by comparing the baseline to postintervention data to determine the intervention's impact toward the goal. Based on analysis, the QI team can now "Act." If the goal was met, the question becomes how to best sustain the improved outcome. If the goal was not met, the team needs to decide what the next intervention, or cycle, will consist of toward reaching the goal.

Because processes are complex, it may take multiple PDSA cycles to accomplish the goal, with each cycle introducing a new intervention, as seen in Figure 11.2. This also occurs if the intervention selected did not have the intended impact. When additional PDSA cycles are needed, the team creates a new PDSA. The PDSA cycles continue until a solution is reached and implemented (Langley et al., 2009). Silver, McQuillan, et al. (2016) discuss how one of the greatest challenges of QI is in sustaining the improved change over time. Silver, Harel, et. all. (2016) offer QI teams ways to sustain their efforts because approximately 70% of QI outcomes are not sustained. Considering the time, effort, and work QI teams incur, lack of sustainment may impact patient safety and cost to the organization. This unfortunate reality may result in reduced leadership support in conducting QI.

Box 11.3 provides an example of how the PDSA model works in an organization. Nurses have an advantage in applying the PDSA model because the PDSA model is closely replicated in the nursing process of assessment (plan), diagnosis (plan), planning (plan), implementation (do), and evaluation (study and act).

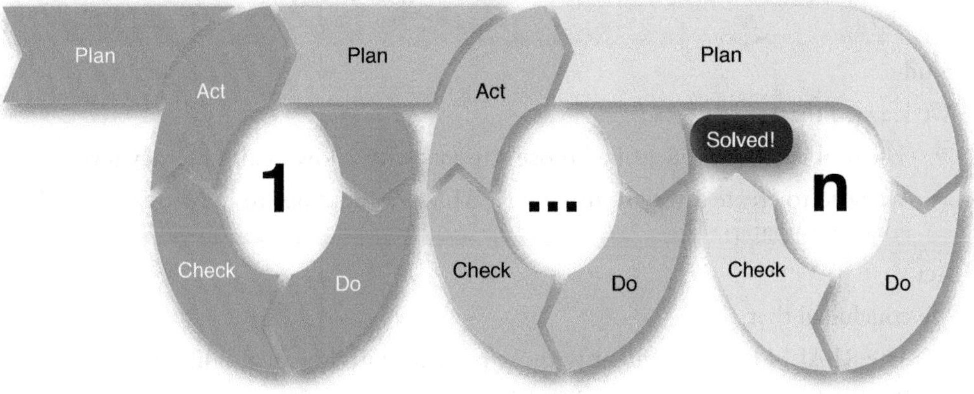

FIGURE 11.2 Multiple PDSA Cycles.

PDSA, Plan-Do-Study-Act.

Source: Courtesy of Christopher Roser at AllAboutLean.com.

BOX 11.3 Example of PDSA

Problem: Patients do not appear to understand health education provided in the hospital as evidenced by high rates of readmissions for the same diagnosis, patients not understanding medications and not taking them as directed, and missing appointments with the physician after discharge.

Solution: Assess the patient's understanding of health information by performing the health literacy assessment using the REALM short-form tool.

Plan

We plan to

- Train nurses to use the REALM health literacy assessment tool to identify those patients with low health literacy. Patients identified as having low health literacy will have education provided at an easier-to-understand level.
- Implement the REALM tool for 1 week on one unit for all patient admissions to assess health literacy.
- Create an area in the computerized charting system to document the results.

Do

We found that:

- Not all patients are directly admitted to the unit; therefore, they did not have a health literacy assessment.
- Completing the REALM tool was time-consuming until the nurses became used to the tool.
- The findings from the use of the REALM tool were not used to individualize health education materials.

(*continued*)

BOX 11.3 Example of PDSA (*continued*)

Study

We learned that:

- The tool accurately identified those patients with a low health literacy level.
- We need to create a way to use the REALM tool findings to individualize health education materials.

Act

We concluded that:

- The REALM tool does identify those patients with low health literacy.
- We need to look at what we do with the information from the REALM health literacy assessment.
- We need to look at ways to meet the patient's individual health education needs by creating an online repository of health education materials designed for low health literacy education.

PDSA, Plan-Do-Study-Act; REALM, Rapid Estimate of Adult Literacy in Medicine.

As mentioned earlier in this chapter, there are many factors that may reduce QI sustainment, such as not considering factors that influence change. Marshall et al. (2016) spoke about their experience conducting an improvement and identified six risks to be aware of that may contribute to QI process failures:

1. The problem may be defined too vaguely or lack clarity.
2. There may be a lack of a clearly defined methodology, such as PDSA.
3. Interventions involve people who function in a social context. Social context may not be considered in the identification or deployment of the intervention.
4. What the intervention is, how it is deployed, and the organizational context are interdependent.
5. Evaluation and actions based on evaluation may occur too rapidly.
6. QI teams may lack a necessary level of expertise. Service users, improvement specialists, clinicians, and potentially academic partners can all contribute.

Also consider that although interprofessional staff are expected to participate in QI activities, not all will bring the QI QSEN KSAs to the project. There are many resources to assist healthcare professionals who may need orientation to QI methods. The IHI Model for Improvement, accessible at www.ihi.org, is an excellent resource.

LEAN

The principles of **Lean** thinking strive to eliminate forms of waste within a process to increase efficiency while enhancing effectiveness (Hallam & Contreras, 2018). According to Shrank et al. (2019), waste accounts for approximately 25% of healthcare spending. Healthcare organizations are applying Lean methodologies to QI projects to increase efficiency and to reduce waste. There are eight identified sources of waste in organizations: unnecessary services/overproduction, mistakes/defects, delays in waiting, unnecessary motion, over processing, excessive inventory, excessive transport, and unused human

CASE STUDY

You are a nurse manager of a long-term care unit. Due to the Coronavirus pandemic, the facility leadership is requiring every unit to develop creative methods that may reduce the risk of transmission or isolation, or improve staff ability to provide palliative care when appropriate among this vulnerable population. Regardless of treatment or vaccination for Coronavirus, leadership is using the pandemic to improve weaknesses the pandemic identified. Leadership has scheduled a poster session where each unit will showcase and disseminate their QI outcomes that must conform to the Institute for Healthcare Improvement's (IHI) Model of Improvement. The units were divided, and your unit was one of three units assigned palliative care. Your staff is not trained on QI models but has received specific training on Coronavirus.

1. *As a nurse manager, what administrative judgments can you make based on the cues in this scenario?*
2. *What actions to improve knowledge on the Model for Improvement should you take? Go to IHI.org. In the search box, type in "Model for Improvement." Review the two brief videos:*

   Model for Improvement (Part 1) www.ihi.org/education/IHIOpenSchool/resources/Pages/AudioandVideo/Whiteboard3.aspx

   Model for Improvement (Part 2) www.ihi.org/education/IHIOpenSchool/resources/Pages/AudioandVideo/Whiteboard4.aspx
3. *After viewing the two videos, you decide to use them for staff training. What actions would be most effective in creating unit-based training?*
4. *To evaluate the effectiveness of the training, you establish a set of standardized questions you will ask participants after the videos are shown. To prepare, you must first answer the questions yourself:*
   a. *What is the first question asked in the Model for Improvement?*
   b. *What is the second question asked in the Model for Improvement?*
   c. *What is the third question asked in the Model for Improvement?*
   d. *How does the Model for Improvement get activated?*
   e. *How would implementing multiple cycles of a PDSA impact the Model for Improvement?*
5. *Once training is completed, you begin to consider who will lead the QI project. You have several ideas. What position would be most effective in leading a QI team on palliative care?*

potential/overburden (Hallam & Contreras, 2018). When these sources of waste occur, employees may figure out work-arounds rather than considering new processes to improve efficiency. A work-around is a deviation from an approved process or procedure often done to increase efficiency or to create a "short-cut" that is perceived to be "more" efficient. There are risks associated with not following approved processes or procedures. For example, the nursing assistant is tasked with changing bed linens for each patient every day. To make the process quicker, the midnight shift nursing assistant collects the linens and places them in each patient's room. This action saves the day shift nursing assistant time in having to gather linens. Although a seemingly innocent and kind gesture, a problem arises when the original patient is discharged before the linens are used. The linens are then sent back to laundry for cleaning, causing an increase in workload for the laundry workers. Even worse, the linens might be used for the newly admitted patient.

The danger of a work-around is the error that may result from creating and applying nonapproved processes. Lean interventions center on improving efficiency, reducing waste, and streamlining processes that are patient and employee centered. Lean thinking builds on the belief that it is the sum or cumulative effect of many small improvements that creates the greatest impact in performance (Evans, 2008). Small, low-cost, and low-risk improvements are easily implemented with the goal to keep the project simple over a short duration of time. Lean addresses visible problems. For example, a nurse can see that items in a clean utility room are orderly or in disarray. Color-coding shelves to hold specific types of equipment or supplies helps to quickly identify an item. Placing items together that are typically needed at the same time such as an indwelling urinary catheter kit next to a clean specimen collection kit is an example of Lean. A nurse searching for supplies is wasted time that can be much better spent. Simple Lean tools, such as the 5S process, can be quickly and easily applied to ensure the work environment is clean and organized, which will reduce nonvalue-added activity that wastes the nurse's time. Lean is easily taught, intuitive, and easy to apply in practice. The improvement process of 5S also impacts patient safety by standardizing the environment, allowing staff to consistently locate the products used to deliver patient care. The 5S process includes the following:

1. Sorting the necessary from the unnecessary; discard unnecessary items.
2. Set items in order; everything has a place and keep everything where it belongs.
3. Shine; keep the area clean, neat, and organized.
4. Standardize the area.
5. Sustain the first four Ss (Hadfield et al., 2009).

Although reducing healthcare waste seems logical, Cohen (2018) provides an excellent overview of Lean in healthcare but identifies that some healthcare organizations may object to Lean principles because Lean was founded in manufacturing. Objection may result in perceptions that patients are not automobiles or healthcare organizations are not assembly lines. Cohen (2018) argues that healthcare and manufacturing do have similarities. Both are in business to produce high-quality products, have limited resources, require complex processes with numerous inputs and outputs to each process, and must meet or surpass customer satisfaction. Applying Lean principles in healthcare to reduce unnecessary waste has a profound impact on patients. For example, patients want efficient and timely care, simplified and timely access, streamlined procedures, continuity of their healthcare management, and coordinated care. These few examples and many more can be improved by applying Lean principles.

SIX SIGMA AND DEFINE, MEAUSRE, ANALYZE, IMPROVE, AND CONTROL

Six Sigma, one of the more advanced methodologies adopted from the business sector, encompasses interventions with the goal to reduce variation in existing processes. In doing so, it often leads to new process design or redesign. When a process is carried out inconsistently, the outcomes of that process vary over time, leading to process variation. The goal is to reduce variation by standardizing the process so that the process's outcomes are consistent over time. Consider a nurse working on a surgical unit with a common nursing intervention of pain reassessment after providing pain medication. Because the

TABLE 11.3 DEFINE, MEASURE, ANALYZE, IMPROVE, AND CONTROL (DMAIC)

Define	Identifies the QI focus. Defines the team, operational definition of the variable, baseline data and improvement aim or expected level of performance when variability is reduced, and the project timeline. Tools such as fishbone diagrams and process maps are used to define the problem.
Measure	Includes identifying the current process, validating the variable to measure, assessing baseline performance, and selecting who will conduct measurement procedures. Tools such as Pareto charts and process control charts are often useful in this step (see Chapter 12).
Analyze	Rigorous analysis to understand top causes of why errors are occurring. Tools such as statistical measurements, control charts, fishbone diagrams, and hypothesis testing are often useful in this step (see Chapter 12 and the fishbone diagram in this chapter).
Improve	Brainstorming what solutions may be useful in reducing variation and conducting small-scale trials of possible solutions.
Control	Methods to sustain improvements, such as employee education, and the process for ongoing measurement to ensure the new and improved processes are sustained over time.

QI, quality improvement.

pain reassessment policy would stipulate the reassessment and documentation requirement post-medication administration, a nurse can measure how consistently that is being accomplished. If the policy stipulates 30 minutes as the time frame from administration to reassessment, outcomes hovering around that 30-minute time frame would demonstrate a stable process. If the average time were found to be 45 minutes with a range of 33 to 48 minutes, the process demonstrates variation. Not only does this example show if staff are following the policy, it also speaks to the risk that patients may continue to experience pain because they are not consistently being reassessed.

Six Sigma incorporates several problem-solving steps to reduce variation in a healthcare process (Evans, 2008). The steps are known as define, measure, analyze, improve, and control, or DMAIC, as defined in Table 11.3.

Although similar, there are appreciable differences between Lean and Six Sigma. Lean focuses on reducing waste while Six Sigma is more focused on variation in performance and requires specialized skills and statistical tools, making it a more sophisticated improvement approach. There are QI professionals who believe it is first necessary to make a process more efficient before attempting to reduce variation, thus combining the two methodologies within QI activities.

APPROACHES TO QUALITY IMPROVEMENT PROBLEMS

The QI process is often a critical response to an adverse event, near miss, or sentinel event. To identify the actual cause of a problem and implement improvement strategies, it is important to know how the problems are identified and resulting specific actions by a QI team. Uncovering the problem can be more difficult than one might expect. Reactive strategies are those actions that occur after an event has taken place, such as peer review (discussed earlier in the chapter) and root cause analysis (RCA). Healthcare Failure Mode and Effect Analysis (HFMEA) is a proactive method to identify risks before they result in errors, allowing the team to prevent problems in high-risk processes before a near miss or adverse event occurs.

RETROACTIVE APPROACH: ROOT CAUSE ANALYSIS

A **root cause analysis** (RCA) is an investigation of what caused a problem and why the problem occurred. Haxby and Shuldham (2018) outline three stages of the RCA process:

1. Identifying the fundamental issues and contributing factors that resulted in an incident.
2. Asking crucial questions of what, how, and why the incident happened.
3. Recommending opportunities for improvement, to mitigate similar future risks.

The most frequent root causes of sentinel events reported to TJC between 2005 to 2018 can be viewed at www.jointcommission.org/resources/patient-safety-topics/sentinel-event/sentinel-event-data----event-type-by-year. Unfortunately, these reports reveal consistent sentinel events to include unintended retention of foreign object, wrong-patient, wrong-site, wrong-procedure, and falls despite efforts to mitigate them.

The RCA process is also a valuable tool that can be used in any instance where the need to know the underlying root cause of a problem exists. RCAs are formal and often interprofessional. Nurses are often invited to participate on RCA teams because nurses are integral and participate in most care delivery as the ones who bring clinical knowledge and skill in identifying the root cause and potential corrective action. Completing the Developing Clinical Judgment box will reinforce the role of the nurse in RCAs.

RCAs are conducted when an actual error has occurred and require **corrective action**, the action taken to eliminate the cause(s) of an error with the goal to prevent recurrence (International Organization for Standardization, 2015b). For example, a patient with insulin-dependent diabetes is given the wrong dose of insulin. Although the patient did not experience any detrimental effects, the medication error is considered an adverse event. The staff determined that an RCA can help determine the contributing factors to the medication error and how to prevent similar errors from occurring. An interprofessional team consisting of nurses, physicians, nursing assistants, quality department representative, central supply representative, and clinical educator is gathered to investigate the problem. To conduct an RCA, the following steps occur:

1. Identify what happened.
2. Review what should have happened.
3. Determine causes.
4. Develop causal statements.
5. Generate a list of recommended changes.
6. Share findings with those who affect or are affected by the outcome.
7. Ensure actions are taken and sustained to prevent or reduce the risk of future recurrence.

The first step, identify what happened, occurs through a dialogue among all team members. The team starts with the statement that a medication error occurred, resulting in 10 times the ordered dose of insulin given to the patient. The clear statement brings all team members to the same starting point to examine the problem.

To understand what happened, the team develops a flow chart (Figure 11.3) of the insulin preparation process. Team members use the flow chart to identify and examine factors in the process that may have contributed to the near miss or sentinel event. The process is mapped out to show each of the steps involved with the insulin preparation process.

Those team members directly involved with the medication error provide information about steps that can highlight process problems. It is important to note here that the RCA looks at process breakdowns rather than the individual person's error. In this scenario, the

CASE STUDY

You are a member of your organization's CPR Committee. One committee responsibility is to review all rapid response team (RRT) documents to determine if the RRT was an appropriate action and what follow-up steps are necessary. The first review is an 80-year-old patient admitted for abdominal pain found to have ulcerative colitis. The patient had a bowel resection with an uneventful postoperative recovery period. On the second postoperative day, however, an RRT was called based on assessment findings of a pulse of 130, blood pressure (BP) 70/30, and PulseOx 87%. The patient had been completely oriented but is now disoriented to place and time. During the RRT, the patient was given a liter of normal saline and transferred to the ICU. The patient's condition worsened in the ICU, leading to intubation. The CPR Committee has asked you as the nurse committee member to present this case to the Committee. In preparation, you begin by reviewing medication administration records in the EMR. Although antibiotics were ordered, three postop doses were not documented as given. Morphine Sulfate was ordered and given consistently every 6 hours for postoperative pain as prescribed. Because of time, your initial preparation ends.

1. *To continue preparation for your presentation to the Committee, what additional clinical information would you evaluate before the Committee meeting to effectively present this case?*
2. *In addition to clinical data, what nonclinical other data would you need to evaluate to determine appropriateness of the RRT?*
3. *After your overview, which includes the nurse who called the RRT and did follow the RRT procedure, the chair of the Committee asks for your judgment and recommendations:*
   a. *What recommendation would you, the nurse, make regarding appropriateness of the RRT based on the RRT procedure?*
   b. *While reviewing the case, what cues did you identify as potential root causes that may have precipitated this outcome? Identify four potential root causes from the scenario.*
   c. *Would you recommend this Committee should refer this case for an official RCA to be conducted?*

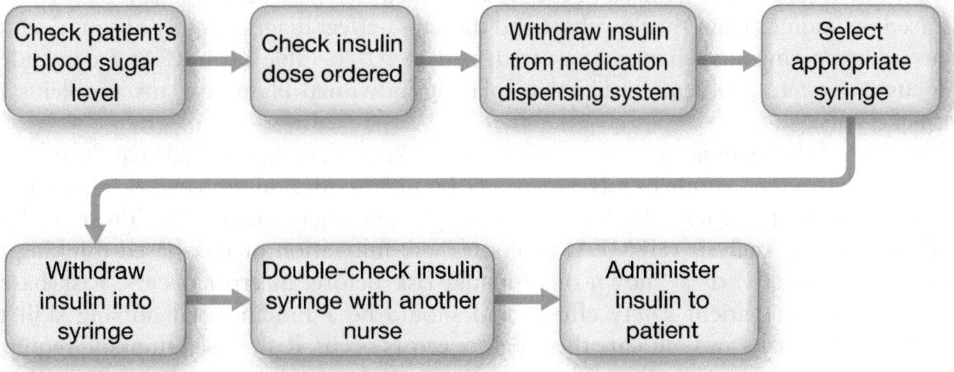

FIGURE 11.3 Flowchart of Insulin Preparation

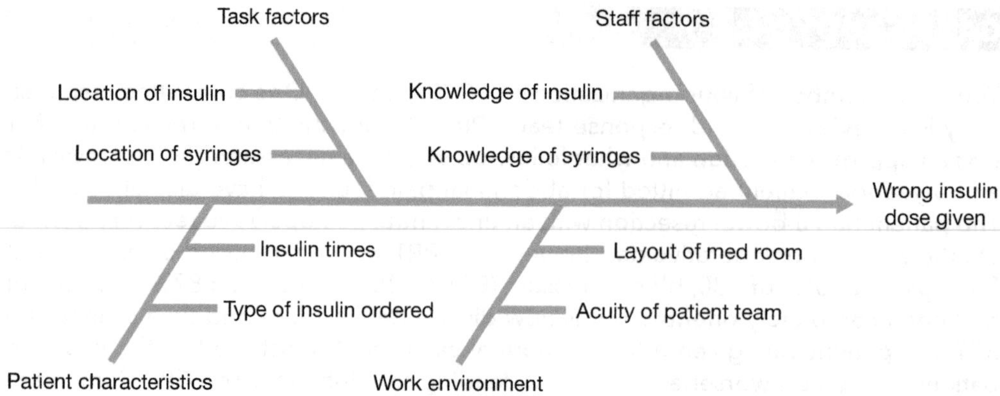

FIGURE 11.4 Fishbone Diagram.

nurse is not viewed as causing the error; rather, a breakdown in the process allowed the error to occur. This encourages all participants to fully engage in identifying contributing factors.

The next step is to determine causes. A cause-effect diagram, or fishbone diagram, helps participants understand the contributing factors to the medication error. The "bones" of the fish, as seen in Figure 11.4, represent the common areas that might contribute to the problem. Common categories seen on cause-effect diagrams are methods or task factors, people or patient/staff characteristics, work environment, and equipment (Institute for Healthcare Improvement, 2017). It is important to note that the categories, or bones of the fish, may have different labels depending on what template is used.

Each area is discussed by team members and examined in terms of what happened during the near miss or sentinel event that contributed to the outcome. During this process, an effective method to get at the core causes of the problem is to ask "Why/" five times. Asking "Wh?" five times helps the team dig deeper into the actual process issues that caused the problem. For example, a problem could be finding time to study for an examination. Asking "Why?" helps clarify what the core of the problem is. By the time the fifth "Why?" is asked, the core root of the problem should become evident.

During the creation of the flowchart, the team identified that the nurse reached for a syringe from a drawer labeled "insulin syringes," but instead the drawer was stocked with tuberculin syringes. This resulted in the nurse giving 10 times the ordered dose of insulin. Another misstep occurred when the nurse asked another nurse to double-check the dose of insulin. The second nurse glanced at the syringe and agreed the dose was correct.

Based on findings from the flowchart and the cause-effect diagram, a list of causal statements and recommended changes is created, as depicted in Table 11.4. RCAs are intended to focus on system problems rather than placing individual blame for any problems or sentinel events.

The goal of the team is to improve the safety of known, complex, high-risk healthcare processes before they result in adverse events by identifying, minimizing, or eliminating high-risk aspects and other vulnerabilities of the process. Therefore, the **Healthcare Failure Mode and Effect Analysis (HFMEA)** promotes risk mitigation or **risk-based-thinking** to eliminate the cause(s) of a known or potential risk before an error occurs. Risk-based thinking enhances patient safety efforts and should be a fundamental nursing skill to identify practice risks and mitigate them before errors occur. Risk-based thinking requires accurate nursing judgment, ethical decision-making to act, and follow through to ensure appropriate actions are implemented timely.

TABLE 11.4 CAUSAL STATEMENTS AND RECOMMENDED CHANGES

CAUSAL STATEMENTS	RECOMMENDED CHANGES
Tuberculin syringes were inappropriately stocked in the insulin syringe drawer.	Move tuberculin syringes to a different location.
Tuberculin and insulin syringes both have orange caps and black markings on the syringe.	Check with other vendors about the availability of different colored syringes.
Verifying the insulin dose with another nurse did not catch the medication error.	Double-checks with another nurse need to include specific steps such as looking at the type of syringe, the amount of medication in the syringe, and the dose ordered.

CASE STUDY

Because healthcare processes are complex and often people-dependent, **risks** or deviation from what the process is expected to accomplish may result (International Organization for Standardization, 2015a). HFMEA is a prospective risk analysis system to identify, assess, and address vulnerabilities in high-risk processes. Failure Mode and Effect Analysis (FMEA) has its roots in the U.S. military, engineering, and aerospace industries, where steps are taken to minimize or eliminate the risk that an accident or failure will occur. In 2001, the U.S. Department of Veterans Affairs, National Center for Patient Safety, developed a hybrid model specific to, and ideal for, the healthcare environment (DeRosier et al., 2002). At the same time, TJC introduced a new leadership standard, still in effect today, that speaks to healthcare leaders ensuring a proactive risk assessment be conducted for identified high-risk processes (TJC, 2020b). Three basic questions are the focus of any proactive failure mode/risk analysis:

1. *What could go wrong?*
2. *Why would the failures occur?*
3. *What would be the consequences of each failure?*

Many errors can be prevented by informal or formal risk mitigation. Many organizations offer HFMEA resources but, in general, flow mapping and fishbone diagrams are commonly used tools by HFMEA teams. For example, the administration of a heparin infusion, a high-risk medication, involves many complex steps including calculating the patient's weight in kilograms, ensuring the correct amount of heparin is in the solution, changing doses, and administering boluses based on laboratory studies. The role of the provider who must order the heparin correctly, the pharmacist who may prepare or deliver the heparin, and the nurse who must administer the heparin are all involved in a process with risk for error. HFMEA allows the team to assess potential risks of each step. Teams prioritize actions based on a severity of risk rating scale. The VA National Center for Patient Safety (accessible at www.patientsafety.va.gov/professionals/onthejob/hfmea.asp) identifies five steps to be completed during a HFMEA:

1. Define the HFMEA topic.
2. Assemble the team.
3. Graphically describe the process.

4. Conduct a hazard analysis.
5. Perform actions and outcome measures.

HFMEA improvement strategies commonly involve redesigning processes to minimize or eliminate identified risks. Of consideration, nurses should maintain an ongoing awareness of those high-risk processes that may serve well for an HFMEA. Nurses are encouraged to participate or lead teams, as many high-risk processes involve nursing judgment and oversight, and will therefore benefit from that nursing expertise. Teams conducting an HFMEA will identify many actions believed to reduce the risk of error from occurring. The team must also prioritize actions based on a risk assessment.

The added value of nurses participating in QI activities is more evident once the basics of QI are learned, including models and improvement methods. Nurses collaborating to improve patient care is an expectation of practice and of your employer. While working toward improvement is rewarding and necessary, challenges may occur. Work through the corresponding Case Study.

CASE STUDY

Each QI methodology discussed in this chapter has value and application depending on the situation. QI tools, mainly discussed in Chapter 12, are often shared within QI methodologies. For example, flow mapping can be used in any QI activity to better understand the process under investigation. Read the corresponding Current Literature feature that demonstrates how one improvement activity utilized many of the methodologies and tools discussed in this chapter.

CURRENT LITERATURE

CITATION

Wilson, J., Swee, M., Mosher, H., Scott-Cawiezell, J., Levins, L., Fort, K., & Kumar, B. (2020). Using lean six sigma to improve pneumococcal vaccination rates in a veterans affairs rheumatology clinic. *Journal for Healthcare Quality, 42*(3), 166–174.

DISCUSSION

The authors clearly make a case for improved vaccination rates against pneumococcal disease. Vulnerable populations, such as immunocompromised patients are at greater risk for pneumococcal disease. A VA Rheumatology Clinic audit result demonstrated a <3% vaccination rate, a definite opportunity for improvement. Rather than one improvement approach, the authors apply multiple improvement methodologies to meet their goal of 70%. The interprofessional QI team describe their use of applying multiple QI methods. A **preintervention process mapping** (flow map) that was used to identify barriers to the time required for vaccination administration. The **Define-Measure-Analyze-Improve-Control** (DMAIC) is presented to outline the QI process. To test interventions, three **PDSA cycles** were conducted where Cycle-1 was provider education, Cycle-2 reinforcement of provider education and voice of the customer, and Cycle-3 Workflow improvements. Pre-intervention (current state) and post-intervention (future state) **process maps** were created. A **control chart** (discussed in Chapter 12) was used to track vaccination rates during the PDSA cycles. **Voice of the Customer** was also used to better understand veteran perceptions of vaccinations, provider awareness, those involved with the actual administration of the vaccination, and medical assistants/schedulers regarding timeliness. Despite these efforts, the authors reported an increase from 3% to 23% vaccinations, well short of the 70% goal. The authors provide rational why the goal was not met and determined 70% was too ambitious when starting at 3%. Educational interventions were not sustained. The QI methods used in the project allowed the interprofessional team a better understand how complex meeting vaccination guidelines can be and how more PDSA cycles will be needed.

IMPLICATIONS FOR PRACTICE

There are several implications. First, establishing realistic goals is necessary in QI. Second, there are valuable lessons learned from QI not meeting goals. In this citation, educational interventions were not sustained. That said, educational interventions may be successful in a different situation or setting. The authors successfully demonstrated how multiple QI methods can be applied within one project. This is important because health care is complex. Flow mapping a process can illustrate where interventions may be used to reduce process steps that may increase outcomes. Studying the process map alone may identify numerous interventions, each serving as a new PDSA cycle toward meeting the goals. Consider various QI methods when you are a member of a QI team and do not be afraid of not meeting goals. Rather, consider that more opportunities for improvement. QI teams should celebrate outcomes even when not meeting goals because of lessons learned and that the team is working to continuously improve. Also note that when conducting QI, voice of the customer does may not only mean patients. Staff involved in the process serve as customers and their voice matters. Staff in the process often have ideas how to improve the process.

CASE STUDY

As important as team members are in QI activities, appreciate that not every improvement requires a formal, full team to be successful. A new nurse brings a great advantage to the work area because they will see opportunities for small-scale changes and daily improvements that other staff may not recognize. Every organization has problems big and small and every process has at least some irritant. It is the staff doing the work every day that is most knowledgeable about what those irritants are, how they affect the workflow, and what the best possible fixes may be. When every staff member makes "seemingly small" improvements every day, a fully engaged workforce emerges that is committed to improvement. Together, over time, that can add up to significant organizational improvements in patient care and outcomes. By encouraging those daily improvements, leaders demonstrate support by recognizing staff knowledge, skills, and commitment toward improving quality and patient safety. Staff is empowered and sees the value of doing "what is possible today." New staff that are sometimes overwhelmed by the complexity, length, and breadth of large formal QI projects that can go on for months or more can appreciate and enjoy the small successes that come from small tests of change. Those successes can then be the impetus for involvement in larger scale QI projects.

THE ROLE OF THE NURSE IN QUALITY IMPROVEMENT

As described earlier in this chapter, the nursing process mimics QI. Nurses collect patient data, analyze the data, plan and implement nursing interventions, and evaluate patient outcomes for decision-making. This foundation in preparing nurses for practice also prepares nurses to participate and lead QI activities.

Nurses can assume a variety of roles when conducting QI activities. Novice nurses committed to improving care can help collect data or assist with literature reviews for more complex improvement interventions; therefore, it is important to know what sources of data and information are available, how to access them, and who the QI resources are. When processes involve multiple disciplines, representatives from each discipline should be included on the QI team. To better understand the importance of selecting QI team members, complete the corresponding Case Study.

In addition to participating or leading QI is the expectation of disseminating QI outcomes. There are many venues to disseminate what was done and improvements from the QI project. Feedback and dissemination of the results of QI projects are essential for improvement. Healthcare and professional organizations offer a variety of mechanisms including newsletters, presentations, posters, new employee orientation, email communication, staff training, staff meetings, and unit-based communication boards. One method of sharing QI data is to use scorecards or dashboards that use a quick-look approach to show where the current standing is on a quality issue in relation to benchmarks. QI outcomes can stimulate other professionals to assess their area of care delivery or processes to determine if improvement is warranted or not. QI outcomes can also identify potential interventions that others can consider and apply when successful or possibly avoid if unsuccessful. The various lessons learned when conducting QI also have value and could help other nurses be more efficient in their efforts. Academic education also utilizes QI, particularly when assessing curriculum to determine if improvement is needed. Read the corresponding Current Literature feature that describes how academic QI utilizes guidelines to standardize dissemination of academic improvements and will introduce another example of an improvement methodology.

CURRENT LITERATURE

CITATION

Ogrinc, G., Armstrong, G. E., Dolansky, M. A., Singh, M. K., & Davies, L. (2019). SQUIRE-EDU (Standards for Quality Improvement Reporting Excellence in Education): Publication guidelines for educational improvement. *Academic Medicine, 94*(10), 1461–1470.

DISCUSSION

Not every change is based on QI, but every successful QI outcome should result in some change. For change to occur, improvement outcomes need disseminated or reported. There are many venues such as speaking at conferences, presenting posters, sharing at staff meetings, etc. In this chapter, many improvement methods have been described. PDSA for example is one model that can easily be used for disseminating QI outcomes. The SQUIRE Guidelines (Standards for QUality Improvement Reporting Excellence) is another, more scholarly example of a standardized means of reporting health care improvements. Standardizing dissemination increases the reader or participant ability to better understand the details of the QI and its potential application to their work. In the citation, the authors nicely outline the SQUIRE Guidelines. As you review the guidelines, you will see how the guidelines include many PDSA concepts but add additional detail. For example, in PDSA, a description of the intervention occurs at step 2, or within the DO of the Plan-Do-Study-Act. For the SQUIRE guidelines, the intervention is also outlined but adds more specifics such as commenting on ethical considerations addressed or mitigated specific to how the QI intervention was implemented. Because academics is also working to continuously improve, the same reporting principles apply to reporting academic QI. The authors describe how the SQUIRE Guidelines can be modified to report on educational QI for standardization of educational QI among health professions (SQUIRE-EDU). For example, the SQUIRE guideline for ethical considerations mentioned above has an educational ethical QI component. For example, did the educational QI intervention consider vulnerable learners, such as learners with English as a second language and if so, how did that impact the intervention.

IMPLICATIONS FOR PRACTICE

Conducting QI without disseminating outcomes, even those unsuccessful outcomes, is necessary for professional growth and to promote patient safety. Just as our colleagues in practice need to hear, read, and share QI outcomes, academic QI is also working to improve and needs to disseminate educational QI outcomes. Standardizing how these outcomes are reported has value for those reading or listening to better analyze, synthesize, and determine applicability of outcomes to their practice or curriculum. Journals, such as the Journal of Nursing Education, is one example where curricular innovations and improvements are published.

Nurses are expected to have the KSAs to assess, analyze, intervene, and evaluate not just patient outcomes, but outcomes that reflect individual and interdisciplinary practice. Salmond and Echevarria (2017) offer some advice. Nurses will need to shift their focus from episodic care to care across the continuum, partner with patients and families, and consider the social context to include resources that support wellness and independence. Assessing care across the continuum to include social context requires a skill set, such as auditing.

AUDITING

The International Organization for Standardization defines **audit** as a documented, systematic process to obtain objective evidence of conformity or nonconformity to established procedures or requirements (International Organization for Standardization, 2015a). In healthcare, determining conformity or nonconformity occurs in several ways. An external audit, such as TJC, is an independent organization that establishes evidence-based criteria, then audits to that criteria to determine if the organization is conforming to the criteria. External audits provide some form of certification or accreditation and often are required for reimbursement. External auditors have no vested interest in the organization they are auditing.

External accreditation not only impacts reimbursement but also implies the organization successfully met the requirements that were surveyed. Confirming requirements are met is important to the organization's patients, families, and staff because it demonstrates a level of reliability. Because accreditation is important, the organization's ability to determine **survey readiness**, or ensuring all staff know and follow regulatory requirements and that established processes to meet requirements are followed, is a priority. Survey readiness speaks to how assured the organization is should an external auditor or surveyor, such as TJC, arrive to inspect the organization. One method an organization may employ to determine their survey readiness is to create a formal Internal Audit Program.

One aim of an internal audit is to self-identify errors or risks and mitigate them before external surveys occur. Internal auditors, or select employees who work for the organization, are trained to audit their own organization's processes to determine conformity to regulatory requirements. The added value of internal audits is to self-identify process errors or risks for potential error and take action to mitigate them. Establishing formal internal audits and teams to conduct them is common practice. For example, many healthcare organizations employ Environment of Care internal audits to assess environmental requirements, such as verifying that no used reusable medical equipment is found in a clean utility room. Earlier in this chapter, TJC tracer methodology was introduced. Conducting internal audits closely replicates tracer methodologies as both assess complex or high-risk processes. Audit teams are typically interprofessional and include subject matter experts. For example, if a mock survey of a complex process such as medication administration was being performed, the audit team should minimally include representatives from pharmacy, nursing, and medicine as these services are all involved in medication administration. Nurses are excellent candidates and are often requested to serve on internal audit teams because nurses are involved in many care delivery processes. For this reason, Review Activity #5 at the end of Chapter 11 was created to further explore principles of auditing. The act of auditing is only one aspect of survey readiness. Internal auditing serves no purpose if results are not mitigated prior to an external audit. More importantly, audit results identify what the organization needs to focus on to improve, which has direct impact on patient safety outcomes.

LEADERSHIP SUPPORT

There are many factors that contribute to successful QI initiatives, including engaged leadership (Kampstra et al., 2018). A supportive and empowering organizational culture and leadership commitment is necessary for optimal QI. Given the ramifications of quality outcome performance for organizational reimbursement, there are financial implications that impact leadership's full support for improving hospital processes. This includes clinical and administrative processes, as well as processes managed by support services. Leaders are the catalyst of change (Sandberg, 2018). Leaders must demonstrate their commitment. For example, visibility by rounding on patient care units and directly talking with staff could lead to identifying quality and safety concerns. Having access to leadership empowers staff to voice strengths and challenges. Effective leaders partner with their employees by empowering them to ask questions, seek new ways of doing business, remove fear of failure and reporting it, and provide the resources needed to try new ideas that may improve organizational performance. Lindberg and Kimberlain (2008) note that if the intent of every healthcare worker is to provide quality care, then the responsibility of executives is to create a culture for that to occur.

Organizational leaders support QI activities by providing a set of clear expectations, providing ongoing and meaningful feedback, ensuring staff are educated on QI methodologies, and providing time away from duties to devote to improvement. When an organization's leadership participates in QI projects, it sends the message that quality is a shared team responsibility. By the same token, nurses, physicians, and the entire interdisciplinary healthcare team must actively engage in QI efforts by bringing issues to leadership's attention from the ground up. If this can occur, improvements are more likely to be meaningful and sustained. Nurse managers and leaders must use caution, however, on the amount of raw data and information shared. Large quantities of unanalyzed data and information can become difficult to understand, overwhelming, and less meaningful for staff. It is best to share concise analyses that highlight how a process was improved or how a quality benchmark was met (Lindberg & Kimberlain, 2008). It is leadership's responsibility to balance QI activities, practice, and dissemination of outcomes.

OVERCOMING QUALITY IMPROVEMENT BARRIERS

In today's complex healthcare organizations, it is the responsibility of both novice and expert nurses to improve quality. It is intuitive to nurses to want to improve and focus on enhanced patient outcomes (Berwick, 2011). In fact, the optimal goal of nursing care is to improve health, improve the processes and systems that contribute to positive outcomes, and reduce harm. Despite everyone's responsibility, limitations or barriers toward nurse's involvement in QI exist. Dunagan (2017) created and tested a nurse QI attitude survey and found nurses were unclear as to their role in QI and not feeling safe in reporting safety risks. Although a small survey sample size, fear of reporting risks must be mitigated to truly create a culture of continual improvement. Risks must be listened to, evaluated, and serve as opportunities for improvement when substantiated. Rather than fear, leadership and the culture must celebrate identified risks. Only then can a just culture and high reliability be realized.

Although it is the goal of many healthcare organizations to engage the healthcare team in QI initiatives, a significant barrier is adequate time for healthcare workers and support staff to participate in improvement projects. Additionally, nurses may want to, or feel obligated to, participate in QI initiatives, but they may lack the knowledge and skills necessary to comfortably and actively participate. Moreover, many of these challenges can be overcome with a style of leadership called shared governance.

Shared governance is a professional practice model founded on the principles of partnership, equity, accountability, and ownership that form a culturally sensitive and empowering framework, enabling sustainable and accountability-based decisions to support an interdisciplinary design for excellent patient care (Cox-Sullivan et al., 2017). It is the shared control over nursing practice and clinical decision-making that empowers staff nurses and managers to work together for successful QI projects. When frontline staff nurses actively participate in QI and take control over their practice, the expected result is a better work environment, better staff satisfaction, improved staff retention, and better patient outcomes, all of which impact the patient's healthcare experience.

Internal auditing may be a potential QI barrier. Auditors who are subjective or unfamiliar with the criteria they are auditing to can miss nonconformities. Auditors may not know how to identify evidence that confirms conformity when assessing complex processes across the organization. They must have interview skills when obtaining information from staff or patients and consider the social context to responses. These examples of auditor barriers indicate training and competency is required that may not be provided. It may also be wrongfully assumed experience equates to auditor skills. In addition, for successful survey readiness, audit results need analyzed, corrective actions implemented when appropriate, and potentially QI activities conducted using the various methods described in this chapter. Without a clear process for reporting audit results to process owners who mitigate them and follow up to ensure mitigated actions have been sustained, survey readiness may not occur. The barriers associated with internal audits and auditors can be overcome with leadership oversight, creating a comprehensive internal audit program, training and assessing auditor competency, and mitigating internal audit findings.

Academic barriers exist in preparing students to apply QI methodologies and in developing student interest and motivation to value their role in QI as professional nurses. A small study conducted by Peterson-Graziose and Bryer (2017) supports the existence of this academic-practice gap regarding QI. The researchers asked 73 undergraduate nursing students their perceptions to the extent they acquired the KSA of the six QSEN competencies. Regarding QI, students reported that QI content was taught the least in the curriculum, was the lowest skill set they felt prepared for, and rated QI the least important of all six QSEN competencies. Organizations desperately seek nurses with the QI KSAs to recognize processes needing improvement, to act, implement improvement interventions, evaluate the outcomes of actions, and determine whether or not the outcome meets the expectation. Faculty can promote the QSEN QI KSAs by creating partnerships. Partnerships with clinical sites can offer students access to real-time QI activities and experienced staff who can mentor on QI methodologies, and potentially create opportunities for students to participate in active projects. Partnerships can shift QI KSAs from being largely theoretical to being more foundational to nursing practice. There is truly a sense of accomplishment, of victory when a problem, outcome, or process is improved. If students can experience victory as students, their interest and ability to continue QI as professional nurses may increase. Learning principles of QI in a classroom is necessary but applying principles of QI in clinical settings may be a barrier for students to appreciate the value and their role in QI.

It is truly an exciting time for nurses and those participating in and leading QI activities. Empowering and preparing nurses to be active participants in QI activities encourages them to make decisions that impact the quality and safety of their patient's care. This chapter highlighted QI methodologies and other essential QI concepts that increase QSEN QI knowledge, skills and attitudes. The essentials are important, but to successfully contribute to QI activities, nurses must be able to understand and utilize a broad array of QI tools that are presented in Chapter 12. Identifying new, improved ways to provide care and services is only one part of the QI equation. Disseminating outcomes from QI projects to other colleagues helps others to improve their own practices. Once the QI KSAs are obtained, the ability to improve patient outcomes and organizational processes is limitless.

END-OF-CHAPTER RESOURCES

KEY CONCEPTS

1. Quality improvement (QI) is defined as to "use data to monitor the outcomes of care processes and use improvement methods to design and test changes to continuously improve the quality and safety of health care systems" (QSEN Institute, n.d.-a, n.d.-b).
2. QI began with the work of the American Medical Association in the early 1900s. Over time, QI changed from standardizing care to include measurements of the process of care and healthcare outcomes in response to accreditation standards of The Joint Commission (TJC). The current focus of QI continues to evolve in response to the Centers for Medicare and Medicaid (CMS) programs such as Value-Based Purchasing.
3. QI is the incorporation of existing information and data into QI activities. EBP focuses on translating evidence into clinical, educational, or administrative practice. The aim of research is to generate new knowledge by testing theories or interventions.
4. Donabedian's Model looks at three areas for QI: structure, process, and outcomes. Deming's model prescribes how QI takes place in a cyclical manner using Plan-Do-Study-Act (PDSA). Six Sigma prescribes five steps for QI to reduce variation in performance: define, measure, analyze, improve, and control (DMAIC). Lean interventions focus on improving efficiency, reducing waste, and streamlining processes through the cumulative effect of small improvements.
5. Patient satisfaction data is collected and reported to the CMS. CMS makes the patient satisfaction data publicly available on their website. The data allows consumers to make an informed decision about where to seek healthcare.
6. A root cause analysis (RCA) is conducted after a near miss or sentinel event has occurred. An RCA is an investigation of what caused a problem and why the problem occurred. Corrective action is expected. TJC requires that an RCA take place whenever a sentinel event occurs.
7. Examine how the RCA process helps understand near miss events or sentinel events.
8. Healthcare Failure Mode and Effect Analysis (HFMEA) is a QI tool that looks at a healthcare process to determine the potential for risk. The goal of a HFMEA is preventative, or to improve the safety of a complex, high-risk healthcare process before an adverse event occurs by identifying and eliminating high-risk aspects of the process.
9. Nurses, both experienced and novice, are expected to have the knowledge, skills, and attitudes (KSA) to assess, analyze, intervene, and evaluate not just patient outcomes, but outcomes that reflect individual and interdisciplinary practice. Nurses approach the processes and systems of care they use every day as variables that constantly need evaluation, recognizing processes that may enhance care or lead to errors and recognizing how such processes can be improved to promote patient safety and performance excellence.
10. Organizational leadership must support staff to conduct QI efforts to enhance patient safety and to support the organization's high-reliability journey. Although QI barriers exist, they can be overcome with leadership support and ensuring staff are educated on QI methodologies and tools.

KEY TERMS

- Audit
- Baseline data
- Corrective action
- Healthcare Failure Mode and Effect Analysis (HFMEA)
- Hospital Value-Based Purchasing
- Improvement sustainability
- Lean
- Malcolm Baldrige Performance Excellence Framework
- Outcome data
- Outcomes
- Plan-Do-Study-Act (PDSA)
- Postintervention data
- Preventive action
- Process
- Quality improvement (QI)
- Risk
- Risk-based-thinking
- Root cause analysis (RCA)
- Six Sigma
- Structure
- Survey readiness
- Tracer methodology

REVIEW QUESTIONS

Answers to Review Questions appear in the Instructor's Manual. Qualified instructors should request the Instructor's Manual from textbook@springerpub.com.

1. You are a staff nurse caring for a patient that TJC surveyor has selected for a tracer. This is the first day you are caring for this patient. Because you are not familiar with this patient, which of the following actions would be best for you and the organization?
   - **A.** Explain to the surveyor that this is your first day caring for the patient.
   - **B.** Request another patient.
   - **C.** Review the EMR to ensure all provider documentation is up-to-date.
   - **D.** Transfer the patient to another unit.
   - **E.** Request the nurse from the previous shift stay to talk with TJC surveyor.
2. What is the *primary* goal of quality improvement?
   - **A.** Improve patient outcomes
   - **B.** Create evidence of a high-reliability organization
   - **C.** Improve cost-effectiveness of care delivery
   - **D.** Identify potential opportunities to reduce waste

3. The emphasis on risk reduction using preventive actions is similar to what improvement methodology?
   A. Lean/Six Sigma
   B. HFMEA
   C. RCA
   D. All of the answers are correct.
4. A group of nurses on a medical-surgical unit noted their readmission rates were higher than those of other units. With further investigation, the nurses identify that patients were readmitted to the hospital based on a lack of understanding of discharge instructions. As a team, the nurses decide to look at how they could assess every patient's health literacy level (understanding of health information) because health literacy was identified as a contributing factor to increased readmissions. The team identifies three tools commonly found in the literature. They decide on one tool that is appropriate for their medical-surgical population of patients. To implement the tool, they teach the staff how to use it, document the patient's literacy level score in the EMR, and brief the rest of the patient's care team on use of that health literacy information during interactions with the patient. Readmissions are reduced from 15% to 8% at the end of a 4-month trial period. Is this considered research, quality improvement, or evidence-based practice?
   A. It is research since the nurses research each tool to find evidence.
   B. It is quality improvement since the nurses used data and identified an intervention to improve their readmission outcome.
   C. It is evidence-based practice since the nurses evaluated three tools and selected the most appropriate tool for their patient population.
   D. None of these answers are correct; the nurses only wanted to find out the patient's literacy level.
5. Which of the following processes using Deming's Plan-Do-Study-Act method for quality improvement is correct?
   A. Collect baseline data, evaluate the improvement, measure outcomes, and redesign the plan.
   B. Collect baseline data, use small-scale trials for change, collect data and compare against desired outcomes, and adjust the plan.
   C. Implement small-scale change, collect data, disseminate the data, and sustain the improvement.
   D. Implement changes, evaluate effects from change, identify data, and readjust the plan.
   E. None of these answers are correct.
6. Many organizations are combining Lean and Six Sigma concepts within their quality improvement efforts. Which of the following options best explains why this combination may be successful?
   A. Lean focuses on optimizing existing processes (e.g., removing non-value-added activities) for cost reduction and efficiency while Six Sigma focuses on minimizing variability to eliminate defects.
   B. Lean focuses on variability reduction over time while Six Sigma focuses on efficiency in the current existing process.
   C. Lean, emphasizing efficiency, and Six Sigma, emphasizing increasing variability, are seldom combined as they both focus on separate improvement methods.
   D. Lean focuses on eliminating existing processes to reduce costs while Six Sigma focuses on eliminating defects to increase variability over time.

7. Which of the following options is true about a fishbone diagram?
   A. It is a useful data analysis tool in determining variability over time.
   B. It visually represents a process, from beginning to end.
   C. It is commonly used to determine definitive cause-and-effect relationships.
   D. It is a quality improvement tool to identify relationships among possible factors.
   E. None of these answers are correct.
8. Healthcare Failure Mode and Effect Analysis (HFMEA) is different from a root cause analysis (RCA) because of which of the following?
   A. HFMEA is a proactive process to assess, eliminate, or reduce the risks related to complex, high-risk processes before they result in adverse events. RCA is a retrospective analysis of an event that has already occurred.
   B. HFMEA is a proactive process of an event that has already occurred. RCA is a retrospective process to identify the most appropriate intervention when developing a PDSA.
   C. HFMEA is an adverse event documentation system commonly employed by organizations to track sentinel events. RCA is an improvement tool that must be done annually on one significant event that occurred within the organization.
   D. HFMEA is one single process used to enhance the quality culture within the organization. RCA is a part of every PDSA and is documented as part of the D ("Do") phase.
9. Which of the following types of problems would likely prompt the initiation of a root cause analysis? *Select all that apply.*
   A. A suicidal patient signs out against medical advice (AMA) in the emergency department.
   B. An adult dose of heparin is given to an infant.
   C. Surgery was performed on the wrong leg.
   D. A staff member fails to resuscitate a patient after an inadvertent morphine overdose in the hospital.
   E. Two different hemostats, one reusable, one disposable, are stocked in the clean utility room within the same bin.
10. As you are walking down the hall of your unit, you hear a patient you have cared for all shift call out for help. When you arrive to the room, the patient is on the floor. After you call for help you see the patient is awake and alert and says they needed to go to the bathroom and "slipped." A physician quickly arrives. After physical assessment and x-rays, the patient is diagnosed with a fractured hip needing surgical intervention. Your manager calls you to their office to complete an incident report. Of the following actions, what initial action would you document on the incident report as your next step?
    A. Conduct an interdisciplinary QI project regarding reducing falls.
    B. Conduct a HFMEA™ to prevent future falls.
    C. Analyze the unit's fall data to determine if falls are a problem.
    D. Revise the fall risk checklist, an approved procedure.

REVIEW ACTIVITIES

1. Go to the Institute for Healthcare Improvement (IHI) website at www.ihi.org.
   - Select EDUCATION.
   - Select IHI Open School.

- Select Take a Course.
- Select course number **PS 201** (Root Cause Analyses and Actions) and complete the course.

2. Consider the following situation: The headline of your school's daily newspaper reads, "Food Services to Increase Prices." The article explains revenue from sales has decreased by 20%, leaving no other option but to increase prices. Now, go to the Institute for Healthcare Improvement (IHI) website at http://ihi.org. Enter PDSA worksheet in the search box. You will find the PDSA worksheet is available in PDF. (Note: You will have to register with IHI to open the PDF document.) Divide into groups of four to five students. Use the PDSA worksheet to develop a small scale of change that could prevent cost increases incurred by students and faculty. Create an AIM and PLAN. Identify an intervention you would DO. Create a measurement plan to STUDY. Whether or not your intervention was successful, describe how you would next ACT. Compare student group ideas for improvement.

3. Go to the Baldrige Performance Excellence Program www.nist.gov/baldrige. Select Award Recipients. Select 2011 as your year option, and in the Search section, select 2011 as the year and Health Care for the Sector. Three healthcare award recipients will be available. Select the Award Application Summary for Henry Ford Health System (HFHS).

   a. Identify examples of innovations that demonstrate performance excellence.

   b. Would you want to be employed by this organization? Why or why not?

   c. View the YouTube video from HFHS: www.youtube.com/watch?v=rw380n-6JhW4
   How does this performance by senior leadership speak to performance excellence?

   d. Is there evidence of Lean/Six Sigma and preventive actions in the HFHS Application Summary?

4. Access the American Society for Quality website at http://asq.org.

   a. Select Learn About Quality. Many quality topics are listed that were discussed in this chapter. As you learned, preventive actions are taken when a risk for error is identified but has not occurred.

   b. From the Quality Topics A to Z list, select Mistake-proofing. Read through this brief explanation including the accompanying flowchart.

   c. Can you apply the restaurant example to an outpatient clinic? What questions could be asked?

   d. Can you think of an operating room procedure that was created using mistake-proofing principles?

5. Audits or inspections are common in healthcare settings. An audit examines if a process follows requirements, such as TJC requirements. External audits occur when auditors come from outside the organization. Internal audits occur from staff within the organization, which supports survey readiness. It is common for nurses to serve as auditors on an internal audit team at their organization. Access the American Society for Quality website at http://asq.org. Select Learn About Quality. From the Quality Topics A to Z list, select Auditing.

a. View the brief video. What are a few benefits of auditing identified by the speaker?
b. Select the three different types of auditing. Scroll down to Performance Audits vs. Compliance and Conformance Audits. What is the major difference between performance and compliance audits?
c. When TJC conducts an audit, would that audit be defined as a first-, second-, or third-party audit?
d. You are a nurse on an internal audit team auditing the environment of care to determine if the environment meets TJC requirements. The Quality Management department has provided the audit team with a checklist of key JC environmental requirements as a reference that must be turned in to verify the audit was conducted. During the audit, you ask a nurse who works in the environment being audited to explain how IV pumps are managed. Is there evidence of compliance, process, or both audit methods in this scenario?
e. Is auditing an essential element of QI?

SPRINGER PUBLISHING CONNECT™ | A robust set of instructor resources designed to supplement this text is located at **http://connect.springerpub.com/content/book/978-0-8261-6145-1.** Qualifying instructors may request access by emailing **textbook@springerpub.com.**

REFERENCES

American Nurses Association. (2015). Code of ethics for nurses with interpretive statements. Author. https://www.nursingworld.org/coe-view-only

Aroh, D., Colella, J., Douglas, C., & Eddings, A. (2015). An example of translating value-based purchasing into value-based care. *Urologic Nursing, 35*(2), 61–75. https://doi.org/10.7257/1053-816X.2015.35.2.61

Berwick, D. M. (2011). Preparing nurses for participation in and leadership of continual improvement. *Journal of Nursing Education, 50*(6), 322–327. https://doi.org/10.3928/0148483420110519-05

Berwick, D. M., & Hackbarth, A. D. (2012). Eliminating waste in US health care. *Journal of the American Medical Association, 307*(14), 1513–1516. https://doi.org/10.1001/jama.2012.362

Carroll, N. W., & Clement, J. P. (2020). Hospital performance in the first 6 years of Medicare's value-based purchasing program. *Medical Care Research and Review, 78*(5), 598–606. https://doi.org/10.1177/1077558720927586

Casarett, D., Karlawish, J. H. T., & Sugarman, J. (2000). Determining when quality improvement initiatives should be considered research. *Journal of the American Medical Association, 283*(17), 2275–2280. https://doi.org/10.1001/jama.283.17.2275

Centers for Medicare & Medicaid Services. (2018a). *CMS Hospital Value-Based Purchasing Program results for fiscal year 2019.* https://www.cms.gov/newsroom/fact-sheets/cms-hospital-value-based-purchasing-program-results-fiscal-year-2019

Centers for Medicare & Medicaid Services. (2018b). *CMS Office of the Actuary releases 2017-2026 projections of national health expenditures.* https://www.cms.gov/newsroom/press-releases/cms-office-actuary-releases-2017-2026-projections-national-health-expenditures

Cohen, R. I. (2018). Lean methodology in health care. *Chest, 154*(6), 1448–1454. https://doi.org/10.1016/j.chest.2018.06.005

Cox-Sullivan, S., Norris, M. R., Brown, L. M., & Scott, K. J. (2017). Nurse manager perspective of staff participation in unit level shared governance. *Journal of Nursing Management, 25*(8), 624–631. https://doi.org/10.1111/jonm.12500

DeRosier, J., Stalhandske, E., Bagian, J. P., & Nudell, T. (2002). Using Health Care Failure Mode and Effect Analysis™: The VA National Center for Patient Safety's prospective risk analysis system. *The Joint Commission Journal on Quality Improvement, 28*(5), 248–267. https://doi.org/10.1016/s1070-3241(02)28025-6

Donabedian, A. (2003). *An introduction to quality assurance in health care.* Oxford University Press.

Dunagan, P. B. (2017). The quality improvement attitude survey: Development and preliminary psychometric characteristics. *Journal of Clinical Nursing, 26*, 5113–5120. https://doi.org/10:1111/jocn.14054

Evans, J. R. (2008). *Quality & performance excellence: Management, organization, and strategy* (5th ed.). Thompson South-Western.

Figueroa, J. F., Tsugawa, Y., Zheng, J., Orav, E. J., & Jha, A. K. (2016). Associations between the value-based purchasing pay for performance program and patient mortality in US hospitals: Observational study. *British Medical Journal, 353*, i2214. https://doi.org/10.1136/bmj.i2214

Gaines, K. (2021). *Nurses ranked most trusted profession 19 years in a row*. https://nurse.org/articles/nursing-ranked-most-honest-profession

Hadfield, D., Holmes, S., Kozlowski, S., & Sperl, T. (2009). *The new Lean healthcare pocket guide: 5S in healthcare-why you need it*. MCS Media.

Haley, D. R., Hamadi, H., Zhao, M., Xu, J., & Wang, Y. (2017). Hospital Value-Based Purchasing. The association between patient experience and clinical outcome. *The Health Care Manager, 36*(4), 312–319. https://doi.org/10.1097/HCM.0000000000000183

Haxby, E., & Shuldham, C. (2018). How to undertake a root cause analysis investigation to improve patient safety. *Nursing Standard, 32*(20), 41–46. https://doi.org/10.7748/ns.2018.e10859

Hallam, C. R., & Contreras, C. (2018). Lean healthcare: Scale, scope, and sustainability. *International Journal of Health Care Quality Assurance, 31*(7), 684–696. https://doi.org/10.1108/IJHCQA-02-2017-0023.

Hughes, R. G. (2008a). Nurses at the "sharp end" of patient care. In R. Hughes (Ed.), *Patient safety and quality: An evidence-based handbook for nurses* (AHRQ Publication No. 08-0043, Chapter 2). Agency for Healthcare Research and Quality. https://archive.ahrq.gov/professionals/clinicians-providers/resources/nursing/resources/nurseshdbk/nurseshdbk.pdf

Hughes, R. G. (2008b). Tools and strategies for quality improvement and patient safety. In R. Hughes (Ed.), *Patient safety and quality: An evidence-based handbook for nurses* (AHRQ Publication No. 08-0043, Chapter 44). Agency for Healthcare Research and Quality. https://archive.ahrq.gov/professionals/clinicians-providers/resources/nursing/resources/nurseshdbk/nurseshdbk.pdf

Institute for Healthcare Improvement. (2017). *Cause and effect diagram*. http://www.ihi.org/resources/Pages/Tools/CauseandEffectDiagram.aspx

Institute of Medicine. (2001). *Crossing the quality chasm: A new health system for the 21st century*. National Academies Press. https://doi.org/10.17226/10027

International Organization for Standardization. (2015a). ISO 9000:2015, Quality Management Systems–Fundamentals and Vocabulary. https://www.iso.org/standard/45481.html

International Organization for Standardization. (2015b). ISO 9001:2015, Quality Management Systems–Requirements. https://www.iso.org/standard/62085.html

The Joint Commission. (n.d.-a). *After the survey*. https://www.jointcommission.org/accreditation-and-certification/health-care-settings/hospital/prepare/after-the-survey

The Joint Commission. (n.d.-b). *History of The Joint Commission*. https://www.jointcommission.org/about-us/facts-about-the-joint-commission/history-of-the-joint-commission

The Joint Commission. (n.d.-c). *Hospital: 2022 National Patient Safety Goals*. https://www.jointcommission.org/standards/national-patient-safety-goals/hospital-national-patient-safety-goals

The Joint Commission. (2020). *Hospital standard (Leadership), edition*. Proactive Risk Assessment.

The Joint Commission. (2016). The SAFER Matrix: A new scoring methodology. *The Joint Commission Perspectives®*, 36(5), 1–3.

Jones, T. L. (2016). Outcome measurement in nursing: Imperatives, ideals, history, and challenges. *The Online Journal of Issues in Nursing, 21*(2), Manuscript 1. https://doi.org/10.3912/OJIN.Vol21No2MAN01.

Kampstra, N. A., Zipfel, N., Van der Nat, P. B., Westert, G. P., Van der Wees, P. J., & Groenewoud, A. S. (2018). Health outcomes measurement and organizational readiness support quality improvement: A systematic review. *BMC Health Services Research, 18*(1), 3–14. https://doi.org/10.1186/s12913-018-3828-9

Kohn, L. T., Corrigan, J. M., & Donaldson, M. S. (Eds). (2000). *To err is human: Building a safer health system.* National Academies Press. https://doi.org/10.17226/9728

Langley, G. L., Nolan, K. M., Nolan T. W., Norman C. L., & Provost L. P. (2009). *The improvement guide: A practical approach to enhancing organizational performance* (2nd ed.). Jossey Bass.

Lindberg, L., & Kimberlain, J. (2008) Engage employees to improve staff and patient satisfaction. *Hospitals & Health Networks, 82*(1), 28–29.

Lloyd, R. C. (2010). Navigating in the turbulent sea of data: The quality measurement journey. *Clinics in Perinatology, 37*, 101–122. https://doi.org/10.1016/j.clp.2010.01.006

Luce, J. M., Bindman, A., & Lee, P. R. (1994). A brief history of health care quality assessment and improvement in the United States. *The Western Journal of Medicine, 160*, 263–268. http://www.ncbi.nlm.nih.gov/pmc/articles/PMC1022402

Marshall, M., De Silva, D., Cruickshank, L., Shand, J., Wei, L., & Anderson, J. (2016). What we know about designing an effective improvement intervention (but too often fail to put into practice). *British Medical Journal Quality & Safety, 26*, 578–582. https://doi.org/10.1136/bmjqs-2016-006143

McLaughlin, M., Houston, K., & Harder-Mattson, E. (2012). Managing outcomes using an organizational quality improvement model. In P. Kelly (Ed.), *Nursing leadership & management* (3rd ed., pp. 474–496). Delmar.

Mitchell, S. E., Martin, J., Holmes, S., Van Deusen-Lukas, C., Cancino, R., Paasche-Orlow, M., Brach, C., & Jack, B. (2015). How hospitals reengineer their discharge processes to reduce readmissions. *Journal for Healthcare Quality, 38*(2), 116–126. https://doi.org/10.1097/JHQ.0000000000000005

Moen, R., & Norman, C. (2009). *Evolution of the PDCA cycle.* Associates in Process Improvement. http://www.cologic.nu/files/evolution_of_the_pdsa_cycle.pdf

Ogrinc, G., Armstrong, G. E., Dolansky, M. A., Singh, M. K., & Davies, L. (2019). SQUIRE-EDU (standards for quality improvement reporting excellence in education): Publication guidelines for educational improvement. *Academic Medicine, 94*(10), 1461–1470. https://doi.org/10.1097/ACM.0000000000002750

O'Rourke, H. M., & Fraser, K. D. (2016). How quality improvement practice evidence can advance the knowledge base. *Journal for Healthcare Quality, 38*(5), 264–274. https://doi.org/10.1097/JHQ.0000000000000067

Owens, L. D., & Koch, R. W. (2015). Understanding quality patient care and the role of the practicing nurse. *Nursing Clinics of North America, 50*, 33–34. https://doi.org/10.1016/j.cnur.2014.10.003

Peterson-Graziose, V., & Bryer, J. (2017). Assessing student perceptions of Quality and Safety Education for Nurses competencies in a baccalaureate curriculum. *Journal Nursing Education, 56*(7), 435–438. https://doi.org/10.3928/01484834-20170619-09

QSEN Institute. (n.d.-a). *Graduate QSEN competencies: Quality improvement.* https://qsen.org/competencies/graduate-ksas/#quality_improvement

QSEN Institute. (n.d.-b). *QSEN competencies: Quality improvement.* https://qsen.org/competencies/pre-licensure-ksas/#quality_improvement

Salmond, S. W., & Echevarria, M. (2017). Healthcare transformation and changing roles for nursing. *Orthopedic Nursing, 36*(1), 12–25. https://doi.org/10.1097/NOR.0000000000000308

Sandberg, K. C. (2018). Leadership in quality improvement. *Current Problems Pediatric Adolescent Health Care, 48*, 206–210. https://doi.org/10.1016/j.cppeds.2018.08.007

Shrank, W. H., Rogstad, T. L., & Parekh, N. (2019). Waste in the US health care system estimated costs and potential for savings. *Journal of the American Medical Association, 322*(15), 1501–1509. https://doi.org/10.1001/jama.201913978

Silver, S. A., McQuillan, R., Harel, Z., Weizman, A. V., Thomas, A., Nesrallah, G., Bell, C. M., Chan, C. T., & Chertow, G. M. (2016). How to sustain change and support continuous quality improvement. *Clinical Journal American Society of Nephrology, 11*, 916–924. https://doi.org/10.2015/CJN.11501015

Silver, S. A., Harel, Z., McQuillan, R., Weizman, A. V., Thomas, A., Chertow, G. M., Nesrallah, G., Bell, C. M., & Chan, C. T. (2016). How to begin a quality improvement project. *Clinical Journal American Society of Nephrology, 11*, 893–900. https://doi.org/10.2015/CJN.11491015

Small, A., Gist, D., Souza, D., Dalton, J., Magny-Normilus, C., & David, D. (2016). Using Kotter's Change Model for implementing bedside handoff: A quality improvement project. *Journal of Nursing Care Quality, 31*(4), 304–309. https://doi.org/10.1097/NCQ.0000000000000212

Squires, D., & Anderson, C. (2015). U.S. health care from a global perspective: Spending, use of services, process, and health in 13 countries. *The Commonwealth Fund, 1819*(15), 1–15. https://www.commonwealthfund.org/publications/issue-briefs/2015/oct/us-health-care-global-perspective

Tolbert, J., Orgera, K., Singer, N., & Damico, A. (2019). *Key facts about uninsured population*. Issue Brief (Dec 13, 2019) Kaiser Family Foundation. https://www.kff.org/uninsured/issue-brief/key-facts-about-the-uninsured-population

Wilson, J., Swee, M., Mosher, H., Scott-Cawiezell, J., Levins, L., Fort, K., & Kumar, B. (2020). Using Lean Six Sigma to improve pneumococcal vaccination rates in a Veterans Affairs rheumatology clinic. *Journal for Healthcare Quality, 42*(3), 166–174. https://doi.org/10.1097/JHQ.0000000000000218

SUGGESTED READINGS

Agency for Healthcare Research and Quality. (2013). *QI guide on improved nursing care*. https://www.ahrq.gov/data/monahrq/myqi/nursing.html

Davies, C., Lyons, C., & Whyte, R. (2019). Optimizing nursing time in a day care unit: Quality improvement using Lean Six Sigma methodology. *International Journal for Quality in Health Care, 31*(1). 22–28. https://doi.org/10.1093/intqhc/mzz087

Hain, D. J. (2017). Focusing on the fundamentals: Comparing and contrasting nursing research and quality improvement. *Nephrology Nursing Journal, 44*(6). 541–543. https://link.gale.com/apps/doc/A523213261/AONE?u=anon~45e64c42&sid=googleScholar&xid=ee5294d8

Johnson, H. (2021). Restorative quality improvement: Novel application of Six Sigma in a skilled nursing facility. *Journal of Nursing Care Quality*, *36*(1). 67–73. https://doi.org/10.1097/NCQ.0000000000000492

Kazana, I., & Dolansky, M. (2021). Quality improvement: Online resources to support nursing education and practice. *Nursing Forum, 56*(2), 341–349. https://doi.org/10.1111/nuf.12533

Mileski, M., Topinka, J. B., Lee, K., Brooks, M., McNeil, C., & Jackson, J. (2017). An investigation of quality improvement initiatives in decreasing the rate of avoidable 30-day, skilled nursing facility-to-hospital readmissions: A systematic review. *Clinical Interventions in Aging, 12*, 213–222. https://doi.org/10.2147%2FCIA.S123362

Strand, K., & Tveit, B. (2020). Planning and implementing quality improvement projects in clinical practice: Third-year nursing students' learning experiences. *Journal of Clinical Nursing, 29*(23/24), 4769–4783. https://doi.org/10.1111/jocn.15521

Toles, M., Colón-Emeric, C., Moreton, E., Frey, L., & Leeman, J. (2021). Quality improvement studies in nursing homes: A scoping review. *BMC Health Services Research, 21*, 803. https://doi.org/10.1186/s12913-021-06803-8

CHAPTER 12

Quality Improvement Tools

Anthony L. D'Eramo

"Modern health care demands continual system improvement to better meet social needs for safety, effectiveness, patient centeredness, timeliness, efficiency, and equity. Nurses, like all other health professionals, need skills and support to participate effectively in that endeavor, and, often, to lead it."

–Donald M. Berwick, 2011

Upon completion of this chapter, the reader should be able to:

1. Describe types of data such as qualitative and quantitative data.
2. Differentiate the four sources of data: internal, external, baseline, and post-intervention.
3. Explain the importance of an operational definition.
4. Discuss how descriptive statistics are used in quality improvement (QI).
5. Differentiate among the three commonly used methods to display data: histogram, scatter plot diagrams, and pareto charts.
6. Explain why statistical process control is used in QI.
7. Discuss the use of Gantt charts and flow maps by QI teams.

CROSSWALK

This chapter addresses the following:

QSEN Competency: Quality Improvement

The American Association of Colleges of Nursing. (2021). *The essentials: Core competencies for professional nursing education.*

Domain 5: Quality and Safety

OPENING SCENARIO

As a day shift nurse on a patient-care unit, the nurse performs assessments on the patients at the beginning of the shift. The first patient that the nurse assesses is an 85-year-old man admitted yesterday with pneumonia. During shift handoff, the night nurse stated the patient had a fever on admission but that the patient's temperature was normal during the night shift. The patient had an elevated white blood cell count of 12.4 (10,000 mm^3) on admission and received three doses of IV antibiotics since admission. As the nurse assesses the patient's vital signs, the patient is noted to have a temperature of 101.1 °F (38.4 °C). The nurse finds upon patient assessment a respiratory rate of 20 and a pulse oximeter reading of 95% on 1.5 L of oxygen delivered through a nasal cannula. His repeat white blood cell count on the morning of care is 13.2 (10,000 mm^3). As the nurse continues the patient assessment, the healthcare team enters the patient's room. One of the providers asks, "Is he improving?"

1. *How should the nurse respond to the physician?*
2. *What questions should the nurse have asked during the handoff shift report when it was reported that the patient had a normal temperature during the night shift?*
3. *Is a temperature finding of 101.1 °F or a white blood cell count of 13.2 (10,000 mm^3) an improvement?*

INTRODUCTION

Quality is whatever patients, family, and the healthcare industry define it to be. Beyond the prevention, reduction, or elimination of harm is the search for innovations and breakthrough improvements that contribute to quality outcomes. Innovative improvements can contribute to advancing average or good performance to performance excellence. Such innovations occur with visionary thinking, being alert to healthcare processes that need to be changed, responding to patient and staff satisfaction concerns, and by understanding and applying **quality improvement** (**QI**) methods into our daily clinical practice. This chapter focuses on the science and process of QI. For nurses to gain the necessary knowledge, skills, and attitudes to continuously improve healthcare quality, safety, and systems used to deliver healthcare, the Quality and Safety Education for Nurses project (QSEN Institute, 2020) defines QI as "Use data to monitor the outcomes of care processes and use improvement methods to design and test changes to continuously improve the quality and safety of healthcare systems."

This chapter includes defining data and commonly used descriptive statistics applied in QI activities. It explores the types and uses of data for QI including how data are displayed for analysis and how data are analyzed to identify both the need for improvement and if improvement occurred. Statistical process control (SPC) is introduced to include the run and control charts. When indicated, interprofessional teams may conduct QI activities. The teams have a variety of improvement tools and methods they can employ. The most basic and effective processes used by teams are described.

WHAT ARE DATA

Nursing practice and organizational healthcare processes all produce outcome data that can be measured, displayed, and compared. So, what are data? **Data** are the raw numbers or results collected to measure processes and outcomes. Data are used to determine if healthcare performance meets the expected goal (e.g., the number of patients with blood pressure in control). Data are used to measure performance quality that is valued by purchasers of care, accreditation agencies, governing bodies, the general public, and providers of healthcare. A clear understanding of the context or goal related to data measurement is necessary for interpretation; for example, understanding goals that can be measured, why the goal was selected, and ways in which the goal can be met. **Qualitative data** is nonnumeric, such as the data gathered during an interview. **Quantitative data** are numeric data and are commonly collected during quality improvement (QI) activities (Williams, 2018a).

By itself, data do not require a nurse to act. Consider the following: A heart rate of 60 is an isolated piece of data from one assessment finding. By itself, the heart rate data point of 60 seems "normal." Nurses do not usually base any changes on one piece of data, unless it indicates a critical change or value. If a nurse looks at heart rate readings over time (e.g., the heart rate is taken twice a shift for 1 day providing six data points) then the nurse can identify if a trend exists. A trend looks at changes in data over time. If the six heart rate readings were 110, 100, 90, 80, 70, and 60, the nurse would have information. **Information** is the analysis of collected data that is used to make decisions. As nurses, information is used to make nursing care decisions. In the heart rate example, the trend provides information that the heart rate has steadily fallen over three shifts. The nurse needs to decide if action is needed, such as informing the provider of the trend, reviewing medications or changes in medications over the past three shifts, or monitoring the patient more closely to watch for any other assessment changes.

Patients can provide both subjective and objective data. **Subjective data** are reported by the patient. For example, a patient may state pain status as "5" on a scale of 1 to 10. **Objective data** may include what the healthcare worker can see or measure, such as the patient's blood pressure or blood glucose results. Both subjective and objective data are collected, analyzed, and interpreted as information. This information is used to make clinical decisions about whether the patient is getting better, worse, or if the information requires provider notification.

SOURCES OF OBJECTIVE DATA FOR QUALITY IMPROVEMENT

There are many sources of data that may trigger QI activities, such as patient, unit, or organization performance outcomes. **Internal data** are those found within a healthcare organization and are generated by staff, such as falls and medication errors. **External data** are data provided from outside sources (e.g., state quality review organizations) that evaluate and report on the organization's internal processes and outcomes. When conducting QI interventions, **baseline data** are the preintervention data measurements that are used to identify a problem needing improvement. **Postintervention data** are the changes from baseline data after an improvement intervention was introduced and confirm the success or failure of that intervention. For example, a team is working to decrease the number of hospital-acquired pressure injuries (HAPIs). The average number of HAPIs was six per month for the last 3 months. Six HAPIs represents baseline data. Because six HAPIs was unacceptable, a QI intervention to reduce HAPIs was instituted. After the QI intervention, the average number of HAPIs was three per month, or a reduction of 50% in HAPIs over a 3-month period. Three HAPIs represents the postintervention data. Although a 50% reduction occurred, the team must analyze the postintervention data into information and decide if three HAPIs is acceptable or if further improvement is needed.

When data are reported, it is important to distinguish between incidence and prevalence data. Both incidence and prevalence data are often collected quarterly. **Incidence data** are the actual counts of every event that occurred during a specific time frame; for example, counting the number of falls that occurred on a medical-surgical unit for one quarter. **Prevalence data** are a snapshot of an event under measure for 1 day. For example, counting the number of falls that occurred on one specific day during the quarter. To illustrate further, suppose the prevalence rate was measured on one specific day and no fall occurred on the specific date of measurement. The prevalence rate would be zero. Now suppose over the same 3-month period, the actual incidence of falls was 11. Based on how the data were collected, either incidence or prevalence, it can result in dramatically different outcomes. It is important to understand the difference between incidence and prevalence data as organizations may report either depending on their preference or on external reporting requirements. For example, the National Database of Nursing Quality Indicators (NDNQI) requires reporting of pressure injuries as prevalence data. In the example regarding HAPIs, because both the baseline and postintervention data were actual numbers of HAPIs over a 3-month period, both data points represent incidence data. If the number of HAPIs was a snapshot on a given day, that would have represented prevalence data. Nurses are inundated with data. Appreciate that, regardless of the type of data, incidence or prevalence, analysis of the data into information for clinical decision-making must occur for data to be useful.

Aggregate Data

When subjective and/or objective data are collected for process improvements or to assess care delivery, such as HAPIs, it is necessary to ensure that no patient identifiers are captured linking outcomes to specific patients, families, or staff. This will help to protect privacy and confidentiality of data. QI projects generally use **aggregate data**, which are large, grouped data without patient identifiers. These aggregate data, often listed in a table format, may be grouped by time, cause, diagnosis, or the specific variable(s) being studied. An example of a study variable can include the staff's adherence to hand hygiene practices, as seen in Table 12.1. In Table 12.1, nursing hand hygiene compliance data are reported in aggregate form that compares three units over a 9-month period. Notice that there is no ability to identify which staff was in or out of compliance during measurement because the data is reported in aggregate.

In Table 12.1, the use of bolding (met the target) and shading (did not meet the target) helps to quickly identify areas needing improvement when looking with large numbers of aggregate data.

TABLE 12.1 PERCENT COMPLIANCE WITH CENTERS FOR DISEASE CONTROL AND PREVENTION HAND HYGIENE GUIDELINES USING OBSERVATIONS (THREE MEDICAL/SURGICAL UNITS)

	JAN	FEB	MAR	APR	MAY	JUNE	JULY	AUG	SEPT
Unit A	**91%**	80%	87%	86%	73%	69%	80%	77%	79%
Unit B	40%	45%	44%	54%	79%	59%	50%	50%	61%
Unit C	87%	88%	84%	88%	**90%**	**93%**	**90%**	79%	89%

Compliance goal is set at 90%. Bolded = Meeting 90% compliance goal; shaded = Not meeting 90% compliance goal.

Operational Definitions

An essential aspect of creating information from data is to have a clear definition of the data source and how the data is measured. An **operational definition** describes in detail what is being specifically measured, how it is being measured, who will measure it, and when measurement should occur.

It is important to know how the data for QI activities are defined and collected, including who can collect the data and use of clearly defined operational definitions. Because many staff may be collecting the data at different time points, having one clear operational definition ensures that the data are collected and measured the same way, regardless of where the data are collected or who collects the data. For example, in Table 12.1, aggregated data on hand hygiene compliance from three different medical-surgical units are presented. To make sure these data are collected and measured the same way on all units, there would need to be clear statements following the operational definition such as the definition for hand hygiene, who is to collect the data, when the data are to be collected, the number of hand hygiene observations expected, and when the results are to be reported and to whom. Once these variables are known, a numerator and denominator can also be defined. In addition, it is essential to have evidence that those staff involved in observations successfully completed CDC hand hygiene education prior to observing for compliance. An example of an operational definition and the numerator and denominator is provided as follows:

> Hand hygiene, a required organizational measure related to patient safety, is defined as compliance with the Centers for Disease Control and Prevention (CDC) hand hygiene guidelines accessible at www.cdc.gov/handhygiene/providers. Each unit will identify a "secret" observer on each shift who will monitor hand hygiene compliance for that unit on the first day of each month. Each observer will assess at least 10 interprofessional staff on the unit by observing their hand hygiene during interactions with patients. Results of compliance with CDC hand hygiene guidelines will be reported to the infection control staff within 48 hours of observations. Infection control staff will aggregate the observations as follows:
>
> **Numerator**: Total number of observations that followed CDC hand hygiene guidelines correctly, for example, 39
> **Denominator**: Total number of hand hygiene observations, for example, 45
> **Example Answer**: 39 hand hygiene observations were correct out of 45 hand hygiene observations (87% compliance)

In this example, there is a clear numerator and denominator for reliable measurement. It can be challenging to develop a clear operational definition to guide a sustainable, consistent process for data collection among the observers. The corresponding Case Study provides an opportunity to review examples of operational definitions to determine which is most comprehensive.

CASE STUDY

While participating on a QI team, the nurse asked to create an operational definition for falls. Several team members offer ideas:

- *A "fall" is defined as the number of patients who fall and for which an incident report is completed. The patient safety officer will collect the aggregate data and report it to the unit practice council annually using a control chart. Major injuries will require a root cause analysis (RCA).*
- *A "fall" is defined as the number of patients admitted to the unit who fall and who suffer no injuries, whether minor (e.g., a laceration), or major (e.g., fractured hip). All such incidents will be reported using electronic incident reporting procedures per policy 101-5.*

- *A "fall" is defined as any patient who falls that results in no injury, a fall that results in a minor injury (laceration) or a fall that results in a major injury (fractured hip). All such incidents will be reported using electronic incident reporting procedures per policy 101-5. The fall numerator is the number of falls and the fall denominator is the total number of patients on the unit during the measurement time period.*

  1. *Of the three options, what operational definition is most comprehensive? Explain why you selected that option.*
  2. *One of the team members is not sure why an operational definition is necessary. How would you respond?*

DATA COLLECTION

Data are only useful when collected rigorously, meaning that data collection tools must be valid (measures what it is supposed to measure) and reliable (consistently measuring what it is supposed to measure). To illustrate, in the hand hygiene compliance example, although all staff are expected and taught to follow hand hygiene compliance, every "secret" observer should complete additional training on the CDC guidelines and demonstrate competency in hand hygiene compliance before monitoring and observing other staff. The additional training can secure validity by helping the observer accurately measure if hand hygiene compliance occurred according to the CDC guidelines (validity). For example, two observers could observe the same area at the same time. Afterwards, their results (numerator/denominator of compliance percent) could be compared. **Interrater reliability** (IRR) refers to the consistency of data collected or measured by different observers (Lee et al., 2019). In the handwashing example, IRR would be used to determine if the observers are applying and interpreting the CDC guidelines correctly. The more accurate observers collect data consistently, the more reliable the data are. Conducting IRR may identify observers who need additional education in the interpretation and application of the CDC hand hygiene guidelines. As a result, education can be provided to reduce observational errors. One risk of data collection is identifying that a problem exists when in fact there is not a problem. For example, hand hygiene compliance may include using both a hand sanitizer and, when indicated, soap and water. If the trained observer misunderstood the definition of hand hygiene compliance and only counted the instances where the healthcare worker used soap and water, the findings would be inaccurate. In this case, the number of healthcare workers that used the waterless hand sanitizer was not counted, causing a decrease in the percent of hand hygiene compliance. When the trained observer reports the observations, one could easily determine the information on hand hygiene compliance needs improvement when it may not! Demonstrating IRR provides trust that data were collected systematically by all those in the data collection process. For more practice on IRR, complete the corresponding Case Study.

CASE STUDY

Two nurses have agreed to collect data on a QI project to decrease the number of patients who cancel their clinic appointments at two different surgical clinics. These patients are called clinic no-shows. The nurse manager over both clinics asks the two nurses to assure interrater reliability. Not being familiar with the concept of interrater reliability, the nurses look to the literature and discover that this term refers to ensuring those collecting data are following the same data collection procedures. Those collecting the data will do so at the same time and same location and compare their findings. The nurse manager requests a written plan to assure IRR between both nurses at the two clinics.

1. *Create an example operational definition that both nurses could use when collecting data.*
2. *Create an example spreadsheet that both nurses could use while collecting data and for providing the results to their nurse manager.*
3. *Should the nurses pilot the spreadsheet before starting data collection?*

Another risk for interpretation error can occur with inaccurate or vague operational definitions. For example, if the trained observer misunderstood the hand hygiene guidelines and interpreted them to say that the only time the healthcare worker had to use the hand sanitizer or wash their hands was if the worker touched the patient, then there would be a problem. The trained observer would then only count compliance when the patient was touched and hand hygiene was completed, missing the fact that hand hygiene should be completed every time the healthcare worker enters and leaves the room. The hand hygiene compliance rates would not clearly identify if any hand hygiene practices need improvement.

DESCRIPTIVE STATISTICS

Descriptive statistics are tools used to analyze and summarize relationships among variables. Statistics can identify significance within the data and relationships between variables (Nelson et al., 2004). **Descriptive statistics** are used to define and describe a set of data. For aggregate data, descriptive statistics are commonly calculated and include the mean, median, mode, range, and standard deviation (SD) of a set of data. Review the Unit A Hand Hygiene data displayed in Table 12.2. Note how the mean, median, mode, and range are calculated given a set of data. The **mean** is determined by an average of a set of numbers. This is done by adding all the numbers together and then dividing by the total number of observations. In looking at hand hygiene compliance for Unit A, there are 9 months of hand hygiene compliance percent ages reported. The mean compliance for Unit A is calculated by adding all findings and dividing by 9, the number of months. Table 12.2 demonstrates the calculation of mean for Unit A.

An example of a mean that a student may be familiar with is in calculating a grade point average (GPA). A common GPA scale: A = 4 points, B = 3 points, C = 2 points, D = 1 points, and F = 0 points. If all the grades earned in one semester over the time spent in college are converted to point values as described, a student could calculate the GPA using the illustration from Table 12.2. For example, if a student took five courses and received one A, two Bs, and 2 Cs, the GPA would be calculated as 4 + 3 + 3 + 2 + 2 = 14/5 = 2.8 GPA.

The **median** of a set of data is determined by listing the hand hygiene findings from lowest to highest values. Once listed, the median is the value at the separation point, where half of the data is above and the other half is below the data point that falls within the middle of the set of data. To illustrate, here are five data points arranged from lowest to highest: 4, 6, 11, 13, and 15. The median is 11 or the middle number of the set as there are two data points before and after 11. When there is an even number of results, the median is the average of the two middle results. For example, if the values were 4, 6, 7, 11, 13, and 15, the median would be 9, the average of 7 and 11, or 18/2 = 9. Table 12.2 illustrates the median, or 80%, for hand hygiene compliance on Unit A. The median statistic is used less frequently than the mean in statistical QI work.

In QI activities, the mode is of less use compared to the other descriptive statistics, but it may be included in analyses; therefore, it is useful to define. The **mode** is simply the value that is repeated most frequently in a set of data or the "typical" value observed. To illustrate this, refer to Table 12.2. Note the value 80 is repeated.

TABLE 12.2 UNIT A DESCRIPTIVE STATISTICS

SUMMARY STATISTIC	ILLUSTRATION
Mean	91+80+87+86+73+69+80+77+79=722 722 divided by 9 (months)=80.22
Median	91, 87, 86, 80, **80**, 79, 77, 73, 69 80 is the middle point
Mode	91, **80**, 87, 86, 73, 69, **80**, 77, 79 80 is repeated
Range	91, 80, 87, 86, 73, 69, 80, 77, 79 69 (lowest value) to 91 (highest value)

The **range** represents the lowest and highest values in the data. Reviewing the range of data is a quick measure of variability. **Variability** refers to the differences between the numbers in a data set. A simple measure of variability can be determined by observing the range of a data set.

Table 12.2 illustrates the range of values for Unit A from 69 to 91. Knowing data variability helps identify just how far apart the data are during one range of values. Consider this: A nurse is working on a QI project to reduce falls. Over 12 months, one unit had a high of 13 falls and a low of zero falls. The variability shows the nurse that the unit is not consistent in reducing falls, unless, of course, it went from 13 to 0 over time as the result of continuous improvement.

The most common method used to describe the variability of a data set is **standard deviation (SD)**, which reflects how "tightly" the data points cluster around the mean, as seen in Figure 12.1. SD is often abbreviated as the Greek letter sigma (σ). In a "normal" distribution of a data set, most measures hover around the mean while a few measures tend to be at opposite extremes from the mean. In a SD curve, the mean is located at the center of the graph and is represented as 0 in Figure 12.1. In a normal distribution, it is expected that 68.3% of outcomes will fall within one SD above or below the mean (+1/-1). Another 27.1% of outcomes should fall within two SD from the mean (+2/-2), accounting for 95.4% of all expected outcomes. An additional 4.2% of outcomes should fall within 3 SD from the mean (+3/-3), which accounts for 99.8% of expected outcomes.

Note that, if 20 students completed a test with a mean score of 80%, it is expected that most of those students (68.3%) would hover around an 80% score. More, or 95.4%, of students would be expected to fall within two SD of 80%, and even more (98.8%) students would fall within three SD from the mean. SD of a set of data can be easily calculated using software such as Microsoft Excel.

As seen in Figure 12.1, outcomes (99.8%) are expected to fall within three SD of the mean. Variability in a data set is an important concept in QI activities and is further examined with charts later in the chapter. For practice calculating basic descriptive statistics, refer to the corresponding Case Study.

DATA DISPLAY

Data are visible in all healthcare settings. It is difficult to walk onto an inpatient or outpatient area without seeing data. It is necessary, however, to analyze and interpret data into usable information. **Data display** refers to a visual picture or graphing of data that best depicts the story of that data to exhibit. Data should be displayed in ways that staff, patients, and families can understand. Figures, graphs, and tables are acceptable methods of displaying data. Whatever the format, data must include a clear title of what is being presented, including the use of footnotes to clarify aspects of the table or figure

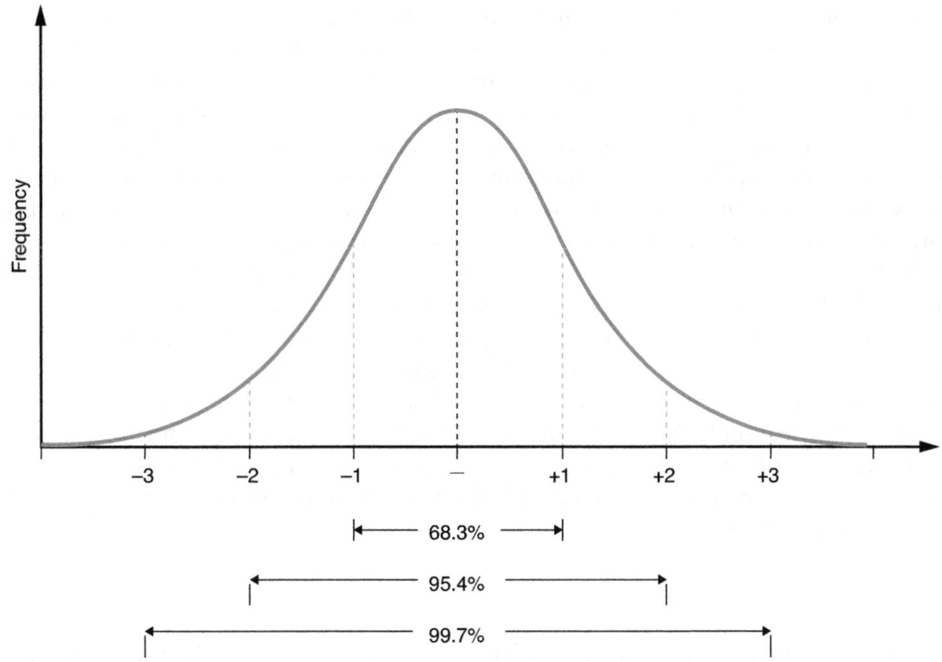

FIGURE 12.1 A Normal Distribution Standard Deviation Curve.

Source: From https://www.google.com/search?q=standard+deviation&tbm=isch&ved=2ahUKEwiQkJzqzqnrAhVGEd8KHUxpD-MQ2-cCegQIABAA&oq=standard+deviation&gs_lcp=CgNpbWcQARgAMgUIABCxAzIFCAAQsQMyBQgAELEDMgIIADICCAAyBQgAELEDMgIIADIFCAAQsQMyAggAMgIIADoECAAQQzoICAAQsQMQgwE6BwgAELEDEENQ8u8CWOKPA2DzqgNoAHAAeACAAeIBiAGnFpIBBjAuMTUuM5gBAKABAaoBC2d3cy13aXotaW1nwAEB&sclient=img&ei=GVY-X9CfIMai_AbM0r2YDg&bih=676&biw=1499&tbs=sur%3Afc&hl=en-US&hl=en-US#imgrc=AUqaaRnDHbGeUM

CASE STUDY

The nurse has just completed data collection on a QI project to reduce calloffs on the unit. To obtain calloff baseline data, the nurse has been asked to document the number of calloffs over a 3-week period to identify the number of calloffs more prominently for each shift. The results are gathered in the following list:

Week 1: (Days) 3	(Evenings) 1	(Nights) 1
Week 2: (Days) 4	(Evenings) 2	(Nights) 2
Week 3: (Days) 1	(Evenings) 3	(Nights) 1

Based on the results, calculate the (a) mean, (b) median, (c) mode, and (d) range of the data set.

(Nelson et al., 2004). For example, footnotes may be useful to define a column title, or to refer the reader to the operational definition of a specific value. Recall Table 12.1, regarding hand hygiene compliance for three nursing units. Those months meeting the targeted goal of 90% were highlighted while those not meeting the goal were shaded for easier and quicker analysis.

Data alone do not always offer guidance regarding improvement priorities. For example, looking at Table 12.1, Unit B lists outcomes for May (79%) and June (59%). Does this decrease in compliance require immediate attention? A "yes" response may be premature. In fact, the answer to that question should not be determined by comparing two results alone as two results may not provide enough data for analysis and decision-making. Fortunately, more sophisticated methods are available to better inform improvement decisions. Visually displaying data over time is useful when assessing outcomes to better inform if interventions are needed, if improvement occurred, or if improvement was sustained.

When data are generated, they must be interpreted as meaningful information. For example, in Table 12.1, if Unit B wanted to improve its hand hygiene compliance rate (mean = 53.5% over 9 months), some change or intervention must be implemented. Recall that 53.5% or the baseline measure will be compared to the postintervention percent compliance to determine if the intervention worked. Displaying data in graphical formats is helpful. This section focuses on commonly used formats including a histogram, scatter plot diagram, and Pareto charts, as well as run and control charts. It is important to note that when data are plotted within a graph, the horizontal axis of the graph is referred to as the *x*-axis and the vertical axis of the graph as the *y*-axis.

Histograms

A **histogram**, as seen in Figure 12.2, is a bar graph that displays the data. Data displayed using a histogram allows for easier visualization of large, aggregate data that may originate from a table. To understand a histogram, it is important to know the *y*-axis and *x*-axis. The *y*-axis is the vertical line and is easily remembered as "*y* to the sky." The *x*-axis is the horizontal line and can be remembered as "*x* to the left." Histograms are useful in determining patterns within historical data or displaying baseline data. In Figure 12.2, the histogram uses a bar to display the lengths of stay for the last 50 admissions.

The number of admissions is located on the vertical *y*-axis. The variable along the horizontal *x*-axis (lengths of stay in days) is sequential starting with the shortest to the longest length of stay. The most frequent average length of stay (14 observations) is between 3 and 4 days. Histograms are easily made with or without software and quickly depict the distribution of a set of data or outcomes.

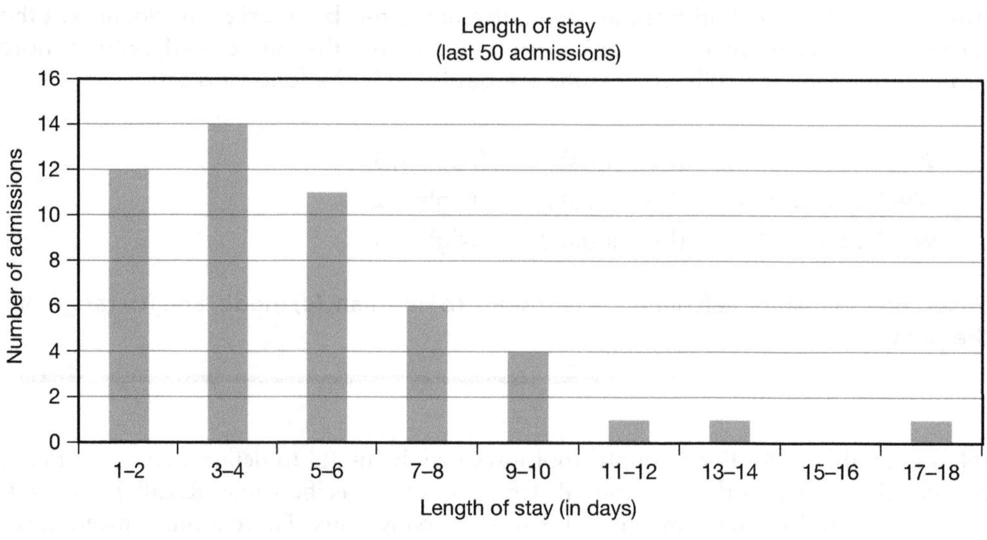

FIGURE 12.2 The Histogram. Length of Stay (Last 50 Admissions).

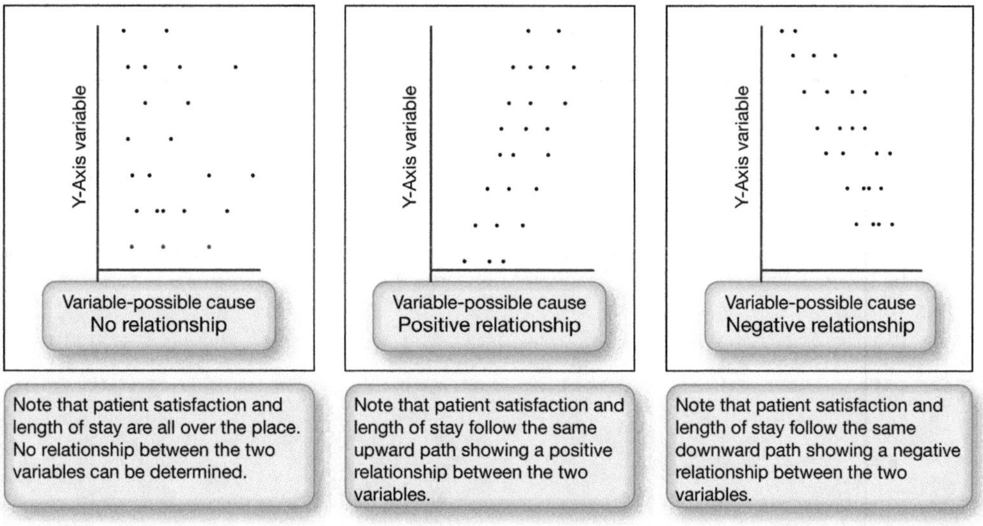

FIGURE 12.3 Basic Scatter Plot Patterns.

Scatter Plot Diagrams

Scatter plot diagrams display relationships between two variables by providing a visual means to test the strength of the relationship between the two variables. The design of the dots within the scatter plot diagram is used for interpretation. Several designs can be depicted when observing the scatter plot diagram, a positive, negative, or no relationship design. Examples of each scatter plot design are depicted in Figure 12.3. The scatter plot looks at two variables, or issues, under investigation. A relationship between the two variables does not indicate that one variable caused the other. The scatter plot assists in determining if a relationship exists.

Consider the length of stay data displayed in the histogram in Figure 12.2. The relationship between the variable of length of stay could be compared to another variable, such as patient satisfaction, using a scatter plot (Figure 12.3).

The scatter plot diagram in Figure 12.4 illustrates the relationship between lengths of stay (in days) and patient satisfaction scores using a Likert scale ranging from 5 to 1, where 5 is most satisfied, 3 is neutral, and 1 is least satisfied. In Figure 12.4, the design of the scatter plots indicates there is no relationship between length of stay and patient satisfaction for the 50 patients in this sample.

PARETO CHART

The Pareto chart is another type of bar graph. It is like the histogram because it depicts how often data represent a value. The difference between a histogram and a Pareto chart is that the **Pareto chart** orders findings in a descending order from high to low with the most frequent issue contributing to the results furthest to the left on the x-axis. Visualizing results from high to low allows prioritizing or identifying what data most impact the variable in question. One benefit of the Pareto chart is in demonstrating the Pareto principle that 80% of the problem comes from 20% of the causes. When the causes of problems are ranked in order of effect on the QI problem, it clearly identifies those causes having the greatest effect. The Pareto chart in Figure 12.5 illustrates that tardiness of the oncoming shift, furthest to the left, is the most common cause of unit overtime during a 1-month period.

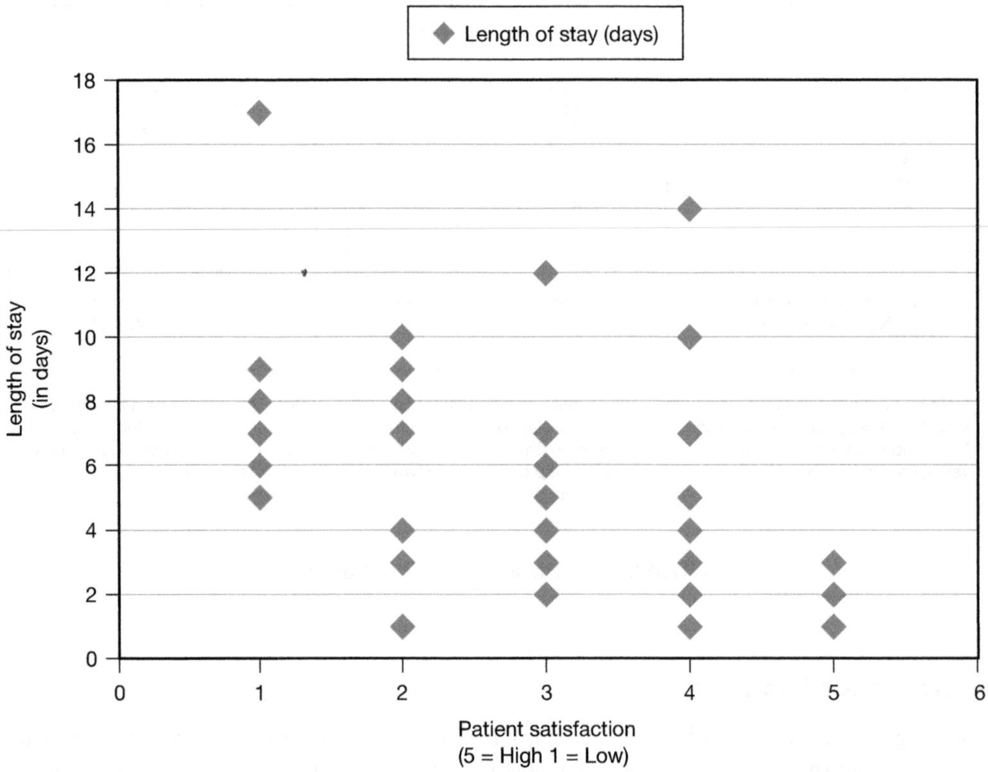

FIGURE 12.4 Scatter Plot Diagram (Variables Patient Satisfaction and Length of Stay).

In Figure 12.5, the four most common causes of overtime, that is, tardiness, turbulence, handoff delays, and staffing pattern, are ranked from high to low reading from left to right. These four causes represent 81% of the problems leading to overtime. Look above the column labeled "staffing patterns" and see where the line marks 81% of the problems. These four causes will serve as target problems needing improvement to reduce overtime costs. The manager can easily visualize, prioritize causes, and plan improvement interventions to reduce overtime usage based on review of the Pareto chart. Appreciate that the leading cause of a problem may not be the focus of improvement. In this example, if meeting with the Employee Health Department has been the greatest cause of overtime, it may not be feasible to address since the manager of the unit may have little control over employees appropriately seeking Employee Health Department services. Or, looking at that scenario from another perspective, if meeting with Employee Health Department services was the greatest cause of the overtime, the manager may want to do an RCA, fishbone diagram, or ask the five Whys discussed in Chapter 11 to determine why there is so many more staff than usual seeking Employee Health Department services and driving up overtime usage.

STATISTICAL PROCESS CONTROL)

In the Pareto chart depicted in Figure 12.5, tardiness is the most significant cause of overtime. However, the chart does not illustrate any change from previous months. Perhaps individuals calling off work were once the most frequent cause of overtime but

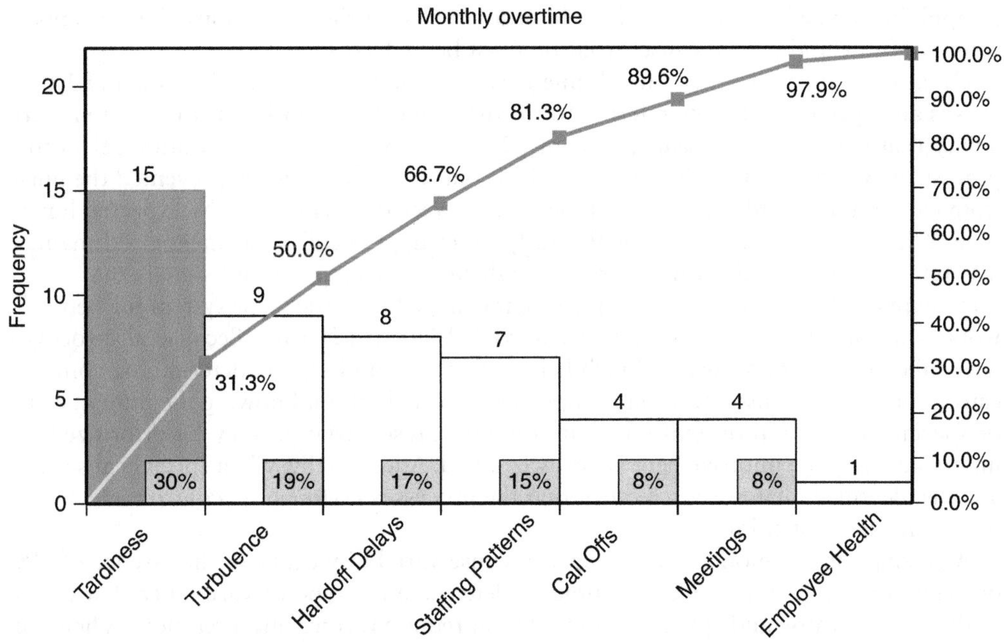

FIGURE 12.5 Pareto Chart on Causes of Overtime for 1 Month.

are now reduced? Perhaps these causes of overtime are changing month to month? The Pareto chart categorizes factors leading to specific outcomes; however, these data are mainly a snapshot of what existed at the time the data were collected (Grube, 2008). Other approaches exist that depict data trends over time that allow for improved decision-making and prioritization. **Statistical process control** (SPC) is an approach for analyzing data through adding science to QI decision-making (Nelson et al., 2004). SPC uses statistical methods to monitor and control quality processes to reduce or eliminate waste. This chapter will only introduce and cover the basics of SPC as they apply to QI projects.

SPC, a branch of statistics, combines sequential time-based measurements using graphical presentation of performance (Vetter & Morrice, 2019). SPC is a type of statistic that, when applied, demonstrates a statistical approach to QI decision-making. SPC is used to monitor a process over time (time-series design) but adds the ability to identify variation within that process by plotting data points within a run chart or control chart.

In Figure 12.5, after identifying tardiness as the major contributing factor to overtime, it would be valuable to apply principles of SPC to assess variability in the causes of overtime and identify the need for change. For example, 15 causes of overtime in Figure 12.5 were from tardiness. Is this a new outcome? Was tardiness noted only twice last month and suddenly increased? Is tardiness a priority to improve or are there other competing processes needing attention first? SPC depicts process variability, the degree to which the process is stable or unstable over time. Think about the hand hygiene data in Table 12.1. Any change in the percent of hand hygiene compliance from one month to the next month is variability. In Table 12.1 data are presented in a time series, from January through September. However, data displayed in tables do not allow for analysis beyond descriptive statistics. Could the hand hygiene data represent an unstable hand hygiene process, meaning the data fluctuate unpredictably over time? These are important questions answered by applying SPC when analyzing data. In order to answer these questions, the concepts of common cause and special cause variation must be understood.

On any given day, a nurse's lunchtime may vary anytime between 11 a.m. and 1 p.m. This is an expected variation, referred to as **common cause variation** or the inherent variability that exists in all systems (Williams, 2018b). Common cause variation refers to a process or system that is stable "in control." If one day an emergency prevented the nurse from eating lunch until 3 p.m., that time point is very different from the expected lunchtime. When a data point varies significantly in an unpredictable or unexpected manner, it is referred to as **special cause variation**, which is not inherent and signals that something happened (an emergency occurred) that changed the process or system for better or worse and that the process is "out of control" (Williams, 2018b). Because all processes have inherent variation, such as lunch between 11 a.m. and 1 p.m., determining common cause from special cause variation is important. The risk of not knowing if common cause or special cause variation exists is that common cause variation may be prioritized for improvement when improvement is not warranted. Additionally, when special cause variation is identified, that raises a red flag that the process is no longer in control, which may need immediate attention.

Assessing for common cause and special cause variability captures the essence of SPC or being able to look at data over time to determine the type of variability that exists. Both common cause and special cause variation require further interpretation. When special cause variation is found, efforts should focus on identifying an explanation of what occurred that resulted in the process being out of control. If the process exhibits common cause variation, it may not need improvement. When common cause variation exists, the analysis must include answering the question if the process is performing at an acceptable or desired level. Just because the process is under control (common cause variation) does not mean the process could not be improved to a higher level of performance. For example, say hand hygiene data that illustrate compliance to the CDC hand hygiene guidelines was measured monthly for a home healthcare team. The annual mean of compliance was reported as 65%, within common cause variation. Although 65% is within common cause variability, the question remains if 65% is acceptable. If it is not, an improvement could be recommended. If it is not but other priorities for improvement take precedence, working to increase hand hygiene compliance may need to wait.

In SPC, assessing variability requires use of formats such as the run chart (Figure 12.6) or Shewhart control chart (Figure 12.7). Because the goal is to reduce process variation and to sustain reduced variation over time, there is considerable movement in healthcare to use SPC as a QI methodology when analyzing outcome data (Brady et. al., 2018). Both the run chart and the Shewhart control chart are tools used to assess process variation.

The Run Chart

The **run chart** is a graphical display depicting data over time (Williams, 2018a). Run charts are frequently used in QI and are an important tool to assess effectiveness of QI changes (Institute for Healthcare Improvement [IHI], 2020). The graph includes data on one outcome variable, for example, compliance to hand hygiene CDC guidelines, on the *y*-axis of the run chart or graph. Intervals or time points based on the frequency of data outputs are plotted along the graph's *x*-axis. Recall that a time-series format refers to the representation of data over consecutive time points. It can be used for any type of data, including measurement and count data created by hand or using software. Characteristic of all-time series charts, the *x*-axis (horizontal) represents the period of time and the *y*-axis (vertical) represents the variable being measured (Figure 12.6).

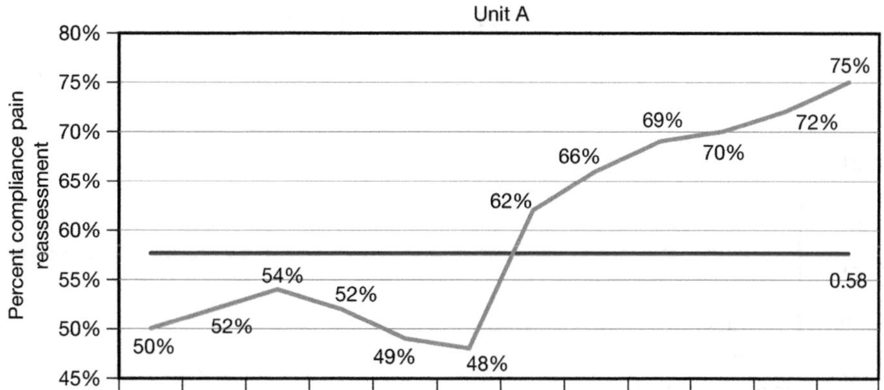

	Oct	Nov	Dec	Jan	Feb	Mar	Apr	May	Jun	Jul	Aug	Sep
Unit A	50%	52%	54%	52%	49%	48%	62%	66%	69%	70%	72%	75%
Median	0.58	0.58	0.58	0.58	0.58	0.58	0.58	0.58	0.58	0.58	0.58	0.58

(a)

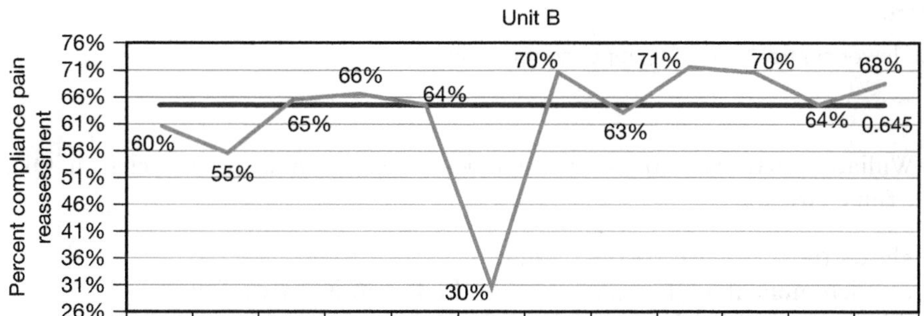

	Oct	Nov	Dec	Jan	Feb	Mar	Apr	May	Jun	Jul	Aug	Sep
Unit B	60%	55%	65%	66%	64%	30%	70%	63%	71%	70%	64%	68%
Median	0.65	0.65	0.65	0.65	0.65	0.65	0.65	0.65	0.65	0.65	0.65	0.65

(b)

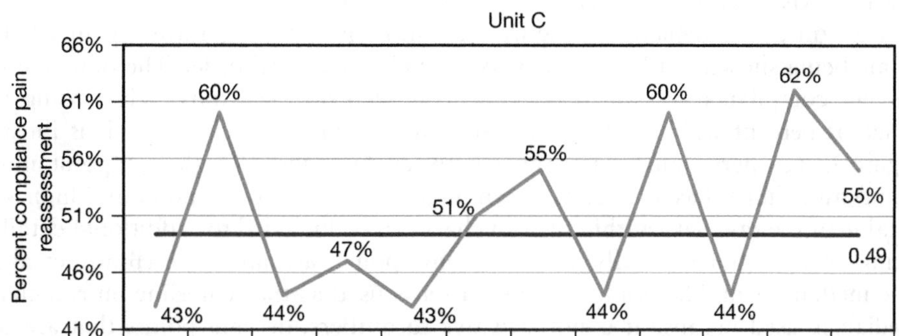

	Oct	Nov	Dec	Jan	Feb	Mar	Apr	May	Jun	Jul	Aug	Sep
Unit C	43%	60%	44%	47%	43%	51%	55%	44%	60%	44%	62%	55%
Median	0.49	0.49	0.49	0.49	0.49	0.49	0.49	0.49	0.49	0.49	0.49	0.49

(c)

FIGURE 12.6 Run Charts Demonstrating Pain Reassessment Compliance Within 60 Minutes of IV Pain Medication Administration for Three Units.

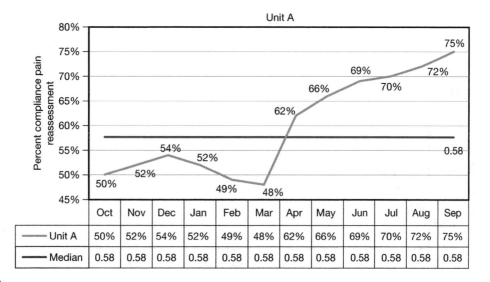

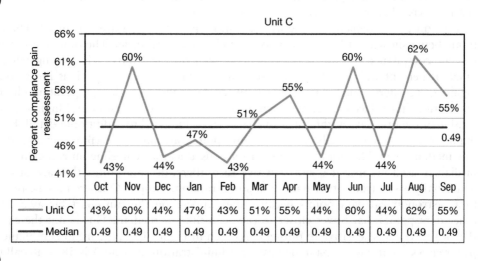

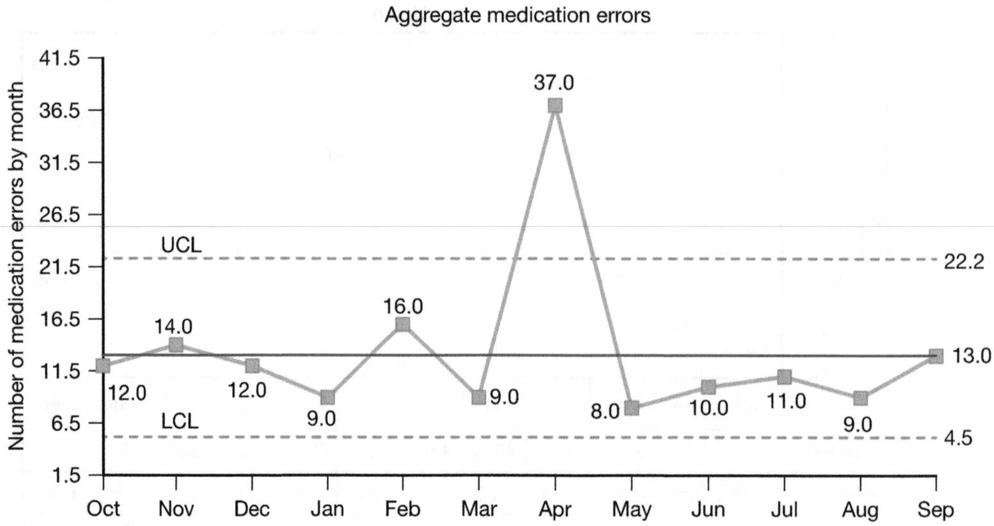

FIGURE 12.7 Aggregate Incident Report Data Over 12 Months Using a Shewhart Control Chart.

LCL, lower control limit; UCL, upper control limit.

Williams (2018a) identifies three significant benefits of using a run chart in QI activities. The run chart:

- allows the process to become visible
- can determine if a QI intervention resulted in an improvement
- if improvement has been sustained post-intervention

Process trends or movement away from a central point, such as the median, can be analyzed using the run chart. The run chart allows teams to assess how a process is working. The process can be routine, such as assessing pain reassessment post IV pain administration or assessing a new process implemented for an improvement. Simply stated, the run chart is a visual graph displaying a processes' performance.

The run charts depicted in Figure 12.6 show how the data are organized. The time frame being shown is 12 months (x-axis) in chronological order. The outcome variable, percent compliance of pain reassessment, is seen on the y-axis. When using SPC, the range of percent will vary by unit based on each unit's outcomes. This is illustrated in Figure 12.6, where Unit A has a range between 48% and 75% (lowest point and highest point) and Unit B has a range between 30% and 71% (lowest point and highest point). A table of the raw data within the run chart can be included for additional detail. Expert opinions vary, but generally 10 to 20 time points are adequate (Brady et al., 2018). The median or middle point of the data set is used as the centerline on run charts. The median is used because it is not sensitive to **outliers**, or data points that are observed abnormally away from other data points in a random sample. Outliers may be referred to as astronomical data points because they appear on the run chart far away from other data points that hover closer to the centerline or median. This is not the case of the mean, which is sensitive to outliers. As seen in Figure 12.6, the mean compliance of pain reassessment post IV pain medication administration for Unit A is 58%. Recall that the median is calculated by first arranging the data from low to high (48, 49, 50, 52, 52, 54, 62, 66, 69, 70, 72, 75). Because the median is the middle point and there are 12 time points on the graph (October to September), the sixth (54%) and seventh (62%) data points are added and divided (54%+ 62% = 116/2 = 58%). In assessing the run chart, first consider if the data are hovering close to the median line or if the data are spread inconsistently from the median. If the data points hover close to the median, the process variation is minimal. If the data are inconsistently away from the median line, that represents greater process variation. When data points fall significantly above or below the median line, an outlier or an unusual finding exists. Now, look at Unit C in Figure 12.6. The median centerline is at 49%, which was determined by the raw compliance percent in chronological order from low to high: 43, 43, 44, 44, 44, 47, 51, 55, 55, 60, 60, and 62. Because we have an even number of data points, the two middle points (47 and 51) are averaged (47 + 51= 98/2 = 49%).

The run chart is useful in determining QI opportunities. When using a run chart, there is no true statistical analysis occurring in comparison to the control chart discussed in the following section. However, the run chart allows for quick analysis and visual review of how a process is performing. Looking back at Figure 12.6, does any unit's data demonstrate an outlier or finding different from the others? With a median of 65% compliance, the 30% compliance observed in March is an outlier. In general, Unit B is relatively stable with most compliance scores hovering around the median line, except for March, which was a drastic drop from February (64%). Unit B should ask, what happened in March? Is there an explanation for this change? Perhaps Unit B was orienting new nurses who were not yet familiar with the pain policy. Also notice the improvement in April (70%). Is this improvement based on a QI intervention or did the new nurses become familiar with the pain policy? Before mobilizing resources to improve an outlier representing special cause variation, first determine if there is an explanation. If so, monitor the unit for the next few months to determine if that outlier was incidental or if there actually is a problem needing QI intervention. If one special cause data point cannot be explained that might place patients at risk, further QI intervention is warranted.

Comparing the three units in Figure 12.6 regarding their compliance with pain reassessment requires thinking about the data. Unit A was below the median for the first 6 months then steadily improved over the last 6 months. What is not known is if the unit implemented a QI intervention in March with the following 6 months demonstrating positive improvement. If an intervention was implemented it should be sustained and celebrated. Also unknown is if the change from March (48%) to April (62%) was special cause variation. With the additional subsequent data points in June and September, it appears that the pain reassessment process changed for the better and that improved performance is being sustained. One challenge when interpreting a run chart is the subjectivity in identifying a data point as an outlier. Subjectivity is eliminated by using the control chart, described in the following section. Unit B's process has been in control except for that one special cause finding in March. Unit C demonstrates lots of variability in outcomes. There is little consistency month to month. Although no special cause can be clearly defined, a QI intervention may be needed to reduce or explain the process variation that is illustrated.

When evaluating outcomes on a graph, such as a run chart, establishing an acceptable outcome goal is necessary for analysis and decision-making. In addition, publishing the goal on the graph ensures accurate interpretation. In Figure 12.6, only Unit A added the goal of 90% compliance to their graph. Adding relative internal and external comparison to the run chart can also provide benchmarking opportunities. For example, organizations may wish to compare their outcomes to other organizations and such comparisons could be used to determine if one organization is performing at a different level than another. Table 12.3 summarizes types of variation, analysis considerations, and potential QI actions. Prioritization is based on the volume and criticality of the outcomes and should include the consensus of QI experts and staff involved in the process. The run chart is helpful to determine improvement priorities and actions

TABLE 12.3 VARIATION INTERPRETATIONS, ANALYSIS, AND QUALITY IMPROVEMENT ACTIONS

TYPE OF VARIATION	ANALYSIS	QI ACTIONS
Common Cause Variation (Process In-Control)	Is the process demonstrating acceptable variation/acceptable level of performance?	No QI actions are required.
	Is the process in control but a widerange or unacceptable variation exists?	QI actions may be required based on QI priorities.
Special Cause Variation (Process Out-of-Control)	Is the process statistically demonstrating a problem, a change that is not desirable?	Action is required.
	Is the process statistically demonstrating improvement based on QI efforts?	Continue to monitor to determine if efforts are sustained over time; if so, spread the lessons learned.

QI, quality improvement.

to be taken based on analysis. Additionally, although Unit C might like to reduce its variation, the reality is other more critical problems may require attention first. At the same time, if the organization only has three units and all three did not meet the compliance goal, that may imply a systemic problem needing further analysis and potential QI action.

One advantage of using a run chart is its ease in interpretation. One disadvantage is that it is not as statistically sensitive as other tools with more specificity (Brady et al., 2018; Lloyd, 2010). There is another type of chart, the Shewhart control chart, commonly referred to as the control chart, described in the following section that adds a statistical advantage to the run chart that clearly detects outliers and eliminates the need for guessing. It takes time and practice to interpret run charts. For a closer look at interpreting a run chart, refer to Box 12.1.

BOX 12.1 Developing Clinical Judgment

At a Unit C QI meeting, a nurse asks for assistance interpreting the run chart on Unit C's pain reassessment compliance presented in Figure 12.6. The nurse wants to know if the unit improved their pain reassessment compliance over the last month. The nurse also is unsure if high or low results are the goal.

1. What **CUES (Assessment)** in Figure 12.6 would you use to provide a brief interpretation of the run chart for this nurse regarding high versus low results, variation over time, and the overall median of the unit's pain reassessment compliance?
2. What **HYPOTHESIS (Diagnosis)** or hypotheses can the nurse consider based on interpretation of the data?
3. What **ACTION (Plan and Implement)** will be most effective based on the data analysis?
4. Would you recommend a QI action based on the run chart **OUTCOME (Evaluation)**?

The Shewhart Control Chart

The Shewhart control chart, often referred to as simply a **control chart**, is similar to a run chart in that it is a graphical display of data but adds statistical control limits to the run chart using SD (Williams, 2018b). Because SD is used, the centerline is represented by the mean of the data set rather than the median that is seen on the run chart. The *x*- and *y*-axis are set up the same on both charts, with the *x*-axis being the time points and the *y*-axis being the variable or process under study. The Shewhart control chart has the same purpose as the run chart, that is, to distinguish common cause from special cause variation.

Recall the discussion about SD and that "sigma" is another term used for SD. The Shewhart control chart, created by software such as QI Macros, will set SD control limits at 1, 2, and 3 SD above and below the mean of the data set. The advantage of the Shewhart control chart is the addition of SD because there is no guessing if an outlier or abnormal data point is present, which will be demonstrated shortly. When analyzing a Shewhart control chart, the **upper control limit** (UCL) is defined as the line 3 SD above the mean while the **lower control limit** (LCL) is the line 3 SD below the mean. The addition of SD represents a clear advantage over the run chart because the control chart defines expected variation by adding the UCL and LCL (Brady et al., 2018). A process that is considered in control or demonstrating common cause variability will have all data points between the UCL (+3 SD from the mean) and LCL (-3 SD from the mean). Together, the upper and lower control limits represent Six Sigma. When a data point falls above or below the UCL or LCL, the process is said to have a statistically significant outcome, referred to as special cause variation, or abnormal finding.

Data can be displayed using a variety of formats, including histograms, Pareto charts, run charts, and Shewhart control charts. Each format has a purpose and a value within QI. Consider the Pareto chart in Figure 12.8. These data represent the annual incident reports of a large multisite organization. Medication errors are the leading cause of incident reports over a 12-month period. That outcome could trigger a QI activity. However, there are more sophisticated SPC methods available to better analyze these incident report data.

In Figure 12.7, aggregate medication errors are shown on a Shewhart control chart using a time-series design over 12 months. A range of outcomes, in this case from eight to 37 medication errors, is depicted, which represents significant variation. In analyzing aggregate medication errors in Figure 12.7, consider the differences in the control chart as opposed to a run chart. The major difference includes the addition of the UCL and LCL, which can be used to analyze the process range. Because nearly 100% (specifically 99.8%) of outcomes are expected to fall within three SD from the mean, as seen in Figure 12.1, using three SD is generally considered acceptable when analyzing for special cause variation. In Figure 12.7, the UCL was automatically calculated at 22.2 and the LCL at 4.5 using the QI Macros software.

Evaluating the UCL and LCL is valuable because these limits specify the process range. As illustrated in Figure 12.7, the mean of aggregated medication errors over the 12-month period was 13. The UCL or 3 SD above the mean is 22.2 while the LCL or 3 SD below the mean is 4.5. The significance or analysis of these results is that between 22 and 4.5 medication errors could occur each month and be considered in control, or within Six Sigma of the mean. In this case, that alone might trigger a QI activity as 22 medication errors a month while being considered in control would be concerning from a patient safety perspective. Also note in Figure 12.7 the centerline is the mean of the data points in a Shewhart control chart, whereas the centerline on a run chart is the median of the data set.

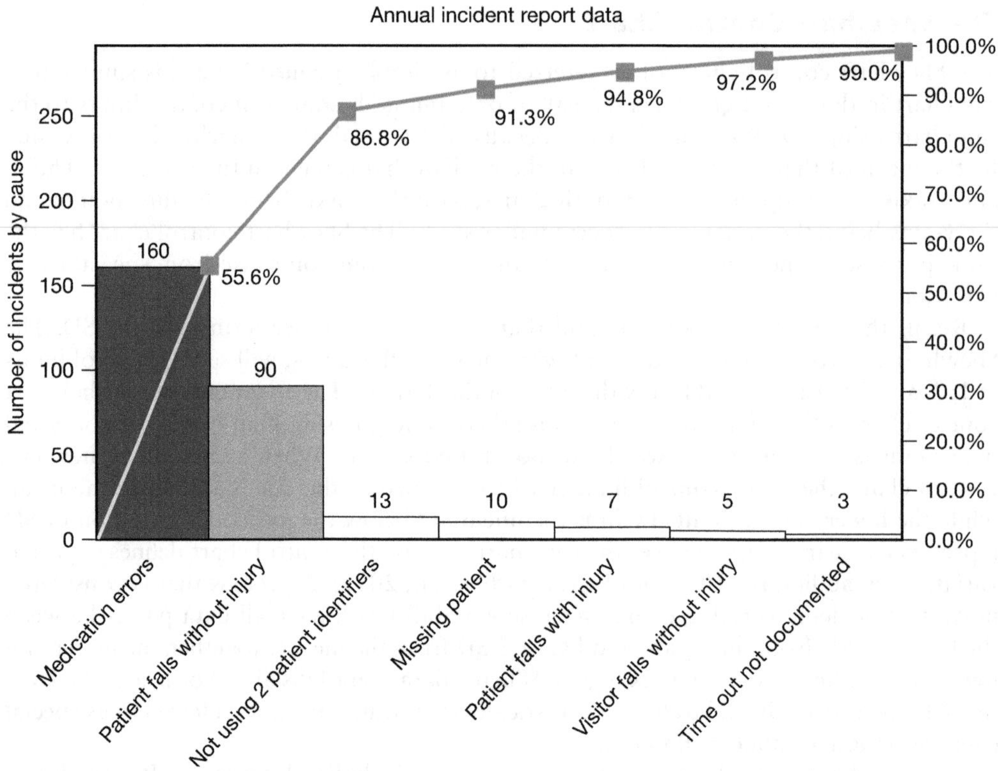

FIGURE 12.8 Incident Report Data Over 12 Months Using a Pareto Chart.

There are several different types of Shewhart control charts beyond the scope of this chapter. At this point, it is important to apply the same rule used with the run chart, that is, identifying if an outlier or astronomical data point exists. With the Shewhart control chart, special cause is evident when a data point appears either above or below the control limits. Analysis and QI actions taken based on the interpretation of the run chart outlined in Table 12.3 also apply to the Shewhart control chart: 37 incidents in April is nicely depicted significantly above the UCL in Figure 12.7. There is no guessing required if the data point represents special cause variation as it is above the UCL of 22. The Shewhart control chart reduces interpretation errors and the risk of not implementing QI activities when necessary or implementing QI activities when not necessary, leading to inappropriate resource utilization. In addition, notice that the number of medication errors was significantly reduced in the month of May to eight and remained hovering around the mean of 13 through September. This is a good example that when an unusual outcome occurs, such as 37 medication errors in April, it may be advantageous not to react and implement a QI activity but rather to acknowledge the outcome, continue to assess it, and follow the trends to determine if the number of medication errors continues to rise over time, which would demonstrate statistical significance by being above the UCL.

In addition to assessing for outliers, or astronomical data points on run or control charts, there are additional basic rules applied for analyzing these charts as illustrated in Box 12.2.

SPC is a common tool used in QI by plotting data over time on a run or control chart. Recall the discussion on rapid cycle PDSA in Chapter 11. Each PDSA cycle introduces a different intervention followed by measurement. A run or control chart can be used to show at what time point the PDSA cycle was introduced (McQuillan et al., 2016). Analysis of the chart can follow measurement to visualize the impact the intervention has on the process measure and subsequently the impact toward the improvement goal (Roberts et al., 2018). There are many examples and resources demonstrating the value of incorporating multiple PDSA cycles to either a run or control chart, such as the resources from the IHI accessible at www.ihi.org/resources/Pages/HowtoImprove/ScienceofImprovementEstablishingMeasures.aspx.

It is, however, feasible to react to data displayed on any of the data display methods described in this chapter rather than conducting thoughtful analysis. In addition, the opposite may occur when data clearly indicates special cause variation and is analyzed as such, but no action is implemented. There is potential to mistakenly introduce many interventions at the same time or an intervention that does not address the root cause of the problem because the actual root cause was not identified. Even those considered "experts" may react, as seen in Box 12.3.

Stratification

Stratification is the process of breaking down large amounts of data into subsets or groups. Using stratification separates data for easier interpretation or to identify patterns within the data (ASQ, 2021). Suppose the patient safety officer (PSO) is studying Figure 12.7 and prioritizes medication errors for a QI project. Before moving forward, stratification of the 160 aggregated medication errors could help target where QI efforts should

CASE STUDY

After a successful QI project, the improvement advisor on the team, a nurse from Quality Management, notices your interest in analyzing control charts. During the conversation, you ask the advisor if there are tips to analyzing control charts. You mention understanding the basics, such as an outlier outside the control limits, but know there must be more to it than that. The advisor agrees there are several easy rules to analyze run and control charts. The advisor offers to send you a simple table with the rules. The advisor also notes rules may vary depending on reference, but simplifying is best when learning to apply these rules for analysis.

RUN CHART	CONTROL CHART
Look for a **SHIFT**: ***6*** or more consecutive data points either above or below the ***median***.	Look for a **SHIFT**: ***8*** or more consecutive data points either above or below the ***mean***.
Look for a **TREND**: ***5*** or more consecutive data points going either up or down.	Look for a **TREND**: ***6*** or more consecutive data points going either up or down.
Look for an outlier or **ASTRONOMICAL** data point: An obvious data point unexpected, either above or below the ***median***.	Look for an outlier or **ASTRONOMICAL** data point: A data point above the UCL or below the LCL.

Sources: Data from McQuillan, R. F., Silver, S. A., Harel, Z., Weizman, A., Thomas, A., Bell, C., Chertow, G. M., Chan, C. T., & Nesrallah, G. (2016). How to measure and interpret quality improvement data. *Clinical Journal of the American Society of Nephrology, 11*, 908-914. https://doi.org/10.2215/CJN.11511015; Williams, E. (2018a). Understanding variation: Part 1- the run chart. *Current Problems in Pediatric Adolescent Health Care, 48*, 186-190. https://doi.org/10.1016/j.cppeds.2018.08.012; Williams, E. (2018b). Understanding variation-Part 2: The control chart. *Current Problems in Pediatric Adolescent Health Care, 48*, 202-205. https://doi.org/10.1016/j.cppeds.2018.08.009

(continued)

CASE STUDY (CONTINUED)

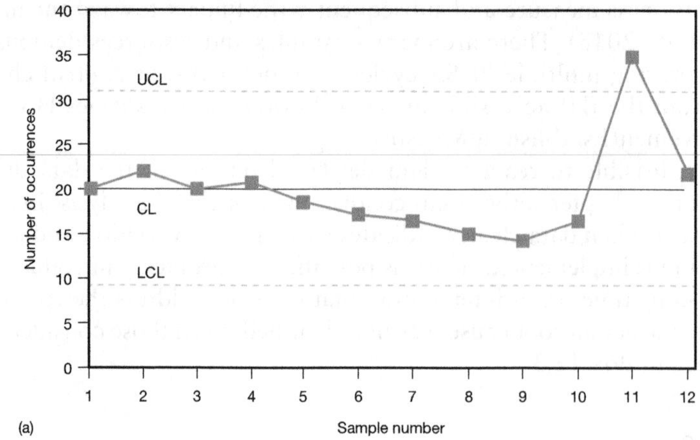

(a)

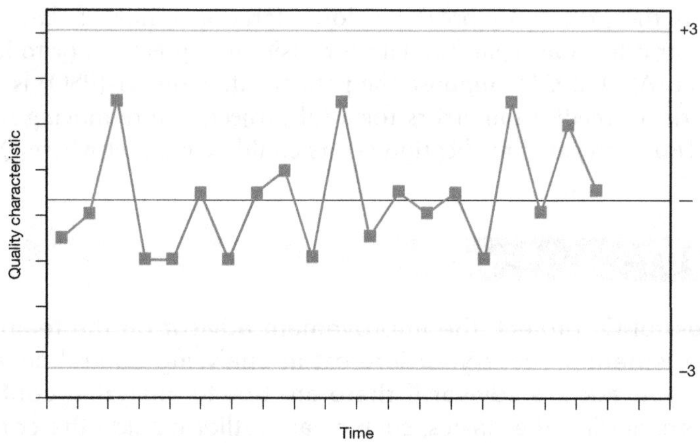

(b)

1. *Using the first example and the cues from the interpretation rules, is there evidence of a shift, trend, or astronomical data point?*
2. *As you look at Example 2, is the graph a run or control chart?*
3. *If Example 2 is a run chart, is there evidence of a shift or trend? If Example 2 is a control chart, is there evidence of a shift or trend?*
4. *After analyzing the example charts sent, you meet with the advisor. You ask what the significance of a shift or trend means when analyzing these charts. The advisor asks you to think about it. How could a shift or trend impact run or control chart analyses?*

CL, control limit; LCL, lower control limit; UCL, upper control limit.

focus. To do so, the 160 medication errors could be stratified into outpatient and inpatient areas. Data could be further stratified among inpatient or outpatient units to better determine if one unit is contributing to the abnormal finding. Additional questions should be considered: Were there truly so few errors, except in April? Does all staff understand the reporting process? Is the operational definition of medication errors clear? Does the organization's culture support reporting medication errors?

CASE STUDY

At a staff meeting, the control chart of aggregate medication errors, Figure 12.7, is presented. The facility PSO is very concerned about the 37 errors that occurred in April. The PSO informs the staff they must do a QI project as 37 errors is unacceptable. In addition, the PSO informs staff several interventions must occur by the end of the week including to read the procedure on medication administration, complete a self-study exercise created by the PSO, and schedule in-services with pharmacy staff to identify what the incidents were related to (the root cause) in April before the QI project is started.

1. *What QI cues could you identify as problematic based on the PSO's intervention recommendations before the QI project began?*
2. *The PSO did not interpret the control chart (Figure 12.7) at the staff meeting. Wanting to confirm the urgency of the problem, you analyze the chart. What analysis of the chart would allow you to agree or disagree with the PSO's level of urgency?*
3. *A QI team is created to reduce the number of medication errors. The three interventions identified by the PSO are considered because the PSO identified them. Before acting by introducing each intervention, the team plans the project by evaluating the 37 incident reports observed in April:*
   - *How would you begin evaluating the specific April data points?*
   - *Does the initial evaluation of April's data points identify the root cause?*
   - *How would you assess the control chart to determine when continued PDSA cycles are no longer warranted?*

Real World Interview

Transitioning from the role of bedside nurse to the role of a quality assurance nurse was quite an adjustment, but I saw it as an opportunity to blend my clinical knowledge with my knowledge of information systems. I'm a problem-solver by nature, and I am passionate about developing ways to apply technology in a meaningful way to better serve our organization. Important tasks of my role as a quality assurance nurse include collecting, analyzing, and presenting data. When I first began in this role, much of this was being done by hand, which was hard for me to believe knowing that we as a facility had the technology available to make this process easier and more efficient. I knew I could immediately improve this process by using Microsoft Excel. Microsoft Excel is my go-to application for data collection and analysis because it is a widely available application and many software packages offer the ability to export their data collected in a format that is easily imported to Excel.

Although I consider myself to be very competent with the use of Excel, I quickly learned that some of the functions that I wanted to execute required me to seek additional training. YouTube and internet search engines like Google are my learning tools of choice. It still amazes me as to how much information is available at my fingertips through the internet. Additionally, I reach out to subject matter experts, colleagues, and participate in training available to me through work.

Some of the challenges I face include ensuring the data collected is meaningful and presented in an organized, clear manner. A way to make the data more meaningful is through standardization. Many times, I can standardize data through the creation of lists in Excel. This data standardization makes it easier for me to analyze the data and choose the right type of graph or chart to present the data in a meaningful way. I also work closely with health information specialists and clinical application coordinators to develop a standardized method of data collection at the end-user level.

In my role as a quality assurance nurse, my knowledge and appreciation for information systems has grown tremendously. I am committed to continued learning and growth, and I am honored that my role as a quality assurance nurse affords me the opportunity to enhance patient safety and quality care through the meaningful use of technology and information systems.

Nichole Coyne, RN, BSN

Quality Assurance Nurse

Sterile Processing Service, Boston VA Healthcare System, Boston, Massachusetts

OTHER QUALITY IMPROVEMENT TEAM TOOLS

Interprofessional teams are often created to bring experts and /or process owners together to address problems and make improvements. QI tools, such as Gantt charts and flow maps, help teams work through projects. These team tools as well as those discussed in Chapter 11, such as cause and effect or fishbone diagrams, Lean thinking, Six Sigma, Plan-Do-Study-Act (PDSA), Health Failure Mode and Effect Analysis (HFMEA), and RCA, are all QI tools used by teams.

Gantt Chart

A **Gantt chart** is a graph depicting the phases of a project over the project's timeline and is used to keep the team on schedule (Figure 12.9). All known project tasks are included in the Gantt chart, from beginning to end. Because QI takes time and effort, line 16 of the Gantt chart in Figure 12.9 nicely reminds us to celebrate and share success, something all teams should include in their planning.

Flow Map

QI is focused on improving the healthcare process; therefore, understanding each step within the process must be considered before interventions are identified. As introduced in Chapter 11, a **flow map**, or process flowchart, is a visual depiction of a process from the beginning of the process to the conclusion or end of the process and allows the QI team to diagram the actual sequence of activities and decisions within the process. Clarifying the sequence of a process reduces redundancy, unnecessary steps, and may illustrate overly complex or unnecessary steps of a process that can be redesigned or eliminated. Because healthcare processes are often complex, reducing the number of steps or decisions within a process is not only more efficient but may enhance patient safety. In addition to identifying inefficient steps in a process, flow maps also provide a visual step-by-step flow of a process that may not need to be more efficient but rather to provide a visual tool outlining the steps of a task or procedure. For example, although a nursing procedure such as blood administration will outline a written step-by-step process that the nurse must follow when administering blood, it is not uncommon to include a visual flow map of that process within the procedure.

Different steps or actions within a healthcare process are represented by specific symbols in a flow map, such as ovals to depict the beginning and end points. Squares are used to identify steps in the healthcare process. Diamonds identify decision points, and arrows

Emergency department microsystem redesign project

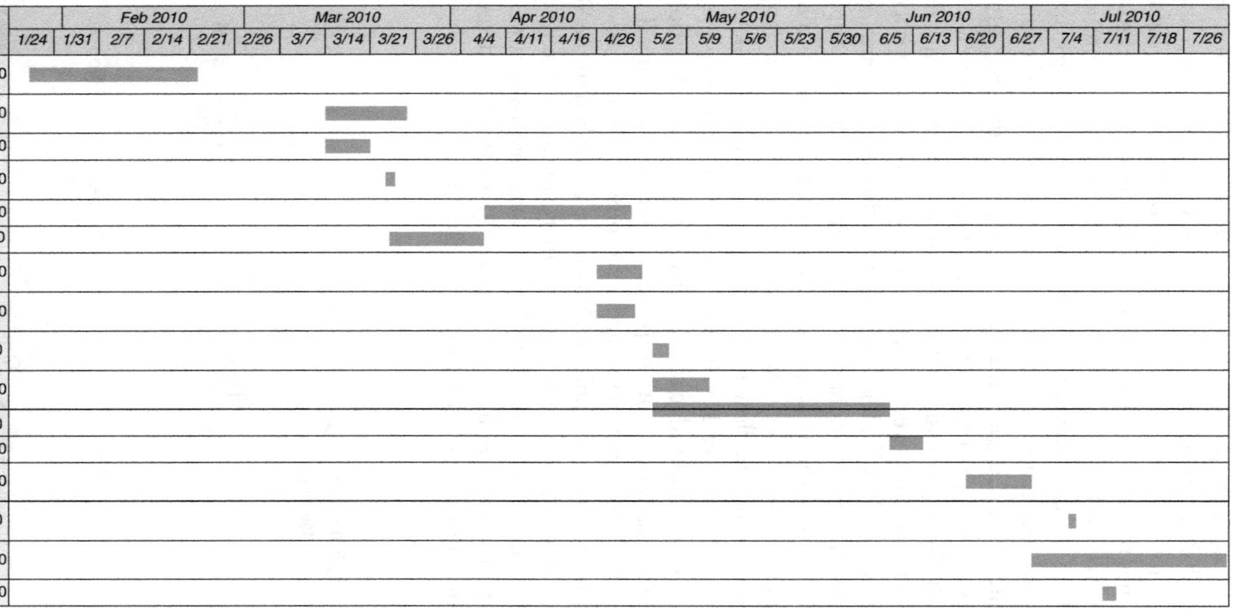

ID	Task name	Start	Finish
1	Defined global aim of the project	1/29/2010	2/21/2010
2	Defined specific aim of the project	3/15/2010	3/24/2010
3	Created ED flow log	3/15/2010	3/19/2010
4	Team coaching regarding the tool	3/24/2010	3/24/2010
5	Data collection (pre)	4/9/2010	4/29/2010
6	Study and evaluate ED tools	3/25/2010	4/8/2010
7	Satisfaction survey (pre) for patients and ED staff	4/26/2010	4/30/2010
8	Created SharePoint access to data and satisfaction survey	4/26/2010	4/29/2010
9	Made changes to computerized triage template	5/7/2010	5/7/2010
10	Team coaching regarding the triage tool	5/7/2010	5/12/2010
11	Data collection (post)	5/8/2010	6/9/2010
12	Analyzed the data	6/10/2010	6/14/2010
13	Satisfaction survey (post) for patients and ED staff	6/23/2010	6/30/2010
14	Displayed the results to the team	7/7/2010	7/7/2010
15	Report to management in PDSA format	7/1/2010	7/30/2010
16	Celebrate and share success	7/14/2010	7/14/2010

FIGURE 12.9 The Gantt Chart.

identify directional flow of the process. Figure 12.10 shows a basic flow map on the flow of patients through an ED. There are different types of flow maps that can be used based on the process complexity, allowing easier examination of the process. Figure 12.11 is a flow map using swim lanes that divides the process into key phases with the steps of each phase outlined. This flow map in Figure 12.11 divides new employee orientation of a sterile processing service, where reusable medical equipment is reprocessed for safe reuse, into four phases. Phase 1 is arrival, general orientation, and completion of computerized required orientation content. Phase 2 depicts the new employee in an observational role learning by watching the preceptor perform the reprocessing tasks. The new employee observes the preceptor in all the reprocessing areas that exist at this facility. Phase 3 replicates Phase 2 but now the new employee is performing the task in all reprocessing areas being observed by the preceptor. Finally, Phase 4 illustrates that the new employee has completed the knowledge components of orientation and is now ready to complete competencies. There are several benefits to this example flow map. It can be used as a recruitment tool to explain to potential new employees how they will be oriented. Should any auditor ask how new employees are oriented, the flow map can easily be used to walk the auditor through the orientation process. Another key benefit is ensuring new employees have adequate time to gain the necessary knowledge to correctly perform the tasks prior to assessing their competency skills and the opportunity to provide additional training if needed.

This chapter examined what data are and how data can be displayed for QI decision-making and monitoring. Tools, such as those described in the SPC section earlier, provide the QI team with the most efficient, systematic means of determining what healthcare process needs improvement or if a QI was sustained over time. **Interprofessional teams** are charged to learn, conduct, and utilize QI methods and tools in practice, as described in the corresponding Current Literature feature.

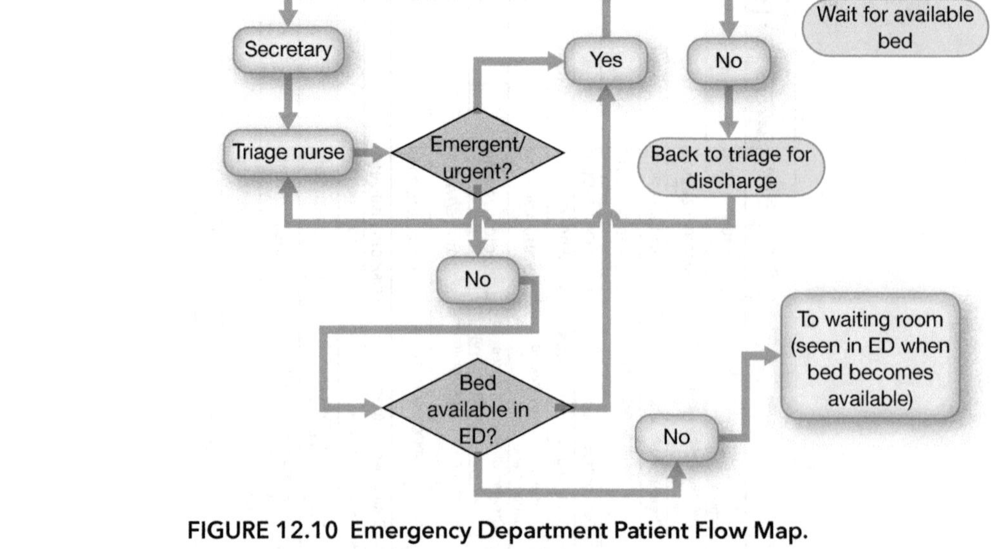

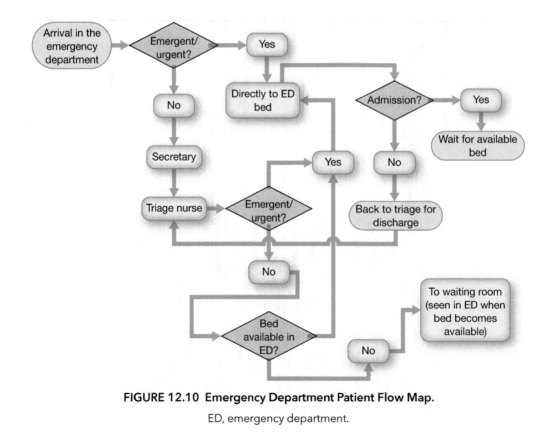

FIGURE 12.10 Emergency Department Patient Flow Map.

ED, emergency department.

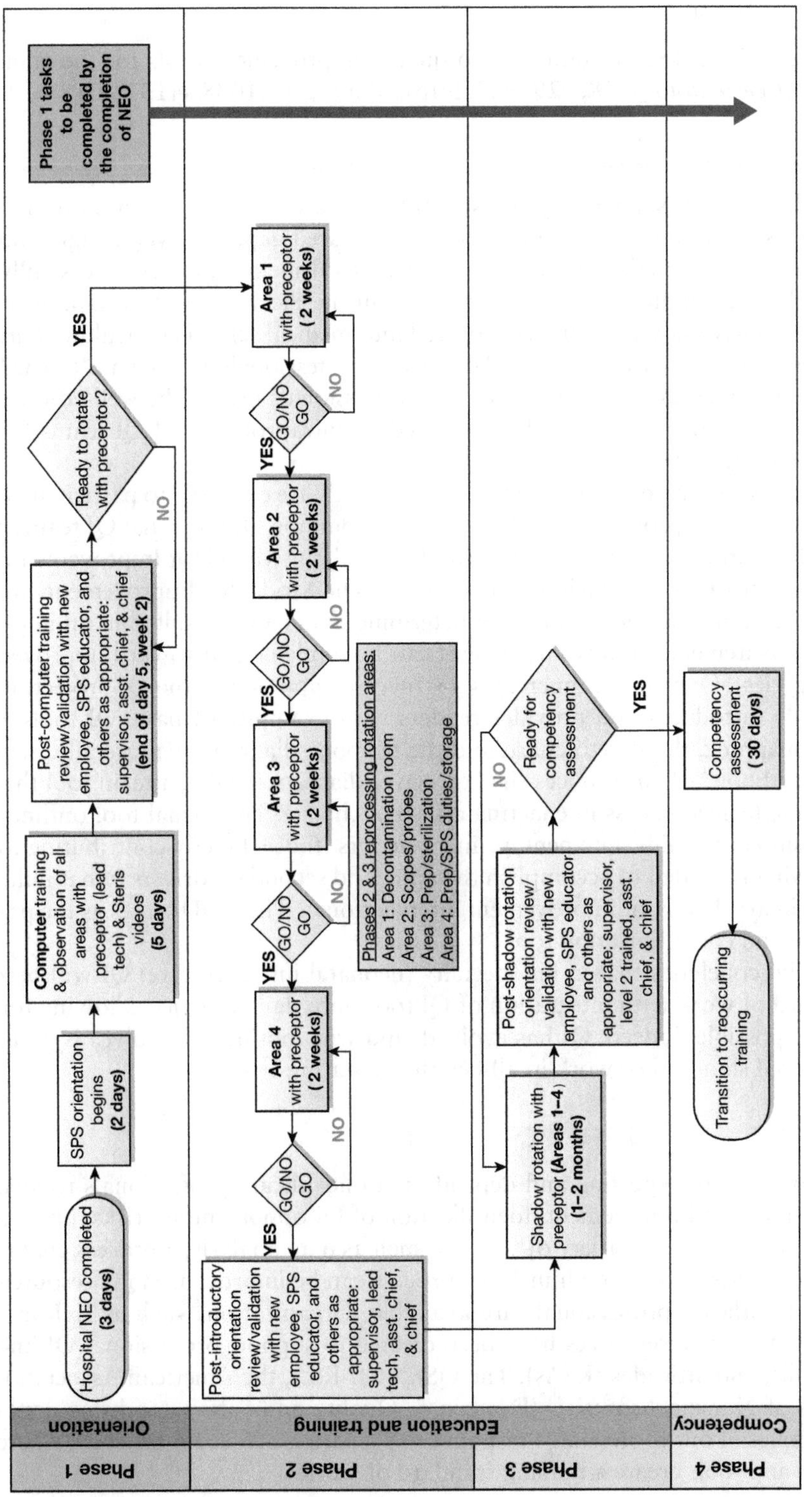

FIGURE 12.11 Flow Map Using Swim Lanes.

CURRENT LITERATURE

CITATION

Picarillo, A. P. (2018). Introduction to quality improvement tools for the clinician. *Journal of Perinatology, 38*, 929–935. https://doi.org/10.1038/s41372-018-0100-4

DISCUSSION

The author describes a gap in professional healthcare workers, attention to measuring processes that impact care delivery. This declared gap, however, is tightening as healthcare professionals embrace the science of QI methodologies successfully applied in business industries, such as manufacturing. Picarillo, a physician, mentions QI methods have slowly been incorporated into medical school curriculum. Furthermore, as expectations rise that all healthcare professionals participate toward the goal of improving care delivery processes, professionals need to be well-educated to the various QI tools and how they are used by intraprofessional QI teams for the gap to be mitigated.

After making a case that healthcare professionals are expected to participate in QI activities, Picarillo provides a brief overview of common QI tools that QI teams must be familiar with. He described a templated QI tool, the Model for Improvement, that creates a structured approach for the QI team. The Model for Improvement emphasizes a clear aim statement, ability to determine if a change resulted in an improvement (measurement), and what changes can be implemented toward improvement (PDSA cycles). Once the team creates a structure approach to the QI project, Picarillo briefly introduces and provides readers with examples of basic QI tools, such as flow mapping, the Pareto chart, and the fishbone diagram, that are all discussed in this textbook. He introduces the key driver diagram (KDD), a team tool that increases the team's success in enacting a system change. This visual tool outlines the relationship of the aim statement, primary drivers (those directly contributing to the aim or what is needed to accomplish the aim), and secondary drivers (what influences the primary drivers or improvement interventions). The KDD serves as the project roadmap and communication tool.

Picarillo concludes that in his specialty (neonatal intensive care) QI will become a standard of work with integration of QI tools into daily practice, allowing for the best care possible. Indeed, QI has evolved, and will continue to evolve, as an intraprofessional standard of work in all healthcare settings.

IMPLICATIONS FOR PRACTICE

Organizations are expecting and depend on all healthcare professionals to identify opportunities for improvement. Identification of QI opportunities, risks, or even errors may occur from a variety of sources, such as data analysis, a process challenge, audits, errors/risks, or just a hunch the process can be improved. Many resources to support healthcare professionals are available. Organizations such as IHI are one example. Academic resources have been created to support professional QI knowledge, skills, and attitudes (KSAs). The QSEN QI KSA, the American Association of Colleges of Nursing *Essentials* (Domain 5: Quality and Safety), and this textbook are examples of our profession's response to preparing nurses for practice, where QI methods and tools create a nursing standard of work.

Academics provide an introductory or fundamental knowledge of QI, but the skills, comfort, and energy gained making improvements are truly realized by doing QI projects at your organization. Although Picarillo was specific to healthcare professionals, do not forget to include support staff in QI activities. A secretary, housekeeper, telephone operator, logistic supply technician, and so on, all provide services we depend on. Support staff can identify issues and interventions, and provide insight we may miss on how their role can impact care delivery. We are all in this together, trying to learn how to create and sustain improved healthcare outcomes. QI KSAs support our professional development, patient safety, and our organization's journey toward excellence. You will soon be working at a healthcare organization that expects you to have QI KSAs. Are you ready?

Given the advantages of SPC, these tools should be applied to healthcare decision-making whenever possible. Creating and analyzing data using run or control charts require time and practice. Collaborating with QI experts for assistance is recommended. The next step in the QI journey is to empower a team who utilizes appropriate QI tools for data-driven QIs.

END-OF-CHAPTER RESOURCES

KEY CONCEPTS

1. Quality improvement (QI) is a continuous process used to prevent, recognize, and reduce harm. It includes the ongoing search for performance excellence.
2. QI is defined using the QSEN definition, to "Use data to monitor the outcomes of care processes and use improvement methods to design and test changes to continuously improve the quality and safety of healthcare systems."
3. Quality initiatives are data driven and patient centered.
4. Many sources of data exist, including internal, external, baseline, postintervention, incidence, prevalence, and aggregate.
5. Data can be displayed using a variety of formats, including histograms, Pareto charts, scatter plot diagrams, and run and control charts.
6. The science of QI, mainly statistical process control, is concerned with minimizing variability within healthcare processes.
7. Teams, often interprofessional, bring expertise and innovation to improving outcomes.
8. Teams can use a variety of tools (e.g., flow maps and Gantt chart) during the improvement process.

CRITICAL DISCUSSION POINTS

1. Data is displayed in various formats. A large healthcare organization conducted an analysis of in-patient complaints ($N = 370$) over the past 3 years. A summary of the top 10 standardized complaint categories included:

   Delay in response-call light not answered timely (56)

   Poor food quality (23)

   Cleanliness failures (30)

   Waiting for tests and procedures to be completed (25)

   Waiting for tests and procedure results (40)

   Lack of staff empathy (51)

   Being asked the same questions by different staff (39)

   Pain management (19)

   Poor communication (66)

   Delay in diagnosis (21)

   Given this data, would the nurse support the use of a Pareto chart?
2. At your next clinical experience, ask a nurse about what data is presented to the staff. Ask to see examples of data. Can the nurse locate data? Can the nurse specify the format the data is displayed in? Can the nurse provide a brief analysis of what the key take-away points are based on the data outcomes? Has the data been used for improvement?
3. Thinking about process variation, describe one clinical or personal process where an outlier within that process occurred. Did you make a change to the process because of the outlier?

4. Consider the table of patient heart rate outcomes over the last 3 days:

Day	8a	12N	4p	8p	12M
1	72	84	88	76	64
2	84	104	68	88	72
3	60	80	72	76	64

Can you use the 15 heart rate outcome measures to construct a run chart on a piece of paper? Should the median or mean be used to calculate the centerline? (Then calculate it and add it to your chart.) Does an outlier exist? How would you describe the variation in this patient's HR?

5. Of the two flow maps presented in this chapter, which one would an interprofessional team find more superior?

KEY TERMS

Aggregate data
Baseline data
Common cause variation
Control chart
Data
Data display
Descriptive statistics
External data
Flow map
Gantt chart
Histogram
Incidence data
Information
Internal data
Inter-rater-reliability
Lower control limit
Mean
Median
Mode
Objective data
Operational definition
Outliers
Pareto chart
Postintervention data
Prevalence data
Quality improvement
Quantitative data
Qualitative data
Range
Run chart
Scatter plot diagram
Special cause variation
Standard deviation
Statistical process control
Stratification
Subjective data
Upper control limit
Variability

REVIEW QUESTIONS

Answers to Review Questions appear in the Instructor's Manual. Qualified instructors should request the Instructor's Manual from textbook@springerpub.com.

1. You are reviewing a control chart that depicts the number of falls over a 24-month period. You observe a special cause variation that occurred at month 6. Which characteristic is indicative of a special cause variation?

   A. The sixth month data point is between the upper and lower control limits.

B. The sixth month data point is 2 SD below the mean.

C. The sixth month data point is 1 SD above the mean.

D. The sixth month data point is above the mean at 3 SD.

2. At a staff meeting, the nurse manager reports patient satisfaction has declined on the unit. In analysis of the patient comments, 30% of the 100 discharged patients surveyed over the last month complained about the noise at night. You are asked to be a participant in an improvement team to increase patient satisfaction. Which of the following questions regarding data are most appropriate to obtain from the manager before the team begins their QI project? *Select all that apply.*

A. How many staff will be invited to participate in the team?

B. Is there evidence this finding is a special cause variation?

C. What time frame is permitted to complete the project?

D. Will there be overtime to attend meetings?

E. How will trends be measured?

F. How will participation affect my performance?

3. Tardiness of evening-shift staff has been a problem on the unit. This has led to excessive overtime to ensure that patient shift handoffs are conducted in a timely manner. The manager invites you to monitor evening-shift tardiness for 1 week. There are eight evening nurses. You just completed data collection and are preparing a spreadsheet to share with your manager. Using the findings in the table that follows, what is the mean time for tardiness and range of minutes that evening staff were tardy over this 7-day time period?

Table: Tardiness of Evening Shift

NURSE	SUN	MON	TUE	WED	THU	FRI	SAT
A	OFF	OFF	OT	3 min	OT	OFF	OT
B	OT	12 min	5 min	OFF	13 min	11 min	OFF
C	OT	OFF	OT	5 min	OT	12 min	OFF
D	OT	OT	OFF	OT	OT	OT	OFF
E	OFF	3 min	OT	OT	3 min	OFF	5 min
F	OFF	OT	ILL	5 min	OFF	OT	15 min
G	OT	OFF	20 min	OT	OT	OT	OFF
H	OFF	OT	4 min	OFF	7 min	OT	OT

OT, On Time

A. Mean = 8.0 minutes Range = 3.0–20.0

B. Mean = 5.0 minutes Range = 3.0–20.0

C. Mean = 5.0 minutes Range = 123

D. Mean = 8.2 minutes Range = 3.0–20.0

4. You are the nurse manager of a busy primary care clinic. The providers are complaining they cannot keep up with the increased volume of patients. You decide to look back over time to review monthly appointments. At the next staff meeting, you present the numbers that follow:

Month	No. of Appointments	Month	No. of Appointments
Jan 19	201	Dec 19	263
Feb 19	168	Jan 20	248
Mar 19	210	Feb 20	264
Apr 19	198	Mar 20	245
May 19	201	Apr 20	263
Jun 19	221	May 20	258
Jul 19	227	Jun 20	260
Aug 19	212	Jul 20	283
Sep 19	202	Aug 20	236
Oct 19	237	Sep 20	295
Nov 19	249	Oct 20	275

The providers argue the primary care data is too difficult to analyze in a table format. You agree to put the data into an SPC chart:

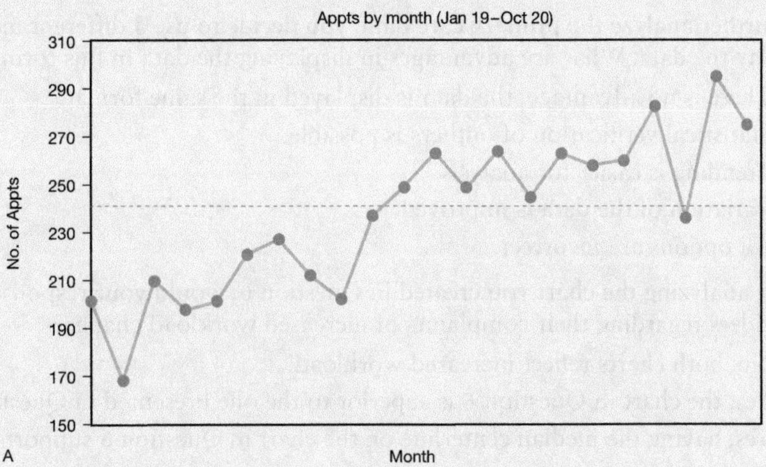

A

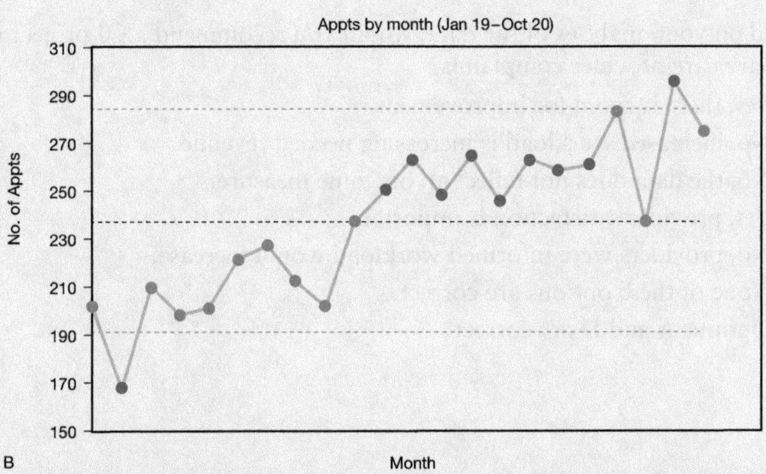

B

How would you best respond to the provider's concerns of increased workload?

A. The mean of the data is 240. Your workload has been consistent over time.

B. The median of 241 is evidence of increased workload.

C. There are several outliers in the data that do not allow for interpretation on workload.

D. Workload has increased but the trends over the last 6 months are decreasing.

E. Options B and C are correct.

F. None of the options are correct.

5. One of the nurse practitioners (NP) at the staff meeting suggested the data should be displayed in a run chart. What would be your response to the NP?
   A. The data displayed is in a run chart.
   B. The data display used will not change the outcome.
   C. The control chart will improve analysis.
   D. The decision how to display data is one for leadership.
   E. Three of the options are correct.
   F. Two of the options are correct.

6. To further analyze the primary care data, you decide to use a different method to display the data. What are advantages in displaying the data in this format?
   A. There is no advantage, the data is displayed in the same format.
   B. Statistical verification of outliers is possible.
   C. Trending is easier for analysis.
   D. Variation of the data is improved.
   E. All options are incorrect.

7. After analyzing the chart you created in Question 6, would your response to the providers regarding their complaints of increased workload change?
   A. No, both charts reflect increased workload.
   B. Yes, the chart in Question 6 is superior to the one presented in Question 4.
   C. Yes, having the median centerline on the chart in Question 6 supports increased workload.
   D. No, workload has increased due to more referrals (data can't answer this).

8. Based on your analyses of the data, would you recommend a QI project to reduce primary care provider complaints?
   A. Yes, there is room for improvement.
   B. No, increased workload is increasing needed revenue.
   C. No, the data does not reflect an outcome measure.
   D. Yes, provider satisfaction is important.
   E. No, providers were informed workload would increase.
   F. None of these options are correct.
   G. Options A and D are correct.

9. Stratification of data refers to which of the following?
   A. Averaging the number of data points
   B. Identifying the lowest and highest data point
   C. Noting 3 standard deviation above or below the mean
   D. Segmenting the data from aggregate to more specific subsets
10. When a QI team wants to document a process from beginning to end, which of the following tools is most helpful?
   A. Flow map diagram
   B. Fishbone diagram
   C. Scatter plot diagram
   D. Pareto chart
11. What is the greatest benefit of using baseline data in QI activities?
   A. It is used to differentiate common from special cause variation.
   B. If an outlier, it will trigger a QI project.
   C. It is used to demonstrate a sustained improvement outcome.
   D. It is used to compare preintervention to postintervention outcomes.

REVIEW ACTIVITIES

1. National Association for Healthcare Quality (NAHQ) http://nahq.org. Read about NAHQ's history and code of ethics. Explore how healthcare professionals, including nurses, can become certified in healthcare quality.
2. The Joint Commission (TJC) www.jointcomission.org. Type in "Sentinel Event" in the search option. Select one of the alerts listed midway down the page. Consider the impact of this alert. What data is presented on the sentinel alert? Conduct a web search on the sentinel alert to identify the prevalence of the problem in healthcare. Consider QI ideas that might eliminate this occurrence from happening. How would you approach preventing this incident in your organization?
3. The Institute for Healthcare Improvement (IHI) www.ihi.org. Create an account to access IHI content. Select the "RESOURCES" tab. Select the "How to Improve" tab. Notice the PDSA cycle is presented with many resources that the improvement team can access. Explore how IHI speaks about "Forming the Team" and examples of effective teams.

EXPLORING THE WEB

1. Robert Wood Johnson Foundation: http://rwjf.org
2. Agency for Healthcare Research and Quality; Data Sources: www.ahrq.gov/research/data/dataresources/index.html
3. The Healthcare Effectiveness Data and Information Set (HEDIS): www.ncqa.org/hedis-quality-measurement
4. Health-Related Datasets: www.healthdata.gov
5. Centers for Medicare & Medicaid Services (Research, Statistics, Data & Systems): www.cms.gov/Research-Statistics-Data-and-Systems/Research-Statistics-Data-and-Systems

A robust set of instructor resources designed to supplement this text is located at **http://connect.springerpub.com/content/book/978-0-8261-6145-1.** Qualifying instructors may request access by emailing **textbook@springerpub.com.**

REFERENCES

American Society for Quality (ASQ). (2021). *What is stratification?* https://asq.org/quality-resources/stratification

Berwick, D. M. (2011). Preparing nurses for participation in and leadership of continual improvement. *Journal of Nursing Education, 50*(6), 322–327. https://doi.org/10.3928/01484834-20110519-05

Brady, P. W., Tchou, M. J., Ambroggio, L., Schondelmeyer, A. C., & Shaughnessy, E. E. (2018). Quality improvement feature series article 2: Displaying and analyzing quality improvement data. *Journal of Pediatric Infectious Disease Society,* 7(2), 100–103. https://doi.org/10.1093/jpids/pix077

Grube, J. A. (2008). Strategy and leadership. In L. R. Pelletier & C. L. Beaudin (Eds.), *Q solutions: Essential resources for the healthcare quality professional* (79–120). National Association for Healthcare Quality.

Institute for Healthcare Improvement. (2020). *Run chart tool.* http://www.ihi.org/resources/Pages/Tools/RunChart.aspx

Lee, K. C., Bamford, A., Gardiner, F., Agovino, A., ter Horst, B., Bishop, J., Sitch, A., Grover, L., Logan, A., & Moiemen, N.S. (2019). Investigating the intra-and inter-rater reliability of a panel of subjective and objective burn scar measurement tools. *Burns, 45*(6), 1311–1324. doi:10.1016/j.burns.2019.02.002

Lloyd, R. C. (2010). Navigating in the turbulent sea of data: The quality measurement journey. *Clinics in Perinatology,* 37, 101–122. https://doi.org/10.1016/j.clp.2010.01.006

McQuillan, R. F., Silver, S. A., Harel, Z., Weizman, A., Thomas, A., Bell, C., Chertow, G. M., Chan, C. T., & Nesrallah, G. (2016). How to measure and interpret quality improvement data. *Clinical Journal of the American Society of Nephrology,* 11, 908–914. https://doi.org/10.2215/CJN.11511015

Nelson, E. C., Batalden, P. B., & Godfrey, M. M. (2004). The model for improvement: PDSA SDSA. In E. C. Nelson, P. B. Batalden, & M. M. Godfrey (Eds.), *Quality by design: A clinical microsystems approach* (pp. 271–283). Jossey-Bass.

Roberts, J. C., Johnston-Walker, L., Parker, K., Townend, K., & Bickley, J. (2018). Improving communication of patient issues on transfer out of intensive care. *British Medical Journal Open Quality,* 7(e000385). doi:10.1136/bmjoq-2018-000385

Vetter, T. R., & Morrice, D. (2019). Statistical process control: No hits, no runs, no errors? *Anesthesia &Analgesia, 128*(2), 374–382. https://doi.org/10.1213/ANE.0000000000003977

Williams, E. (2018a). Understanding variation: Part 1- the run chart. *Current Problems in Pediatric and Adolescent Health Care, 48*, 186–190. https://doi.org/10.1016/j.cppeds.2018.08.012

Williams, E. (2018b). Understanding variation–part 2: The control chart. *Current Problems in Pediatric and Adolescent Health Care, 48*, 202–205. https://doi.org/10.1016/j.cppeds.2018.08.009

SUGGESTED READINGS

Baker, A. W., Haridy, S., Salem, J., Ilies, I., Ergai, A. O., Samareh, A., Andrianas, N., Benneyan, J. C., Sexton, D. J., & Anderson, D. J. (2018). *British Medical Journal Quality and Safety, 27*, 600–610. doi:10.1135/bmjqs-2017-006474

Berwick, D. M. (1991). Controlling variation in health care: A consultation from Walter Shewhart. *Medical Care, 29*(12), 1212–1225.

Berwick, D. M., Nolan, T. W., & Whittington, J. (2008). The triple aim: Care, health, and cost. *Health Affairs, 27*(3), 757–769. doi:10.1377/hlthaff.27.3.759

Crockett, C. J., Donahue, B. S., & Vandivier, D. C. (2018). Distraction-free induction zone: A quality improvement initiative at a large academic children's hospital to improve the quality and safety of anesthetic care for our patients. *International Anesthesia Research Society, 129*(3), 794–803. doi:10.1213/ANE.0000000000003879

Donaldson, M. S. (2008). An overview of To Err is Human: Re-emphasizing the message of patient safety. In R. G. Hughes (Ed.), *Patient safety and quality: An evidence-based handbook for nurses* (pp 1–9). Rockville, MD: Agency for Healthcare Research and Quality.

Duclos, A., & Voirin, N. (2010). The p-control chart: A tool for care improvement. *International Journal for Quality in Health Care, 22*(5), 402–407. doi:10.1093/intqhc/mzq037

Flood, D., Douglas, K., Goldberg, V., Martinez, B., Garcia, P., Arbour, M., & Rohloff, P. (2017). A quality improvement project using statistical process control methods for type 2 diabetes control in a resource-limited setting. *International Journal for Quality in Health Care, 29*(4), 593–601. doi:10.1093/intqhc/mzx051

Goldmann, D. (2011). Ten tips for incorporating scientific quality improvement into everyday work. *British Medical Journal of Quality and Safety, 20*(Suppl 1), i69–i72. doi:10:1136/bmjqs.2010.046359

Ilies, I., Anderson, D. J., Salem, J., Baker, A. W., Jacobsen, M., & Benneyan, J. C. (2020). Large-scale empirical optimization of statistical control charts to detect clinically relevant increases in surgical site infection rates. *British Medical Journal Quality and Safety, 29*, 472–481. doi:10.1136/bmjqs-2018-008976

Iman, N., Spelman, T., Johnson, S. A., & Worth, L. J. (2019). Statistical process control charts for monitoring *staphylococcus aureus* bloodstream infections in Australian health care facilities. *Quality Management Health Care Journal, 28*(1), 39–44. doi:10.1097/QMH.0000000000000201

Neuburger, J., Walker, K., Sherlaw-Johnson, C., Van der Meulen, J., & Cromwell, D. A. (2017). Comparison of control charts for monitoring clinical performance using binary data. *British Medical Journal Quality and Safety, 26*, 919–928. doi:10.1136/bmjqs-2016-005526

Øvretveit, J. (2011). Understanding the conditions for improvement: Research to discover which context influences affect improvement success. *British Medical Journal of Quality and Safety, 20*(Suppl 1), i18–i23. doi:10.1136/bmjqs.2010.045955

Pocha, C. (2010). Lean six sigma in health care and the challenge of implementation of six sigma methodologies at a veterans affairs medical center. *Quality Management in Health Care, 19*(4), 312–318. doi:10.1097/QMH.0b013e3181fa0783

Radner, W. (2019). Standardization of reading charts: A review of recent developments. *Optometry and Vision Science, Journal of the American Academy of Optometry, 96*(10), 768–779. doi:10.1097/OPX.0000000000001436

Robinson, S. N., Neyens, D. M., & Diller, T. (2017). Applied use of safety event occurrence control charts of harm and non-harm events: A case study. *American Journal of Medical Quality, 32*(2), 285–291. doi:10.1177/1062860616646197

Russell, T. A., Chung, H., Riad, C., Reardon, S., Kazanjian, K., Cherry, R., Hines, O. J., & Lin, A. (2018). Sustaining improvement: Implementation and spread of a surgical site infection bundle. *The American Surgeon, 84*(10), 1665–1669. http://visn1kis.idm.oclc.org/login?url=https://search-proquest-com.visn1kis.idm.oclc.org/docview/2136868645?accountid=29039.

Schmidtke, K. A., Watson, D. G., & Vlaev, I. (2017). The use of control charts by laypeople and hospital decision-makes for guiding decision making. *The Quarterly Journal of Experimental Psychology, 70*(7), 1114–1128. doi:10.1080/17470218.2016.1172096

Schuh, A., Canham-Chervak, M., & Jones, B. H. (2017). Statistical process control charts for monitoring military injuries. *Injury Prevention of the British Medical Journal, 23*, 416–422. doi:10.1136/injuryprev-2016-042089

Shewhart, W. A., with Deming, W. E. (1939). *Statistical method from the viewpoint of quality control*. Washington, DC: Department of Agriculture.

Vest, J. R., & Gamm, L. D. (2009). A critical review of the research literature on six sigma, lean, and studer-group's hardwiring excellence in the United States: The need to demonstrate and communicate the effectiveness of transformation strategies in healthcare. *Implementation Science, 4*(35), 1–9. doi:10.1186/1748-5908-4-35

UNIT III

Application for Practice

CHAPTER 13

Implementation Science

Brant J. Oliver, Kolu Baysah Clark, and Christine Rovinski-Wagner

"To him who devotes [his/her] life to science, nothing can give more happiness than increasing the number of discoveries, but this cup of joy is full when the results of [one's] studies immediately find practice applications."

–Louis Pasteur

Upon completion of this chapter, the reader should be able to:

1. Define innovation, improvement, and implementation science approaches.
2. Describe major implementation science frameworks including the Consolidated Framework for Implementation Research (CFIR); (b) the Reach, Effectiveness, Adoption, Implementation, and Maintenance (RE-AIM) framework; and (c) the Dynamic Sustainability Framework (DSF).
3. Discuss the three main types of hybrid research designs (type I, type II, and type III).
4. Apply Quality and Safety Education for Nurses (QSEN) competencies to implementation science.
5. Explore implementation science and bedside clinical care, patient education, professional development, and research aspects of nursing practice.
6. Analyze examples of implementation science in nursing practice.

CROSSWALK

This chapter addresses the following:

QSEN Competency: Evidence-Based Practice, Quality Improvement

The American Association of Colleges of Nursing. (2021). *The essentials: Core competencies for professional nursing education.*

Domain 7: Systems-Based Practice

OPENING SCENARIO

Kim is a charge nurse on an inpatient general-surgical unit and recently learned at a conference that healthcare-associated infections (HAIs) are significant in the acute care setting and affect hundreds of thousands of patients annually. In addition to the burden/risk placed on the patient, these kinds of infections are associated with high costs. One of these HAIs is catheter-associated urinary tract infection (CAUTI). From the knowledge gained at the conference, she realized her unit often had inappropriate use of urinary catheters following surgery; from checking with other nurses at the hospital, she found the practices within the hospital varied widely. She therefore found risk for CAUTI was a problem in her unit and the hospital at large.

When she voiced her concern to her unit manager, Kim was invited to the next leadership meeting, where she presented what she learned at the conference to the committee. In this same meeting, the hospital chief nursing officer shared that the hospital had just received new Centers for Medicare and Medicaid Services (CMS) guidelines, where the hospital would no longer be reimbursed for preventable HAIs such as CAUTI, since research suggests these are highly preventable. Kim and the head of infectious disease (ID), Dr. Hopkins, were then tasked with formulating an interprofessional team to help address this problem.

1. Which professionals should be represented on the interprofessional team?
2. What are some reasons these team members would be either for or against any practice change?

INTRODUCTION

This chapter defines implementation and implementation science in healthcare, and compares and contrasts implementation with two other approaches commonly used to optimize healthcare delivery and outcomes: innovation and improvement. Three commonly used implementation science frameworks are introduced: (a) the Consolidated Framework for Implementation Research (CFIR); (b) the Reach, Effectiveness, Adoption, Implementation, and Maintenance (RE-AIM) framework; and (c) the Dynamic Sustainability Framework (DSF), as well as three implementation hybrid research designs. The Quality and Safety Education for Nurses (QSEN) competencies, quality improvement (QI), evidence-based practice (EBP), patient-centered care, safety, teamwork and collaboration, and informatics are applied to implementation science. Implementation science is explored as an important part of bedside clinical care, patient education, professional development, and research aspects of nursing practice. Examples of implementation science in nursing practice will be discussed.

INNOVATION, IMPROVEMENT, AND IMPLEMENTATION SCIENCE APPROACHES

Healthcare is a complex system for both producers of healthcare, such as nurses, doctors, and hospital leadership, and users of healthcare, such as patients and their families. It is in the best interest of both producers and users of healthcare to improve the ways in which care is delivered. The complexity of the healthcare system requires a systematic method of organization to guide any changes toward success. It is crucial for nurses at the bedside to understand some basic concepts that play a vital role in taking an evidence-based idea, getting it into practice, and sustaining it. These concepts include the 3 I's, that is, innovation, improvement, and implementation. While the terms are often used interchangeably, the 3 I's are different (Table 13.1).

TABLE 13.1 CHARACTERISTICS, MODELS, METHODS, AND EXAMPLES OF THE "3 I'S"

CHARACTERISTICS	METHODS, MODELS, & FRAMEWORKS	EXAMPLE
INNOVATION Evidence-based, Solution-focused, Progressive	Diffusion of Innovations	A new checklist for nurses determining the continued need for a urinary catheter in postop patients, with the goal of reducing CAUTI.
IMPROVEMENT Evidence-based, Adaptive, Measurable, Clearly Defined Aims, Iterative	IHI Model for Improvement, PDSA, Lean Six Sigma, ISO 9001	The occurrence of CAUTI decreases as the number of nurses trained to use the urinary catheter checklist increases.
IMPLEMENTATION SCIENCE Acceptability, Adoption, Appropriateness, Cost, Feasibility, Fidelity, Reach, Sustainment	Consolidated Framework for Implementation Research (CFIR) Reach, Effectiveness, Adoption, Implementation, and Maintenance (RE-AIM) Dynamic Sustainability Framework (DSF)	The catheter checklist proves to be effective at reducing CAUTI and becomes standard hospital policy with continued evaluation of nursing use and CAUTI rates.

CAUTI, catheter-associated urinary tract infection; IHI, Institute for Healthcare Improvement; ISO, International Organization for Standardization; PDSA, Plan-Do-Study-Act.

Innovation is the creation of a novel idea, service, process, or product not previously used in a particular setting, with the goal of helping to solve an identified problem. There are many evidence-based innovations in healthcare, yet there are no guarantees that they will be used or make it to the bedside as standard practice. In fact, the majority of evidence-based interventions with proven efficacy to optimize patient care takes many years, even decades, to become accepted and maintained as standard practice. Even when innovations are successfully proven in one location, they might be slowly adopted elsewhere. Not every evidence-based intervention will be widely accepted by all healthcare organizations.

To better understand this concept, consider how new ideas naturally spread through society, in a process termed "diffusion," the passive spread of an idea without controlling factors such as planning or targeting. Through studying aspects of diffusion, it is apparent that some ideas will spread faster and easier, while others will seem to stall. Six traits affect how quickly a new idea will diffuse: cost, effectiveness, simplicity/complexity, compatibility, observability, and trialability (Rogers, 1995). Even with all of these traits maximized, it is important to consider that individuals and organizations differ in how much they embrace new ideas. There are early adopters who are more open to and excited by change, laggards who will resist change at all costs, and the vast majority who fall somewhere between these extremes. Rogers expressed this concept as the Diffusion of Innovations, where he consolidated and focused on much of the diverse aspects of diffusion theory (Rogers, 1995). There are Diffusion of Innovations examples from everyday life. Imagine when cell phones were introduced. First there were just a few people using them, then more people, then the vast majority. Yet even today there are likely to be people who cling to their house phone and do not want to change. A similar transition is occurring today with electric vehicles. Consider all of the diffusion traits (cost, effectiveness, and so on) and the effects of these traits on how quickly and easily this (or any) innovation will be adopted by society. This same adoption pattern happens any time there is a change, including in healthcare, as seen in Table 13.2.

TABLE 13.2 DIFFUSION TRAITS, DEFINITIONS, AND EXAMPLES

TRAIT	DEFINITION	EXAMPLE
Cost	A measure of the perceived resources to adopt an innovation, not all of which are monetary.	How much time and effort will be required to train nurses in the use of a new medication-dispensing machine?
Effectiveness	A comparison of how the innovation is perceived as better than the current practice being replaced.	Do patients, nurses, and hospital leadership agree that the new discharge process is better?
Simplicity	The ease with which the innovation is understood.	Are the new intravenous pumps easy to use or will they require extensive training?
Compatibility	Similarity of the innovation to the current practice, which influences how much an individual can relate to the innovation.	How much would the new electronic health record program disrupt the flow of the existing routine of the hospital unit?
Observability	The extent to which outcomes can be seen.	A new nurse watches how a more experienced nurse organizes tasks to provide care to patients and then organizes work in the same way.
Trialability	Whether the innovation can be tried on a smaller scale first, to see how well it works.	A new intravenous pump is used on one nursing unit to evaluate whether it should be used throughout the hospital.

Understanding these traits can help to overcome any potential barrier. A **barrier** is a structure, process, belief system, cultural aspect, or behavior that inhibits or limits progress toward successful innovation, improvement, or implementation. The opposite of a barrier is referred to as a facilitator. A **facilitator** is a structure, process, belief system, cultural aspect, or behavior that enables, empowers, accelerates, or maximizes progress toward successful innovation, improvement, or implementation.

Nurses need to understand this concept, so ways to motivate both early and late adopters to the proposed innovation can be identified, aiding success. With nurses' key role being between the patients and various providers/staff, they have an excellent vantage to gather information, including which groups are more open to change. By doing an in-depth analysis and understanding the challenges, nurses have the needed information to begin the process of innovation in the care setting, which typically involves people changing their behavior. The Quality and Safety Education for Nurses (QSEN) competencies can guide nurses in selecting the right innovation to improve practice by incorporating the attitudes and skills associated with teamwork and collaboration, safety, quality improvement (QI), evidence-based practice (EBP), person-centered outcomes, and informatics.

Improvement activities iteratively refine, optimize, or standardize an existing process, product, method, or approach to improve performance and outcomes. While improvement is the topic of Chapter 11, it must be briefly discussed here, as it intertwines with other concepts of this chapter, such as innovation and implementation. Improvement is an applied science that uses innovation, rapid-cycle testing in the field, and spread in order to create learning about what changes and conditions lead to an improved outcome. It involves the combination of subject matter experts along with improvement methods and tools. Improvement starts with identifying a clear aim and developing a measurement plan, which will ultimately lead to small iterative tests of change through cycles. Over time, these changes are refined and put into practice. When successful, these cycles increase in scope and scale.

Before an organization can make a permanent large-scale change to a practice, policy, or method, it is important to have proof that the change would be an improvement and is achievable. This proof can be through the evidence collected by a review of the literature (including methods implemented at similar institutions) or achieved through testing of the innovation in the proposed environment. Since both of these methods for proof complement each other, the more evidence obtained by one method means that less evidence is required of the other, to ultimately provide this proof. If the improvement team finds extensive quality evidence in the literature that the innovation has been proven effective in similar environments, fewer testing cycles will be needed to confirm the evidence. Conversely, an innovation that has a smaller amount of evidence in the literature can still be considered, but the testing cycles will need to begin at a much smaller scale, requiring additional cycles in order to provide adequate proof that it is indeed an improvement and that it is achievable.

Implementation science is the study of adopting, installing, or integrating evidence-based interventions into an existing practice of healthcare to beneficially affect outcomes. Implementation has significant importance and implications for nurses. It is used to change systems of care to create better conditions for effective nursing practice and improve health outcomes for patients. Implementation is used to integrate better, faster, or more effective evidence-based care approaches into the delivery of healthcare. It can also be used to introduce new methods of educating health professionals and studies about scientific approaches for implementation.

Implementation is based, in part, on testing approaches for increasing the use of and sustaining evidence-based interventions. While dissemination is the increase of evidence-based interventions to the target population, implementation differs in that it focuses on ways to increase the use of those interventions in a particular healthcare setting, such as an in-patient medical unit, an ambulatory care clinic, or a surgery center.

Implementation frameworks are conceptual models developed to help implementation science researchers to (a) learn how to conduct successful implementation efforts; (b) determine what elements are essential to and resultant from a successful implementation; and (c) discover how to sustain implementation efforts over time. Frameworks are used as a systematic way of providing structure for development, management, and evaluation in the implementation of interventions. The frameworks link the study aim, design, measurements, and analysis.

Along with frameworks providing structure, **implementation strategies** specifically aid the process of adoption, implementation, sustainment, and scale-up of an innovation. There are 73 distinct implementation strategies identified, categorized in nine broad clusters, built along common themes (Waltz et al., 2015). Implementation strategies are not simply a checklist of things which must be done. They provide insight for ways to overcome barriers to achieving implementation of an innovation. More than one strategy is usually needed for successful implementation but using multiple strategies does not promise success. There is no one-size-fits-all. Strategies should be chosen based on the innovation and the identified barriers to its implementation. Since barriers often vary by setting, appropriate strategies will also vary by setting. For example, different units within the same hospital will have different barriers to implementation and will need different implementation strategies to overcome the barriers. Understanding these challenges prior to implementing a project informs the process and helps the team choose the best implementation strategies. The framework used can also help guide the selection of implementation strategies. Implementation strategies support widespread adoption and use of innovation in healthcare. The example in Table 13.3 demonstrates this.

TABLE 13.3 IMPLEMENTATION STRATEGIES WITH EXAMPLES FOR CATHETER-ASSOCIATED URINARY TRACT INFECTION BUNDLE

STRATEGY CLUSTER WITH ASSOCIATED IMPLEMENTATION STRATEGIES	EXAMPLES FROM CAUTI BUNDLE SCENARIO
Use Evaluative and Iterative Strategies. Assess readiness, identify barriers/facilitators. Audit and provide feedback. Conduct cyclic small tests of change. Conduct local needs assessment. Develop a formal implementation blueprint. Develop and implement tools for quality monitoring. Develop and organize quality monitoring systems. Obtain and use patients/consumers and family feedback. Purposely reexamine the implementation. Stage implementation scale up.	Kim **conducted a local needs assessment** by personally observing inappropriate use of urinary catheters on her unit as well as having discussions from nurses of other units about their catheter practices.
Provide Interactive Assistance Centralize technical assistance. Facilitation. Provide clinical supervision. Provide local technical assistance.	In order to ensure the proposed innovation is conducted properly, additional training is given to nurses in leadership roles so they in turn can support front-line nurses in the implementation of the innovation by **providing clinical supervision.**
Adapt and Tailor to Context Promote adaptability. Tailor strategies. Use data experts. Use data warehousing techniques.	Before expanding the urinary catheter protocol to other units, Kim and her interprofessional team should assess facilitators and barriers to implementing the protocol in each of those units, so they can **tailor strategies** for successful implementation on each new unit.
Develop Stakeholder Interrelationships Build a coalition. Capture and share local knowledge. Conduct local consensus discussions. Develop academic partnerships. Develop an implementation glossary. Identify and prepare champions. Identify early adopters. Inform local opinion leaders. Involve executive boards. Model and stimulate change. Obtain formal commitments. Organize clinician implementation team meetings. Promote network weaving. Recruit, designate, and train for leadership. Use advisory boards and workgroups. Use an implementation advisor. Visit other sites.	Kim and her team can **identify and prepare champions,** such as nurses who have a strong motivation for the implementation to be a success, who will help encourage their colleagues to carry out the protocol.
Train and Educate Stakeholders Conduct educational meetings. Conduct educational outreach visits. Conduct ongoing training. Create a learning collaborative. Develop educational materials. Distribute educational materials. Make training dynamic. Provide ongoing consultation. Shadow other experts. Use train-the-trainer strategies. Work with educational institutions.	Kim and her interprofessional team can **conduct educational meetings,** sessions where nursing staff will learn about the new measures in the protocol, along with how they will improve patient care and health outcomes.

(continued)

TABLE 13.3 IMPLEMENTATION STRATEGIES WITH EXAMPLES FOR CATHETER-ASSOCIATED URINARY TRACT INFECTION BUNDLE (*continued*)

STRATEGY CLUSTER WITH ASSOCIATED IMPLEMENTATION STRATEGIES	EXAMPLES FROM CAUTI BUNDLE SCENARIO
Support Clinicians Create new clinical teams. Develop resource sharing agreements. Facilitate relay of clinical data to providers. Remind clinicians. Revise professional roles.	The Information Technology department can set up a reminder in the electronic health records to **remind clinicians** such as nurses when the patient is due to have their urinary catheter removed per the protocol.
Engage Consumers Increase demand. Intervene with patients/consumers to enhance uptake and adherence. Involve patients/consumers and family members. Prepare patients/consumers to be active participants. Use mass media.	Having a patient as a member of the interprofessional team would be an excellent way to **involve patients/consumers and family members,** ensuring their interests are represented.
Utilize Financial Strategies Access new funding. Alter incentive/allowance structures. Alter patient/consumer fees. Develop disincentives. Fund and contract for clinical innovation. Make billing easier. Place innovation on fee for service lists/formularies. Use capitated payments. Use other payment schemes.	While the new protocols should not require much funding to maintain, Kim and her team may need to **access new funding** from the hospital or through grants/endowments to pay for the training sessions.
Change Infrastructure Change accreditation or membership requirements. Change liability laws. Change physical structure and equipment. Change record systems. Change service sites. Create or change credentialing and/or licensure standards. Mandate change. Start a dissemination organization.	By Kim's team getting hospital leadership to pledge their support for the new protocol, the leadership may **mandate change,** requiring that the protocol be followed.

CAUTI, catheter-associated urinary tract infection.

Source: Data from Waltz, T. J., Powell, B. J., Matthieu, M. M., Damschroder, L. J., Chinman, M. J., Smith, J. L., Proctor, E. K., & Kirchner, J. E. (2015). Use of concept mapping to characterize relationships among implementation strategies and assess their feasibility and importance: Results from the Expert Recommendations for Implementing Change (ERIC) study. *Implementation Science, 10*, Article 109. https://doi.org/10.1186/s13012-015-0295-0

MAJOR IMPLEMENTATION FRAMEWORKS

Implementation frameworks organize how to successfully conduct an implementation effort, identify what elements are essential to a successful implementation, and how to successfully sustain an implementation effort. Three implementation science approaches are commonly used to influence implementation in practice and the scientific study of implementation in research: the **Consolidated Framework for Implementation Research (CFIR)**, the **Reach, Effectiveness, Adoption, Implementation, and Maintenance (RE-AIM) framework**, and the **Dynamic Sustainability Framework (DSF)**. Each serves a different purpose; CFIR focuses on *how*, RE-AIM focuses on *what*, and DSF focuses on *sustaining* (Table 13.4).

TABLE 13.4 CHARACTERISTICS OF IMPLEMENTATION SCIENCE FRAMEWORKS

FRAMEWORK	KEY USE(S)	COMPONENTS
Consolidated Framework for Implementation Research (CFIR) Recommended Resource: https://cfirguide.org	Assessment of barriers and facilitators for implementation Learning how to best conduct an implementation Determining the optimal conditions for successful implementation	Individuals Inner Setting (the front line) Outer Setting (environment) Intervention (exposure) Processes (how it happens)
Reach, Effectiveness, Adoption, Implementation, and Maintenance (RE-AIM) Recommended Resource: www.re-aim.org	Describes what can be used to build an effective implementation strategy. Helps to assess the intended or actual results of an implementation effort.	Reach (scope) Effectiveness (impact) Adoption (will and spread) Implementation (fidelity) Maintenance (staying power)
Dynamic Sustainability Framework (DSF) Recommended Resource: Chambers, D. A., Glasgow R. E., & Stange, K. C. (2013). The dynamic sustainability framework: Addressing the paradox of sustainment amid ongoing change. *Implementation Science*, 8, 117. http://www.implementationscience.com/content/8/1/117	Focuses specifically on sustaining an existing or planned implementation Can help to identify factors which contribute to degradation of the implementation over time Uses PDSA improvement methods to adapt intervention and context to achieve better sustainability	Intervention Practice Setting (context) Ecological System (environment) Plan-Do-Study-Act (PDSA) improvement cycles

CONSOLIDATED FRAMEWORK FOR IMPLEMENTATION RESEARCH

The CFIR was initially designed by the Department of Veterans Affairs Diabetes Quality Enhancement Research Initiative (QUERI) to provide a method to study implementation approaches to improve diabetes care outcomes in veterans (CFIR Research Team, 2020; Damschroeder et al., 2009). It is the most widely used implementation science approach with over 400 published implementation research studies having used it to date. CFIR is often used because of its ability to help healthcare professionals and researchers determine how to best conduct an implementation and under what conditions an implementation is most likely to be successful.

Real World Interview

Prior research demonstrates the feasibility and acceptability of telehealth for perinatal women fortunate enough to have access to technology. However, little research has explored solutions to the real-world challenges of engaging in telehealth for low-resource pregnant and postpartum people. We used a hybrid implementation-effectiveness approach to evaluate the feasibility of deploying prepaid cell phones and data cards to low-resource pregnant people in remote rural communities, and to evaluate the impact of this program on outcomes. The CFIR was used to develop interviews of clinic staff involved in implementing the program at all levels, as well as patients receiving phones and/or data cards. Engagement in care was tracked through the number and type of appointments attended (in-person vs. telehealth) as well as missed appointments, along with standard obstetrical outcomes. As this work continues, one important lesson has been the profound impact of context (that this work is occurring during the COVID-19 pandemic), both on the ability to engage in care for already vulnerable rural populations, and the eagerness of staff to implement new procedures perceived as beneficial to patients, even in the midst of a rapidly changing clinical environment.

Daisy Goodman, CNM, DNP, MPH, CARN-AP
Director of Women's Health Services
Dartmouth-Hitchcock Perinatal Addiction Program
Assistant Professor of Obstetrics and Gynecology
The Dartmouth Institute for Health Policy and Clinical Practice, Geisel School of Medicine at Dartmouth, Lebanon, New Hampshire

The CFIR provides an interactive understanding of five components which are critical to facilitating effective implementation: (a) **individuals**—the population of interest; (b) the **inner setting**—the context and lived experience of the frontline healthcare environment; (c) the **outer setting**—the external policy, systems, economic, social, and other environmental factors influencing and interacting with the inner setting; (d) the **intervention**—the EBP, method, technology, or other exposure that will be applied to make a beneficial change (and how it is adapted and optimized over time during implementation); and (e) the **processes** that are used in the existing system of care that can be used to facilitate implementation. Within each of these categories, assessments of barriers and facilitators to implementation can be conducted, aiding planning for a successful implementation. In the following example, the opening scenario is revisited to apply a CFIR approach to assess barriers and facilitators of a CAUTI bundle implementation (Table 13.5). In this scenario, the implementation team is planning to implement the CAUTI bundle in a single unit as an initial proof of concept test case, or pilot study, and is using the CFIR to carefully assess barriers and facilitators.

CASE STUDY

A hospital with several outpatient clinics decides to directly implement a vastly proven evidence-based intervention of co-locating mental health (MH) providers with primary care providers (PCP), their nurses, and administrative support personnel to boost collaboration and make it easier for patients to receive timely mental healthcare. Currently, MH providers, PCPs and nurses are located on two different floors of the hospital. The administrative support personnel are located in a different part of the hospital. The hospital leadership believes co-locating these personnel would make it more competitive with other hospitals and more patients would use the hospital's services. The anticipated improvement in patient care experience might also result in increased revenue. Although PCP and MH teams have worked together for a long time, they are accustomed to the old referral system in the electronic medical records, which is creating resistance. Both PCP and MH providers feel they will have their workdays constantly interrupted because the new process requires the PCP to do a warm handoff, that is, taking the patient to where the MH provider is. They believe there should be more staff hired to help with this change. The providers are all committed to providing quality healthcare but believe this change is only motivated by leadership's concern with increasing revenue.

1. *Describe possible barriers and facilitators of the inner settings that might be impacted by the co-location.*
2. *What are the elements of the outer setting?*
3. *What processes are already used in the existing system of healthcare that could be used to facilitate implementation of warm handoffs?*

TABLE 13.5 CONSOLIDATED FRAMEWORK FOR IMPLEMENTATION RESEARCH ANALYSIS OF BARRIERS AND FACILITATORS TO CATHETER-ASSOCIATED URINARY TRACT INFECTION BUNDLE IMPLEMENTATION

CFIR COMPONENT	BARRIERS	FACILITATORS
Inner Setting	Workflow and electronic health record (EHR) not currently configured for bundle implementation. Senior nursing staff ambivalent about the need for "one more thing," thinks it is a "problem that has been around forever and can't be solved."	There is an EHR redesign effort currently underway. Recent influx of new nurses who are graduates of a nurse residency program and have a strong evidence-based practice mentality. Some have quality improvement experience. Support from unit nurse manager and physician champion.
Outer Setting	Current human resources and career ladder policies do not reward implementation work. During the COVID pandemic admissions are increased and staffing is limited.	CMS does not reimburse hospitals for preventable CAUTI incidences; the hospital has lost revenue due to poor CAUTI outcomes, and wants a better reputation for preventing CAUTI events. Nursing leadership is considering adding participation in improvement work as a job performance element.
Intervention	Implementation will cause disruptions in the shortterm, including changes to workflow. It will take some time to optimize efficiency and consistency of the implementation of the intervention.	The CAUTI bundle is evidence-based. The effort invested in implementation of the bundle could result in better outcomes. The nurses with QI experience can help to optimize the implementation and reduce disruptions.
Processes	Admission and discharge processes are strained by increased demand and short staffing. Staff feel rushed at times, and are worried that adding "another bundle" will just make their work harder.	Current workflow will be integrated already with the EHR as CAUTI events are documented in EHR form fields. The staff perception of "adding one more thing," may be erroneous, and improvement may make work easier.

CAUTI, catheter-associated urinary tract infection; CFIR, Consolidated Framework for Implementation Research; CMS, Centers for Medicare and Medicaid Services; QI, quality improvement.

REACH, EFFECTIVENESS, ADOPTION, IMPLEMENTATION, AND MAINTENANCE (RE-AIM)

RE-AIM (Glasgow et al., 1999) is another commonly used implementation science framework and is featured in over 140 published implementation studies. It was originally

BOX 13.1 Developing Clinical Judgment

The nurses on the medical-surgical unit noted a high readmission rate related to hypoglycemia in type 2 diabetes (T2D) patients, including those newly diagnosed and patients who were newly transitioned to insulin management. Given this, the charge nurse met with the nursing team to discuss the discharge protocol for all T2D patients. The nurses discovered there were many T2D patient education materials but no guidelines for selecting the most appropriate materials according to patient needs. The team also discovered that not all of the nurses felt comfortable discharging diabetics. One new nurse shared her experience of discharging a newly diagnosed patient at 5 p.m. on a Friday afternoon. The patient was going home on insulin for the first time but did not have his first endocrinologist appointment until 2 weeks after discharge. The nurse discovered none of the nurses working with the patient before her had initiated diabetic teaching. The patient's discharge was delayed until the next day.

1. What **CUES (Assessment)** can the nurses, using the RE-AIM framework, assess about the lack of a standard approach to teaching patients with diabetes about their disease?
2. What **HYPOTHESIS (Diagnosis)** could the nurse form about innovations that could be effective to address the discharge preparation of T2D patients?
3. What **ACTION (Plan and Implement)** will be most effective for the nurses to take to ensure safe quality healthcare for patients with type 2 diabetes who have been newly transitioned to insulin or newly diagnosed?
4. How will the nurses evaluate the **OUTCOME (Evaluation)** of the team's work for the purpose of arriving at a satisfactory clinical outcome?

designed to standardize the reporting of research results, especially in studies of health promotion, health behavior, and disease management approaches in public health. Over time, it has also proved useful in informing methods to translate research evidence into frontline practice, including implementation efforts and implementation science research. RE-AIM emphasizes the essential program elements required for successful implementation, or, in other words, what components are needed. RE-AIM can also be used to assess the results of implementation.

The RE-AIM acronym has five essential components. Reach is the engagement of people in an implementation effort, its scope, and the ability of the implementation effort to connect with people. Effectiveness is the impact, for example, positive and negative outcomes, of the implementation and its implications. Adoption is the magnitude of participation, organizational support, and will to facilitate the implementation. Implementation (not to be confused with the general definition of implementation) is the fidelity of the intervention, that is, the degree to which the planned implementation is carried out as designed, and the degree to which it is consistently applied. Lastly, maintenance is the degree to which the implementation is formally adopted into standard practices and policies and sustained over time.

In Table 13.6, the RE-AIM framework is applied to the opening scenario to assess the CAUTI bundle implementation effort. In this example, the CAUTI bundle effort is now in the early stages of implementation in a single hospital unit and the implementation team is using the RE-AIM approach to assess its current and future potential for success.

TABLE 13.6 REACH, EFFECTIVENESS, ADOPTION, IMPLEMENTATION, AND MAINTENANCE ANALYSIS OF CATHETER-ASSOCIATED URINARY TRACT INFECTION BUNDLE IMPLEMENTATION

RE-AIM COMPONENT	ANALYSIS AND DISCUSSION
Reach	There is strain on the current system due to increased care demands. Initial implementation is limited to one unit for "proof of concept" with a plan to scale hospital-wide once implementation here is successful. Leadership has budgeted for improvement coaching to help the team with planning, executing, and evaluating the implementation. The EHR upgrade includes a feedback function that will allow the nursing team to track CAUTI performance over time.
Effectiveness	Workflows have been modified and the CAUTI bundle implemented, but as of a month postimplementation, CAUTI rates have not yet significantly changed. Fidelity (consistency) of bundle application is not readily measurable; there is a need to develop a reliable and practical way to regularly assess this.
Adoption	Senior leadership, middle management, physician colleagues, information technology, and frontline nurses with evidence-based practice and QI experience are engaged. Senior nurses are ambivalent but are not obstructing the work. There is a clear perception "from top to bottom" that implementation of the bundle is a priority and "will be done." The staff is appreciative of the coaching support, but feels more burdened by the implementation effort thus far. They are requesting some release time from clinical duties in order to participate in the implementation more meaningfully.
Implementation	An assessment conducted by the implementation team reveals that many on the frontline staff are unfamiliar with the new workflow process and the EHR upgrade is not yet completed. Although the administration can readily access unit level CAUTI outcomes data, the frontline staff cannot see these in realtime, only via monthly summary reports provided to the unit manager. The QI team thinks that intervention fidelity (consistent use of the bundle) needs improvement and that education efforts are needed to help the front-line team acclimate to the bundle. "Buddy-systems" have been considered to pair nurses experienced with the bundle with nurses new to it.
Maintenance	The bundle implementation is in an early stage of maturation and is currently being pilot tested in a single unit. If successful there, additional planning and resources will be needed to scale to additional units effectively and efficiently, benefiting from the lessons learned from the initial pilot effort. Current hospital policies include some expectations regarding evidence-based prevention practices for CAUTI and other hospital-acquired conditions, but may need to be revisited and updated if the CAUTI bundle becomes the new standard of care practice expectation for the hospital. Leadership may need to revisit resource allocation to provide ongoing education and implementation support to monitor and sustain the implementation over time once the initial implementation phase is completed.

CAUTI, catheter-associated urinary tract infection; EHR, electronic health record; RE-AIM, Reach, Effectiveness, Adoption, Implementation, and Maintenance; QI, quality improvement.

CASE STUDY

The nurse has been asked by the hospital's new clinical dietitian to join an interprofessional team that wants to start a support group for patients with diabetes. The purpose of forming the group will be to increase self-management in patients with type 2 diabetes and improve their diabetic control. One of the team members is an endocrinologist who has worked at the hospital for many years and does not think the team is necessary. Hospital leadership wants to open the support group to the community.

1. *What barriers might confront the interprofessional team with implementation of the support group?*
2. *Based on the identified barriers, which implementation strategies could be used?*
3. *How can the team measure the fidelity of the new processes?*

DYNAMIC SUSTAINABILITY FRAMEWORK

The DSF (Chambers et al., 2013) is a newer implementation science framework developed to help healthcare professionals and researchers address voltage drop, a commonly occurring problem in implementation efforts. **Voltage drop** refers to the gradual degradation of the implementation over time, causing a loss of its fidelity and/or effectiveness. The DSF focuses specifically on how to prevent or remedy voltage drop and sustain an established or planned implementation over time.

The DSF can be thought of as a combination framework because it utilizes some elements featured in the CFIR and RE-AIM frameworks and also incorporates a popular

BOX 13.2 Developing Clinical Judgment

The improvement team in the opening scenario conducted medical record reviews and many interviews with nurses and other interprofessional staff on the preoperative and postoperative units, operating rooms, and the post-anesthesia recovery unit. The team identified that the physician orders for many postoperative patients returning to the unit did not state why the urinary catheter was needed, that the nursing staff didn't question why, and that these patients often had indwelling catheters for the duration of their hospital stays. The team also learned that the decision to insert an indwelling urinary catheter was based on the physician's discretion since the hospital did not have a standard protocol to guide who needed a catheter.

1. What **CUES (Assessment)**, using the RE-AIM framework, can the nurse and the improvement team assess about adoption of the indwelling urinary catheter protocols?
2. What **HYPOTHESIS (Diagnosis)** can the nurse and the improvement team make about causes of improper catheter use from their initial findings?
3. What **ACTION (Plan and Implement)** will be most effective for the nurse and the improvement team to take to ensure that use and management of indwelling urinary catheters provides safe quality patient care?
4. How could the nurse and the improvement team evaluate the **OUTCOME (Evaluation)** of the team's work for determining the effectiveness of the urinary catheter protocols?

improvement method, the Plan-Do-Study-Act (PDSA) cycle, as part of its approach to optimize sustainability. The DSF has three main components: (a) the intervention; (b) the **practice setting**—refers to the context in which an intervention or implementation is being conducted or studied, such as the frontline practice environment (similar to the "inner setting" in the CFIR); and (c) the **ecological system**—the context of the implementation effort such as external policy, regulatory, economic, and social factors influencing the implementation (similar to the "outer setting" in the CFIR). DSF differs from CFIR and RE-AIM in that it emphasizes the study of the interactions between these components and the identification of factors therein which could contribute to voltage drop. The DSF integrates the PDSA cycle as an approach to repeatedly and sequentially test strategies which modify and optimize the context and/or intervention in order to maintain or improve implementation sustainability over time. In Table 13.7, the CAUTI bundle implementation case study is again revisited using the DSF framework. In this scenario, the initial implementation effort previously discussed has been successful and is now being scaled to additional units across the hospital. At the same time, in the initial implementation pilot unit, work is underway to develop an approach to sustain the implementation of the bundle.

HYBRID RESEARCH DESIGNS

Frontline nurses working in collaboration with nurse scientists or other researchers engaged in formal studies of implementation in clinical settings will need to be knowledgeable of the three major categories, or hybrid research designs, of implementation science. **Hybrid research designs** are research designs that focus on the implementation of an evidence-based intervention and its effectiveness and/or utility (Curran et al., 2012). The three major hybrid research designs are effectiveness (Type I), feasibility (Type III), and a combination of effectiveness and feasibility (Type II; Table 13.8).

BOX 13.3 Developing Clinical Judgment

The nurse is a member of the hospital's infection control team. The hospital initiated a robust re-education effort about hand hygiene and ensured that all staff had ready access to alcohol-based hand rub, as well as soap and water for visibly soiled hands. The increased compliance with recommended hand hygiene practices was evident during the initial months of the initiative. As time passed, the infection control committee members observed decreased compliance with hand hygiene recommendations.

1. What **CUES (Assessment)** can the nurse and the infection control team assess, using the DSF framework, about the lack of sustained compliance with hand hygiene recommendations?

2. What **HYPOTHESIS (Diagnosis)** can the nurse and the infection control team consider about reasons compliance would decrease over time?

3. What **ACTION (Plan and Implement)** will be most effective for the nurse and the infection control team to take to ensure increased compliance with hand hygiene and the provision of safe quality healthcare that protects patients and staff?

4. How will the nurse and the infection control team evaluate the **OUTCOME (Evaluation)** of the team's work for the purpose of arriving at sustained compliance to the hand hygiene recommendations?

TABLE 13.7 DYNAMIC SUSTAINABILITY FRAMEWORK ANALYSIS FOR SUSTAINABILITY OF THE CATHETER-ASSOCIATED URINARY TRACT INFECTION BUNDLE IMPLEMENTATION

DSF COMPONENT	ANALYSIS AND DISCUSSION
Intervention	New workflow is in place and QI efforts during initial implementation were successful in optimizing intervention fidelity (how consistently the bundle is applied and documented). Unit-level CAUTI rates have dropped and now the unit has the lowest rates in the hospital. However, the "fidelity metric" has been dropping in recent months (a "voltage drop") and the implementation team is worried that this will translate into increased CAUTI rates. The implementation team is now running small tests of change (PDSA cycles) aimed at testing small adjustments to the intervention workflow and processes to assess if they will increase fidelity. These tests target specific areas of the workflow. The team is hoping to design an "enduring fix to the problem" that will not require frequent review by staff and ongoing demand on staff to monitor.
Practice Setting	The new workflow is working fairly well and has not resulted in additional perceived workload. It has resulted in removing unneeded workflow elements. The new EHR build has made related documentation easier and included ready feedback of unit-level CAUTI and fidelity metrics that the frontline team could use in real time to guide work on the implementation efforts. Coaching supports have been withdrawn and reallocated to scale-up efforts at other units of the hospital. Without the coaches involved, the team feels overwhelmed trying to keep a focus on sustaining the implementation effort. The hospital is relying more on traveling nurses to address staffing shortages. The travelers are not well acclimated to the hospital culture or the current prioritization of the CAUTI implementation effort. The nurse manager is advocating to leadership for additional support to help with the effort. The nurse manager is worried that if the current effort does not sustain, the ongoing scale-up effort currently underway hospital-wide will also fail in the long-run.
Ecological System	Leadership is pleased with the success of the initial implementation effort in the pilot unit and is now moving to scale the effort hospital wide, anticipating considerable positive impact on revenue and reputation for doing a better job on managing preventable CAUTI events. However, at present, the hospital has not yet realized substantial financial benefit from the effort and resources are stretched due to the COVID pandemic. No policy changes have yet been made to accommodate the effort because, at present, it has only been successfully tested on one unit.

CAUTI, catheter-associated urinary tract infection; DSF, Dynamic Sustainability Framework; EHR, electronic health record; QI, quality improvement.

TABLE 13.8 CHARACTERISTICS OF HYBRID RESEARCH DESIGNS

HYBRID DESIGN TYPE	EMPHASIS	TYPICAL RESEARCH QUESTIONS
Type I	Effectiveness of an intervention	"Will this intervention (implementation) work in this setting and population?"
Type II	Effectiveness and feasibility of an intervention	"Will the intervention work in this setting and population and does the approach show promise in implementing it?"
Type III	Feasibility of an implementation strategy	"Which implementation method works best for facilitating the intervention?"

Type I implementation research is designed specifically to evaluate the effectiveness of a specific evidence-based intervention when it is implemented. It is concerned entirely with assessing the degree to which the intervention works as expected when it is implemented. Type III implementation research is focused on determining the best way to implement an intervention that has already been studied and has been shown to be effective. It is concerned with determining feasibility, the best way to implement the intervention so that it will be most acceptable, usable, and helpful to clinical care. Type II implementation research is considered by many to be the most "hybridized" approach in that it has a combined focus on assessing effectiveness (a Type I characteristic) and feasibility (a Type III characteristic). This is very attractive to a research team because both issues can be addressed simultaneously using less time than doing each sequentially. However, this approach is also the most complicated to design and may be the most resource intensive to conduct.

In Table 13.9, the CAUTI bundle implementation scenario is revisited a final time. In this scenario, scale-up efforts in the hospital have progressed across the hospital with mixed results. In some cases, they have failed initially; in others, they have succeeded but

TABLE 13.9 USE OF HYBRID RESEARCH DESIGNS FOR IMPLEMENTATION SCIENCE RESEARCH OF A CATHETER-ASSOCIATED URINARY TRACT INFECTION BUNDLE INTERVENTION

HYBRID DESIGN	ANALYSIS AND DISCUSSION
Type I	This is of interest to the research team because CAUTI outcomes are the ultimate objective of the work. The team wants to know if the intervention works. How successful was the CAUTI bundle in reducing CAUTI rates? Did the intervention work?
Type III	Finding out why some units succeeded and sustained and others did not could inform a better and standardized strategy that all of the units could use to successfully implement the intervention. Why did the implementation of the CAUTI bundle work on one unit and not another? How can the implementation process be improved?
Type II	This design focuses on effectiveness and fidelity, providing a "Type I + Type III" approach (effectiveness and utility). However, it is also the most complicated design. The research team will have to weigh if this approach is feasible at this time given current resources and constraints.

CAUTI, catheter-associated urinary tract infection.

have not sustained, and in others they have succeeded and sustained. The nurse scientists on the research team are considering a study approach that will best serve a formal inquiry into what works best for CAUTI bundle implementation. They hope that the results of the study will better inform future implementation efforts at this hospital and others.

APPLYING QUALITY AND SAFETY EDUCATION FOR NURSES COMPETENCIES TO IMPLEMENTATION SCIENCE

Nurses work with interprofessional teams to apply the QSEN competencies of QI, patient-centered care, EBP, teamwork and collaboration, safety, and informatics to enhance the provision of care and improve outcomes for patients. Knowledge of QI increases as caregivers learn how to appreciate the value of what individual staff and interprofessional teams can do to positively impact care. A nurse becomes more skilled in applying evidence-based care by collaborating with the interprofessional team to structure the work environment and use processes that integrate new evidence into standards of practice to achieve desired outcomes of patient care. For example, the nurse can participate in an informatics project by providing visual layout suggestions, discovered in a literature search, that facilitate capture of relevant clinical information in a new electronic document. The nurse can also be an opinion leader by focusing on an area of special interest to the nurse such as patient and healthcare staff safety initiatives. Applying QSEN competencies is key to the nurse's understanding of implementation science. Implementation science typically begins with an EBP that is underutilized, and then identifies and addresses resultant quality gaps at the provider, unit, or healthcare system level (Bauer et al., 2015). QSEN competencies are the underpinning for the processes that accomplish that work.

IMPLEMENTATION SCIENCE AND BEDSIDE CLINICAL CARE, PATIENT EDUCATION, PROFESSIONAL DEVELOPMENT, AND NURSING RESEARCH

Implementation science provides structures and processes that lead to outcomes which inform caregivers how to get the best care to as many patients as possible who need it. It influences how quickly and efficiently an EBP is adopted and followed. EBP implements a clinical intervention designed to improve care and is thoroughly discussed in Chapter 9 but will be reviewed here in terms of implementation. The adoption of EBP is supported by combinations of strategies identified through implementation science frameworks that overcome barriers and facilitate EBP use. Implementation science provides implementation interventions, factors, and contextual variables that result in knowledge uptake and subsequent improvement in the provision of patient-centered safe care.

For example, a nursing unit has a high fall rate, and the nurse manager asks a staff nurse to assume a leadership position by becoming the unit's fall risk reduction champion. The nurse joins the hospital's interprofessional fall reduction committee. The goal of the committee is to reduce each nursing unit's overall fall rate and revise the procedure for preventing patient falls. At the meetings, EBPs are discussed, and the Patient-Centered Fall Prevention Toolkit, Fall TIPS (Agency for Healthcare Research and Quality, 2021), is selected for use. The hospital's fall prevention procedure is revised to include the Fall TIPS toolkit. The committee uses the hospital's improvement method of PDSA cycles for the improvement work and monitors the data at its monthly meetings. Dashboards are prominently displayed on hospital bulletin boards. Over the next

TABLE 13.10 EXAMPLES OF BARRIERS TO IMPLEMENTING EVIDENCE-BASED PRACTICE IN HEALTHCARE

Uncertainty	Belief perseverance: "This is the way I learned it."
Professional norms	Favoring individual professional judgment: "This is a practice guideline so I can choose to use it or not."
Multilevel influences	Constraints on healthcare practices: "We don't have enough staff or time to do it."

several months, the fall rate on the unit declines but then begins to increase. The nurse and the nurse manager continue to analyze the data and realize that the staff is not consistently implementing all the interventions in the new fall prevention procedure. This is called an implementation gap.

The implementation gap can be examined by identifying what helps, or facilitates, implementation of the procedure changes and what serves as obstacles or barriers to implementation. There are three basic characteristics of barriers in healthcare: uncertainty, professional norms, and multilevel influences (Table 13.10). Uncertainty is when the clinician questions the validity of the EBP and uses that as the reason for not using the EBP. Professional norms can interfere with implementation of an EBP because the clinician believes that the EBP is optional. For example, if an EBP is not incorporated within a hospital's procedure, clinicians may believe it is not necessary to use the EBP. Multilevel influences interfere with EBP implementation through lack of leadership support, healthcare staff not understanding the impact of the EBP on achieving an improved healthcare outcome, and through miscommunication about why the EBP is necessary.

As the fall reduction champion, the nurse can observe which staff members are involved in the implementation of the new procedure and how they must adjust their work to implement the procedure. Do they follow the procedure as written or do they change something in the procedure? Strategies to support the implementation that the nurse can use include providing the evidence-based literature about the new procedure to the staff, discussing the new procedure at staff meetings, and asking about reasons for choosing to not follow the new procedure. Doing a literature search and sharing the results of that search with colleagues is a path of professional development. An open discussion will help the staff understand why the new procedure is better than one they learned earlier in their careers.

If the reasons for non-use reflect professional norms, there is a way to compromise. Sometimes parts of an EBP can be changed without eroding the intended positive outcome. This decision must be done in consultation with clinical experts, such as the clinical nurse specialist and the patient's physician. Consultation with experts is a skill that demonstrates the QSEN teamwork and collaboration as well as the EBP competency. Multilevel influences, such as reduced staffing or lack of necessary equipment, will require the assistance of hospital leaders to obtain enough resources to enable implementation of the new procedure. Nurses who can respectfully and professionally assert their own perspectives in discussions with leadership about patient care are demonstrating the QSEN competency of teamwork and collaboration and applying one of the strategies recommended by implementation science. Additionally, the nurse can search electronic sources of healthcare information to inform a decision about changing an EBP. Sometimes the compromise is necessary because the patient is resistant to the change or is unable to participate in the changed procedure. Discussions among the interprofessional team, including the patient and family, that build consensus about patient care achieve effective teamwork and collaboration and contribute to safe patient outcomes.

CURRENT LITERATURE

CITATION

Boehm, L. M., Stolldorf, D. P., & Jeffery, A. D. (2020). Implementation science training and resources for nurses and nurse scientists. *Journal of Nursing Scholarship, 52*(1), 47–54. https://doi.org/10.1111/jnu.12510

DISCUSSION

Implementation science programs, organizations, and literature were analyzed to determine the roles of nurses and nurse scientists in translating evidence into routine practice. The role of implementation scientists is to evaluate how nurses use an implementation strategy to implement a new intervention in their clinical setting and determine if the selected strategy results in greater implementation of the intervention. The role of nurses frequently is to bring together colleagues to address an issue needing improvement, evaluate the literature related to the issue, and suggest interventions and strategies that are best suited for their setting. Implementation scientists measure outcomes specific to implementation efforts, such as acceptability and sustainability of the intervention. Nurses at the frontline of healthcare measure the clinical outcomes of their improvement efforts.

IMPLICATIONS FOR PRACTICE

Nurses can use implementation science in their daily work by understanding their practice settings and selecting strategies that will facilitate use of acceptance and use of evidence-based processes. Nurses who can successfully facilitate implementation efforts have the opportunity to improve health and healthcare of their patients.

Nurses can also participate in helping with **de-implementation** of do-not-use practices, such as not placing or maintaining an indwelling urinary catheter in a patient unless there is a specific indication to do so. De-implementation is the process of removing a process, intervention, technology, or other element previously implemented into a healthcare process or system. Barriers to de-implementation of old practices may include staff support for the status quo, beliefs that the current practice is working fine, and a general lack of recognition or openness to exploring a practice change (Tucker & Gallagher-Ford, 2019). Identifying the barriers to changing a procedure guides the identification of facilitators and behaviors that will support practice changes based on the newest evidence and help the nurse gain proficiency in the attitudes necessary to achieve QSEN competencies (Table 13.11).

Implementation science helps the nurse understand why the new procedure is not being used and how the nurse can increase its use through the best-suited strategies. Having creative and easy-to-interpret dashboards to help monitor outcomes is an important factor in the implementation process but alone is not sufficient to motivate change in healthcare practices. A systematized approach to addressing barriers and strengthening facilitators to system change will help the interprofessional team understand, accept, and adopt the new procedure.

Implementation science is supported by theoretical frameworks, requires contextual analysis, builds on patient and stakeholder involvement, applies implementation strategies, and focuses on both clinical and implementation outcomes (Zullig et al., 2020). Nurses who understand the theoretical frameworks of implementation science gain skill in how to improve and sustain improvements in patient healthcare. Nurses who understand the healthcare organizations where they work can provide critical insight for contextual

TABLE 13.11 BARRIERS, FACILITATORS AND BEHAVIORS, AND QUALITY AND SAFETY EDUCATION FOR NURSES COMPETENCY ATTITUDES THAT SUPPORT SYSTEM CHANGE IN HEALTHCARE

BARRIER	FACILITATOR AND BEHAVIOR	QSEN COMPETENCY ATTITUDE
Uncertainty	Training and education: hands-on experience; case review including how to apply the procedure for special populations (such as patients with dementia)	Value own and others' contributions to outcomes of care in local care settings.
	Performance feedback: ongoing, timely audits and reminders	Appreciate the cognitive and physical limits of human performance.
	Feedback on progress: posting data graphs (audit/feedback) benchmarking, internal and external comparisons	Value measurement and its role in good patient care.
Professional norms	Leadership: Experienced nurses providing support and guidance for less experienced nurses	Value the perspectives and expertise of all health team members.
	Emphasizing the benefit to the patient: Sharing positive outcomes and recognizing coworkers by storytelling during staff meetings	Value local change (in individual practice or team practice on a unit) and its role in creating joy in work.
	Ownership: Identifying a champion: Identifying staff who have a passion for the healthcare issue and its improvement (these staff are also called opinion leaders)	Acknowledge own potential to contribute to effective team functioning. Respect the unique attributes that members bring to a team, including variations in professional orientations and accountabilities.
Multilevel influences	Resources: Commitment by senior leadership to provide staff, supplies, and equipment Commitment among colleagues to work together	Value nurses' involvement in design, selection, implementation, and valuation of information technologies to support patient care. Respect the unique attributes that members bring to a team, including variations in professional orientations and accountabilities.

QSEN, Quality and Safety Education for Nurses.

analysis regarding which implementation strategies will work best and how they can be applied. Nurses at the bedside can participate in implementation science to improve nursing quality indicator outcomes by applying QSEN competencies when using strategies demonstrated to be effective in promoting EBP (Table 13.12).

IMPLEMENTATION SCIENCE IN NURSING PRACTICE

Staff education and patient education are the most frequently used strategies to implement nursing guidelines in practice (Spoon et al., 2020). However, neither a single strategy, nor a combination of strategies, can be linked directly to successful implementation of nursing guidelines (Spoon et al., 2020). Speroni et al. (2020) found that 90% of nursing research leaders in their study specified that their hospital used an EBP model and implemented findings into practice. Implementation facilitators were identified as nursing leadership,

TABLE 13.12 QUALITY AND SAFETY EDUCATION FOR NURSES COMPETENCY SKILLS AND IMPLEMENTATION STRATEGIES THAT CAN IMPROVE NURSING QUALITY INDICATOR OUTCOMES

NURSING QUALITY INDICATOR	QSEN COMPETENCY SKILL	IMPLEMENTATION STRATEGIES
Patient Falls	Patient-centered care: Elicit patient values, preferences, and expressed needs as part of clinical interview, implementation of care plan, and evaluation of care. Teamwork and collaboration: Communicate with team members, adapting personal style of communicating to needs of the team and situation. Assert own position/perspective in discussions about patient care.	Engagement of patients in fall risk assessment and management Clear and routine communication among team members Leadership interest and provision of necessary resources
Infection	Teamwork and collaboration: Assume the role of team member or leader based on the situation. Solicit input from other team members to improve individual, as well as team, performance. Evidence-based practice: Participate in structuring the work environment to facilitate integration of new evidence into standards of practice.	Clinical champion role Ongoing education, audit, and feedback integrated in nurses' routine practice Education strategies such as posters and using a scenario-based quiz
Pain Management	Safety: Use national patient safety resources for personal professional development and to focus attention on safety in care settings. Informatics: Use information management tools to monitor outcomes of care processes.	Education of key staff Changing the infrastructure by revising the vital sign form to include pain assessment
Stroke Care	Quality improvement: Use quality measures to understand performance. Safety: Use national patient safety resources for own professional development and to focus attention on safety in care settings.	Frequent and sustained audit and clinician-led feedback High-level management support
Pressure Injuries	Safety: Demonstrate effective use of technology and standardized practices that support safety and quality. Quality improvement: Design a small test of change in daily work (using an experiential learning method such as Plan-Do-Study-Act [PDSA])	Collaborative learning PDSA cycles

QSEN, Quality and Safety Education for Nurses.

Sources: Data from Jolliffe, L., Morarty, J., Hoffmann, T., Crotty, M., Hunter, P., Cameron, I. D., Li, X., & Lannin, N. A. (2019). Using audit and feedback to increase clinician adherence to clinical practice guidelines in brain injury rehabilitation: A before and after study. *PLOS One, 14*(3), e0213525. https://doi.org/10.1371/journal.pone.0213525; Lin, F., Marshall, A. P., Gillespie, B., Li, Y., O'Callaghan, F., Morrissey, S., O'Callaghan, F., & Marshall, A. (2020). Evaluating the implementation of a multi-component intervention to prevent surgical site infection and promote evidence-based practice. *World Views on Evidence-Based Nursing, 17*(3), 193–201. https://doi.org/10.1111/wvn.12436; Quality and Safety Education for Nurses. (2020). *QSEN competencies*. https://qsen.org/competencies/pre-licensure-ksas; Tequare, M. H., Huntzicker, J. J., Mhretu, H. G., Zelelew, Y. B., Abraha, H. E., Tsegay, M. A., Kesatea Gebretensaye, K. G., Tesfay, D. G., Sotomayor, J. G., Nardos, R., Yosses, M. B., Cobbs, J. E., Pui, J., Schmidt, L., Weisman, W., & Breitner, K. (2020). Pain management and its possible implementation research in North Ethiopia: A before and after study. *Advances in Medicine,* Article ID 531735. https://doi.org/10.1155/2020/5317352; Tucker, S., Sheikholeslami, D., Farrington M, Picone, D., Johnson, J., Matthews, G., Evans, R., Gould, R., Bohlken, D., Comried, L., Petrulevich, K., Perkhounkova, E., & Cullen, L. (2019). Patient, nurse, and organizational factors that influence evidence-based fall prevention for hospitalized oncology patients: An exploratory study. *Worldviews on Evidence-Based Nursing*, *16*(2), 111–120. https://doi.org/10.1111/wvn.12353; Wood, J., Brown, B., Bartley, A., Cavaco, A. M. B. C., Paul Roberts, A., Santon, K., & Cook, S. (2019). Reducing pressure ulcers across multiple care settings using a collaborative approach. *BMJ Open Quality*, 8, e000409. https://doi.org/10.1136/bmjoq-2018-000409

dissemination of findings, and engaged and educated nurses. To champion implementation science, nurses working in healthcare organizations that have academic affiliations can partner with nurse researchers who are studying the use and impact of implementation strategies to help build knowledge in this critical area. Researchers value collaboration with nurses who are working on the front lines of clinical care. Bedside nurses are more familiar with the hands-on provision of care. As a result, they may be able to identify implementation gaps that lead to new research projects. The trust patients and caregivers have in bedside nurses puts nurses in an opportune position to facilitate implementation of EBP.

CASE STUDY

The bedside nurse is working with a nurse researcher who is planning an implementation science research study of an intervention to prevent falls in an inpatient neurology unit. The nurse is interested in learning how to best conduct the implementation and is most interested in determining if the intervention works.

1. ***Which implementation science framework could the nurse use? Why?***
2. ***Which hybrid research design could the nurse use? Why?***
3. ***What actions could the bedside nurse take to assist the nurse researcher?***

Bedside nurses with any amount of experience can demonstrate leadership by collaborating with their nurse managers to incorporate implementation science into daily practice. They can volunteer to teach about implementation science at a staff meeting. They can offer to find articles about implementation strategies and successful EBP projects that address patient care issues on their units and can lead discussions about these at a journal club meeting. They can volunteer to lead an interprofessional team which uses RE-AIM or CFIR to improve patient or work environment-related outcomes. Most importantly, bedside nurses participate in implementation science by adopting, implementing, and integrating evidence-based interventions to deliver quality, evidence-based healthcare.

Real World Interview

In today's healthcare environment, change is a constant which requires nurses to be at the forefront of implementing new clinical practices and stopping the use of obsolete practices. It can often take years for only a fraction of new evidence-based knowledge to be translated into real world settings. Frontline nurses play an essential role in interdisciplinary teams across all settings with a healthcare organization and are expected to carry out these evidence-based changes. Implementation science focuses on the adoption and integration of evidence-based practices into routine care by applying behavioral science principles to change organizational behavior across healthcare settings and clinical disciplines. Training in implementation science theories, frameworks, evaluation designs, outcomes, and change strategies complements standard quality improvement knowledge by strengthening a nurse's ability to identify multilevel organization barriers to practice change and develop appropriate interventions to reduce these barriers so that the improved practice can be spread throughout a given health system.

David E. Goodrich, EdD

Implementation Scientist

VA Center for Evaluation & Implementation Resources (CEIR), VA Ann Arbor Healthcare System, Ann Arbor, Michigan

END-OF-CHAPTER RESOURCES

KEY CONCEPTS

1. Implementation science typically begins with an evidence-based practice (EBP) that is underutilized or has not yet been utilized.
2. Implementation science identifies and addresses resultant quality gaps at the provider, unit, or healthcare system levels.
3. Implementation science is the study of implementation interventions, factors, and contextual variables that cause learning and use of the learning in the provision of healthcare.
4. There are three basic characteristics of barriers in healthcare: uncertainty, professional norms, and multilevel influences.
5. Implementation science frameworks help frontline nurses and researchers engaged in the study of implementation to understand: (1) *how* to best implement; (2) *what* elements are necessary for successful implementation; and (3) strategies to *sustain* implementation.
6. Three commonly used implementation science frameworks are: (a) the Consolidated Framework for Implementation Science (CFIR); (b) Reach, Effectiveness, Adoption, Implementation, and Maintenance (RE-AIM); and the Dynamic Sustainability Framework (DSF).
7. Implementation science is often developed following one of three hybrid research designs: (a) Type I (effectiveness); (b) Type II (effectiveness + feasibility); and (c) Type III (utility).
8. Implementation science relates to bedside clinical care, patient education, professional development, and research aspects of nursing practice.
9. Implementation science is aligned with the six QSEN competencies: patient-centered care, quality improvement, teamwork and collaboration, evidence-based practice, safety, and informatics.
10. Nursing practice offers many opportunities to participate in implementation science.

CRITICAL DISCUSSION POINTS

1. Attend a clinical council meeting and ask if there are any barrier(s) to implementing EBP, and what the rationales are for these barriers. Identify strategies that might be used to overcome the barrier(s).
2. What innovation(s) have you seen in your clinical setting? How is this innovation helping to improve the healthcare of patients?
3. Cross your arms. Once you are settled, cross your arms the other way. Why is the second crossing more uncomfortable? Discuss this experience in relation to barriers in de-implementation of the provision of non-EBP healthcare practices.
4. Review the American Academy of Nursing's list of Twenty-Five Things Nurses and Patients Should Question found at www.choosingwisely.org/wp-content/uploads/2015/02/AANursing-Choosing-Wisely-List.pdf. Think about your clinical experiences. How would knowing about this "do-not-do" list influence your provision of interprofessional healthcare to patients?

5. Think of a clinical problem in frontline nursing practice and how you might use the elements of implementation science frameworks to help you to design an implementation approach. Which frameworks would you use to figure out *what* is important in the implementation, *how* to implement it, and how to *sustain* it? What elements from the frameworks seem most helpful and useful? Are there places where they overlap?

KEY TERMS

- Adoption
- Barriers
- Consolidated Framework for Implementation Research (CFIR)
- De-implementation
- Dynamic Sustainability Framework (DSF)
- Ecological system
- Effectiveness
- Facilitators
- Hybrid research designs
- Implementation
- Implementation framework
- Implementation science
- Implementation strategies
- Improvement
- Individuals
- Inner setting
- Innovation
- Intervention
- Maintenance
- Outer setting
- Practice setting
- Processes
- Reach
- Reach, Effectiveness, Adoption, Implementation, and Maintenance (RE-AIM)
- Voltage drop

REVIEW QUESTIONS

Answers to Review Questions appear in the Instructor's Manual. Qualified instructors should request the Instructor's Manual from textbook@springerpub.com.

1. Surgeons notified the nurse manager on the orthopedic floor about too many calls during the overnight shift for interventions that don't require a physician's judgment, such as patients requesting a lozenge for a sore throat (after intubation). In working to resolve this concern, an interprofessional team suggests a comfort list of things the nurse can initiate without contacting a physician. The comfort list is approved by the hospital leadership team as a pilot project on the surgical unit. Which one of the following best describes the new comfort list?

   A. It is an improvement because patients will receive comfort items more quickly.

   B. It is an implementation because it was approved for use on the surgical unit.

   C. It is an innovation because the order set has not been tested before in this setting.

   D. It is a sustainability process because it was approved by the leadership team.

2. Nursing staff at a hospital have been informed of an increased use of inappropriate indwelling catheter placements and the hospital is looking to improve this. Applying the CFIR framework to assess barriers and facilitators, what are some ways of demonstrating that the nursing staff is ready to help with the project? *Select all that apply.*

   A. A nurse volunteers to search for new practices on indwelling catheters in peer-reviewed journals.

   B. A nurse states that she is not prepared to go against the doctor's orders, even if they are improper.

   C. A nurse states that working with patients who have urinary issues is a particular interest area.

   D. One nurse suggested they start a committee on indwelling catheters for best practices that meets weekly

   E. A nurse suggests the problem is not new and is happening due to limited staffing, so there is no need for a new team.

3. At a staff meeting, the idea of bedside shift reports was presented as an evidence-based way to reduce time required for nurse-to-nurse reports, as they keep the conversation more objective, concise, and relevant to patients' care. The nurse manager assigned a team to evaluate and implement this intervention. Which one of the following is consistent with a potential barrier to the implementation process?

   A. A recent influx of new nurses has a strong evidence-based practice mentality.

   B. The project has support from the nurse manager and the hospital leadership.

   C. The staff says there isn't enough time to go to each patient's bedside to give a report.

   D. The nurses with quality improvement experience can optimize changed processes.

4. Which of the following reflect essential characteristics of innovations in order for them to be implemented in clinical care? *Select all that apply.*

   A. Innovations can challenge the status quo.

   B. Innovations must focus on the clinical team's work.

   C. Innovations must be supported by research.

   D. Innovations do not have to be supported by research.

   E. Innovations are always widelyaccepted.

5. Which of the following factors can be barriers to the implementation process in a hospital? *Select all that apply.*

   A. Lack of support exists from executive leadership.

   B. The hospital nursing staff is looking for change.

   C. Limited resources are available to do the implementation.

   D. Monitoring of the implementation is necessary.

   E. The interprofessional team thinks it is too much work.

6. An interprofessional team reviews submissions for clinical improvements. A particular innovation is selected to implement on all the medical-surgical units. Which of the following would increase the likelihood of adoption and diffusion of the innovation? *Select all that apply.*

A. The innovation must be simple to understand.
B. The innovation must be launched on a largescale.
C. The innovation must be perceived as effective.
D. The innovation must be similar to the current way of doing things.
E. The impact of the innovation must be kept hidden.

7. A team is assigned to look at interventions which could be implemented to reduce long wait times in the emergency department (ED), but the task is daunting, with many interrelated variables. It is suggested the team use the Consolidated Framework for Implementation Research (CFIR) as the variables can be separated into different categories (components) to better understand the big picture. Which of the following statements describe the inner setting? *Select all that apply.*
A. Due to flu season, visits to the ED have increased.
B. Reduction in long wait times will be beneficial for hospital leadership.
C. The nurse manager and one of the ED physicians have agreed to be on the team.
D. Admission and discharge processes are strained by increased demand and short staffing.
E. A patient who has been receiving care at the hospital has volunteered to work with the team.

8. A nurse on the safety team was assigned to evaluate the hospital's medication safety protocol, which was implemented 6 months ago, using the RE-AIM framework to fully cover all aspects and present them in ways easy for everyone to follow. What types of information might the nurse include to demonstrate the protocol's effectiveness?
A. Increase or decrease in adverse drug event rates
B. The percentage of staff who have been trained in the new protocols
C. The medication safety protocols incorporated into the nurses' workflow
D. The medication safety protocols that are still being pilot tested

9. At an interprofessional meeting focused on discussing ways to improve response time in code teams when a code blue is called, one of the team members stressed that previous interventions had suffered from voltage drop. What actions could the nurse take in this situation to address voltage drop?
A. Ensure defibrillators are fully charged so they do not lose voltage.
B. Examine why previous interventions may have lost fidelity.
C. Remove obstacles to implementing any improvement.
D. Begin the new code blue intervention on one hospital unit.

10. The nurse has been working for the past 6 months with an interprofessional team focused on reducing the rates of catheter-acquired urinary tract infections (CAUTI). The team has applied many Plan-Do-Study-Act (PDSA) cycles to achieve the desired improvement in patient care. Which implementation science framework uses the PDSA cycle as part of its structure?
A. Consolidated Framework for Implementation Research (CFIR)
B. Diffusion of Innovation Framework (DIF)
C. Dynamic Sustainability Framework (DSF)
D. Reach, Effectiveness, Adoption, Implementation, and Maintenance (RE-AIM)

REVIEW ACTIVITIES

1. A nurse working in the hospital asthma clinic discovered that many clinic patients called to request early refills on their inhalers 60 days before their refills were due. In talking with some of these patients, the nurse discovered that the early refills were not necessarily due to poor asthma control, but were sometimes due to people wanting extra inhalers for places like their gym bags, cars, and so on. Wanting to identify patients who needed better asthma symptom control, the management of the clinic budgeted for training and coaching of all staff who take calls to ask probing yet nonjudgmental questions during these phone encounters, to understand why the patient needed the early refill. Management knew this would help the clinicians understand when patents were actually using their inhaler more than expected, which would help to guide their plan of care. The clinic workflow was modified to include the new call protocol but a month after implementation, only a few poorly controlled asthma patients had been identified. An assessment was conducted by the implementation team which revealed that many of the clinic staff were unfamiliar with the new call protocol and that the training questions were not readily available when needed for consultation. Based on post-implementation findings, clinic management decided to allocate resources to provide ongoing education and implementation support to monitor and sustain the implementation over time once the project was fully implemented. Use this scenario to briefly describe each component of the RE-AIM framework.
2. The nurse working with the hospital interprofessional team was tasked to identify some ways he can help the team implement a new hand hygiene protocol. In doing research, the nurse discovered some practice environments are better suited to successful implementation of projects, while some present barriers. The nurse then made a list of the barriers and reported back during his team's weekly meeting. He found that stakeholders do not see the relative advantage of the new system, there isn't an urgency for change because the old way works "well enough," and there is a belief the cost of the new dispensers would be too high. What are some implementation strategies with rationales that might help to overcome these barriers?
3. The nurse scientist on the interprofessional team has been tasked with increasing nursing involvement on the hospital implementation team. After a few weeks of recruiting nurses who expressed interest to join the team, the nurse scientist decided to call a first meeting to discuss the nursing role. The team expectation is that frontline nurses' involvement will better inform future implementation efforts at this hospital. From information gathered in this chapter, describe possible roles of bedside nurses in implementation efforts.

EXPLORING THE WEB

1. Go to the QSEN website (www.qsen.org) and under tags select "Evidence-Based Practice." Click on Policy Review. Review the learning strategy. How could implementation science be included in a policy review?

2. Go to the QSEN website (www.qsen.org) and select the Resources tab. Scroll down to implementation methods. Select "Continue Reading" under AHRQ Implementation Methods. Click on and review the booklet *Implementation Science at a Glance: A Guide for Cancer Control Practitioners*. Discuss how this tool could be used in your clinical setting.

3. Go to the *Implementation Science Journal* site (https://implementationsciencecomms.biomedcentral.com). Select the About tab, and read the second paragraph under Aims and Scope. Think about your clinical setting and discuss what difficulty might be encountered if someone suggested de-implementation of a clinical process.

4. Go to the CFIR website (https://cfirguide.org) or the RE-AIM website (www.re-aim.org). Select one of the published articles listed on the website which use that framework. Try to identify elements of the framework in the article. How did the authors apply them and how did it help them conduct and study the implementation? How would you apply the same elements in your practice setting if you were planning an implementation initiative?

SPRINGER PUBLISHING CONNECT™ | A robust set of instructor resources designed to supplement this text is located at **http://connect.springerpub.com/content/book/978-0-8261-6145-1.** Qualifying instructors may request access by emailing **textbook@springerpub.com.**

REFERENCES

Agency for Healthcare Research and Quality. (2021). *Fall TIPS: A patient-centered fall prevention toolkit.* https://www.ahrq.gov/patient-safety/settings/hospital/fall-tips/index.html

Bauer, M. S., Damschroder, L., Hagedorn, H., Smith, J., & Kilbourne, A. M. (2015). An introduction to implementation science for the non-specialist. *BMC Psychology, 3*, Article 32. https://doi.org/10.1186/s40359-015-0089-9

CFIR Research Team-Center for Clinical Management Research. (2020). Home page: What is the CFIR? https://cfirguide.org

Chambers, D. A., Glasgow R. E., & Stange, K. C. (2013). The Dynamic Sustainability Framework: Addressing the paradox of sustainment amid ongoing change. *Implementation Science, 8*, Article 117. https://doi.org/10.1186/1748-5908-8-117

Curran, G. M., Bauer, M., Mittman, B., Pyne, J. M., & Stetler, C. (2012). Effectiveness-implementation hybrid designs: Combining elements of clinical effectiveness and implementation research to enhance public health impact. *Medical Care, 50*(3), 217–226. https://doi.org/10.1097/MLR.0b013e3182408812

Damschroeder, L., Aron, D., Keith, R., Kirsh, S. R., Alexander, J. A., & Lowery, J. C. (2009). Fostering implementation of health services research findings into practice: A consolidated framework for advancing implementation science. *Implementation Science, 4*, Article 50. https://doi.org/10.1186/1748-5908-4-50

Glasgow, R. E., Vogt, T. M., & Boles, S. M. (1999). Evaluating the public health impact of health promotion interventions: The RE-AIM framework. *American Journal of Public Health, 89*(9), 1322–1327. https://doi.org/10.2105/ajph.89.9.1322

Rogers, E. M. (1995). *Diffusion of Innovations* (4th ed.). Free Press.

Speroni, K. G., McLaughlin, M. K., & Friesen, M. A. (2020). Use of evidence-based practice models and research findings in Magnet-designated hospitals across the United States: National survey results. *Worldviews on Evidence-Based Nursing, 17*, 98–107. https://doi.org/10.1111/wvn.12428

Spoon, D., Rietbergen, T., Huis, A., Heinen, M., van Dijk, M., van Bodegom-Vos, L., & Ista, E. (2020). Implementation strategies used to implement nursing guidelines in daily practice: A systematic review. *International Journal of Nursing Studies, 111*, Article 103748. https://doi.org/10.1016/j.ijnurstu.2020.103748

Tucker, S. J., & Gallagher-Ford, L. (2019). EBP 2.0: From strategy to implementation. *American Journal of Nursing, 119*(4), 50–52. https://doi.org/10.1097/01.NAJ.0000554549.01028.af

Waltz, T. J., Powell, B. J., Matthieu, M. M., Damschroder, L. J., Chinman, M. J., Smith, J. L., Proctor, E. K., & Kirchner, J. E. (2015). Use of concept mapping to characterize relationships among implementation strategies and assess their feasibility and importance: Results from the Expert Recommendations for Implementing Change (ERIC) study. *Implementation Science, 10*, Article 109. https://doi.org/10.1186/s13012-015-0295-0

Zullig, L. L., Deschodt, M., & DeGeest, S. (2020). Embracing implementation science: A paradigm shift for nursing research. *Journal of Nursing Scholarship, 52*, 3–5. https://doi.org/10.1111/jnu.12507

SUGGESTED READINGS

Balasubramanian, B. A., Cohen, D. J., Davis, M. M., Gunn, R., Dickinson, L. M., Miller, W. L., Crabtree, B. F., & Stange, K. C. (2015). Learning evaluation: Blending quality improvement and implementation research methods to study healthcare innovations. *Implementation Science, 10*, Article 31. https://doi.org/10.1186/s13012-015-0219-z

Birken, S. A., Powell, B. J., Shea, C. M., Scott, J., Leeman, J., Grewe, M. E., Alexis Kirk, M., Damschroder, L., Aldridge II, W. A., Haines, E. R., Straus, S., & Presseau, J. (2017). Criteria for selecting implementation science theories and frameworks: Results from an international survey. *Implementation Science, 12*, Article 124. https://doi.org/10.1186/s13012-017-0656-y

Boehm, L. M., Stolldorf, D. P., & Jeffery, A. D. (2019). Implementation science training and resources for nurses and nurse scientists. *Journal of Nursing Scholarship, 52*(1), 47–54. https://doi.org/10.1111/jnu.12510

Boulton, R., Sandall, J., & Sevdalis, N. (2020). The cultural politics of "implementation science" *Journal of Medical Humanities, 41*, 379–394. https://doi.org/10.1007/s10912-020-09607-9

Dang, D., & Dearholt, S. (2018). *Creating a supportive EBP environment: Johns Hopkins nursing evidence-based model & guidelines* (3rd ed.). Sigma Theta Tau International. https://sigma.nursingrepository.org/bitstream/handle/10755/623549/FreeDownload_JohnsHopkinsEBPModelGuidelines3rdEdition_DangDearholt.pdf;jsessionid=143BBB3E558CF9A2BF2165AA6228EBB2?sequence=1

Raderstorf, T., Barr, T. L., Ackerman, M., & Melnyk, B. M. (2020). A guide to empowering frontline nurses and healthcare clinicians through evidence-based innovation leadership during COVID-19 and beyond. *Worldviews on Evidence-Based Nursing, 17*, 254–257. https://doi.org/10.1111/wvn.12451

Zullig, L. L., Deschodt, M., & De Geest, S. (2020). Embracing implementation science: A paradigm shift for nursing research. *Journal of Nursing Scholarship, 52*, 3–5. https://doi.org/10.1111/jnu.12507

CHAPTER 14

Quality Improvement and Project Management

Marianne K. Schallmo

"If you fail to plan, you plan to fail."

–Benjamin Franklin

Upon completion of this chapter, the reader should be able to:

1. Describe how project management techniques improve the delivery of quality improvement (QI) projects.
2. Explain the nurse's role as an interprofessional team member on a QI project.
3. Examine the five phases of project management.
4. Apply the five phases of project management to a healthcare problem.
5. Discuss leadership and management characteristics required during project management.
6. Examine the benefits and limitations of project management.

CROSSWALK

This chapter addresses the following:

QSEN Competency: Teamwork and Collaboration and Quality Improvement

The American Association of Colleges of Nursing. (2021). *The essentials: Core competencies for professional nursing education.*

Domain 4: Scholarship for the Nursing Discipline

Domain 5: Quality and Safety

OPENING SCENARIO

Roberto is the nurse manager on a medical-surgical floor. He recently received the monthly report on nursing overtime and noticed overtime costs have been rising. He walks to the nursing station to discuss the issue with the staff. He notices several incoming nurses waiting to receive change-of-shift report. When he inquires about the situation, the incoming shift nurse states the shift report delay occurs when they wait to receive report from four different nurses. The outgoing shift nurse states the problem occurs when healthcare providers want to complete hospital rounds during shift change. Another nurse attributes the problem to disruptions from other staff, such as when the dietary delivers morning trays during change of shift or the emergency department transfers a patient during change of shift. Roberto realizes there are multiple reasons for the delay in shift report. He quickly appreciates everyone's viewpoint and realizes the solution involves many different hospital departments. Resolving the problem requires an interprofessional team approach. Another hospital unit resolved their overtime costs by implementing a quality improvement project designed to streamline the change-of-shift report. Before he can recruit team members to help implement a quality improvement project, he has questions needing answers. For example:

1. *How does he identify the scope of the project and who should participate on the project team?*
2. *How will he organize the project steps?*
3. *How can he ensure the project is completed on time?*

INTRODUCTION

In a healthcare environment that is constantly changing, it is essential organizations deliver care based on the most recent and best available evidence. However, this can only be realized if the best available evidence on clinical practice issues is translated for use at the bedside. An organization dedicates time and money to translate the best available evidence into quality improvement (QI) projects that will benefit their organization. These QI projects are complex, requiring a precise project plan, which includes a purpose statement, aims, and outcomes. A designated project leader is charged with assembling the team members and directing the project plan. The project leader uses project management (PM) techniques to coordinate team effort, ensure proper sequencing of project events, and assure project completion. Without PM techniques, even important projects may be destined to fail.

This chapter explores how effective PM techniques can guide improvement in healthcare quality, safety, and patient outcomes. Project management will be defined and key concepts explored. In today's healthcare environment, every healthcare member is responsible for and contributes to QI translation and sustainability. This chapter introduces the nurse as an integral interprofessional team member and discusses how frontline workers are crucial in QI projects.

Using PM techniques increases QI project success. The PM techniques include the five phases of initiating, planning, executing, monitoring and controlling, and closing. In this chapter, each phase will be defined. In addition, this chapter will demonstrate how the nurse answers a current healthcare problem using PM techniques. The chapter then highlights nursing leadership skills central to managing interprofessional teams and QI projects. Finally, PM benefits and limitations will be examined.

PROJECT MANAGEMENT TECHNIQUES IMPROVE THE DELIVERY OF QUALITY IMPROVEMENT PROJECTS

Healthcare costs have increased every year and this trend continues to rise (Keenhan et al., 2020). The 2020 National Health Expenditure is $4.01 trillion, and this is projected to grow an average of 5.4% annually through 2028 (Keenhan et al., 2020). Strained healthcare budgets create a critical need for healthcare organizations to better manage costs while striving for high-quality patient care outcomes. Recent research indicates QI projects lower healthcare costs while maintaining or improving patient outcomes (Agency for Healthcare Research and Quality [AHRQ], 2020; de la Perrelle et al., 2020).

Projects are defined as "a temporary endeavor undertaken to create a unique product, service, or result" (Project Management Institute, 2020). Project attributes include:

- Projects are temporary with a defined beginning and end. A team assembles to complete a project, then dissolves after project completion.
- Projects are unique. Ongoing operations are the day-to-day work, whereas projects have a one-time specific purpose.
- Projects require input from multiple perspectives. Projects require innovation and diverse teams foster better innovation.

Quality for Safety Education for Nurses (QSEN) defines **quality improvement (QI)** when nurses "use data to monitor the outcomes of care processes and use improvement methods to design and test changes to continuously improve the quality and safety of healthcare systems" (QSEN, 2020). Healthcare agencies use QI projects to optimize care delivery and reduce costs. Chapter 11 covers content on QI and Chapter 12 reviews QI data.

Every QI project takes time, energy, and costs to develop, implement, and sustain. When QI project deadlines are missed, budgets are underestimated, or time is wasted, the chance of the QI project being developed, implemented, or sustained is reduced and patient outcomes may not meet the healthcare organization's expectations. To contain costs while maintaining quality patient care outcomes, healthcare organizations must employ nursing leaders who are able to develop and implement QI projects on time and on budget.

Project management (PM), as defined by the Project Management Institute (PMI, 2020), is "the application of knowledge, skills, tools, and techniques to project activities to meet the project requirements." PM involves a variety of methods, techniques, skills, and processes that are designed to identify potential project obstacles and to develop strategies to overcome challenges. PM techniques save time, costs, and eliminate wasteful processes by standardizing and optimizing current work processes. Using PM strategies helps minimize or mitigates obstacles and improves project completion success (Project Management Institute, 2018). Healthcare organizations need nurses with PM and leadership skills who use reliable and proven PM techniques to develop and deliver successful QI projects.

In the opening scenario, the medical-surgical unit manager needs to decrease overtime costs. The unit manager recognizes he needs a QI project aimed at reducing costs. This QI project is unique to this specific problem, meaning the project's single purpose is to decrease overtime costs on the medical-surgical unit. Since the problem has multiple causes, the solution will require input from multiple perspectives. The unit manager will assemble an interprofessional team. The unit manager will use PM techniques to lead the team through developing, implementing, and sustaining the QI project. The team will be convened temporarily during the QI project and charged with analyzing the problem, creating an action plan, and implementing the plan. After the QI project is sustained, the team will disband.

Real World Interview

New registered nurse graduates play a critical role in QI projects. Their critical role is inserting a fresh voice at the table. New registered nurses are immersed in the latest evidence-based practice and can assist in steering the QI team in an appropriate direction. In addition to bringing the most current evidence-based practice to the table, they are able to share what is really happening at the bedside, including what they perceive will work seamlessly in the current workflow and what problems may arise. The PM team leader must set the expectations for the new graduates who will be on the team. In addition, the team leader will need to meet with the new graduate team members prior to the initial project kick off. The initial interaction will allow the team leader to outline expectations for the new graduates and to empower the new graduate team members to speak up and speak out.

–Lisa Grubb, DNP, MSN, RN, WOCN, C/DONA, CPHQ

Senior Director of Quality Improvement, Deputy Director Johns Hopkins Armstrong Institute at Howard County General Hospital, Howard County General Hospital, Part-Time Faculty at The Johns Hopkins University School of Nursing, Core Faculty at The Johns Hopkins Armstrong Institute for Patient Safety and Quality

NURSE'S ROLE AS AN INTERPROFESSIONAL TEAM MEMBER

The demand for hospitals to report quality measures and achieve benchmarks for quality care has impacted the nurse's role in QI projects. In today's healthcare environment, interprofessional teamwork is necessary for optimal patient care. Interprofessional teams may consist of nurses, physicians, therapists, dietitians, pharmacist, housekeeping, and others with skill sets that are deemed necessary for the success of the project. No matter the level of nursing title, from the chief nursing officer to the direct care nurse, every nurse plays an equally important role in QI. Nurses may be the project leader, a project team member, or participate in implementing or sustaining the project.

Frontline workers, such as bedside nurses, are often in the best position to identify patient care process problems as this is where they spend the majority of their time. Middle nursing managers, such as unit directors, have access to daily operation data. At this level, they can determine the impact of the problem on nursing care and patient outcomes. They can recruit an interprofessional project team to address a specific problem. Executive nursing managers, such as the chief nursing officer, also play an important role. It is their role to encourage a culture of support and openness, ensuring all nurses are comfortable voicing patient safety concerns and encouraging and supporting implementing QI initiatives. While the involvement of nursing leadership is crucial in QI, bedside nurses play a more direct role in the implementation and sustainability of QI activities.

SYSTEMATIC PHASES OF PROJECT MANAGEMENT

Nursing leadership and interprofessional teams use PM techniques to translate QI initiatives. PM approaches help the nurse leader to consider key issues with the identified problem and maintain the trustworthiness of the project. PM is similar to the nursing process in that both are tools which use a systematic stepwise approach to problem-solving. Nurses use the nursing process to solve clinical problems. The nursing process includes the stages of assessment, nursing diagnosis, planning, implementing, and evaluation. These stages are closely

CASE STUDY

Mikayla is a bedside nurse on a same-day surgery unit. Mikayla noticed that when she discharges a patient the physician does not consistently order a postoperative office visit. Often, the patient is discharged home without a scheduled postoperative visit with the surgeon. Mikayla discusses the problem of postoperative patients not having a follow-up appointment with the surgeon at the next monthly unit meeting. The unit manager assumed all patients received a follow-up office visit appointment, as she assumed it was part of the postoperative protocol and no one raised this problem previously. The unit manager listens to Mikayla's concerns and decides the postoperative discharge protocol needs to be updated. The unit manager assembles an interprofessional team to address the problem.

Because Mikayla provides direct patient care to this population of patients, she is able to identify a problem and call attention to her concerns about the quality of patient care processes. In this example, Mikayla identified a situation that could detrimentally affect patient care outcomes. Mikayla recognizes her role in QI and felt supported in voicing her concerns. The unit manager has created an environment of openness and encourages her staff to discuss patient-safety concerns. Because direct care nurses have a unique perspective on patient care, they can identify problems in providing quality patient care. Nurses have an obligation to question current nursing practices when a process does not meet the expected outcomes.

1. *Why are bedside nurses in a good position to discover clinical problems?*
2. *How did the unit manager's attitude toward QI encourage Mikayla to speak up about a clinical problem?*
3. *If the unit manager displayed a negative attitude toward QI, what other avenues could Mikayla pursue to resolve the clinical problem?*

BOX 14.1 Developing Clinical Judgment

Fara is a staff nurse working in an outpatient cardiovascular clinic. Today she is working in the hypertensive clinic. During her assessment of a patient, the patient's blood pressure is 170/90. When Fara reviewed the patient's medication, the patient states he forgot to take his morning medication. Fara realizes forgetting to take medication is a common clinical problem. In the last few months, Fara remembers several patients who admitted to sometimes forgetting to take their medication. Fara wants to help her patients achieve a healthy blood pressure. She recalls reading in a nursing journal about a new phone app that sends patient medication reminders via their cell phone.

1. What clinical judgment might the nurse make based on the **CUES** (**Assessment**) in the scenario?
2. What **HYPOTHESIS** (**Diagnosis**) will the nurse consider?
3. What **ACTION** (**Plan and Implement**) will be most effective for the nurse to take to assure the best outcome?
4. How will the nurse evaluate the **OUTCOME** (**Evaluation**) for the purpose of arriving at a satisfactory clinical outcome?

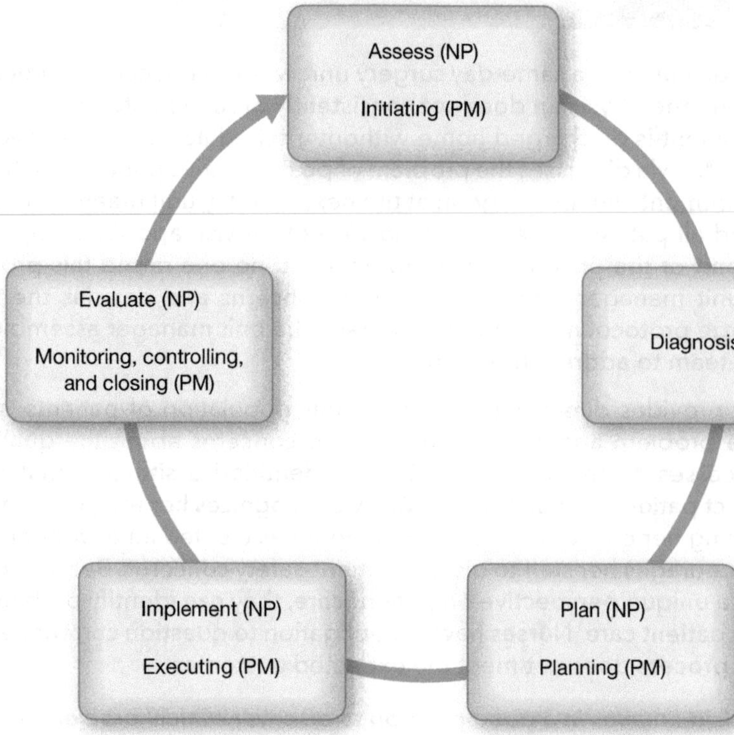

FIGURE 14.1 Nursing Process and Project Management Phases Comparison.

NP, nursing practice; PM, project management.

related to the five PM phases of initiating, planning, executing, monitoring and controlling, and closing. See Figure 14.1 for a comparison between the nursing process and PM. The following section will detail each PM phase, including tools to assist in facilitating the phase.

Project Management Phase 1: Initiating

The first PM phase is initiating. In PM, the first phase is one of the most important as it influences the success of the project. This phase includes recruiting an interprofessional team to work on the QI project, defining the project problem on a broad level, and articulating the problem statement, project purpose, and project aims. The last step of the initiating phase is outlining the project scope.

The first phase involves identifying and recruiting the individuals who must be included on a PM team. While seemingly easy, this phase requires careful thought and planning to ensure the right individuals are brought in to participate on the team. The team will be most effective when they collectively have the necessary knowledge, skills, and attitudes (KSA) to solve the problem (Rosen et al., 2018). This often involves assembling a diverse interprofessional team. Diversity fosters creativity, and innovation, and broadens the team's skill set. The result includes increased project performance and outcomes (PMI, 2020). All projects involving patient care should have a direct care nurse on the team.

Individuals who either affect or are affected by the problem are called **stakeholders**. Stakeholders are vital on the PM team since they can directly influence the success of the project. **Stakeholders** can include persons, groups, or organizations who have an interest in, are affected by, or can affect a practice change (Verzuh, 2016). Stakeholders should be engaged in the PM process based on the stakeholder's influence on the project success. For example, if a PM team was assembled to address an increase in fall rates on a medical-surgical unit, it would be expected that a representative from each of the following would be included: nursing, nursing assistant, physical therapy, physician, pharmacist, dietary, informatics, quality department, and a charge nurse. If the team was assembled and a representative from informatics was not included it may not appear to be a problem. If the team decided that electronic charting should include a new prompt to complete a fall risk assessment and an informatics representative was not on the team it could cause delays and problems in making changes to the charting. While the influence of informatics might not be apparent at first, when a change in the electronic documentation system is needed for a project, the informatics representative becomes critical to making this change happen. A stakeholder assessment should be undertaken to determine the stakeholder's project influence and support. Table 14.1 is a tool to assist the team in determining the stakeholder's influence and support for a project. Those stakeholders with high project influence and high project support should be engaged first. Table 14.1 also includes strategies to engage stakeholders in the project.

When assigning responsibilities for project tasks, two roles need to be identified at the beginning of any project: project manager and project leader. Although these two terms are similar, they are not the same. The project manager is the top project authority, and

TABLE 14.1 STAKEHOLDER SUPPORT, INFLUENCE, AND STRATEGIES FOR ENGAGEMENT

STAKEHOLDER INFLUENCE AND SUPPORT GRID (WITH GENERIC STRATEGIES FOR ENGAGEMENT)		
INFLUENCE	LOW	
High	• Will positively affect dissemination and adoption • Need a great deal of attention and information to maintain buy-in **Strategies:** • Collaborate • Involve and /or provide opportunities where they can be supportive • Support and nurture • Encourage feedback • Prepare for change management • Empower High Support High Influence	• Can positively affect dissemination and adoption if given attention • Need attention to maintain buy-in and prevent development of neutrality **Strategies:** • Collaborate • Encourage feedback • Empower with professional status • Encourage participation • Prepare for change management • Involve at some level High Support Low Influence
Low	Low Support High Influence • Can negatively affect dissemination and adoption in a big way • Need great amount of attention to obtain support and /or neutrality • Work toward buy-in **Strategies:** • Consensus • Build relationships • Recognize needs • Use external stakeholders and consultants • Involve at some level • Don't provoke into action • Monitor	Low Support Low Influence • Least able to influence dissemination and adoption • Could have negative impact on plans • Some attention to obtain support and /or neutrality • Work toward project buy-in **Strategies:** • Consensus • Guild relationships • Recognize needs • Use external stakeholders and consultants • Involve at some level • Monitor

Source: From Registered Nurses' Association of Ontario. (2012). *Toolkit: Implementation of best practice guidelines* (2nd ed., Figure 1). Author. https://rnao.ca/sites/rnao-ca/files/RNAO_ToolKit_2012_rev4_FA.pdf

their responsibility includes overseeing project production, maintenance, and completion. The project leader communicates between the project manager and the team members. The project leader is the main point of contact for day-to-day project problems, and they focus on managing and motivating the team members. The leader collaborates between the team and the manager using their leadership skills (Rowe, 2020).

During the initiating phase of PM, the project problem is identified, and the problem statement is clearly identified. The project problem is defined as the gap between the institution's current situation and the ideal situation. For example, a hospital's inpatient hospice unit recently closed and the hospice patients who are diagnosed with heart failure will now be transferred to the general medical cardiac unit. The general medical cardiac unit nurses voice concern as they feel they do not possess the knowledge to care for hospice patients. Ideally, all cardiac nurses should possess the knowledge to care for patients with heart failure receiving hospice care. The problem, or gap, is the difference between the general medical cardiac nurses' actual hospice care knowledge and the ideal hospice care knowledge level. Comparing the institution's identified problem to local data establishes the project's background and significance. Local data may include admission or discharge data, billing information, patient satisfaction statistics, QI measurements, or morbidity and mortality statistics. The project problem should also be established in a larger context using national or global data, to compare current institutional performance to national or global goals.

Once the problem has been clearly identified, the problem statement can be established. The problem statement details the background and significance of the problem. The problem statement must be grounded in strong research evidence and should answer the following question, "Based on the best available evidence, what should the project team do in order to solve the current problem?"

Once a problem statement is created, the project purpose and project aims are drafted. The project purpose clearly justifies the institution's need for the project and describes the project end result. The project purpose guides the PM team to make informed decisions throughout the project life cycle. Project aims must be clearly stated in a way that is both attainable and measurable. Providing specific, clear project aims helps all team members understand the expected outcomes. The project aims will guide the project work and provide measurement of project success during the monitoring and controlling phase. Exhibit 14.1 is an example of a project problem, purpose statement, project purpose, and project aims. It is important the project problem, project purpose, and project aims are clearly communicated among the project manager, project leader, team members, and stakeholders. Without clear communication, project ambiguity can occur and the QI project may fail (see Figure 14.2).

The final step of the initiating phase is outlining the project **scope**, which is the essential work needed to accomplish the project (PMI, 2020). Current processes can be detailed using a flowchart. The flowchart simply illustrates the steps of the current process including decision points. Once the team is assembled, roles are defined, and the project goals and scope are outlined, the team is ready to begin the planning phase.

Project Management Phase 2: Planning

The planning phase includes creating the project roadmap that will guide the team from project execution through project closure. The project roadmap ensures project fidelity, or adherence to the project plan, by detailing every step/task and assisting the team to critically think about possible roadblocks that may derail the project. The team will also plan how to avoid such roadblocks and how to overcome them if they occur. The desired outcome at the end of the project is achieving the project aims and delivering the project on time and on budget. There are several important processes developed during the planning phase of the project, including:

EXHIBIT 14.1 PROJECT PROBLEM, PROBLEM STATEMENT, PROJECT PURPOSE, AND PROJECT AIMS EXAMPLE

Project Problem: Although international clinical practice guidelines recommend healthcare providers discuss PC options with patients, HF patients are not offered PC as often as those with other life-limiting diseases because nurses did not possess sufficient knowledge to offer PC to patients with HF.
Problem Statement: HF is a common, complex, life-limiting syndrome with a poor prognosis. Palliative care improves quality of life in those with life-limiting illnesses. Palliative care is optimized when it is initiated at the time of diagnosis and HF patients receiving PC experience improved symptom control and better quality of life. Although international clinical practice guidelines recommend nurses discuss PC options with patients, HF patients are not offered PC as often as other life-limiting diseases. Research revealed nurses did not possess sufficient knowledge to offer PC to patients with HF. To increase PC utilization, it is essential PC education combine knowledge and communication techniques to improve nurse's knowledge, attitude, and confidence to practice PC.
Project Purpose: The purpose of this project is to expand the cardiac nurses' skill set to include comprehensive PC to the patient with HF and their family.
Project Aims: 1. Measure the percentage of nurses completing the Palliative Care Education Training Program. 2. Evaluate the effectiveness of a PC education program on changing cardiac nurses' knowledge level of PC in HF. 3. Evaluate the effectiveness of a PC education program on changing cardiac nurses' confidence level of providing care for patients diagnosed with HF.

HF, heart failure; PC, palliative care.

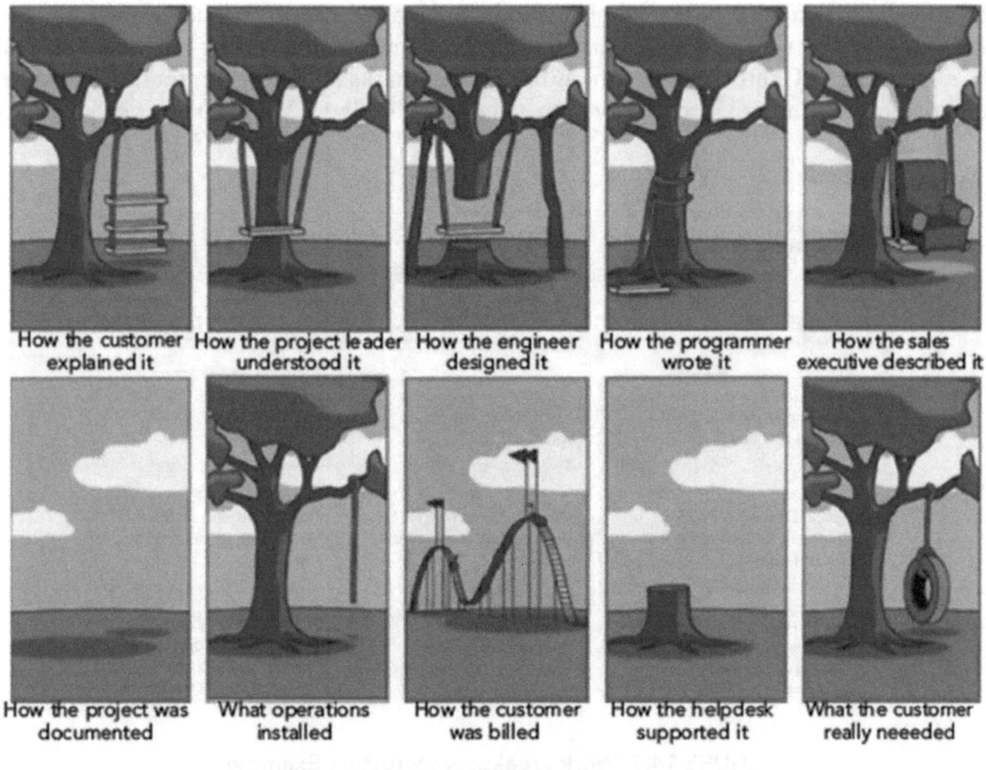

FIGURE 14.2 Project Management Tree.

CASE STUDY

In a nursing course, students are required to submit all class assignments as a hard copy before class. The students would like to submit the papers electronically so there will be documentation of the submission. The students decide to discuss the situation with their professor.

1. *Using the information in Table 14.1, who are the stakeholders for this project?*
2. *What is each stakeholder's level of influence on the project?*
3. *What strategies will assist the students in engaging the stakeholders in this project?*

- Work breakdown. Break down each project aim into steps and tasks.
- Time schedule. Place every project step and task in time sequence of execution.
- Budget. Determine and estimate project costs.
- Risk management. Predict possible future risks and establish a plan to reduce possible future risks.
- Communication. Draft a project communication plan for all team members and stakeholders.

There are several planning tools to assist the team. Each of the tools are described in the text that follows.

Work Breakdown and Time Schedule.

The team must first break down each project aim into smaller, manageable tasks. This breakdown records the detailed steps and tasks needed to achieve each aim. Tools, such as a work breakdown structure (WBS), are designed to help the project team drill down each aim. See Figure 14.3 for a WBS example. Once the WBS is complete, the project time schedule will be established. A Gantt chart uses the WBS steps and tasks and incorporates time schedule, task ownership, and task progression into a chart (see Table 14.2). Each task is given a start

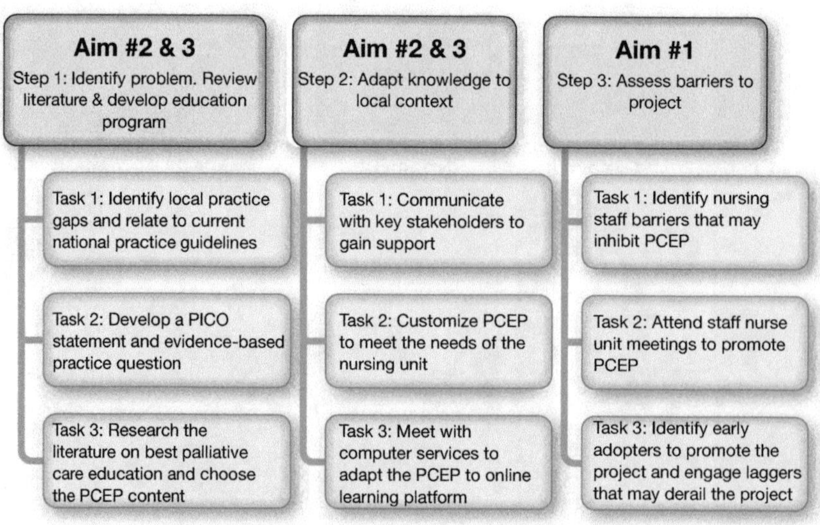

FIGURE 14.3 Work Breakdown Structure Example.

PCEP, Palliative Care Education Program; PICO, problem, intervention, comparison, outcome.

TABLE 14.2 GANTT CHART EXAMPLE

TODAY'S DATE 02.28.20	TASK OWNERSHIP	START DATE	END DATE	TASK PROGRESSION:	TIME SCHEDULE MONTH 1			
				PERCENT COMPLETE	02.01-02.07	02.08-02.14	02.15-02.21	02.22-02.28
AIM #2 & 3								
Step 1: Identify problem. Review literature and develop education program	Project lead	02.01.20	02.21.20	100%	x	x	x	
1a Task: Identify local practice gaps & relate to current national practice	Project lead	02.01.20	02.07.20	100%	x			
1b Task: Develop a PICO statement & evidence-based practice question	Project lead	02.01.20	02.15.29	100%	x	x		
1c Task: Research the literature on best palliative care education & choose the PCEP content	Unit educator	02.01.20	02.21.20	100%	x	x	x	
AIM #2 & 3								
Step 2: Adapt knowledge to local context	Unit educator	2.01.20	3.15.20	25%	x	x	x	x
2a Task: Communicate with key stakeholders to gain support	Project manager	2.01.20	2.28.20	100%	x	x	x	x
2b Task: Customize PCEP to meet the needs of the nursing unit	Unit educator	2.15.20	3.15.20	75%			x	x
2c Task: Meet with computer services to adapt the PCEP to online learning platform	Unit educator	02.15.20	3.15.20	50%			x	x

PCEP, palliative care education program; PICO, problem, intervention, comparison, outcome.

date and an end date within the project time schedule. Once the steps and tasks are determined, the project manager assigns the steps and tasks to groups or individual people. Steps and tasks are typically assigned according to each team member's personal and professional strengths. A Gantt chart is periodically updated to monitor and record the team's progress.

Budget

Cost management includes all necessary expenses needed to deliver the project. Since every project has a monetary limit, it is essential the actual costs do not exceed the budgeted cost. All costs associated with the project need to be approved by senior management. Projects that exceed the budgeted cost limit may be delayed, derailed, or never completed. Although a budget review is typically performed by the project manager, everyone on the team is responsible for being aware of project cost constraints.

Risk Management

A good project plan does not mean a project will not experience problems. Every project has the potential to become derailed. A good project plan has processes in place to deal with problems as they occur. A Strengths, Weaknesses, Opportunities, and Threats (SWOT) analysis predicts both positive and negative events that can impact the project (Brandenburger, 2019). Strengths are pertinent activities and assets the company does well. This may include knowledgeable and skilled staff, engaged administration, or strong financial capital. Weaknesses are deficiencies in the company's attributes. This may be high staff turnover, outdated processes, or financial limitations. Opportunities are potential growth areas, such as being the only company which developed a new product. Threats are anything that can potentially pose a risk to the company, such as a new competitor moving nearby the company. After the SWOT analysis is completed, the team will carefully develop strategies to augment strengths and opportunities and mitigate weaknesses and threats. Table 14.3 is an example of a SWOT analysis.

Communication

All team members and key stakeholders need clear communication. Updating the Gantt chart and making it available to all team members has several advantages. It provides clear communication, improves time management, promotes personal accountability and task responsibility, and increases transparency among the team. Placing the Gantt chart in a congregate area, such as a break room, is one example of making the Gantt chart available to all team members and key stakeholders.

TABLE 14.3 STRENGTHS, WEAKNESSES, OPPORTUNITIES, THREATS ANALYSIS EXAMPLE

HELPFUL	HARMFUL
Strengths • Project aligns with hospital mission • Hospital values evidence-based practice	Weakness • Lack of unit nurse educator to support project • Lack of current palliative care resources • Nurse time constraints to attend education program
Opportunities • Hospital leaders want palliative care • Nurses will be paid to attend education • Nurses will earn continuing education units after completing education	Threats • Unsure if hospital technology will support education program • Nurses may not value palliative care education

Project Management Phase 3: Executing

Once the project planning is complete, it is time for action. The PM next phase is executing. The executing phase involves carrying out, or translating into actions, the project plan to achieve the project aims. This phase generally lasts the longest and consumes the most resources. Project managers use a PM method to guide the team in the executing phase. There are various PM methods and the project manager selects a PM method based on the type of project, the context or setting for the project, and the project aims to implement the executing phase. Understanding the different types of PM methods is important to project success. Table 14.4 is a comparison of three commonly used PM methods—Lean, Six Sigma, and Five-Step (5S)—along with their process use and outcomes. Each of these

CURRENT LITERATURE

CITATION

Kendig, N. E., Cubitt, A., Moss, A., & Sevelius, J. (2019). Developing correctional policy, practice, and clinical care considerations for incarcerated transgender patients through collaborative stakeholder engagement. *Journal of Correctional Health Care, 25*(3), 277–286. https://doi.org/10.1177/1078345819857113

DISCUSSION

Stakeholder engagement is widely accepted as important for the success of any project. This study organized a meeting of 27 key stakeholders to focus on developing a correctional policy, practice, and clinical care considerations for incarcerated transgender persons. This meeting assembled stakeholders from a diverse range of individuals and organizations. Every individual stakeholder brought their own unique expert perspective pertaining to the topic of interest. The team leader intentionally engaged with each stakeholder with the intent to foster meaningful relationships among the members, eventually leading to a highly interactive team discussion. Key stakeholders included previous incarcerated transgender persons, correctional leaders, government authorities, academia members, general transgender advocates, and healthcare providers.

Three interrelated themes arose from the stakeholder meeting:

1. Stakeholders expanded their own perspective and added new insights after engaging with other stakeholders in the group;
2. Individual networks developed, which led to ongoing discussion; and
3. The advancement of the management and care of incarcerated transgender through the development of a correctional policy, practice, and clinical care procedure occurred.

IMPLICATIONS FOR PRACTICE

The study demonstrates how conversation between key stakeholders is crucial when developing and implementing a project. During the stakeholder meeting, gaps in current knowledge and practice were identified and consensus was achieved when developing policies and procedures. Intentionally engaging multiple viewpoints allowed project leaders to create a team culture that fostered meaningful conversation between the stakeholders.

TABLE 14.4 COMPARISON OF PROJECT MANAGEMENT METHODS, PROCESS USE, AND OUTCOMES

METHOD	PROCESS USE	OUTCOME
Lean	Makes processes more efficient by streamlining them	Eliminated waste in processes
Six Sigma	Improves the quality and efficiency of processes by streamlining them using statistical methods	Optimized process
Five-Step	Reorganizes the workplace	Standardized workplace organization process

three PM methods are briefly discussed in the text that follows. Chapter 11 in this book introduced and explored each of the translation PM methods in depth.

Lean Method for Project Management

The Lean method has been around for at least 100 years, and while Henry Ford first applied this method of thinking to Ford manufacturing, it was Taiichi Ohno from Toyota who perfected the Lean methodology. The Lean method streamlines work processes by making them more effective. The goal of the Lean methodology is to systematically eliminate waste and optimize work processes. In the Lean methodology, waste is considered any task or step that does not add value to a service or product. For example, any employee idle time, such as hospital change of shift delays, wastes both employee time and institute revenue. When applying the Lean method to the change of shift delay, the project manager asks, "What outside processes are necessary to effectively streamline the shift report?"

Six Sigma Method for Project Management

Six Sigma is a PM method used to optimize performance and improve quality and productivity through the measurement and collection of data. When using Six Sigma, institutions continuously collect data and compare the data against the institution's established thresholds (Fernandes et al., 2019). When the data exceeds the threshold, the institution must find the root cause of the problem, then develop and implement a QI project aimed at returning the data to its baseline. For example, the hospital baseline postsurgical hip replacement surgery length of stay is measured at 2 days. If the average length of stay increases to 3 days, the hospital administration will be prompted to investigate the root cause of the increase and develop a QI project. A complete explanation of Six Sigma, including techniques and methodologies, has been discussed in Chapter 12.

Five-Step Method for Project Management

The Five-Step Methodology (5S) was developed in Japan to assist in optimizing processes found in the workplace. It is referred to as 5S because it has five steps: Seiri, Seiton, Seiso, Seiketsu, and Shitsuke (United States Environmental Protection Agency, n.d.). Translated into English, the steps are Sort, Set in Order, Shine, Standardize, and Sustain. Sort refers to sorting out what is needed and not needed in a work area. Set in Order is arranging items so they are easily accessible and ready to use. Shine is cleaning the workspace on a regular basis. Standardize is to routinely revisit the first three steps of the 5S to ensure consistency. Sustain is following the rules to maintain standards. Ideally, when the 5S is implemented correctly, efficiency and effectiveness in reorganizing the workplace and eliminating waste are achieved. Chapter 12 explains the 5S in further detail.

CASE STUDY

Kristen is a unit director at a hospital experiencing an increasing quantity of mislabeled laboratory specimens. She decides to assemble a team to design a QI project to decrease the number of mislabeled specimens. The project aim is to evaluate the effectiveness of an intervention on decreasing mislabeled specimens. The PM method needs to be chosen to best fit the project. Based on the information provided:

1. *Identify two PM methods that can be used to guide and implement this project.*
2. *Compare and contrast both PM methods.*
3. *Explain which PM method best fits the project.*

Project Management Phase 4: Monitoring and Controlling

Monitoring and controlling comprise a dynamic phase that is a continuous process occurring throughout PM. Gathering data during the monitoring and controlling phase allows tracking, reviewing, and regulating the executing phase and provides valuable information concerning project effectiveness. Continuously monitoring allows for rapid problem identification and risk management. Monitoring and controlling compares planned results with actual results, identifies project areas that may need modification, and, if change is necessary, determines the correct change. In the beginning of any new project, frequent monitoring helps identify a small problem before it becomes a major problem. All project changes are recommended and approved by the project team. Typically, the project manager or leader may assign a particular group of team members the responsibility of monitoring and controlling.

BOX 14.2 Developing Clinical Judgment

A QI team is currently working on a project to reduce patient falls. To determine if their intervention will have the desired effect, the QI team piloted the project on one unit. The team chose to pilot the project on one unit so they could make adjustments to the intervention before initiating the change throughout the entire hospital. The QI team needs to measure the following project aim: the effect the intervention has on reducing patient falls. The interventions for reducing falls in high-risk patients include wearing colored socks, signage on the door, call light within reach, and hourly rounding. The QI team assigns the nurse the responsibility to develop a tool to effectively measure the project aim.

1. What clinical judgment might the nurse make based on the **CUES (Assessment)** in this scenario when deciding which information to gather when measuring the project aim?
2. What **HYPOTHESIS (Diagnosis)** will the nurse consider when deciding which information to gather when measuring the aims?
3. What **ACTION (Plan and Implement)** will be most effective for the nurse to take?
4. How will the nurse evaluate the **OUTCOME (Evaluation)** for the purpose of arriving at a satisfactory clinical outcome?

Project Management Phase 5: Closing

The final phase in PM is closing. The closing of a project is vital because it confirms the completion of a project and communicates the final project status to all stakeholders and team members. Activities occurring during the closing phase include documenting a reflection on the project process and what changes may need to occur in future projects. The entire PM team discusses project sustainability, or maintaining the changes, and designs triggers which provide a warning if the newly implementated changes are not performing correctly. For example, for the falls example mentioned earlier, triggers could be built in such as monthly quality audits for compliance with the implementation of high fall risk patients wearing colored socks. The audits could be done by a nurse on the unit and reported to the unit director. Another trigger could be reporting data that exceeds established thresholds. For example, if the total number of patient falls exceeds the established threshold, it would trigger the QI team to reassemble to look at the fall risk process. The closing of a project also allows time for team members to reflect and refine their PM skills. Leadership can use this time to mentor and guide new team members. The final closing step is to celebrate project success.

APPLICATION OF SYSTEMATIC STEPS OF PROJECT MANAGEMENT

To demonstrate how PM techniques improve the delivery of QI projects, an example of a current healthcare quality issue will be examined. The following scenario takes a deeper look into the chapter opening scenario. Hospital leadership has identified labor costs exceeding the established threshold. In order to contain costs, wasteful practices in the hospital must be contained and controlled without sacrificing quality of care. The nurse manager noticed one area for improvement is the shift change report given between the nursing staff. The problem has been identified that nurses are staying past their shift completion time due to lengthy shift reports, therefore causing an increase in overtime expenses. The project purpose is to improve the efficiency of the nursing shift change report and the project aim is to measure the effectiveness of an intervention on changing the amount of time nurses are in shift report. Leadership has decided to use the Six Sigma methodology following the Define, Measure, Analyze, Improve, and Control (DMAIC) method to execute the QI project (see Chapter 12 for an in-depth Six Sigma and DMAIC explanation). Leadership assigned the nurse manager as project manager and a medical-surgical nurse as the project leader. The team is composed of the following interprofessional stakeholders: three medical-surgical nurses, a nursing assistant from the medical-surgical unit, the emergency department nursing supervisor, a healthcare provider, and representatives from both the laboratory and dietary departments. The following section shows how PM techniques are used to improve the delivery of QI projects.

Define

The first step in the DMAIC approach is defining the problem. The shift change report is a tool to ensure continuity of care as patient care staff changes shift. The shift change report contains patient information that is essential to patient care and is given from the nurse completing the shift to the nurse coming on duty and taking the assignment. Typically, the incoming nurses may have to receive shift report from more than one outgoing nurse. The incoming nurse may have to wait for multiple outgoing nurse to receive report. The waiting period is idle and unproductive time for the nurses and the outgoing nurse may not leave in a timely manner, causing an increase in overtime. As directed by the hospital leadership, the shift change report should take no more than 30 minutes to complete. Anything longer than 30 minutes is considered wasteful. During the shift change, every time the incoming nurse receives report from a different outgoing nurse, there is an increase in the total time of the shift report.

Measure

Measure is the next step in the DMAIC approach. In order to measure improvement, the average current time it takes to complete a shift change report needs to be documented to establish a baseline. The project leader randomly observed 30 different nurses' shift reports. The project leader used a smartphone to ensure the time measurement was accurate and consistent. Nurses were timed at a distance so they did not feel the pressure of being timed and the observation could happen in an unhampered way. Both the morning and evening shifts were timed and averaged. The average report time was 43 minutes.

The next step is to determine how much of the 43 minutes accounted for nonvalue added (NVA) steps. NVA steps are those parts of the shift report process that did not contribute to completing the task. The team decided NVA is defined if the nurses were idle and not delivering or listening to the report. To identify the NVA time during reports, the team mapped out the report process from beginning to end. The report process mapping revealed 23 minutes was NVA and was associated with incoming nurses waiting for report from the previous shift. It was noted that one incoming nurse waited for report from three different nurses leaving their shift before she could start her work.

Analyze

The next step in the DMAIC approach is to analyze the data. In order to begin addressing potential solutions for NVA time, the project leader can complete a Healthcare Failure Mode and Effects Analysis or HFMEA chart audit. The Joint Commission requires healthcare providers to select a minimum of one high-risk process annually and complete a proactive risk assessment, such as an HFMEA. An HFMEA provides a mechanism to evaluate for the risk of patient injury and provide a proactive and preventive technique to gauge the severity of the risk before it happens. Conducting an HFMEA helps a PM team identify and prioritize problems.

For the problem concerning shift report, an HFMEA is conducted with input from all committee members. There are steps involved in an HFMEA discussed in Chapter 12 that are applied to the shift change reporting problem:

Define the HFMEA topic.

1. Assemble an interprofessional team.
2. Describe the process via a flowchart.
3. Conduct a risk analysis.
4. Identify actions and outcome measures.

Improve

Improve is the next step in the DMAIC process. After the team defines and measures the data, the key area for most effectively eliminating waste was identified. The most controllable source of unnecessary costs exists in the NVA wait times of nurses to get report. To fully understand the problem, the team looked at other organizations and the literature, and talked with others about best practices in restructuring the unit layout to improve nurses' efficient use of time. The team decided to redesign the layout so assignments are created in clusters based on geographical location on the unit as well as bed assignments based on patient acuity level.

Control

The final step in the DMAIC process is the control step. During a 30-day pilot phase, the new assignments created in clusters were trialed and nurses were surveyed. The shift report time decreased to 25 minutes and the nursing staff survey results were highly favorable of the new assignments. Under the new assignment layout, any given nurse would have no more than two nurses to provide shift change report to. To disseminate the new shift report procedure, the project leader communicated with the entire nursing staff via unit meetings, emails, and informal discussion.

LEADERSHIP AND MANAGEMENT SKILL FOR PROJECT MANAGEMENT

As a direct care nurse develops and gains QI project experience, they may eventually serve as a project leader. A successful project leader must possess both leadership and management skills. The project leader skill set is similar to a managerial role and is outlined in the list that follows.

- **Cognitive Skills:** Understand complex behaviors and patterns, including speaking, active listening, active learning, writing, and critical thinking.
- **Business Skills:** Understand basic business principles, such as personnel management, financial management, and material resource management.
- **Interprofessional Skills:** Obtain professional skills, including social perception, negotiation, and persuasion.
- **Strategic Skills:** Understand the big picture, involving conceptualization of the mission and vision of the organization—vision, system evaluation, key cause identification, problem identification, and solution appraisal (Guzman, 2020; White, Dudley-Brown, & Terhaar, 2019; Sipes, 2020).

The project leader is charged with coordinating and managing a project. In this role, the nurse will need effective communication skills as they liaison between team members and the project manager. The project leader must be able to clearly communicate with nurses

BOX 14.3 Developing Clinical Judgment

A QI nurse has been asked to be the project leader on a project addressing compliance with hourly patient rounding. The QI nurse will lead the team, which includes administration, such as the chief nursing officer, supervisor, and unit manager, as well as two direct care nurses and one certified nursing assistant (CNA). During a team meeting, the direct care nurses and CNA were discussing potential solutions to the problem. The nurses and CNA have opposing viewpoints. Administration wants 100% compliance with hourly rounding. Considering the different viewpoints involving the problem, how can the project leader bring the interprofessional team together?

1. What clinical judgment might the lead nurse make based upon the **CUES (Assessment)** in this scenario?
2. What **HYPOTHESIS (Diagnosis)** will the lead nurse consider?
3. What **ACTION (Plan and Implement)** will be most effective for the lead nurse to take?
4. How will the lead nurse evaluate the situation **OUTCOME (Evaluation)** for the purpose of arriving at a satisfactory conclusion?

delivering bedside care as well as any other stakeholder affected by the project. A project leader must be able to ascertain what skills each team member brings to the project and capitalize on these strengths and mentor other team members in developing their skills. By supporting and growing an individual's skills, buy-in to a project is higher and satisfaction is increased. The project leader must empower team members and be a strong agent for change by supporting their work and championing the project. The project leader should be cognizant of project budget constraints and adhere to the project plan.

BENEFITS AND LIMITATIONS FOR PROJECT MANAGEMENT

While PM in healthcare can help lessen risks and improve the chances of achieving goals, there are other clearly defined benefits. PM can help clarify both the project purpose and goals. The initiating and planning phase of PM helps define not only immediate goals, but also future goals. Effective PM forces team leaders to ask two important questions: Are we doing the right things and are we doing things right? The "right things" refers to the sequence of activities or tasks to accomplish a goal. On the other hand, "doing things right" looks at the quality of the work. Other PM benefits include allocating resources and budget management.

Teamwork is a critical component of PM as collaborating with others who have differing perspectives of a project is essential to understanding the issue. By participating on a QI project, each team member has the opportunity to expand their professional skills. Successful PM gets the most out of each worker and fosters a sense of belonging. The tangible benefit of teamwork leads to an intangible benefit of a productive workforce, which is fundamental to a successful organizational culture.

Limitations can exist with any methodology and a project manager needs to be aware of these limits. There are also limitations arising from unexpected changes during the project, such as changes to team members' jobs, available resources, budget allocation, or leadership changes. These changes may require re-centering the project team by bringing the team back together and reviewing the project purose and aims. Team member disagreements can affect project progression and the project manager should set expected standards for performance. For example, a stakeholder may show some dissatisfaction with the project and ultimately try to sway or undermine the project. If this occurs, the project manager needs to meet privately with the individual and discuss the situation and the impact on the project.

Another PM limitation is the human element limitation. Team members are individuals and some variability in performance, commitment, and conflicts in personalities does happen. These limitations can be avoided by good communication skills, including both speaking as well as good listening skills. Limitations may also include being unable to complete the project with in the proposed budget and/or time schedule. Taking a step back and continually reviewing the project plan can help mitigate limitations.

END-OF-CHAPTER RESOURCES

KEY CONCEPTS

1. Projects are unique, one-time tasks that produce an outcome.
2. Project management (PM) is an essential leadership skill set using a systematic approach to complete projects. Healthcare professionals use PM to improve the quality of care through designing and implementing QI projects.
3. Effective PM requires an interprofessional team effort with each member having distinct roles and responsibilities. The team leader is the project manager.
4. PM utilizes a systematic approach consisting of five phases: initiating, planning, executing, monitoring and controlling, and closing.
5. The three most common project methodologies are Lean, Six Sigma, and Five-Step (5S) methodology.
6. Benefits of PM include ensuring project fidelity, increasing project success, decreasing expenditures, and streamlining processes.
7. Limitations of PM include unexpected changes occurring during the project, team member disagreements, human element limits, and budget and time schedule limitations.

CRITICAL DISCUSSION POINTS

1. Identify a QI initiative that could be implemented. What evidence or data would the nurse need to gather to support the need for the project?
2. When implementing the QI initiative from Question 1, which PM step may be the most difficult for the nurse to implement? As the project manager, what steps could be utilized to overcome the difficulty?
3. New nurses may be involved on an interprofessional QI project. Describe how a new graduate nurse can contribute as a team member. How will this role evolve as the new graduate nurse gains experience?
4. Project managers use a leadership skill set as described in the chapter. What leadership skills does a new graduate nurse possess? What leadership skills will a new nurse need to further develop? What resources can assist the new nurse to gain these skills?
5. How does the nursing unit culture affect project completion and sustainability? What steps can the unit manager do to improve the nursing unit culture?

KEY TERMS

Project
Project management
Quality improvement
Scope
Stakeholders

REVIEW QUESTIONS

Answers to Review Questions appear in the Instructor's Manual. Qualified instructors should request the Instructor's Manual from textbook@springerpub.com.

1. Which of the following are examples of a project? *Select all that apply.*
   - A. Decreasing the call light wait time during change of shift
   - B. Improving patient throughput in the emergency department
   - C. Designing a family waiting room for the same day surgery department
   - D. Completing a chart audit on patient satisfaction
   - E. Redesigning the staff lounge communication board to improve communication

2. Which action demonstrates a nurse utilizing a PM approach to a clinical problem? *Select all that apply.*
   - A. The nurse completes a root cause analysis to determine the cause for an increase in pressure injury in the emergency department.
   - B. The nurse measures and compares recent patient satisfaction scores to the scores achieved a year ago.
   - C. The nurse identifies patient transfers to the rehabilitation center are following the usual protocol.
   - D. The nurse notices a delay in receiving medication from the pharmacy and inquires how the delivery system can improve.
   - E. The nurse reads a journal article about a new medication.

3. The project team completed the project plan. According to the PM phases, what is the project team's next course of action?
   - A. Initiating
   - B. Planning
   - C. Executing
   - D. Closing

4. Which of the following would be considered a process for PM? *Select all that apply.*
   - A. Patient wait time in the emergency department has been increasing over the last several months.
   - B. Patient satisfaction scores as provided by Hospital Consumer Assessment of Health Plans Survey (HCAHPS) are above the national average.
   - C. The nurses report the patient supply room inventory consistently is missing several important items.
   - D. Patient dietary requests are being fulfilled correctly 100% of the time.
   - E. At the completion of orientation, all new hired nurses complete an employee satisfaction survey.

5. Organizations use a Failure Mode and Effect Analysis (FMEA) to detect process errors before they occur. Which of the following are examples of FMEA processes? *Select all that apply.*
   - A. Assembling a team of direct care nurses to address the problem
   - B. Completing a root cause analysis to determine failure frequency
   - C. Determining the impact the failure has on a patient
   - D. Describing the process steps to correctly change a dressing
   - E. Having a unit manager complete a staff nurse's yearly employee evaluation

6. The project team is in the controlling and monitoring phase of PM. How does this phase assist with project success? *Select all that apply.*
   A. It identifies the local data to support the project.
   B. It allows tracking, reviewing, and regulating the implementation process.
   C. It provides information concerning project effectiveness.
   D. It communicates the final project status to all stakeholders and team members.
   E. It assists in recruiting the interprofessional team.
7. The project team is developing the work breakdown structure. Once it is completed, what is the next step in the planning phase?
   A. Developing a timeline for each task and subtask
   B. Crafting the problem statement
   C. Providing the stakeholders with an estimated budget
   D. Starting the pilot study
8. Which statement by the nurse indicates the nurse correctly understands the Lean methodology?
   A. The Lean methodology is taught using levels of "belts" to signify completion of training.
   B. Hospitals use the Lean methodology as a way that patients can rate their satisfaction and hospital experience.
   C. In the Lean methodology, waste is considered any task or step that does not add value to a service or product.
   D. Lean is a process used to identify potential healthcare failures and their causes.
9. The project manager decides to use the Six Sigma methodology for a quality improvement (QI) project. Which of the following statements describes the "I" in DMAIC? *Select all that apply.*
   A. The team members create a process map to understand the problem.
   B. The unit manager collects baseline data to describe the problem.
   C. The project leader schedules a team meeting to brainstorm and create a solution to the problem.
   D. The team conducts a pilot study to evaluate a solution to the problem.
   E. The project leader retrains the staff on a new procedure.
10. PM limitations can hinder the QI process. Which of the following is an example of how a project manager can minimize PM limitations? *Select all that apply.*
   A. During the first meeting, the project manager openly and clearly communicates the project timeline.
   B. If the project begins to exceed the expected budget, the project manager chooses where to minimize costs.
   C. When a project misses an important due date, the project manager schedules a team meeting to discuss the situation.
   D. When a stakeholder attempts to sway a project's scope, the project manager reports the stakeholder's actions to the other team members.
   E. During a meeting the project manager takes time to listen to every team member.

REVIEW ACTIVITIES

1. During a clinical experience, ask a nurse to describe a potential clinical problem on their unit. Based on the identified potential clinical problem, develop a problem statement, a project purpose, and project aims. During postconference, discuss and compare the identified clinical problem with the class.
2. Reflect on a past clinical rotation and recall a potential clinical process that could improve patient outcomes. Record several possible causes of the problem. How would a team manager lead a QI initiative to resolve the problem and improve patient outcomes? Compile a list of stakeholders and potential team members.
3. During a clinical experience, ask a nurse to recall the last QI project on their unit. Discuss the project and the nurses' perception of the project. Develop several questions specific to the management of the project. Example questions include: What was the reason for the project? What was the project purpose and aims? Who was on the project team? What were the implementation steps? How did the team communicate with the nursing staff before, during, and after the project? Was the project successful? During postconference, discuss the findings with other classmates.

EXPLORING THE WEB

1. Practice using PM skills by streamlining a current process. Go to the website Institute for Healthcare Improvement and access the Quality Improvement Essentials Toolkit (http://www.ihi.org/resources/Pages/Tools/Quality-Improvement-Essentials-Toolkit.aspx). Choose two tools not discussed in this chapter. How can each of these QI tools assist a project manager?
2. Enhance your PM skills by accessing free PM templates at Project Management Institute (PMI)—Project management documents. Go to the website: www.projectmanagementdocs.com and download a template. Which template did you choose and how will the template assist the PM team?
3. Go to the website: www.mindtools.com/pages/article/newPPM_60.htm. Read the article, "How Good Are Your Project Management Skills?" Complete the PM Skills Self-Assessment located on the website. Use the "Calculate My Total" at the bottom and calculate your score. Next determine your score and read the "Score Interpretation." Compare your findings to others in your class. What are your PM strengths? What areas are your opportunities for improvement? Based on findings from your class, who would be the project best leader?

REFERENCES

Agency for Healthcare Research and Quality. (2020). *Topic: Quality improvement.* https://ahrq.gov/topics/quality-improvement.html

Brandenburger, A. (2019, August 22). *Are your company's strengths really weaknesses?* Harvard Business Review. https://hbr.org/2019/08/are-your-companys-strengths-really-weaknesses

de la Perrelle, L., Radisic, G., Cations, M., Kaambwa, B., Barbery, G., & Laver, K. (2020). Costs and economic evaluations of quality improvement collaboratives in health care: A systematic review. *BMC Health Services Research, 20*, Article 155. https://doi.org/10.1186/s12913-020-4981-5

Fernandes, M. M., Hurst, J., Antony, J., Turrioni, J. B., & Silva, M. B. (2019). 18 Steps to six sigma project success. *Quality Progress, 52*(2), 16–23.

Guzman, V. E., Muschard, B., Gerolamo, M., Kohl, H., & Rozenfeld, H. (2020). Characteristics and skills of leadership in the context of industry 4.0. *Procedia Manufacturing, 43*, 543–550. https://doi.org/10.1016/j.promfg.2020.02.167

Keenhan, S. P., Cuckler, G. A., Poisal, J. A., Sisko, A. M., Smith, S. D., Madison, A. J., Rennie, K. E., Fiore, J. A., & Hardesty, J. C. (2020). National health expenditure projections, 2019–28: Expected rebound in prices drives rising spending growth. *Health Affairs, 39*(4), 704–714, https://doi.org/10.1377/hlthaff.2020.00094

Project Management Institute. (n.d.). *What is project management?* https://www.pmi.org/about/learn-about-pmi/what-is-project-management

Project Management Institute. (2018). Success in disruptive times: Expanding the value delivery landscape to adding the high cost of low performance. *Pulse of the Profession*. https://www.pmi.org/learning/thought-leadership/pulse/pulse-of-the-profession-2018

Project Management Institute. (2020). A case for diversity. *Pulse of the Profession*. https://www.pmi.org/learning/thought-leadership/pulse/a-case-for-diversity

Quality and Safety Education for Nurses. (2020). *Quality improvement (QI)*. https://qsen.org/competencies/pre-licensure-ksas/#quality_improvement

Registered Nurses' Association of Ontario. (2012). *Toolkit: Implementation of best practice guidelines* (2nd ed.). Author.

Rosen, M. A., Diaz Granados, D., Dietz, A. S., Benishek, L. E., Thompson, D., Pronovost, P. J., & Weaver, S. J. (2018). Teamwork in health care: Key discoveries enabling safer, high-quality care. *The American Psychologist, 73*(4), 433–450. https://doi.org/10.1037/amp0000298

Rowe, S. F. (2020). *Project management for small projects* (3rd ed.). Berrett-Koehler.

Sipes, C. (2020). *Project management for the advanced practice nurse* (2nd ed.). Springer Publishing.

United States Environmental Protection Agency. (n.d.). *Lean thinking and methods–5S*. https://www.epa.gov/sustainability/lean-thinking-and-methods-5s

Verzuh, E. (2016). *The fast forward MBA in project management* (5th ed.). Wiley.

White, K. M., Dudley-Brown, S., & Terhaar, M. F. (2019). *Translation of evidence into nursing and healthcare* (3rd ed.). Springer Publishing.

SUGGESTED READINGS

Al-Mansour, L. A., Dudley-Brown, S., & Al-Shaikhi, A. (2020). Development of an interdisciplinary health care team for pressure injury management: A quality improvement project. *Journal of Wound, Ostomy & Continence Nursing, 47*(4), 349–352. https://doi.org/10.1097/WON.0000000000000652

Baccei, S. J., Henderson, S. R., Lo, H. S., & Reynolds, K. (2020). Using quality improvement methodology to reduce costs while improving efficiency and provider satisfaction in a busy, academic musculoskeletal radiology division. *Journal of Medical Systems, 44*(6), 1–7. https://doi.org/10.1007/s10916-020-01569-8

Centers for Disease Control and Prevention. (n.d.). *CDC unified process project management guide*. https://www2a.cdc.gov/cdcup/default.htm

Chartier, L. B., Cheng, A. H. Y., Stang, A. S., & Vaillancourt, S. (2018). Quality improvement primer part 1: Preparing for a quality improvement project in the emergency department. *CJEM: Canadian Journal of Emergency Medicine, 20*(1), 104–111. https://doi.org/10.1017/cem.2017.361

Chartier, L. B., Stang, A. S., Vaillancourt, S., & Cheng, A. H. Y. (2018). Quality improvement primer part 2: Executing a quality improvement project in the emergency department. *CJEM: Canadian Journal of Emergency Medicine, 20*(4), 532–538. https://doi.org/10.1017/cem.2017.393

Chartier, L. B., Vaillancourt, S., Cheng, A. H. Y., & Stang, A. S. (2019). Quality improvement primer part 3: Evaluating and sustaining a quality improvement project in the emergency department. *CJEM: Canadian Journal of Emergency Medicine, 21*(2), 261–268. https://doi.org/10.1017/cem.2018.380

Cronenwett, L., Sherwood, G., Barnsteiner, J., Disch, J., Johnson, J., Mitchell, P., Sullivan, D., & Warren, J. (2007). Quality and Safety Education for Nurses. *Nursing Outlook, 55*(3), 122–131. https://doi.org/10.1016/j.outlook.2007.02.006

Dawson, A. (2020). A practical guide to performance improvement: Change acceleration process and techniques to maintain improvements. *AORN Journal, 111*(1), 97–102. https://doi.org/10.1002/aorn.12895

Fagnan, L. J., Walunas, T. L., Parchman, M. L., Dickinson, C. L., Murphy, K. M., Howell, R., Jackson, K. L., Madden, M. B., Ciesla, J. R., Mazurek, K. D., Kho, A. N., & Solberg, L. I. (2018). Engaging primary care practices in studies of improvement: Did you budget enough for practice recruitment? *Annals of Family Medicine, 16* (Suppl. 1), S72–S79. https://doi.org/10.1370/afm.2199

Jones, B., Vaux, E., & Olsson-Brown, A. (2019). How to get started in quality improvement. *British Medical Journal, 364*(k5408), 1–4. https://doi.org/10.1136/bmj.k5437

Laycock, A., Bailie, J., Matthews, V., & Bailie, R. (2019). Using developmental evaluation to support knowledge translation: Reflections from a large-scale quality improvement project in Indigenous primary healthcare. *Health Research Policy & Systems, 17*, Article 70. https://doi.org/10.1186/s12961-019-0474-6

Parizh, D., Ascher, E., Raza Rizvi, S. A., Hingorani, A., Amaturo, M., & Johnson, E. (2018). Quality improvement initiative: Preventative surgical site infection protocol in vascular surgery. *Vascular, 26*(1), 47–53. https://doi.org/10.1177/1708538117719155

Project Management Institute. (2017). *PMBOK guide* (6th ed.). Project Management Institute. https://www.pmi.org/pmbok-guide-standards/foundational/pmbok

Rew, L., Cauvin S., Cengiz, A., Pretorius, K., & Johnson, K. (2020). Application of project management tools and techniques to support nursing intervention research. *Nursing Outlook, 68*(4), 396–405. https://doi.org/10.1016/j.outlook.2020.01.007

Smith, C. M. (2019). Preparing nurse leaders in nursing professional development: Project planning and management. *Journal for Nurses in Professional Development, 35*(3), 160. https://doi.org/10.1097/NND.0000000000000549

CHAPTER 15

Population Health and the Role of Quality and Safety

Rita M. Sfiligoj, Jesse Honsky, Shannon Wong, Rebecca L. Mitchell, and Mary A. Dolansky

"A population-focused nurse will move beyond the individualistic, downstream approach, viewing individuals and families in the context of their environment, and assessing how their community affects them."

–Storfjell et al., 2018

Upon completion of this chapter, the reader should be able to:

1. Define population health and its evolution.
2. Examine the intersections between population health and nursing practice.
3. Identify the overlapping concepts between population health and public health.
4. Compare Key Population-Focused Nursing Competencies and Quality and Safety Education for Nurses (QSEN) Competencies.
5. Explain the registered nurse's role in population health related to the QSEN competencies.
6. Analyze the role of interprofessional teams in population health.
7. Identify emerging roles for registered nurses in population health.
8. Apply quality improvement (QI) to population health.

CROSSWALK

This chapter addresses the following:

QSEN Competency: Patient-Centered Care, Evidence-Based Practice, Safety, Informatics, Teamwork and Collaboration, and Quality Improvement.

The American Association of Colleges of Nursing. (2021). *The essentials: Core competencies for professional nursing education.*

Domain 3: Population Health
Domain 5: Quality and Safety
Domain 6: Interprofessional Partnerships
Domain 7: Systems-Based Practice.

OPENING SCENARIO

A school nurse in a large high school in Chicago, Illinois, has noticed teens coming to the clinic with unusual mouth sores and/or an unexplained cough. After researching potential causes of these findings, the nurse recognizes that these symptoms are common side effects of vaping (i.e., the use of electronic vapor products). She brings her concerns to the school administration and finds out that the administration has also noted an increase in student use of electronic vapor products. In the past 6 months, the school has had a 15% increase in student discipline issues related to vaping or the use of electronic vapor products. Wanting to research more statistical information, the nurse reviews the report of the local Community Health Needs Assessment (CHNA), an assessment process in which local health departments, hospitals, and community partners collect, analyze, and summarize health data and prioritize the health-related needs of the community. The CHNA report notes the reported use of electronic vaping products has increased between 2017 and 2019 based on survey results from the Centers for Disease Control and Prevention (CDC) Local Youth Risk Behavior Surveillance Survey (YRBS; Alliance for Health Equality, 2019. The nurse decides to investigate further by reviewing YRBS data directly on the CDC website. She reviews data for Chicago and finds an increase from 6.6% of students reporting current electronic vapor use in 2017 to 12.4% reporting current use in 2019. The nurse also finds that the concern is not just local; vaping among high school students has increased from 13.2% in 2017 to 19.9% in 2019 in the state of Illinois (CDC, n.d.-a). This finding supports the school nurse's clinical observations. It inspires the nurse to create some initiatives at the school to educate the teens about the risks of electronic vapor products; inform parents, teachers, and administrators of signs of electronic vapor use; and explore ways to motivate the student population to either stop the behavior or never start using the vapor products in the first place.

1. Use the website: www.cdc.gov/healthyyouth/data/yrbs/results.htm. Scroll to the "State and National Comparisons" section and check the Youth Risk Behavior Surveillance Survey data for your state. What population health needs did you find for your state?
2. Do a web search for a CHNA done in your community. Nonprofit hospitals and local health departments typically make the reports available online to community members. What are some of the population health issues identified in your community?
3. How can CHNA and the YRBS assist nurses to address community population health needs?

INTRODUCTION

Population health is defined by the Centers for Disease Control and Prevention (CDC, n.d.-b) as an interdisciplinary, tailored approach that connects health departments, healthcare institutions, and policy to achieve positive health outcomes locally. Population health was developed to ensure a more integrated delivery system to improve the health of a specified population and is different from public health. Nurses, trending back to Florence Nightingale and Lillian Wald in the late 1800s to early 1900s, worked with populations (soldiers during the Crimean War and lower income families of New York) to influence their healthcare outcomes. Assuming a variety of roles within healthcare systems and their communities, nurses utilize population health knowledge and skills to realize the goal of creating a culture of health and wellness, rather than concentrating on treating illness. A focus on population health requires nurses to work closely with interprofessional teams to improve health outcomes. The role of the nurse in population health includes identifying groups of at-risk patients, examining the effect of the Social Determinants of Health on their outcomes, and then shifting the focus of nursing care from chronically ill care to patient self-management care for improved healthcare outcomes. The *Future of Nursing 2020–2030* report emphasizes the importance of the nurse's role in addressing the diversity of all the populations they serve with the target to improve health (Wakefield et al., 2021). The Quality and Safety Education for Nurses (QSEN) competencies and population health competencies are important to the role of the nurse in improving health outcomes. The role of the RN in population health is emerging to meet the needs of patients in the community and the application of quality improvement (QI) ensures high quality and safe care.

EVOLUTION OF POPULATION HEALTH

Florence Nightingale, branded for her continuous advocacy of health promotion, cared for soldiers during the Crimean War in 1853. Nightingale and a small crew of nurses tended to the sick and injured soldiers. The nursing quarters where the injured soldiers were cared for were horrid, with poor sanitation, food scarcity, and a shortage of the most necessary supplies. Many more soldiers were dying from infectious diseases than from injuries. Nightingale focused on improved environmental sanitation to care for the sick soldiers. She implemented her environmental theory focusing on the "client." Her environmental theory places the client at the center, surrounded by aspects of the environment. In this theory, Nightingale emphasized, "when one aspect of the environment is out of balance, the client will be stressed" (Zborowsky, 2014).

Lillian Wald, like many nurses, started her career in the hospital caring for patients, but she often knew little about where her patients went after discharge (Anthony, 2019). In 1893, Wald settled in a home on the lower east side of New York, later known as the "House on Henry Street." She moved to this home to live in the community where she cared for children and families, often with low incomes. It was in this community that Lillian Wald and her colleagues established the first Visiting Nurse Association. Wald was acknowledged and well respected for her contributions of recognizing that the community affects the health of individuals.

Florence Nightingale and Lillian Wald worked to improve the health outcomes of the at-risk populations in the late 1800s to early-1900s while working to overcome the Social Determinants of Health (SDoH) in the population. The U.S. Department of Health and Human Services defines the **Social Determinants of Health** as "the conditions in the environment where people are born, live, learn, work, play, worship, and age that affect a wide range of health, functioning, and quality-of-life outcomes and risks" (n.d., para. 1). SDoH include socioeconomic status, education, employment, access to transportation, access to healthcare, social support, physical environment (green space, worksites, recreation sites, and exposure to toxins), housing, and access to healthy foods. Social determinants affect a population's everyday immediate health concerns and are an important consideration when caring for a population's health (Wakefield et al., 2021). See Table 15.1

The healthcare team must understand and respond to the SDoH when developing and implementing healthcare interventions. Reviewing the patient's whole being including reviewing areas such as the patient's economic status, zip code, education, race and ethnicity, gender, age, transportation access, and healthcare access, to name a few areas, often forces a healthcare team to acknowledge "non-medical" factors known as the SDoH (Gamache et al., 2018). For example, Coughlin (2019) reviewed healthcare disparities in a breast cancer population. It is well documented that there are healthcare disparities in breast cancer staging and survival related to SDoH including socioeconomic status, race,

TABLE 15.1 EXAMPLES OF SOCIAL DETERMINANTS OF HEALTH AND COMMON INTERVENTIONS

SDOH	SDOH INTERVENTIONS
PHYSICAL ENVIRONMENT	
Air Quality	• Decrease transportation pollution. • Assist with putting air filters in homes.
Water Safety	• Supply and educate about water kits and clean drinking water. • Decrease the amount of standing water in the environment.
Safe Living and Work Environment	• Provide healthy play spaces. • Provide sanitized work environments. • Provide access to personal protective equipment as needed.
Safe Transportation	• Develop accessible public transportation.
SOCIAL AND ECONOMIC ENVIRONMENT	
Education	• Provide safe/accessible education.
Employment	• Refer to support agencies such as family and job services for employment opportunities. • Develop fair wage practices.
Family and Social Support	• Provide guidance to free clinics and counseling.
Community Safety	• Provide accessible safety seminars. • Increase the presence of the law.
CLINICAL CARE	
Access to Medical Care	• Provide accessible transportation. • Assist with medical insurance. • Provide assistance with Medicaid application.
Quality Care	• Provide access to PCP. • Connect the patient with the care coordinator. • Provide access to mental health services. • Attend to disparities in care.
HEALTH BEHAVIORS	
Tobacco Use	• Provide smoking education. • Provide smoking cessation classes.
Diet and Exercise	• Provide nutrition education. • Develop a guide to affordable fresh produce. • Provide accessible farmers market.
Alcohol & Drug Use	• Provide alcohol and drug education. • Offer in the school curriculum. • Provide addiction services.
Sexual Activity	• Provide safe sex education. • Offer in the school curriculum. • Guide to free clinics.

PCP, primary care provider; SDoH, Social Determinants of Health.

education, poverty, racial discrimination, and access to healthcare. Those that are in the low-income bracket may have limited access to healthcare and are at an increased risk for poor health outcomes and an increased chance of premature death. Activities including increased physical activity, healthy eating, and use of healthcare services can lessen the chance of chronic disease but are often impacted by SDoH such as education and income. To address these SDoH, effective interventions are needed. To make an appropriate plan of care, nurses and the entire healthcare team must make informed decisions based on an inclusive assessment of patients' SDoH.

The work of Nightingale and Wald focused on improving SDoH. Their work compares to what is now known as population health while not labeled that at the time. The term "population health," was first defined by David Kindig and Greg Stoddart (2003) as "the health outcomes of a group of individuals, including the distribution of such outcomes within the group" (p. 381). Any group of individuals with something in common can be a population. For example, a population may include all the people who live in a certain neighborhood or town; it could be all the employees of a large corporation; it could be people who identify as a certain ethnicity; or it could be people who all live with the same chronic disease. In order to understand how health outcomes are distributed within a population, health professionals must compare outcomes among different demographic groups in that population. For example, the **infant mortality rate (IMR)** is the number of infant deaths for every 1,000 live births, and it is a measurable outcome. The data in the Ohio IMR by Race between 2016 and 2018 (Table 15.2) indicates that although Black IMR in Ohio has slightly decreased over time, the IMR of Black infants was almost 2.5 times higher than the IMR of White infants from 2016 to 2018 (Ohio Department of Health, 2020). Infant mortality is a complex health concern impacted by many factors such as access to quality prenatal care, poverty, maternal age, maternal health status, and environmental exposures (Reno & Hyder, 2018). Healthcare professionals must understand how health outcomes are affected by the disparities among populations and many other contributing factors.

Figure 15.1 is a model developed at the University of Wisconsin Public Health Institute in 2014 and updated in 2020. The County Health Rankings and Roadmaps Model explores the many health factors and policies and programs that affect health outcomes. Health outcomes measure the length of life and quality of life of a county. Length of life identifies if people are dying prematurely, promoting investigation into the cause of premature deaths. Quality of life identifies if people feel healthy, comfortable, and are able to participate in and enjoy life.

The health factors that affect the health outcomes of a community include health behaviors (i.e., tobacco use, diet, exercise, alcohol and drug use, and sexual activity), access and

TABLE 15.2 OHIO INFANT MORTALITY BY RACE 2016–2018 PER 1,000 LIVE BIRTHS

YEAR	2016	2017	2018
All Races	7.4	7.2	6.9
White	5.8	5.3	5.4
Black	15.2	15.6	13.9

Note. Data from the Ohio Department of Health, 2018 Infant Mortality Annual Report (Ohio Department of Health, 2020)

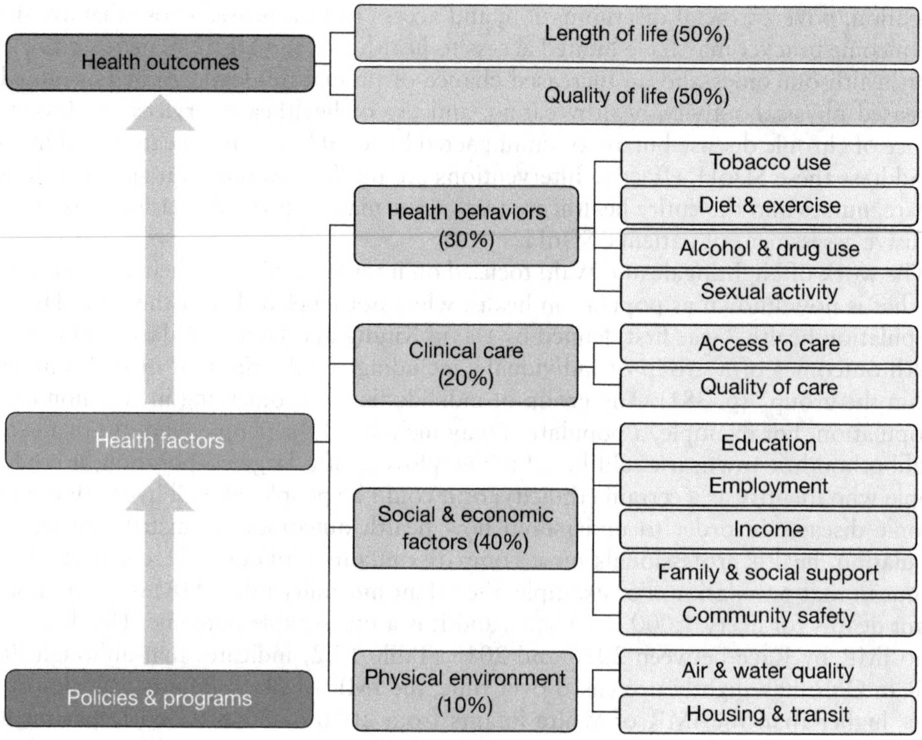

FIGURE 15.1 County Health Rankings & Roadmaps 2020 Model.
Source: From The University of Wisconsin Population Health Institute. County Health Rankings & Roadmaps 2021. www.countyhealthrankings.org Reprinted by permission.

quality of clinical care, social and economic factors (i.e., employment, income, education, family and social support, and community safety), and the physical environment (i.e., air and water quality, housing, and transit).

Policies and programs are at the local, state, and/or federal level and will affect the health factors and health outcomes (University of Wisconsin Population Health Institute, 2020); for example, a local intervention limiting the number of grocery stores in a geographical region may eliminate the amount of car traffic in a community, promoting environmental safety, but marginalizing those who do not have access or transportation outside of their walking community, thus limiting their food sources.

POPULATION HEALTH AND NURSING PRACTICE

Caring for groups, communities, and populations is a longstanding practice in the nursing profession, though often this care was commonly identified as part of the role of public health nurses. The passage of the Patient Protection and Affordable Care Act (ACA) in 2010 has played an important role in aligning healthcare services with public health by requiring nonprofit hospitals to collaborate with local public health departments to conduct Community Health Needs Assessment (CHNA) and incentivizing the Institute for Healthcare Improvement (IHI) **Triple Aim** of "improving the patient experience of care (including quality and satisfaction); improving the health of populations; and reducing the per capita cost of health care" (IHI, n.d., "What Is the Triple Aim?").

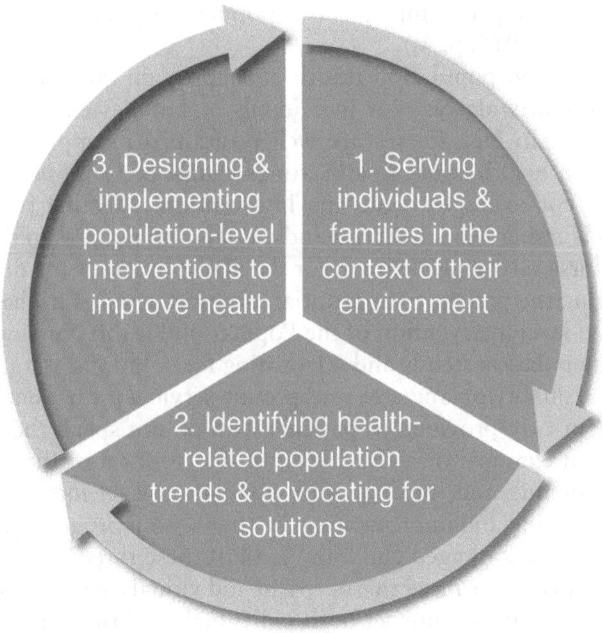

FIGURE 15.2 Population Health Nursing Model.
Source: Reproduced with permission from The Population Health Nursing Model as described in Storfjell, Winslow, & Saunders, 2018, Fig. 1. Copyright 2018. Robert Wood Johnson Foundation. Used with permission from the Robert Wood Johnson Foundation. Storfjell & Cruise, 1984.

Population health requires nurses to look not only at the patient, but also at the SDoH upstream factors that contribute to disease. **Upstream factors** are the SDoH that encompass government, societal, economic, and environmental factors that impact health (Bharmal et al., 2015). In order to address upstream factors, interventions must be targeted upstream as well. A classic illustration of the upstream factor concept is a factory located on a river upstream from a town. The waste of the factory contaminates the river and the people downstream become sick after drinking the water (Braveman et al., 2011). Population health concepts direct the nurse, the interprofessional healthcare team, and the community to identify the source of the contamination and to advocate for it to be stopped in order to prevent illness. It is not enough to just treat those who become ill from drinking the water! Population health considers the root causes of health and disease and the nursing role is to implement interventions to address those root causes or upstream factors.

Although nurses have played a significant role in population health since the time of Florence Nightingale, the ACA has re-invigorated the importance of the role of nurses in population health in all care settings (Cleveland et al., 2019). For example, registered nurses are now being integrated into primary care practices as care coordinators who assist patients with transitions of care from home to hospitals and back again. Additional examples of the nurses' role in population health are described in the Population Health and the Interprofessional Team and Emerging Nursing Roles in Population Health sections of this chapter. Nurses of all education levels and practice areas have population health responsibilities (Storfjell et al., 2018). The **Population Health Nursing Model** (Figure 15.2) encompasses nursing interventions targeted at three levels (i.e., "1) serving and coordinating care for individuals and families in the context of their environment; 2) identifying determinants of health and gaps in resources (trends) and advocating for remedies [solutions]; and 3) designing and implementing population-level interventions [to improve health]" [Storfjell et al., 2018, p. 4]).

The increased focus on population health and upstream factors does not mean that nurses will no longer provide care for individuals or families experiencing illness, such as in hospital settings. In fact, nurses are well positioned to apply the nursing process to address population health issues in all settings (Engle & Campbell, 2019; Fawcett & Ellenbecker, 2015). For example, a nursing intervention reflecting the first level of the Population Health Nursing Model, serving individuals and families in the context of their environment, is a nurse screening a patient for the SDoH before being discharged from the hospital and referring the patient to appropriate support services in their community. An example of a second level intervention of the Population Health Nursing Model, identifying health-related population trends and advocating for solutions, is a nurse working in a clinic to improve the quality of language interpreting services for patients, after identifying gaps in the quality of care provided to patients who do not speak the primary language used in the clinic. An example of a third level of intervention of the Population Health Nursing Model, designing and implementing population-level interventions to improve health, is a nurse designing and implementing an after-school program focused on increasing physical activity in school-aged children. In all of these three population health interventions, the nurse works to meet the needs of individuals within the population and develops interventions that may impact both individuals and the population as a whole.

OVERLAPPING CONCEPTS BETWEEN POPULATION HEALTH AND PUBLIC HEALTH

Population health and public health concepts overlap in many ways. They are closely related concepts and the distinction between the two concepts is blurry. The terms are sometimes used interchangeably since both monitor health trends with an aim to protect and promote health. The IOM in *The Future of Public Health* (1988), defines **public health** as "what we, as a society, do collectively to assure the conditions in which people can be healthy" (p. 1). While this is a broad definition that encompasses many activities, as population health might, the key distinction between population health and public health is that public health commonly refers to government run agencies, programs, and policies. Population health does not exclude public health nor is population health entirely separate; in fact, population health helps to build bridges between public health, healthcare systems (hospitals, clinics, and so on), community organizations, and the populations they serve (CDC, n.d.-b). Population health includes the study of and actions to address health outcomes and the patterns of the SDoH that have historically fallen outside of the public health authority and responsibility in the United States (Kindig & Stoddart, 2003). For example, local and state health departments are not typically charged with monitoring education outcomes and trends, though education level is linked to health outcomes (Hahn & Truman, 2015). Population health also "explicitly includes the health care delivery system, which is sometimes seen as separate from or even in opposition to governmental public health [in the United States]" (Stoto, 2013, p. 2). Ultimately, though, public health and population health share the common goals of maintaining and improving the health of the population and addressing health inequities (Diez Roux, 2016; Kindig & Stoddart, 2003).

Three Levels of Prevention

In population health and public health, prevention of health concerns is a priority. Prevention is aimed at reducing the risks to the health of a population, with an overall goal of wellness and avoidance of illness. The *Future of Nursing 2020–2030* report concludes that our nation will not fully thrive until everyone has the ability to live the healthiest life possible and prevention strategies are key. It is the responsibility of nurses at every level and all settings to promote the fullest health and well-being of all individuals and populations (Wakefield et al., 2021). While planning care for populations, it is important to consider the current health status of a population and implement primary, secondary, or tertiary prevention. Primary prevention is an upstream approach with a goal of disease or injury prevention (British Columbia Health Link, 2016). Examples of primary prevention level activities include health education, vaccination, and policy changes to increase physical activity in a community. Secondary prevention level activities include detecting disease early and preventing it from getting worse. Examples of secondary prevention level activities include screenings (i.e., mammograms, mental health screening), routine laboratory assessments, and implementing interventions to address any problems. Tertiary prevention level activities relate to the correction and prevention of deterioration of a disease state and limiting debilitation. This includes improving quality of life and reducing symptoms of disease. Examples at the tertiary prevention level include health education focused on disease management or rehabilitation services.

CURRENT LITERATURE

CITATION

Farmanova, E., Baker G. R., & Cohen, D. (2019). Combining integration of care and a population health approach: A scoping review of redesign strategies and interventions, and their impact. *International Journal of Integrated Care, 19*(2), Article 5. https://doi.org/10.5334/ijic.4197

DISCUSSION

This review of existing literature explores the benefits of integrated care when extended to the general population. Fifteen organizations using an integrated care model and incorporating a population health approach were identified in 57 articles and reports. The authors reviewed each article and report for specific organizational actions, interventions, and partnerships. They found that each of the 15 organizations attempted to improve population health by addressing the multiple determinants of health outcomes with more than one intervention. The interventions were similarly focused and occurred at both the individual and population levels, whereas, health coaching might be used to move an individual toward weight loss efforts. The development of farmer's markets and safe spaces for physical activity and socialization might be developed as a population health approach to address obesity in the community. Interprofessional teams and linking services provided by community organizations supported the success of the population health interventions. These interventions reduced emergency department visits and hospital admissions; increased disease screening and immunizations; and reduced morbidity and mortality in populations.

IMPLICATIONS FOR PRACTICE

A population health approach that includes evidence-based initiatives administered by interprofessional healthcare teams that also include non-healthcare members and organizations improve individual patient and population health outcomes. This population health approach also leads to equitable and effective health promotion and wellness initiatives.

CASE STUDY

Mr. Thomas is a 55-year-old male who presented to the emergency department (ED) with a gunshot wound. Due to the immediate situation's urgency, little information was exchanged regarding the patient's identifying information upon ED admission. An RN case manager, part of the patient interprofessional team in the ICU, began gathering information about the patient and his health history. A chart review noted that the patient had been seen in the ED seven times in the past 5 weeks. Three of these visits had taken place in the last 3 days. During each of the past three visits, the patient asked for a referral to an inpatient sobriety program to "become clean." However, the social worker notes indicated that the patient was told he was not eligible for an inpatient sobriety program until he attended a 30-day outpatient program.

Mr. Thomas lives with his mother, Mrs. Thomas. She is his emergency contact. Mrs. Thomas indicated that her son lost his job 3 years ago and has been struggling with alcohol abuse since then. He does not have a car or a driver's license. Mr. Thomas is Medicaid eligible but missed his last appointment with the Medicaid Family Services Department, leaving his Medicaid currently inactive. As a result, he cannot afford his medication and he is currently not taking any prescribed medications. His medical history is significant for prior suicidal ideation, depression, diabetes mellitus type 2, hypertension, and hyperlipidemia.

Later in the day, at the weekly scheduled interprofessional team meeting, the ED physicians, the assistant RN manager from the ED, social workers, and RN case managers from the ED and ICU discussed an agenda item focusing on the increase of patients arriving to the ED with alcohol and/or drug intoxication. The main topic of discussion focused on improving strategies to help this patient population, noting that some patients arrive seeking help and others do not.

1. *What SDoH may be impacting Mr. Thomas's health?*
2. *Identify two SDoH interventions that could be addressed for Mr. Thomas.*
3. *What SDoH interventions could be considered for the entire patient population presenting to the ED with alcohol and/or drug intoxication?*

Real World Interview

Population health addresses how we manage a group of patients or a population from a community. It is the concept of managing a large group of patients through their continuum of care. You care for the population in sickness and in health. You maintain their health, make sure they have their immunizations, check that their nutritional needs are met, and provide or encourage well visits. You are familiar with the risks of the community. (It is not only health but the precursors of disease that cause problems for patients.) For example, if high school graduation rates are poor, this could be a precursor of poor health and future life outcomes, including employment and success rates. Employment and success rates are often directly related to how an individual cares for their health and body. We all may know someone who did not graduate from high school and may have had children in their teens or are living unhealthy lifestyles, such as alcoholism or drug abuse. It is unfortunate that these individuals may be somewhat illiterate or do not have the skills for IT [information technology] employment and turn to other unfavorable behaviors.

Over the last several years, I have seen a huge paradigm shift in patient care. It is not just documenting by checking off the box when you move a patient from hospital to home with home care or from home into a skilled nursing facility. It is about building the continuum of quality of care. If the patient needs intravenous (IV) antibiotics at home, you need to be sure the home care agency made contact with the patient and that the IV medications were delivered. You need to confirm that the PCP is aware of the plan of care posthospitalization so they can provide care in the community.

Considering the SDoH, (i.e., transportation, housing, food, medications, and so on), I think we are learning that a lot of times, it may not be an adherence issue on the part of the patient. It may be that there is a barrier to their achievement of health goals. For example, when a patient does not take their medication, they are often labeled as "noncompliant." In actuality, the patient may not have transportation to obtain the medication, or may not have the funds to purchase the medication, or may not have understood the directions about the medication.

With the new population health model, you cannot sacrifice quality of care. Everyone knows that cost containment has to be maintained. You need a balance between cost effectiveness and quality. Years ago, when teaching patients with heart failure, we may have just documented by checking a box indicating it was done (i.e., did I tell them to take their medications and to get exercise, and so on). The result often was the patient coming right back into the hospital a short time after discharge. Now we need to assess the whole patient and ask ourselves, what can we do so they really understand what we are teaching them? We need to offer the patient available resources. Tell the patient where they can go to get their medications and have their blood pressure monitored, where there is an exercise program, where to get help with planning a good diet, and so on. In previous years, it was about "box checking" and now it is about the continuum of care ensuring good population health, patient safety, and quality outcomes.

Mary McLaughlin Davis, DNP, ACNS-BC, NEA-BC, CCM

Senior Director, Care Management Nursing
Cleveland Clinic, Cleveland, Ohio

POPULATION-FOCUSED NURSING COMPETENCIES AND QUALITY AND SAFETY EDUCATION FOR NURSES COMPETENCIES

The knowledge, skills, and attitudes (KSA) required to provide population health nursing care are not new to the nursing profession and they align with the competencies required of all nurses, including the QSEN Competencies. Both the QSEN Competencies and population health emphasize the continuum of individual (patient) interventions to systems interventions (Dolansky & Moore, 2013; Storfjell et al., 2018). For example, with population health, nurses provide quality care to individual patients as well as advocate to improve access to health and remove barriers to care for all people within a healthcare organization or community. Storfjell et al. (2018) reviewed population health competencies from public health nursing and other population health-focused health professions and identified Key Population-Focused Nursing Competencies (Table 15.3). In addition to competencies, QSEN and population health share broader values such as patient-centered care, evidence-based practice, and systems thinking (Dolansky & Moore, 2013). For

TABLE 15.3 KEY POPULATION-FOCUSED NURSING COMPETENCIES

Key Population-Focused Nursing Competencies	
BASIC*	
Wholeness (Whole Person & Whole Community) Providing holistic care to individuals and populations; recognizing strengths and challenges	**Assessment/Analysis** Gathering and interpreting relevant data about individual patients or populations
Coordination Coordinating individual patient care with the healthcare team or coordinating programming and relationships with community organizations	**Cultural Competency/Diversity** Providing culturally appropriate care for individuals and populations and recognizing benefits of diversity
Collaboration (Teamwork/Partnering) Working in partnership with patients, populations, the healthcare team, and/or community organizations	**Attention to Determinants of Health** Assessing for and addressing the SDoH in care planning and/or program planning
Advocacy Advocating for individual patients and for policy change for communities and populations	**Relationship Building** Developing relationships with individuals, populations, and community organizations
Communication Communicating effectively with individual patients, other health professionals, and the general public	**Leadership** Leading within a healthcare team, in organizations, and/or communities
ADVANCED†	
Data Fluency, Assessment, & Analytic Skills (Including Use of Epidemiological Data) Understanding, evaluating, and effectively using population level data and research	**Financial Planning and Management** Understanding and overseeing budgets, understanding the financial impact of health concerns and solutions
Systems Thinking Looking at the big picture, seeking to understand how processes, policies, and actions can impact healthcare and health outcomes	**Policy Development/Program Planning** Developing, implementing, and evaluating policies and programs that impact health
Public Health Science Understanding and integrating research from public health disciplines such as epidemiology, health behavior, and environmental health to address population health issues	**Ethical Principles** Understanding and adhering to ethical principles in nursing and healthcare

Source: Key Population-Focused Nursing Competencies as summarized by Storfjell, Winslow, & Saunders, 2018, p. 28. Copyright 2018. Robert Wood Johnson Foundation. Used with permission from the Robert Wood Johnson Foundation.
*Basic population health competencies required of all RNs.
†Advanced population health competencies required for all BSN and Graduate-level RNs.
SDoH, Social Determinants of Health.

examples of how the six QSEN Competencies apply to nursing in population health, see Table 15.4. When nurses provide population-focused care, they positively impact both individual patient outcomes and population health outcomes within a clinical healthcare mesosystem and healthcare macrosystem, including the healthcare system, non-healthcare agencies, and the community (see Table 15.4 for definitions).

POPULATION HEALTH AND THE INTERPROFESSIONAL TEAM

Addressing both individual patient needs and population health issues requires the skills and expertise of multiple health professions. **Interprofessional collaborative practice** (IPCP) is "when multiple health workers from different professional backgrounds provide comprehensive services by working with patients, their families, [caregivers] and communities to deliver the highest quality of care across settings" (World Health Organization, 2010, p. 13). Improving individual patient outcomes and population health are essential elements of IPCP (Interprofessional Education Collaborative, 2016). Health professionals in many settings have developed programs and practices to foster IPCP and improve the health of the populations they serve.

The Telemedicine IMPACT Plus (TIP) Model was developed for primary care settings to help primary care providers (PCPs) not affiliated with a primary care team to connect with other healthcare professionals in order to access team-based care with their patients (Pariser et al., 2019). The TIP Model is coordinated by a dedicated TIP RN who meets with a PCP and the patient to identify the patient's priority concerns and then leads a coordinated synchronous live-video telehealth visit between the patient, PCP, and other healthcare specialists. Members of the TIP team may include nurses, healthcare providers in psychiatry and internal medicine, social workers, pharmacists, home care workers, occupational therapists, dietitians, and others, based on the patient's needs. The TIP nurse also collaborates with the PCP to assist with follow through on the team's recommendations (Pariser et al., 2019).

An example of population health-focused IPCP in an inpatient setting is the Systems Addressing Frail Elders (SAFE) Care Model. SAFE is a geriatric model of care that consists of a team of an RN, a social worker, and a pharmacist (Borenstein et al., 2016; Peig et al., 2021). The SAFE Care Model is designed to identify and address the specific needs of high-risk hospitalized older adults and to ensure a safe transition back to the community. Patients age 65 and older are screened for issues that are common among older adults; patients identified as high risk are then further screened by the nurse, social worker, and pharmacist for additional issues. After the patient screening, the team meets to discuss and make recommendations for the plan of care (Peig et al., 2021).

ICPC includes all professions and can occur in community settings outside of clinics and hospitals. For example, in Philadelphia, an RN, clinical social worker, and librarian collaborated in a public library to address barriers to healthcare access among individuals experiencing homelessness (Mariano & Harmon, 2019). The nurse and social worker walked around the library and engaged patrons who indicated they had health or social needs. The librarian interacted with patrons within the scope of their regular librarian role and consulted with the nurse and/or social worker if a patron's needs were outside of their expertise. All members of the team provided patient referrals internally among each other, or externally to outside organizations that provided health or social services (Mariano & Harmon, 2019).

These interprofessional care models are all examples of how nurses and other healthcare team members practice ICPC to improve patient outcomes, address the SDoH, and address the health concerns of an identified population. The interprofessional team plays an important role in quality, safety, and population health.

EMERGING NURSING ROLES IN POPULATION HEALTH

The nursing profession and individual nurses have a unique opportunity to expand the role of the nurse as the healthcare focus shifts from individual care to population health with its full continuum of healthcare delivery. While all nurses must expand their current

TABLE 15.4 QUALITY AND SAFETY EDUCATION FOR NURSES COMPETENCIES AND THE ROLE OF THE REGISTERED NURSE IN POPULATION HEALTH

QSEN COMPETENCY	CONTINUUM OF REGISTERED NURSE PH ROLES: PH ROLE WITH AN INDIVIDUAL PATIENT TO PH ROLE WITHIN A MACROSYSTEM				
	PH ROLE WITH AN INDIVIDUAL PATIENT	PH ROLE WITH AN RN PEER GROUP	PH ROLE AS AN HCT MEMBER MICROSYSTEM*	PH ROLE WITHIN AN HEALTH-CARE SYSTEM MESOSYSTEM†	PH ROLE WITHIN A COMMUNITY MACROSYSTEM‡
Patient-Centered Care Recognize the patient or designee as the source of control and full partner in providing compassionate and coordinated care based on respect for the patient's preferences, values, and needs.	Engage the patient in conversation related to healthcare preferences, values, needs, and the patient's SDoH. Document assessment and align care with assessment data.	Support/complete RN-modified PH interventions which are based on patient preference, values, and needs. Monitor patient outcomes and safety during modified interventions.	Communicate patient-specific preferences, values, and PH needs to the HCT. Discuss modified interventions, safety, and outcomes with HCT.	Collaborate with an intra-agency team to publish reasons for practice modifications and improved outcomes of patients with modified PH interventions. Report safety concerns and poor outcomes. Advocate for patient and family preferences, values, and needs during care transitions.	Join the interprofessional team to complete CHNA. Advocate for public policies and education that support the diversity of healthcare preferences, values, and needs as well as address SDoH. Support or initiate healthcare policy change that identifies and resolves recognized SDoH, healthcare barriers, and biases.
EBP Integrate best current evidence with clinical expertise and patient/family preferences and values for delivery of optimal healthcare.	Collect and document data for research, and monitoring quality, safety, performance, and patient outcomes. Consistently use EBP healthcare protocols across racial and ethnic groups, unless patient preferences and values differ.	Establish an RN journal club, discussing the strength of evidence, innovations in nursing care, and best practices. Organize ad hoc meetings with RN colleagues to discuss culturally based requests for patient protocol modifications.	Question patient care resulting in poor outcomes or adverse events. Review policies and procedures, integrating best practices and initiating practice changes based on available evidence. Discuss conflicting healthcare evidence and PH protocols with the HCT.	Initiate ethics consult to resolve conflicts between healthcare evidence and patient values and preferences. Establish an intra-agency HCT team to review data related to poor patient outcomes and adverse events and suggest evidence-based practice changes. Work with librarians to gain access to new and developing PH care evidence.	Join a community team responding to CHNA findings. Update healthcare education materials to reflect current research, population level evidence, and SDoH. Lead a team to review healthcare policies, ensuring that they address community needs, reflect current research, and consider population level evidence and SDoH.

Teamwork and Collaboration Function effectively within nursing and inter-professional teams, fostering open communication, mutual respect, and shared decision-making to achieve quality patient care.	Respectfully provide education to empower the patient in self-care and foster shared decision-making. Consider SDoH and ensure that education includes PH actions available to the patient and caregivers. Integrate patient and HCT member recommendations into the patient plan of care.	Advocate for a full RN scope of practice, including PH. Build a nursing culture based on the Nursing Code of Ethics. Request support from RN peers. Provide support to RN peers.	Clarify team member roles to increase accountability, identify barriers to team functioning, and decrease conflict. Establish HCT huddles to foster transparency, communication, and respect. Lead group discussions related to attributes that foster respect, collaboration, and efficient processes within HCTs.	Create an intra-agency HCT team to review system processes, performance, and patient outcomes, and initiate systems redesign as needed to achieve high-quality PH. Advocate for a just culture, that encourages open reporting of adverse events and risk situations, yet holds people and organizations accountable in a just manner, providing support and respect to HCT members. Consult with appropriate healthcare providers to establish coordinated intra-agency individual patient care and PH.	Partner with non-healthcare groups to complete community level health screenings to identify patients with health-protective and health-risk behaviors. Form a community team to plan interventions that mitigate health-risk behaviors and enhance health-protective behaviors. Collaborate with macrosystem members to change legislative inequities and biases that affect PH health outcomes and maintain social inequities.
Safety Minimizes risk of harm to patients and providers through both system effectiveness and individual performance.	Discuss nursing interventions, planned care, ordered medications, and expected outcomes. Be transparent with the patient and family if an error occurs. This increases public trust and decreases litigation.	Establish standardized PH processes that support safe nursing care. Discuss evidence-based solutions to unsafe practices. Lead a journal club that looks for publications related to the influence of SDoH on safety.	Standardize processes to mitigate error. Utilize available technology as a strategy to decrease reliance on memory and human-generated error. Implement QI initiatives based on unit and PH safety data.	Organize an intra-agency HCT to resolve the root causes of reported safety errors, unmet benchmark performance, and patient outcome measures as well as establish standard patient care processes. Establish a committee to determine, and respond to, barriers to the employee and patient self-care and PH. Practice the principles of a just culture.	Monitor social media and healthcare reporting systems for quality and safety errors. Discuss findings with clinical mesosystem administrators. Use clinical mesosystem and CHNA data to identify at-risk populations, then coordinate with macrosystem members, groups and agencies to plan PH interventions.

(continued)

TABLE 15.4 QUALITY AND SAFETY EDUCATION FOR NURSES COMPETENCIES AND THE ROLE OF THE REGISTERED NURSE IN POPULATION HEALTH (*continued*)

QSEN COMPETENCY	CONTINUUM OF REGISTERED NURSE PH ROLES: PH ROLE WITH AN INDIVIDUAL PATIENT TO PH ROLE WITHIN A MACROSYSTEM				
	PH ROLE WITH AN INDIVIDUAL PATIENT	PH ROLE WITH AN RN PEER GROUP	PH ROLE AS AN HCT MEMBER MICROSYSTEM*	PH ROLE WITHIN AN HEALTH-CARE SYSTEM MESOSYSTEM†	PH ROLE WITHIN A COMMUNITY MACROSYSTEM‡
QI Use data to monitor the outcomes of care processes and use improvement methods to design and test changes to continuously improve the quality and safety of healthcare systems.	Discuss QI measures with patients and families. Follow evidence-based nursing care protocols, modifying care of patients who do not respond to established interventions.	Consider the need to modify patient interventions based on patient preference, values, SDoH, and PH. Determine and resolve potential root causes for poor patient outcomes.	Organize a committee to collect, analyze, and respond to practice errors, near miss reports, poor performance, and patient outcome data. Lead QI initiatives for patient outcomes that are trending down, are below the benchmark, or pose a high safety risk.	Establish an intra-agency quarterly review of patients who do not respond to evidence-based interventions or who returns unexpectedly to the healthcare system. Participate in, or lead, intra-agency QI initiatives based on below benchmark patient, process, performance outcome, and PH measures.	Review the CHNA. Collaborate with healthcare providers, non-healthcare groups, and government agencies to establish a plan to improve population health outcomes below target which were identified in the CHNA.
Informatics Use information and technology to communicate, manage knowledge, mitigate error, and support decision-making.	Use available technology to deliver and immediately document patient assessment, nursing care, and plan future nursing care. When providing patients information, provide printed and verbal information.	Review policies and procedures related to telehealth and telecommunications. Advocate for technology and resources (e.g., UpToDate) that provide a quick reference for evidence-based nursing care. Rehearse the use of new technology with peers. Ask for coaching, as needed.	Compile an electronic list of resources with the HCT that includes HCT names, phone numbers, and email. Include frequently used services and resources on the list (e.g., translators, IT help lines, and so on.	Give feedback to the IT staff and EHR managers to avoid actual and potential breaches in confidentiality by staff or patients. Collaborate with IT staff to build practical institutional and unit dashboards that contain patient outcome and assessment data.	Obtain information from local internet/Wi-Fi providers related to security measures for PHI. Advocate for improvement of systems that do not provide adequate safety measures.

	For individuals who are hard of hearing or who have a different primary language, provide a translator. Instruct patient and family in the use of technology for health monitoring and assistance (e.g. BP machine, C-PAP).	Use technology to monitor patient care and outcomes.	Arrange review courses related to new technologies for the HCT. Identify patient data that needs to be accessible to all HCT members. Collaborate with IT to design a system that allows data sharing and access.	Participate on a Technology Acquisitions Committee or complete surveys related to the use and efficacy of institutional technology. Identify technology practices that may lead to poor outcomes (e.g. copy feature for vital signs).	Partner with local internet/ Wi-Fi providers to produce and provide educational materials related to steps patients can take to secure PHI during virtual/video visits. Join the board of directors of the local library. Integrate library and hospital resources to provide patients with private, secure space for virtual/video visits.

*May also be called a **microsystem** or interprofessional team; includes the patient and their caregivers, a medical provider, RN, and administrative support person. May also include a number of other healthcare staff (e.g., LPN, MA, social worker, behavioral health specialists, clinical pharmacist) involved in the patient's care.
†Includes the healthcare institution, or institutional network, as well as their responsibilities to, and influences from, the community.
‡includes the mesosystem, community members and agencies, regional culture and values, and regulatory and governmental agencies.
CHNA, community health needs assessment; C-PAP, continuous positive airway pressure; EBP, evidence-based practice; EHR, electronic health record; HCT, healthcare team; IT, information technology; PH, population health; PHI, protected health information; QI, quality improvement; QSEN, Quality and Safety Education for Nurses; SDoH, Social Determinants of Health.

Source: Adapted from Dolansky, M. A., & Moore, S. M. (2013). Quality and Safety Education for Nurses (QSEN): The key is systems thinking. *OJIN: The Online Journal of Issues in Nursing, 18*(3), Manuscript 1. https://doi.org/10.3912/OJIN.Vol18No03Man01, Table 2.

TABLE 15.5 CURRENT EXAMPLES OF REGISTERED NURSES WORKING IN POPULATION HEALTH*

Public Health Nurse	Long-Term Care Facility Nurse
School Nurse	Nurse Care Coordinator
Visiting/Homecare Nurse	Correctional Facility Nurse
Primary Care Nurse	Infectious Disease Nurse
Nurse as Community-Based Facilitator	SANE
Hospice Nurse	

*All nurses must expand their current role to include concepts of population health
SANE, sexual assault nurse examiner.

professional role to include concepts of population health, some nurses today work with populations and population health in many well-defined roles. See Table 15.5. For example, nurses have emerging roles in school nursing in which population health competencies are needed such as patient care coordination and data analytics. Data analytics examines data from a population of patients in order to find trends and draw conclusions about the patient populations. Data analytics helps nurses and organizations make sense of data. It uses various tools and techniques to help organizations make decisions and succeed.

The school nurse's role traditionally was viewed as patient centered, providing urgent care and current trends such as high-tech nursing care (i.e., straight catheterization, tracheostomy care, routine medication administration). The National Association of School Nurses (NASN, 2018) reports that school nurses should work as interprofessional team members to improve student and community health outcomes. School nurses are critical resources for the students experiencing food insecurity, homelessness, lack of healthcare, and many more SDoH. The *Future of Nursing 2020–2030* highlights the school nurse as the healthcare provider who provides health equity for these children (Wakefield et al., 2021). School nurses are a link to the community and often able to assess needs in the community, develop a plan, and evaluate health outcomes. All of this is being done in conjunction with the student, the community, and the family, which the school nurse routinely intervenes with while at the same time addressing SDoH.

There are also a variety of emerging roles for nurses to expand their professional roles in population health settings and improve patient care delivery. For example, many nurses currently work as primary care nurses. With a focus on population health, a nurse can expand the nurse's traditional role in primary care clinics to become true primary care partners with the healthcare team (HCT) and work to the full scope of their nursing licensure. The current primary care system in the United States relies heavily on primary care physicians to deliver primary care (Kerns & Willis, 2020). However, over the next decade, the primary care physician workforce is expected to decline, while at the same time the United States will see a growth in population, an increase in the aging population, and an expansion of adequately insured individuals (Bodenheimer & Bauer, 2015). Registered nurses in America must become a full partner in the primary care setting to achieve healthcare improvements throughout the population (Salmond & Echevarria, 2017). To realize this, nurses in primary care must balance their time between traditional roles, like triaging patients and administering vaccines, while also expanding into emerging population health roles such as nurse care coordination and panel management (Bodenheimer & Bauer, 2015).

A **nurse care coordinator** is a nurse who deliberately organizes patient care activities between participants involved in a patient's care to facilitate the appropriate delivery of healthcare services (Scholz & Minaudo, 2015). A nurse care coordinator works closely with patients with complex chronic illnesses to coordinate care services with the goal of promoting positive patient outcomes and containing healthcare costs (Biernacki et al., 2015). A nurse care coordinator, for instance, might recommend a patient with hypertension to join a shared healthcare visit with other similar patients with hypertension. The shared healthcare visits offer the patient the opportunity to learn about their disease from both the healthcare team and other patients with hypertension. Ultimately, nurse care coordinators work to improve patients' health through the development of therapeutic relationships with chronically ill patients (Biernacki et al., 2015), working to anticipate the patient's needs and prevent gaps in their care.

Another role for nurses in population health is **panel management**. In this role, a nurse working as a team member in a primary care setting shares responsibility for a **panel,** or a group of patients assigned to each care team in the practice (Agency for Healthcare Research and Quality [AHRQ], 2013). According to the AHRQ (2013), the average panel size for a care team is between 1,500 to 2,000 patients. Primary care nurses work with the interprofessional team to proactively manage the care for all patients within this panel of patients. The team oversees and tracks the needs of the panel of patients to ensure that all patients receive the services needed to optimize their health and well-being (AHRQ, 2013). Panel management includes the use of data, and nurses need to have advanced informatics competence. **Nursing informatics,** defined as "the specialty that integrates nursing science with multiple information and analytical sciences to identify, define, manage and communicate data, information, knowledge and wisdom in nursing practice" assists with this need (American Nurses Association, 2015). Nursing informatics specialists and nurses contributing to population health use data to predict health behaviors and promote clinical interventions to improve health outcomes (Reynolds et al., 2016).

Population health nurses can also play a role in a **patient-centered medical home (PCMH) model.** The PCMH is a model of care in which patients are engaged in a direct relationship with a chosen healthcare provider who coordinates a cooperative team of healthcare professionals, takes collective responsibility for the comprehensive integrated care provided to the patient, and advocates and arranges appropriate care with other qualified providers and community resources as needed. PCMH practices develop care teams to improve care coordination and care management of patient populations aiming to improve safety, efficiency, and quality in patient care. By becoming a recognized PCMH, practices can improve care delivery and take advantage of private or public incentive payments that reward PCMH. The Patient Protection and ACA offers enhanced federal funding to states for PCMH serving Medicaid beneficiaries (Association of Clinicians for the Underserved, 2015).

Nurses in the PCMH model of care assist with the delivery of primary care services while following five principles: accessible care, coordinated care, quality care, comprehensive care, and patient-centered care (Perez Jolles et al., 2019). In PCMH, the primary care team uses data to understand patterns, recognize gaps in care, and engage in quality improvement. Data can help predict appropriate healthcare needs and promote clinical interventions for patients to ensure that optimal health is achieved for the population (Kaminetzky & Nelson, 2015). For example, the PCMH team monitors patient data, noting when individuals within their panel are due for basic preventive care, like cancer screenings or immunizations. These individuals are then contacted and encouraged to receive this care and any necessary follow-up care.

CASE STUDY

Student nurses in a community clinical experience in an urban school district are tasked with performing capillary blood draws via fingersticks for lead screenings on 4- and 5-year-old students. The school district is in a city where children have a higher risk of lead exposure due to aging and deteriorating houses that are poorly maintained. At one lead screening, a 4-year-old boy is brought to the lead screening table, accompanied by his teacher. The boy seems much smaller than the other students from the same class, so his paperwork is reviewed again to verify that he is indeed 4 years old. The teacher mentions that the boy is quite restless and impulsive, and the teacher offers assistance for the procedure. The boy sits on the teacher's lap, but he is having difficulty following simple instructions. He can't focus on a nearby children's picture book that a student nurse partner has been reading to other preschoolers to distract them from the procedure. Eventually the finger stick is completed, but it took a significant effort by all the helpers in the room. The boy's behavior seems different from the other 4-year-old students who have already been screened that morning. The clinical nursing instructor with the student nurse team points out that these behaviors and clinical findings might indicate that he has an increased lead level in his blood.

The results from the lead screening are released the following day, revealing that this child's blood lead level is 12 mcg/dL. This level exceeds the blood level that is considered acceptable for lead (<3.5 mcg/dL). A venous lead level is then obtained, and the results of this new test show a lead level of 10 mcg/dL. This level remains higher than acceptable.

1. *Identify three possible SDoH that children in this population may encounter.*
2. *What are the risk factors for this child related to elevated lead levels?*
3. *Why are young children living in urban settings more susceptible to environmental lead exposure?*

BOX 15.1 Developing Clinical Judgment

A nurse, working part-time in a three-unit long-term care (LTC) facility with two other RNs on New Year's Day, begins the morning with assessments of all assigned patients. The nurse first assesses Mr. Malcom Green, who is with his wife, Mrs. Rosa Green, celebrating the last day of Kwanzaa. Mr. Green is a 75-year-old obese male admitted after a series of falls at home. He is cognitively intact and able to perform a majority of his own activities of daily living (ADL). Mrs. Green is concerned about Mr. Green's problems, which she states "have been obvious some times and not so obvious at other times, since he came here" and "have been getting worse over the last two weeks."

After a review of Mr. Green's electronic health record (EHR), it is noted that he was transported to his PCP's office 2 days ago for blood pressure (BP) above 140/90 and he was transported to the local emergency department (ED) 6 days ago with complaints of chest pain. Other past symptoms listed in the LTC facility transport notes include complaints of dizziness, a bloody nose, intermittent headache, heart palpitations, tiredness, chest pain, and blurred vision. The PCP's notes, from prior visits, are in the EHR but the ED report cannot be located.

(continued)

BOX 15.1 Developing Clinical Judgment (*continued*)

According to Mr. Green, his current symptoms include dizziness, headache, tiredness, and blurred vision. Looking back over the past 2 months, you find the following BP readings in the LTC facility EHR (oldest to newest BP readings): 130/90, 120/80, 140/80, 120/80, 130/90, 120/52, and 148/96. The reading of 148/96 resulted in Mr. Green's most recent visit to his PCP. Readings recorded in the PCP's office were 156/102, 140/80, and 128/74. Today's BP reading is 112/60. There is no documented change in medication, or other orders, after Mr. Green's PCP's office appointment or after his visit to the local ED. His medications have not changed in 7 months.

The unit's care team today includes three medical assistants who usually work on other units. Mr. Green's care is discussed with the unit's care team, but nothing new related to his activities of daily living, dietary intake, mobility, or symptoms is mentioned. Mr. Green's complaints and BP readings are discussed at the facility's RN huddle with the two other RNs at the facility. The full-time department heads are not working.

Orders for Mr. Green indicate that his BP be taken weekly. Protocols for the LTC facility indicate (a) a call to the PCP when the patient's BP reading is above 140/90 after three consecutive readings separated by 1 or 2 minutes and (b) transport to the local ED, if the BP is above 180/110. Facility protocols are based on available evidence and include the Guideline for the Prevention, Detection, Evaluation, and Management of High Blood Pressure in Adults (Whelton et al., 2018).

1. What **CUES (Assessment)** can the nurse assess (a) for Mr. Green? (b) for a population similar to Mr. Green?
2. What **HYPOTHESIS (Diagnosis** will the nurse consider (a) for Mr. Green? (b) for a similar population?
3. What **ACTION (Plan and Implement)** will be most effective for the nurse to take to assure (a) Mr. Green's safety in this situation? (b) the safety of a similar population?
4. For (a) Mr. Green and (b) a similar population, how will the nurse evaluate the **OUTCOME (Evaluation)** for the purpose of arriving at a satisfactory clinical outcome?

QUALITY IMPROVEMENT AND POPULATION HEALTH

Quality improvement (QI) is the use of data to monitor outcomes and apply tests of change to continuously improve healthcare outcomes, taking into consideration the system in which care is delivered (Cronenwett et al., 2007). QI is essential in population health. Quality outcomes of interest include the six aims from the IOM Framework for Quality Assessment sometimes referred to as STEEEP (IOM, 2001):

- Safe (i.e., harm avoidance when care is intended to help);
- Timely (i.e., reduced delays for patients and provider)
- Effective (i.e., provision of services based on scientific knowledge to those who will benefit);
- Efficient (i.e., avoidance of waste);
- Equitable (i.e., provision of consistent, quality care); and
- Patient-centered (i.e., respectful and responsive care based on patient preferences, needs, and values).

See www.ahrq.gov/talkingquality/measures/six-domains.html for complete definitions of each STEEEP aim. When gaps in STEEEP are identified, QI projects need to be initiated.

Real World Interview

Management of a population of veteran patients at our VA medical center who have chronic diseases is facilitated by panel management. Panel management allows me to evaluate how well each veteran is doing. Are self-care strategies and our healthcare interventions effective, or are some veterans on the panel having issues with managing their chronic disease? I have four different databases to assist me with panel management. They tell me different things [about the veterans on our panel]. Sometimes I use the Electronic Quality Metrics (EQM), a database on our veteran patients over time. The EQM contains quality metrics such as BP and HbA1C which are collected from electronic health records. Other times I may collect data from the Primary Care Almanac, a Veterans Administration specific database with patient diagnoses, previous labs, and other patient information. The databases help me manage my patients by comparing each patient with the population of veterans in our panel.

The databases allow me to get metrics that I would not necessarily be able to get if I were using things like pencil and paper. The databases give me a snapshot of all the patients I manage very quickly. This allows me to see if what we are doing is effective or if our team needs to make individual or systems level changes.

The databases help our team manage our patients' BP or HbA1C. For example, when out of range values are observed, we reach out to patients and get them back on track with their disease management. The database information helps us keep engaged with our panel of patients, keep them focused, and help them reach their healthcare goals.

Anisa Hilliard, BS, MS, RN

Masters in Nursing Informatics

RN Care Manager Patient Aligned Care Team (PACT)

Louis Stokes VA Medical Center, Cleveland, Ohio

For example, if the data demonstrate that patients in the population are experiencing timely delays in seeing their physician after a hospitalization, then the nurse as a part of an interprofessional team can identify the potential causes and test strategies to effect improvements. It may take many strategies to eventually decrease the wait time to see a physician, but the nurse who is skilled in QI understands that determination and perseverance are needed and works to ensure that patients receive timely care.

Equitable care, another STEEP aim (i.e. the provision of consistent, quality care), is an important quality outcome and can be addressed by QI implemented by the larger hospital system. As an example, a patient's homelessness or housing foreclosure may impact a patient's health. Using an SDoH framework re-focuses the traditional role of the hospital from an institution designed to cure and treat illness, to one that supports population health. Hospitals are now required to complete a CHNA every 3 years to help identify the resource needs of their community and develop programming to address these needs (Gruber et al., 2019), Many of the SDoH factors such as education, food, and housing are addressed directly with local stakeholders to improve healthcare. By using QI methods to address the needs of the community, hospitals are taking a primary role to improve the outcomes of the communities or populations that they serve (Craig et al., 2020).

CASE STUDY

An RN works in a primary care clinic affiliated with the local community hospital. Using the PCMH Model, each care team manages a panel of 1,200 patients. In preparation for the weekly team meeting, the RN accesses the BP measurement data for the team's panel of patients. While discussing the available panel data, the team notices the:

- *Percentage of patients at or below their target/goal BP is 69%, while the hospital benchmark is 85%.*
- *Percentage of African American patients at or below their target/goal BP is 63%.*
- *Percentage of patients who do not attend appointments as scheduled is 28%, while the national average is 23.5%.*
- *One hundred eleven patients on the panel have a last recorded BP above the target/goal: 60 patients were seen more than 6 weeks ago and 51 patients were seen more than 3 months ago. The next available face-to-face provider visit is in 6 weeks.*

The team decides to implement a QI initiative.

1. *In addition to the RN, what care team members will participate in the QI initiative?*
2. *What interventions, including referrals and links to population-based interventions, might the QI team use to increase the number of patients on their panel of 1,200 patients who are at or below their target/goal BP?*
3. *What dimensions of quality (STEEEP) are reflected in the data?*

END-OF-CHAPTER RESOURCES

KEY CONCEPTS

1. Population health is "the health outcomes of a group of individuals, including the distribution of such outcomes within the group" (Kindig & Stoddart, 2003). Florence Nightingale began advocating for health promotion for populations of patients as she cared for the soldiers during the Crimean War in 1853. Lillian Wald moved into a home, the "House on Henry Street," in 1893 to care for children and families living in poverty. It was from this beginning that Wald and colleagues began the first Visiting Nurse Association. Both of these women worked to improve the health outcomes of the at-risk populations in the late 1800s to early 1900s.
2. Nurses of all education levels and specialties can integrate population health into their care. The Population Health Nursing Model describes three different levels in which nurses can do this by "1) serving and coordinating care for individuals and families in the context of their environment; 2) identifying determinants of health and gaps in resources (trends) and advocating for remedies [solutions]; and 3) designing and implementing population-level interventions [to improve health]" (Storfjell et al., 2018, p. 4).
3. Population health and public health overlap in many ways and they are closely related concepts. The terms are often used interchangeably because both monitor health trends and aim to protect and promote health. Population health helps to build bridges between public health, healthcare systems (hospitals, clinics, etc.), community organizations, and the populations they serve. Population health includes movement to incorporate broader population health concepts into both individual patient care and the healthcare of the community.
4. Key Population-Focused Nursing Competencies and the QSEN Institute's prelicensure competencies share multiple competencies (i.e., patient-centered care, QI, and evidence-based practice).
5. The QSEN Institute's prelicensure competencies guide role development for nurses in population health. For an explanation of the RN' role based on these competencies, please refer to Table 15.4.
6. Interprofessional collaborative practice is one strategy to address SDoH and other population health needs.
7. RNs currently have the opportunity to expand the role of the nurse as the healthcare focus shifts to the population.
8. QI is an essential function in population health.

CRITICAL DISCUSSION POINTS

1. Think about a recent clinical experience. What type of SDoH can be identified in the patient population served during this experience?
2. Considering the identified SDoH(s) in Question 1, what population-focused interventions could assist with the plan of care?
3. How can interprofessional healthcare teams impact population health outcomes?
4. How does population health fit into all nursing practices?
5. How does the collection and documentation of patient data support the assessment of populations?

6. How can population level data be used to promote a culture of health and wellness?
7. Consider QI in a variety of populations. What measures might be useful to monitor health outcomes of the following populations: (a) schools (K-12), (b) colleges and universities, (c) the community, (d) a primary care clinic, (e) long-term care facilities, (f) homeless shelters, (g) correctional facilities, and (h) adult acute care unit?
8. What population health initiatives can be identified (a) during your clinical experiences and (b) in your community?

KEY TERMS

- Infant mortality rate
- Interprofessional collaborative practice
- Macrosystem
- Mesosystem
- Microsystem
- Nurse care coordinator
- Nursing informatics
- Panel
- Panel management
- Patient-centered medical home model
- Population health
- Population Health Nursing Model
- Public health
- Quality improvement
- Social Determinants of Health
- Triple Aim
- Upstream factors

REVIEW QUESTIONS

Answers to Review Questions appear in the Instructor's Manual. Qualified instructors should request the Instructor's Manual from textbook@springerpub.com.

1. A school nurse is demonstrating the use of a peak flowmeter to help children with asthma recognize when they need to use a rescue inhaler. Which of the following levels of prevention is being used by the nurse?
   A. Primary prevention
   B. Secondary prevention
   C. Tertiary prevention
   D. Both primary and secondary prevention

2. A nurse care coordinator is working with a patient who has been struggling to control her type 2 diabetes. Which of the following describes the role of the nurse care coordinator with this patient?
   A. Pick up necessary prescriptions for the patient and deliver them to the patient during office visits.
   B. Take the patient's blood sugar during weekly visits to the clinic and monitor her labs monthly.
   C. Coordinate care services, anticipating the patient's needs and helping the patient access necessary resources.
   D. Call the patient at home to remind her of upcoming appointments and scheduled procedures.
3. Molly has type 1 diabetes. She states she does not feel safe in her neighborhood because there is a lot of crime. She is currently unemployed and does not have any health insurance. She walks to her medical appointments, but when the weather is bad, she has no transportation and usually does not go to the appointment. Which of the following SDoH may affect Molly's health outcome? *Select all that apply.*
   A. Zip code
   B. Access to transportation
   C. Medication side effects
   D. Gender
   E. Employment status
4. An interdisciplinary approach that connects health departments, healthcare institutes, and policy to achieve positive health outcomes locally is an example of which of the following?
   A. Social Determinants of Health
   B. Population health
   C. Care coordination
   D. Policy development
5. A nurse working in a pediatric clinic screens three siblings from one household for lead exposure and all three have elevated blood lead levels. The nurse then refers the family to a social worker to connect them to a program to help the family find lead-safe housing. This is an example of which of the following?
   A. Assurance, one of the three core functions of public health
   B. A first level intervention from the Population Health Nursing Model, serving individuals and families in the context of their environment
   C. Policy development/program planning, one of the Key Population-Focused Nursing Competencies
   D. Interprofessional population health management for pediatric patients
6. The concepts of population health and public health overlap in many ways. What are the distinctions between the two concepts? *Select all that apply.*
   A. Public health works to improve health inequities.
   B. Public health typically refers to government run agencies, programs, or policies.
   C. Population health addresses the Social Determinants of Health.
   D. Population health only focuses on specific patient populations.
   E. Population health explicitly includes the healthcare delivery system.

7. At a regional correctional facilities' meeting, nurses reviewed the types of cases they had been seeing in their facilities' health clinics over the last few months. Sexually transmitted infections (STI) seemed to be trending upward. To begin a quality improvement initiative, what will the nurses decide are their priority actions? *Select all that apply.*

   A. Inform the medical director at their correctional facilities of the nurse's observations related to STIs.

   B. Collect baseline data related to STI cases seen during health service hours and discuss findings at the next local correctional facility meeting.

   C. Call the local news agencies' investigative reporters and leave anonymous tips suggesting an increase in STIs in the correctional facilities.

   D. Contact the health information technology staff for the county and state, asking for the reported STI cases over the past 2 years for comparison.

   E. Check to see if each of the correctional facilities has a protocol related to STI assessment/testing, care/medication, and reporting/contact tracing.

8. The nurse working in primary care performs her daily panel management and notices that there is an increase in the HbA1c levels on her team's panel of patients. She calls a few of the patients to determine possible reasons for the increase and quickly determines that there are knowledge gaps in understanding insulin doses and blood sugar levels. What is the best next step for the nurse?

   A. Continue to monitor the data to see if the trend continues.

   B. Call each patient and individually review diabetic teaching.

   C. Convene her patient-centered medical home team and initiate a QI project.

   D. Ignore the finding as it is probably an error in the data.

9. A 57-year-old male patient is admitted to the hospital for an exacerbation of COPD symptoms. The bedside nurse conducts an SDoH screen with the patient and the patient indicates two areas of concern (i.e., due to his illness he has been unable to work so he cannot afford to pay his utility bills plus his car broke down and he does not have reliable transportation). Which of the following are the best steps for the nurse to take next? *Select all that apply.*

   A. Refer the patient to the social worker on the unit for further screening and to discuss potential community resources available for the patient.

   B. Ask the patient follow-up questions to help him identify his priority issue and share this information with the interprofessional team.

   C. Call the patient's son to set up a care coordination conference with the family and prepare a detailed agenda to use everyone's time efficiently.

   D. Refer the patient to all members of the interprofessional team by phone; avoid recording the SDoH screen in the EHR as it does not apply to his care in the hospital.

   E. Talk with the patient to identify people who can offer him support both while he is in the hospital and when he returns home.

10. A community assessment reveals a higher than expected rate of hypertension among older adults. To help decrease the rates of hypertension, the community assessment team applies for a small grant that will be awarded based on the development of primary prevention interventions for this population. Choose the best options for primary prevention interventions. *Select all that apply.*
    A. Offering an educational series at the local senior center on, "What is hypertension (high blood pressure)?"
    B. Creating flyers to be distributed at the senior center and local businesses on, "How exercise can help reduce high blood pressure"
    C. Offering a class on, "How a low sodium diet may prevent high blood pressure"
    D. Offering blood pressure screenings once a month at the senior center
    E. Educating healthcare professionals on the purpose of the most popular hypertension medications

REVIEW ACTIVITIES

1. Explore your county rankings at the following website: www.countyhealthrankings.org/explore-health-rankings. Review the population demographics, health outcomes, and health factors (health behaviors, clinical care, social and economic factors, and physical environment). What is your county ranking? Identify three health outcomes for your community. What are the identified outcomes and reflect on what surprised you about your community and why?
2. The Population Health Nursing Model in Figure 15.2 describes three levels of nursing interventions: "1) serving and coordinating care for individuals and families in the context of their environment; 2) identifying determinants of health and gaps in resources (trends) and advocating for remedies [solutions]; and 3) designing and implementing population-level interventions [to improve health]" (Storfjell et al., 2018, p. 4). Table 15.4 illustrates five RN population health roles: (a) PH role with an Individual Patient, (b) PH role with an RN peer group, (c) PH role as an HCT member, (d) PH role within a clinical mesosystem, and (e) PH role within a macrosystem. Match each of these five population health roles to the most appropriate nursing intervention level.
3. Using Table 15.4 as a guide, complete Table 15.6 by creating specific nursing roles or interventions based on the QSEN Competency and Case description in each row, and the RN PH role in each column.

EXPLORING THE WEB

1. Population Health Management (PHM): Registered Nurses' Essential Role in Value-Based Care (https://qsen.org/population-health-management-phm-registered-nurses-essential-role-in-value-based-care) describes the emerging nursing roles in PHM through in-depth learning modules.
2. Geriatrics (https://qsen.org/faculty-resources/geriatrics) provides the user with the knowledge and resources needed to support nursing initiatives that improve the quality and safety of care for older adults.
3. Project Implicit: Health, Mental and Physical (https://implicit.harvard.edu/implicit/user/pih/pih/preliminaryinfo.html), has multiple *Implicit Association Tests* which are designed to assess implicit attitudes, identities, and beliefs that people are either unwilling or unable to report.

TABLE 15.6 Quality and Safety Education for Nurses Competencies and the Role of the Registered Nurse in Population Health

QSEN COMPETENCY	REGISTERED NURSE PH ROLES: CONTINUUM FROM AN INDIVIDUAL PATIENT TO WITHIN A MACROSYSTEM				
	PH ROLE WITH AN INDIVIDUAL PATIENT	PH ROLE WITH AN RN PEER GROUP	PH ROLE AS AN HCT MEMBER MICROSYSTEM*	PH ROLE WITHIN A HEALTH-CARE **MESOSYSTEM**†	PH ROLE WITHIN A **MACROSYSTEM**‡
Patient-Centered Care **Case:** Patient and family experiencing pregnancy					
Evidence-Based Practice **Case:** Patient with chronic kidney disease					
Teamwork and Collaboration **Case:** Patient with type 2 diabetes					
Safety **Case:** Patient with asthma who uses daily and rescue medications					
Quality Improvement **Case:** Patient within the prison system who has not received all current CDC recommended vaccinations					
Informatics **Case:** Patient who has a virtual well care visit					

***Microsystem** may also be called a interprofessional team; includes the patient and their caregivers, a medical provider, RN, and administrative support person. May also include a number of other healthcare staff (e.g., LPN, MA, social worker, behavioral health specialists, clinical pharmacist) involved in the patient's care.
†**Mesosystem** Includes the healthcare institution, or institutional network, as well as their responsibilities to, and influences from, the community.
‡**Macrosystem** includes the mesosystem, community members and agencies, regional culture and values, and regulatory and governmental agencies.
CDC, Centers for Disease Control and Prevention; HCT, healthcare team; PH, population health; QSEN, Quality and Safety Education for Nurses.

4. The Youth Risk Behavior Surveillance System (YRBSS; www.cdc.gov/healthyyouth/data/yrbs/index.htm) monitors six health-related behaviors that contribute to the leading causes of death and disability among youth and adults. Review the YRBSS data for your home state available on the previously noted website. What behavior was most surprising to you?
5. *Healthy People 2030* (https://health.gov/healthypeople). *Healthy People 2030* objectives are organized into topics. Pick a topic of interest on the website and review the objectives. Then explore the Tools for Action and identify an evidence-based resource related to what you learned.
6. Panel Management: Provide Preventative Care and Improve Patient Health (https://edhub.ama-assn.org/steps-forward/module/2702192#:~:text=Panel%20management%20is%20the%20process,practice%20is%20responsible%20for%20receive) is a learning module that describes the steps to implement panel management and the benefits of using panel management.

SPRINGER PUBLISHING CONNECT™

A robust set of instructor resources designed to supplement this text is located at **http://connect.springerpub.com/content/book/978-0-8261-6145-1.** Qualifying instructors may request access by emailing **textbook@springerpub.com.**

REFERENCES

Agency for Healthcare Research and Quality. (2013). *Module 20. Facilitating panel management.* Practice Facilitation Handbook. http://www.ahrq.gov/ncepcr/tools/pf-handbook/mod20.html

Alliance for Health Equity. (2019). *Community health needs assessment for Chicago and suburban Cook County.* https://allhealthequity.org/wp-content/uploads/2019/06/FINAL_2019_CHNA-Report_Alliance-for-Health-Equity.pdf

American Nurses Association. (2015). *Nursing informatics: Scope and standards of practice* (2nd ed.). Nursebooks.org.

Anthony, M. (2019). The legacy of Lillian Wald: *Home Healthcare Now*, *37*(4), 189. https://doi.org/10.1097/NHH.0000000000000806

Association of Clinicians for the Underserved. (2015). *What is a patient-centered medical home (PCMH)?* https://www.pcpcc.org/resource/patient-centered-medical-home-what-patient-centered-medical-home-pcmh

Bharmal, N., Derose, K. P., Felician, M., & Weden, M. M. (2015). *Understanding the upstream Social Determinants of Health* (p. 20). RAND Corporation. https://www.rand.org/content/dam/rand/pubs/working_papers/WR1000/WR1096/RAND_WR1096.pdf

Biernacki, P. J., Champagne, M. T., Peng, S., Maizel, D. R., & Turner, B. S. (2015). Transformation of care: Integrating the registered nurse care coordinator into the patient-centered medical home. *Population Health Management*, *18*(5), 330–336. https://doi.org/10.1089/pop.2014.0131

Bodenheimer, T., & Bauer, L. (2015). Rethinking the primary care workforce—An expanded role for nurses. *New England Journal of Medicine*, *375*(11), 1015–1017. https://doi.org/10.1056/NEJMp1606869

Borenstein, J. E., Aronow, H. U., Bolton, L. B., Dimalanta, M. I., Chan, E., Palmer, K., Zhang, X., Rosen, B., & Braunstein, G. D. (2016). Identification and team-based interprofessional management of hospitalized vulnerable older adults. *Nursing Outlook*, *64*(2), 137–145. https://doi.org/10.1016/j.outlook.2015.11.014

Braveman, P., Egerter, S., & Williams, D. R. (2011). The social determinants of health: Coming of age. *Annual Review of Public Health*, *32*(1), 381–398. https://doi.org/10.1146/annurev-publhealth-031210-101218

British Columbia Health Link. (2016). *Tertiary prevention.* https://www.healthlinkbc.ca/physical-activity/tertiary-prevention

Centers for Disease Control and Prevention. (n.d.-a). *Adolescent and school health: YRBSS results.* https://www.cdc.gov/healthyyouth/data/yrbs/results.htm

Centers for Disease Control and Prevention. (n.d.-b). *Population health training. What is population health?* https://www.cdc.gov/pophealthtraining/whatis.html

Cleveland, K. A., Motter, T., & Smith, Y. (2019). Affordable care: Harnessing the power of nurses. *The Online Journal of Nursing Issues, 24*(2), 2. https://doi.org/10.3912/OJIN.Vol24No02Man02

Coughlin, S. S. (2019). Social determinants of breast cancer risk, stage, and survival. *Breast Cancer Research and Treatment, 177*(3), 537–548. https://doi.org/10.1007/s10549-019-05340-7

Craig, K. J. T., McKillop, M. M., Huang, H. T., George, J., Punwani, E. S., & Rhee, K. B. (2020). U.S. hospital performance methodologies: A scoping review to identify opportunities for crossing the quality chasm. *BMC Health Services Research, 20*(1), Article 640. https://doi.org/10.1186/s12913-020-05503-z

Cronenwett, L., Sherwood, G., Barnsteiner J., Disch, J., Johnson, J., Mitchell, P., Sullivan, D., & Warren, J. (2007). Quality and Safety Education for Nurses. *Nursing Outlook, 55*(3), 122–131. https://doi.org/10.1016/j.outlook.2007.02.006

Diez Roux, A. V. (2016). On the distinction—Or lack of distinction—Between population health and public health. *American Journal of Public Health, 106*(4), 619–620. https://doi.org/10.2105/AJPH.2016.303097

Dolansky, M. A., & Moore, S. M. (2013). Quality and Safety Education for Nurses (QSEN): The key is systems thinking. *OJIN: The Online Journal of Issues in Nursing, 18*(3), Manuscript 1. https://doi.org/10.3912/OJIN.Vol18No03Man01

Engle, T., & Campbell, L. A. (2019). *Key action areas for addressing social determinants of health through a public health nursing lens.* Quad Council Coalition of Public Health Nursing Organizations. https://www.cphno.org/wp-content/uploads/2020/09/QCC-Report-to-NAM-FON2020-2030_2019.11.21-1.pdf

Fawcett, J., & Ellenbecker, C. H. (2015). A proposed conceptual model of nursing and population health. *Nursing Outlook, 63*(3), 288–298. https://doi.org/10.1016/j.outlook.2015.01.009

Gamache, R., Kharrazi, H., & Weiner, J. (2018). Public and population health informatics: The bridging of big data to benefit communities. *Yearbook of Medical Informatics, 27*(01), 199–206. https://doi.org/10.1055/s-0038-1667081

Gruber, J. B., Wang, W., Quittner, A., Salyakina, D., & McCafferty-Fernandez, J. (2019). Utilizing community health needs assessments (CHNAs) in nonprofit hospitals to guide population-centered outcomes research for pediatric patients: New recommendations for CHNA reporting. *Population Health Managments, 22*(1), 25–31. http://doi.org/10.1089/pop.2018.0049

Hahn, R. A., & Truman, B. I. (2015). Education improves public health and promotes health equity. *International Journal of Health Services*, *45*(4), 657–678. https://doi.org/10.1177/0020731415585986

Institute for Healthcare Improvement. (2020). *Triple Aim for populations: IHI - Institute for Healthcare Improvement.* http://www.ihi.org:80/Topics/TripleAim/Pages/default.aspx

Institute of Medicine. (1988). *The future of public health.* National Academies Press. https://doi.org/10.17226/1091

Institute of Medicine. (2001). *Crossing the quality chasm: A new health system for the 21st century.* National Academies Press. https://doi.org/10.17226/10027

Interprofessional Education Collaborative. (2016). *Core competencies for interprofessional collaborative practice: 2016 update.* https://ipec.memberclicks.net/assets/2016-Update.pdf

Kaminetzky, C. P., & Nelson, K. M. (2015). In the office and in-between: The role of panel management in primary care. *Journal of General Internal Medicine, 30*(7), 876–877. https://doi.org/10.1007/s11606-015-3310-x

Kerns, C., & Willis, D. (2020, March 16). *The problem with U.S. health care isn't a shortage of doctors*. Harvard Business Review. https://hbr.org/2020/03/the-problem-with-u-s-health-care-isnt-a-shortage-of-doctors

Kindig, D., & Stoddart, G. (2003). What is population health? *American Journal of Public Health, 93*(3), 380–383. https://doi.org/10.2105/AJPH.93.3.380

Mariano, M. A., & Harmon, M. J. (2019). Living libraries: Nurse integration in interprofessional homeless health care team. *Public Health Nursing, 36*(2), 172–177. https://doi.org/10.1111/phn.12561

National Association of School Nurses. (2018). *Healthy communities—The role of the school nurse* (Position Statement). https://www.nasn.org/advocacy/professional-practice-documents/position-statements/ps-healthy-communities

Ohio Department of Health. (2020). *2018 infant mortality annual report*. https://odh.ohio.gov/wps/portal/gov/odh/know-our-programs/infant-and-fetal-mortality/reports/2018-ohio-infant-mortality-report

Pariser, P., Pham, T. T., Brown, J. B., Stewart, M., & Charles, J. (2019). Connecting people with multimorbidity to interprofessional teams using telemedicine. *The Annals of Family Medicine, 17*(Suppl. 1), S57–S62. https://doi.org/10.1370/afm.2379

Peig, N. N. A., Ansryan, L., Mamais, F., Appleby, R., dela Cruz, K., Caffarini, E., Yoo, J., Holden, K., Brasel, J., Gorman, E., Guy, T., Duong, B., Furukawa, M., Chhan, K., Ward, C., & Miller, P. S. (2020). Implementing SAFE™ care: Evaluation of a geriatric model of care for real-world practice. *Geriatric Nursing , 42*(1), 167–172. https://doi.org/10.1016/j.gerinurse.2020.09.009

Perez Jolles, M., Lengnick-Hall, R., & Mittman, B. S. (2019). Core functions and forms of complex health interventions: A patient-centered medical home illustration. *Journal of General Internal Medicine, 34*(6), 1032–1038. https://doi.org/10.1007/s11606-018-4818-7

Reno, R., & Hyder, A. (2018). The evidence base for Social Determinants of Health as risk factors for infant mortality: A systematic scoping review. *Journal of Health Care for the Poor and Underserved, 29*(4), 1188–1208. https://doi.org/10.1353/hpu.2018.0091

Reynolds, A., Rubens, J., King, R., & Machado, P. (2016). *Technology and engagement: How digital tools are reshaping population health*. https://populationhealthalliance.org/wp-content/uploads/2018/02/pha_paper_techandengagement.pdf

Salmond, S. W., & Echevarria, M. (2017). Healthcare transformation and changing roles for nursing. *Orthopedic Nursing, 36*(1), 12–25. https://doi.org/10.1097/NOR.0000000000000308

Scholz, J., & Minaudo, J. (2015). Registered nurse care coordination: Creating a preferred future for older adults with multimorbidity. *Online Journal of Issues in Nursing, 20*(3), 4. https://doi.org/10.3912/OJIN.Vol20No03Man04

Storfjell, J. L., Winslow, B. W., & Saunders, J., S. D. (2018). *Catalyst for change: Harnessing the power of nurses to build population health in the 21st century*. Robert Wood Johnson Foundation. https://www.rwjf.org/en/library/research/2017/09/catalysts-for-change--harnessing-the-power-of-nurses-to-build-population-health.html

Stoto, M. A. (2013). *Population health in the Affordable Care Act era—Digital Collections—National Library of Medicine*. Academy Health. http://resource.nlm.nih.gov/101655439

University of Wisconsin Population Health Institute. (2021). *County health rankings & roadmaps*. https://www.countyhealthrankings.org

U.S. Department of Health and Human Services. (n.d.). *Social determinants of health*. https://health.gov/healthypeople/objectives-and-data/social-determinants-health

Wakefield, M. K., Williams, D. R., Le Menestrel, S., & Flaubert, J. L. (Eds.). (2021). *The future of nursing 2020–2030: Charting a path to achieve health equity*. National Academies Press. https://doi.org/10.17226/25982.

Whelton, P. K., Carey, R. M., Aronow, W. S., Casey, D. E., Collins, K. J., Dennison Himmelfarb, C., DePalma, S. M., Gidding, S., Jamerson, K. A., Jones, D. W., MacLaughlin, E. J., Muntner, P., Ovbiagele, B., Smith, S. C., Spencer, C. C., Stafford, R. S., Taler, S. J., Thomas, R. J., Williams, K. A., … & Wright, J. T. (2018). 2017 ACC/AHA/AAPA/ABC/ACPM/AGS/APhA/ASH/ASPC/NMA/PCNA Guideline for the Prevention, Detection, Evaluation, and Management of High Blood Pressure in Adults. *Journal of the American College of Cardiology, 71*(19), e127–e248. https://doi.org/10.1016/j.jacc.2017.11.006

World Health Organization. (2010). *Framework for action on interprofessional education and collaborative practice*. http://apps.who.int/iris/bitstream/handle/10665/70185/WHO_HRH_HPN_10.3_eng.pdf

Zborowsky, T. (2014). The legacy of Florence Nightingale's environmental theory: Nursing research focusing on the impact of healthcare environments. *HERD: Health Environments Research & Design Journal, 7*(4), 19–34. https://doi.org/10.1177/193758671400700404

SUGGESTED READINGS

Fernandez, M. E., Ruiter, R. A. C., Markham, C. M., & Kok, G. (2019). Intervention mapping: Theory- and evidence-based health promotion program planning: Perspective and examples. *Frontiers in Public Health, 7*, Article 209. https://doi.org/10.3389/fpubh.2019.00209

Kelly, C., Templeton, M., Allen, K., & Lohan, M. (2020). Improving sexual healthcare delivery for men in prison: A nurse-led initiative. *Journal of Clinical Nursing, 29*, 2285–2292. https://doi.org/10.1111/jocn.15237

Long, K. N. G., Kim, E. S., Chen, Y., Wilson, M. F., Worthington, E. L., & VanderWeele, T. J. (2020). The role of hope in subsequent health and well-being for older adults: An outcome-wide longitudinal approach. *Global Epidemiology, 2*, 100018. https://doi.org/10.1016/j.gloepi.2020.100018

Lönnberg, L., Damberg, M., & Revenäs, Å. (2020). "It's up to me": The experience of patients at high risk of cardiovascular disease of lifestyle change. *Scandinavian Journal of Primary Health Care, 38*(3), 340–351. https://doi.org/10.1080/02813432.2020.1794414

Nanna, M. G., Wang, T. Y., Xiang, Q., Goldberg, A. C., Robinson, J. G., Roger, V. L., Virani, S. V., Wilson, P. W. F., Louie, M. J., Koren, A., Li, Z., Peterson, E. D., & Navar, A. M. (2019). Sex differences in the use of statins in community practice: Patient and provider assessment of lipid management registry. *Circulation: Cardiovascular Quality and Outcomes, 12*(8), e005562. https://doi.org/10.1161/CIRCOUTCOMES.118.005562

Philbin, M. M., Parker, C. M., Flaherty, M. G., & Hirsch, J. S. (2019). Public libraries: A community-level resource to advance population health. *Journal of Community Health, 44*, 192–199. https://doi.org/10.1007/s10900-018-0547-4

Plumer, B., & Popovich, N. (2020, August). How decades of racist housing policy left neighborhoods sweltering. *New York Times*. https://www.nytimes.com/interactive/2020/08/24/climate/racism-redlining-cities-global-warming.html

Szanton, S. L., Han, H., Campbell, J., Reynolds, N., Dennison-Himmelfarb, C. R., Perrin, N., & Davidson, P. M. (2019). Shifting paradigms to build resilience among patients and families experiencing multiple chronic conditions. *Journal of Clinical Nursing, 29*(19–20), 3591–3594. https://doi.org/10.1111/jocn.15145

Wardecker, B. M., & Matsick, J. L. (2020). Families of choice and community connectedness: A brief guide to the social strengths of LGBTQ older adults. *Journal of Gerontological Nursing, 46*(2) 5–8. https://doi.org/10.3928/00989134-20200113-01

Whitehouse, P., & George, D. (2018). From intergenerational to intergenerative: Towards the futures of intergenerational learning and health. *Journal of Intergenerational Relationships, 16*(1–2), 196–204. https://doi.org/10.1080/15350770.2018.1404862

CHAPTER 16

Professional Role Development in Patient Safety and Quality: Transitioning to Practice

Loraine Hopkins Pepe

"Believe you can and you're halfway there."

–*Theodore Roosevelt*

Upon completion of this chapter, the reader should be able to:

1. Describe professional development through the lens of the Novice to Expert Model.
2. Discuss the role nursing orientation has in the transition to practice.
3. Analyze how present-day Transition to Practice Programs complement traditional orientation methodologies.
4. Compare and contrast the influence of mentors and preceptors in clinical practice.
5. Describe the impact of regulatory agencies and national initiatives on quality and safety and how these influence nursing transition into practice.
6. Discuss nursing's role with nursing-sensitive indicator outcomes to understand how individual nursing practice impacts patient care and the financial well-being of organizations.
7. Describe the integration of quality and safety competencies into nursing orientation programs and the impact on nursing practice.
8. Explore strategies to foster nursing professional development that support high quality and safe care in clinical practice.
9. Identify pathways for transitioning to leadership roles after orientation.

CROSSWALK

This chapter addresses the following:

QSEN Competencies: Quality and Safety, Evidence-Based Practice, Safety, Informatics, Teamwork and Collaboration

The American Association of Colleges of Nursing. (2021). *The essentials: Core competencies for professional nursing education.*

Domain 5: Quality and Safety
Domain 9: Professionalism
Domain 10: Personal, Professional, and Leadership Development

OPENING SCENARIO

Javier, a new-to-practice nurse, graduated from nursing school 3 months ago. He has since passed his National Council Licensure Examination (NCLEX-RN®) and has accepted his first nursing position. Javier's new position is in a busy, 800-bed academic medical center, where he will be working on a fast-paced, high acuity medical-surgical unit. Although he is nervous, Javier is excited to begin this next chapter in his nursing journey. He has completed all the hospital's pre-hire requirements and is ready to begin the Nurse Residency Program.

1. How will Javier's nursing orientation program influence his success in his new position?
2. How can Javier's completion of a Nurse Residency Program foster his successful transition into practice?
3. How does a nursing preceptor and mentor influence transition into practice?

INTRODUCTION

This chapter describes the influence nursing orientation programs have on the successful transition of new nurses into the practice setting. It describes the role or orientation and how Transition to Practice Programs are integral in meeting the ever-changing demands of contemporary nursing practice. The influence and important role of mentors and preceptors is also highlighted. This chapter includes a discussion of the impact regulatory agencies have on the nursing profession, recognizing that nurses play a vital role in patient outcomes. A review of current nursing-sensitive indicators is included. Nursing-sensitive indicators provide nurses with a blueprint for the delivery of high-quality nursing care, ultimately achieving the goal of preventing patient harm. Integration of quality and safety competencies into nursing orientation programs, and the impact this can have on the perceptions of newly hired RNs, is examined. Lastly, this chapter includes a discussion about nursing professional development and leadership focusing on the role these have in quality and safety.

BENNER'S PROFESSIONAL DEVELOPMENT MODEL

The healthcare environment is fast-paced and constantly evolving. Technological advances, coupled with the complexity of patients' conditions, require the skills of highly functioning, knowledgeable practitioners. As critical members of the healthcare team, nurses are frequently confronted with challenging scenarios. Prompt, efficient responses are often needed. The critical thinking abilities and technical skills of the nurse are the underpinnings of excellent patient care delivery. Patients rely on expert nurses to anticipate their needs, to prevent adverse events, and to provide exceptional, safe care. Hospitals also depend on highly functioning expert practitioners. When the workforce is composed of technically proficient, critically thinking, customer service-oriented professional nurses, positive patient outcomes ensue. Acquiring the necessary skills and confidence to perform at this high level takes time to develop.

Patricia Benner, a nursing theorist who applied the Dreyfus Model of Skill Acquisition to the nursing profession, identified and categorized levels of nursing competency in clinical nursing practice (Benner, 1984). This model posits that in order to acquire and develop clinical skills of an expert nurse, a nursing student or new nurse passes through five levels of proficiency over time, specifically, moving from novice, to advanced beginner, to competent, to proficient, and finally expert (Benner, 1984). It is important to note that the acquisition of clinical knowledge and progression through the five levels takes years to achieve. Benner defines a novice as anyone, nursing student or inexperienced nurse, working in a new setting or with an unfamiliar population of patients where the new nurse or nursing student has little to no experience (Benner, 1984). Competence is achieved over time, usually within 2 to 3 years after consistently practicing in the same setting (Benner, 1984). Nursing students or new nurses can also function at the advanced beginner stage, where they can demonstrate beginning levels of satisfactory performance (Benner, 1984). Despite the level of proficiency demonstrated by new-to-practice nurses, it is clear that entering the high-stress, rapidly changing environment of healthcare requires support in order to gain the confidence and skills to succeed. Foundational needs related to knowledge and skill must be effectively identified and addressed to successfully provide quality, safe care.

Transition from the academic setting to clinical practice is frequently filled with anxiety and challenges for many novice nurses. Often overwhelmed, new-to-practice RNs struggle to acquire vast amounts of knowledge while working to achieve technical competence. At the same time, novice nurses are expected to improve self-efficacy skills, increase confidence levels, and develop a strong professional identity. Fortunately, there are many ways to promote success for novice nurses.

An initial step to bridge the gap from academia to practice is to provide newly practicing RNs with orientation and Transition to Practice Programs, framed by quality and safety competencies. Providing quality- and safety-framed orientation and Transition to Practice Programs allows new graduate nurses to enhance their competence, while offering new knowledge to RNs who have not yet been exposed to the core content of quality and safety competencies. Having a full understanding of the competencies of person-centered care, interprofessional teams, evidence-based practice (EBP), quality improvement, safety, and informatics promotes a smoother transition into the practice setting and fosters quality care delivery.

THE ROLE OF NURSING ORIENTATION IN TRANSITION TO PRACTICE

Nursing orientation is a formal program offered to all newly hired RNs and is influential in the success, retention, and transition of new RNs. Nursing orientation is a crucial component of the onboarding process that occurs in hospitals across the United States An effective, structured orientation program is a safeguard built into the practice setting that promotes the preparation of new nurses. The goals of nursing orientation are varied and have many emphases, with essential components including introducing new RNs to the mission, vision, and philosophy of the organization while providing the skills needed for nursing competence.

Orientation programs are divided into different levels, specifically, the initial classroom-based hospital-wide nursing orientation program followed by a unit-based clinical orientation. Newly hired RNs begin their journey by attending a 4- to 7-day program occurring in the classroom setting, where new nurses are welcomed into the organization. Information provided focuses on policies, procedures, protocols, and skills needed for new nurses to safely begin practicing. Typically, orientation programs begin with presentations from senior nursing leaders who introduce the organization's mission, vision, and professional nursing practice model. Senior nursing leaders effectively link those important concepts to nursing services and nursing care delivery. In most settings, many topics are presented ranging from descriptions of quality initiatives to demonstration and return demonstration of high-risk skills. To prevent harm and enhance safety, instruction is provided on the correct and safe use of the electronic medical record (EMR), point-of-care testing equipment, resuscitation carts, and safe patient handling equipment.

After completion of the initial hospital-wide nursing orientation program, unit-based orientation begins and takes place in the clinical setting. During this time, newly hired RNs are assigned **clinical preceptors**, skilled nurses who are responsible for assessing, supporting, and evaluating the learning and skill acquisition of newly hired RNs. Unit-based orientation programs are individualized to meet the needs of newly hired RNs and vary in length from 12 weeks to 12 months, depending on the nursing specialty and the experience level of the new RN. The goal of the unit-based orientation is to develop clinical competency, enhance critical thinking abilities, and fortify clinical decision-making skills.

The unit-based orientation is guided by the clinical preceptor who provides close supervision and promotes knowledge and skill acquisition while influencing the socialization of new nurses into the practice setting (Mathen & Hoke, 2020). Clinical preceptors are competent nurses with additional training for the role that allows them to teach clinical skills, provide robust feedback, demonstrate effective communication skills, and exemplify professionalism while supporting the new-to-practice nurse to gain confidence and comfort in the nursing role. Dimino et al. (2020) found that for newly graduated nurses, nurse preceptors were a source of significant support, often creating a welcoming and supportive environment. Preceptors are influential in fostering the acceptance of new nurses into the unit culture and helping them to become members of the team.

As a final point, nursing orientation is a time for newly hired RNs to acclimate to their new positions. Transition into practice is enhanced when new nurses become knowledgeable about the nursing specialty in which they practice, while also acquiring new skills for the clinical setting. To enhance a successful transition, it is imperative for new-to-practice nurses to ask questions, stay informed, engage in unit activities, and seek advice from trusted colleagues.

CURRENT LITERATURE

CITATION

McPhee, K. (2018). Deliberate practice mock codes for new graduate nurses. *Journal for Nurses in Professional Development, 34*, 348–351. https://doi.org/10.1097/NND.0000000000000494

DISCUSSION

New-to-practice nurses frequently lack confidence in their skills, often feeling inadequately prepared for the practice setting. One of the most anxiety provoking situations described by new nurses is responding to emergency situations when a patient's clinical condition is deteriorating. Mock code simulations are provided to assist with learning these important skills; frequently new nurses request repeat mock code sessions and additional simulation time. In order to meet the requests and educational needs of the new-to-practice nurse, one academic medical center implemented a process called "deliberate practice" to further enhance the skills of their staff. Rapid cycle deliberate practice involves having the learner practice a skill in a simulation setting, receive immediate feedback, and continue to practice the skill repeatedly until competence is demonstrated. Educators and learners have found that this method enhances the skill of the learner, improves teamwork, allows challenging concepts and skills to be broken down into smaller components, and increases retention of information.

IMPLICATIONS FOR PRACTICE

Deliberate practice mock codes are an evidence-based educational method which enables new-to-practice nurses to gain the confidence and skills needed to successfully care for a patient during an emergency. Immediate feedback and repetition of skills provide a safe environment in which to make mistakes, learn the correct procedure, and implement suggested changes to individual practice. Mock codes teach new nurses teamwork skills and provide an opportunity to evaluate their progress, so they may successfully care for a patient during a critical emergency.

TRANSITION TO PRACTICE PROGRAMS AS NURSE RESIDENCIES

Nursing orientation programs are the initial step in what creates a robust organizational culture supporting transition into practice. **Transition to Practice Programs**, often referred to as **Nurse Residency Programs**, are structured programs of active learning for newly licensed nurses, designed to support the transition from education to practice. Van Patten and Bartone (2018) have identified that the effectiveness of Nurse Residency Programs impacts competency and confidence of the nurse and is a significant predictor of outcomes related to job performance. They have become the gold standard for supporting the transition of new-to-practice nurses into the practice arena (Slate et al., 2018).

New-to-practice nurses often have unique concerns as they begin their nursing careers. Transitioning into practice is a challenging time, frequently filled with confusion, as new RNs grapple with acquiring new skills and assuming new roles. Novice nurses can find themselves feeling ill-prepared to tackle the challenges of contemporary nursing, resulting in increased stress, anxiety, and patient safety issues (Dimino et al., 2020). Complex patient populations, lofty performance expectations, little confidence, and the practice-knowledge mismatch can hamper the successful transition of new graduate nurses into clinical practice (Dimino et al., 2020).

The academic-practice gap has been an enduring problem for decades. Academic partners criticize their practice partners for having unrealistic expectations, while practice partners hold academe responsible for inadequately preparing new nurses for the practice environment (Huston et al., 2018). The effect of this perceived gap on newly practicing nurses has been described in the literature. New nurses may become disheartened as they transition from the controlled clinical environment experienced during nursing school to the hectic environment often found in nursing practice. New-to-practice nurses may feel disillusioned as they adapt to higher acuity patients, staffing concerns, and heavier workloads (Huston et al., 2018). As a way to foster a smoother transition into the practice setting and to better meet the needs of newly practicing RNs, academic practice partnerships have been formed to close this perceived gap and to develop well-prepared practitioners.

The need to support new-to-practice nurses has served as the impetus for developing strategies to address the academic-practice gap. High-quality safe nursing care can be promoted and enhanced by having new-to-practice RNs enroll in a Transition to Practice Program. The genesis of Transition to Practice Programs came from the Institute of Medicine's (IOM; now the National Academy of Medicine) report titled, *The Future of Nursing Leading Change, Advancing Health* (2011). In this report, the IOM challenged healthcare organizations to take action to improve patient care by developing and implementing Transition to Practice Programs, specifically designed for nurses to be implemented across all practice settings, regardless of specialty. The IOM also charged healthcare organizations to develop plans to ensure that these programs be sustainable with metrics evaluating their effectiveness.

The National Council of State Boards of Nursing (NCSBN; 2008) was one of the first organizations to respond to the IOM's call for reform by developing the original Transition to Practice Program. Hospitals have used the NCSBN's program as the model for creating Nurse Residency Programs ever since. The NCSBN recognized that new graduate nurses in beginning practice roles described the experience as stressful, with it often resulting in high attrition rates (NCSBN, 2017). Additionally, nursing stress has been linked to increased patient safety risks and decreased nurse engagement (NCSBN, 2017). Early on, the NCSBN recognized the value of quality and safety and utilized the Quality and Safety Education for Nurses (QSEN) competencies of Person-Centered Care, Communication and Teamwork, Evidence-Based Practice, Quality Improvement, Safety, and Informatics as the foundation for development of their Transition to Practice Program (Huston et al., 2018; NCSBN, 2017). Subsequently, they conducted the Transition to Practice Study, investigating whether their newly developed program effected a change in new graduate nurses' transition into practice as well as quality and safety outcomes (NCSBN, 2017). Results indicated the program positively impacted new nurses' performance, outcomes in care delivery, and confidence levels (NCSBN, 2017).

Many hospital systems have established evidence-based Nurse Residency Programs and they all share common goals. Most essential of these goals is to form a bridge from the academic setting to the practice setting for new-to-practice nurses, promoting a successful transition into their first role as a professional nurse. Other goals include supporting delivery of quality and safe care, optimizing patient outcomes, and fostering job satisfaction. Achieving these goals can result in a decrease in nurse turnover and an increase in nurse retention after 1 year. Nurse retention is important for many reasons, including the financial well-being of healthcare organizations. With the average cost of replacing a bedside RN being more than $50,000, it is estimated that RN turnover will cost hospitals millions of dollars per year (Nursing Solutions, Inc., 2020). Losses such as these can have a significant impact on the financial well-being of healthcare organizations.

Nurse Residency Programs teach strategies to enhance the critical thinking, clinical decision-making, and interprofessional teamwork abilities of new nurses (Slate et al., 2018). There is an increased focus on quality and safety with discussions highlighting how quality and safety are intimately tied to patient outcomes. The curriculum for most programs includes activities where technical skills are taught. Simulations of emergent situations provide opportunities to learn useful tools for navigating through a rapid response call or a cardiac arrest situation. Many nontechnical, self-care skills are also included. Often new-to-practice nurses are grouped as a cohort and view their time together as a safe space where they share experiences encountered in the clinical setting. This provides them with a certain degree of camaraderie with other new nurses who may be experiencing similar situations and who are able to provide needed feedback and support. New nurses working in complex environments may experience stress and anxiety. As a result, many programs offer seminars on stress management and resilience. Learning stress management techniques, along with support and continued training, have been found to promote successful transition into practice (Chesak et al., 2019).

Each Nurse Residency Program differs in the delivery method of the content with some using a virtual learning platform, others providing in-person presentations, and others using a hybrid of virtual learning and in-person presentations. Frequently, Nurse Residency Programs are 1-year in duration and include monthly educational seminars. Most programs include education on conducting an EBP project with the expectation that the new-to-practice nurse will implement a project on their nursing unit. New nurses may complete an EBP project individually or choose to partner with another new nurse. Since they are novice nurses who may have never completed a project like this before, support and guidance are provided by senior nurses and nurse educators throughout the process.

Nurse Residency Programs have a positive impact on multiple stakeholders. For new-to-practice nurses, tools are provided to promote and fortify their success as they develop enhanced clinical skills, improved decision-making capabilities, and gain a fuller understanding of EBP. For hospital administrators, new-to-practice RNs bring the latest evidence in nursing science and a refreshing and positive energy to the organization. Additionally, successful completion of Nurse Residency Programs has shown demonstrated improvement in retention rates and nurse satisfaction scores. Lastly, and most importantly, patients are positively impacted as they receive high-quality nursing care from confident new-to-practice nurses.

Real World Interview

Nurse Residency Programs assist new-to-practice nurses in transitioning to their new positions by providing a strong foundation at this beginning stage of their professional development. The curriculum offers a broad view of healthcare both from the clinical and business standpoint. The Nurse Residency Program educates the new-to-practice nurse on skills like performing tracheostomy care but also provides opportunities to participate in situational learning, such as with a simulation of a decompensating patient that requires the nurse to respond in an urgent manner. New-to-practice nurses are also enlightened about the business and financial aspects of healthcare and understand the impact of their role in quality outcomes. The completion of EBP initiatives captures the essence of the Nurse Residency Program because it validates new-to-practice nurses' development of leadership skills at the point of care, their understanding of quality outcomes, and their professional role as a nurse.

The best strategy for helping new-to-practice nurses succeed is to align them with people who are willing to take them under their wing and create opportunities to support their professional development that build their confidence and competence within the profession. To succeed, new-to-practice nurses must be proactive in their professional role development and must embrace the philosophy of lifelong learning. Engagement through the participation in unit- or hospital-based committees is a vital part of the transition-to-practice journey. Nurses need to seize every opportunity to advance themselves. These are the avenues that keep nurses excited about the profession and propel them to a life of purpose.

Susan Margaret Benjamin-Mlynarczuk

Nurse Residency Coordinator & Clinical Nurse Educator

Albert Einstein Medical Center Philadelphia,Philadelphia, Pennsylvania

THE ROLE OF PRECEPTORS AND MENTORS

Orientation is a time when a new nurse can feel uncomfortable and need encouragement, guidance, and direction (Mathen & Hoke, 2020). Many variables influence the success of new-to-practice nurses with clinical preceptors and mentors playing vital roles (Van Patten & Bartone, 2018). Although often discussed interchangeably, preceptors and mentors have different roles that emphasize different characteristics (Table 16.1).

TABLE 16.1 DIFFERENCES BETWEEN PRECEPTING AND MENTORING

PRECEPTING	MENTORING
Preceptor is assigned by a nurse manager or clinical nurse specialist/clinical nurse educator.	Mentor is sought out by mentee–can be a colleague within or outside of the nursing discipline.
Follows a formal program of preparing new nurses.	Mentee establishes personal and professional goals. Mentor shares expertise and advice.
Relationship has an ending; exists during the time of the orientation period.	Relationship is long-term; can continue for an indefinite period of time.
Focus is on helping orientee develop a specific set of skills.	Focus is on fostering the mentee's growth and professional development.
Evaluates competencies in practice setting.	Provides personal, professional, and career advice and support.

ROLE AND CHARACTERISTICS OF PRECEPTORS

Preceptorship is a widely used clinical learning method for practice-based professions such as nursing that involves the selection of a clinical preceptor who is willing to teach and work with a new nurse, also known as an orientee (Quek & Shorey, 2018). This pairing of the orientee with the experienced, skilled preceptor is assigned by the nurse manager with input from the unit's clinical nurse specialist and/or clinical nurse educator. Ideally, a new nurse orientee should have two preceptors who expose the new nurse to multiple teaching styles, clinical skill sets, and approaches to the work (Mathen & Hoke, 2020). When matching the nurse preceptor with the orientee, the pairing is based on multiple considerations. Because the preceptor is the first nurse who intensely devotes time and energy to the new nurse, the preceptor should be a clinical role model who possesses competency in the required unit-based skills. Professionalism of the preceptor is significant because it is a core value strongly influencing the success of the orientee. Preceptors role model behavior and attitudes that socialize new orientees into their new roles, the unit culture, and workplace traditions. Socialization is one of the underpinnings needed for new nurses to gain a sense of belonging in their new environment.

A common misconception in nursing is that any competent RN can function in the role of a preceptor. This is simply untrue. It is important to select only those nurses who express an interest in serving as a preceptor, since those without an interest can have a damaging effect on new-to-practice nurses, often causing frustration and dismay in the orientee (Quek & Shorey, 2018). For these reasons, experienced RNs interested in becoming a preceptor are provided with a formal course through which they learn the roles and responsibilities of being a preceptor. Within the course, preceptors learn about the tools necessary for assessing competency, understanding diverse learning styles, providing constructive feedback, promoting clear communication, and implementing appropriate styles of conflict management and resolution.

Upon completion of the course, the preceptor is eligible to begin functioning in the role. As educators, preceptors identify the learning needs of the orientee and, by seeking out additional learning opportunities, they enhance the knowledge and skills of the orientee. Preceptors offer new nurses one-to-one support as they provide guidance with care delivery (Quek & Shorey, 2018). Most important to the learning process of the orientee is that, while affording these opportunities in the clinical setting, preceptors demonstrate significant patience (Mathen & Hoke, 2020). By nurturing competence and confidence, preceptors are influential in increasing skill sets, improving job satisfaction, and enhancing retention of new-to-practice nurses (Quek & Shorey, 2018).

Preceptors need to know the background and experience level of the new nursing orientee. According to Benner (1984), many new-to-practice nurses or nurses new to a specialty are at the advanced beginner stage of proficiency. Preceptors need to appreciate the level of competency of orientees since it influences selection of teaching methods and provision of appropriate learning opportunities. A novice nurse struggles to predict what might happen in various clinical scenarios because of limited clinical exposures. Without experience, clinical judgment, and prioritization skills, novice nurses are frequently unable to discern relevant from irrelevant facts (Benner, 1984), finding themselves overwhelmed by most clinical circumstances and preoccupied with missing something of importance. But advanced beginners may be more adept at recognizing components of situations even if they lack sufficient in-depth experiences from which to draw upon. Advanced beginners rely on rules, guidelines, and policies to determine what is required in various situations. The advanced beginner depends on the skill of the experienced preceptor to assist with identifying priorities and fully understanding situations (Benner, 1984). In order to increase their skills, advanced beginners work best with a nonjudgmental preceptor, who provides a safe environment in which to ask questions. Preceptors should also recognize that these groups of new nurses thrive in an environment filled with simulation sessions, skills labs, and observational experiences to best foster their learning (Mathen & Hoke, 2020).

Professional development meetings are an important component of orientation, where the preceptor(s), new nurse, nurse manager, clinical nurse specialist, or clinical nurse educator meet routinely to discuss clinical progress and professional development. The frequency of these meetings may vary; however, most facilities hold these meetings every 2 to 3 weeks. During the meetings, knowledge acquisition is discussed, and assessment, communication, and technical skills are reviewed. These meetings provide time to examine strengths of the new nurse, identify opportunities for enhancing clinical decision-making, and develop plans for educational support. After reviewing the progression of the orientation, competency achievement is documented, and goals are established for the upcoming weeks. Based on the new nurse's progress, recommendations are made regarding increasing the acuity and volume of the patient assignments. Professional development meetings are instrumental in determining the necessary length of orientation and deciding when the new nurse can safely anticipate practicing independently. The formal preceptor-orientee relationship comes to a close at the end of the orientation period, but the comradery developed between preceptor and orientee can continue for many years.

ROLE AND CHARACTERISTICS OF MENTORS

Many people confuse precepting and mentoring. Although they share a few common traits, there are distinct differences (Table 16.1). A **mentor** is an experienced, trusted, respected professional who possesses expert knowledge and skill in their field and provides personal, professional, and career support to another, often referred to as the mentee. The relationship, based on trust, is formed between a novice and an experienced professional with the goal of providing support and strategies for personal and professional growth (Van Patten & Bartone, 2019). This relationship includes the sharing of expertise and advice with the goal of positively influencing the career of the mentee. Frequently mentors provide guidance to mentees in navigating challenging situations or frustrations (Kowalski, 2019). The process of mentoring provides benefits to both parties. For mentees, this relationship can lead to increased professional opportunities and increased career success (Abbajay, 2019). For mentors, there is satisfaction in influencing the growth of a colleague. Organizations that promote mentoring and have robust mentoring programs reap the benefits of enhanced employee engagement and retention (Abbajay, 2019). In order for this to be a successful relationship, there are multiple attributes that must be found in both the mentor and the mentee.

Strong mentors possess the desire to help others grow and learn. During the mentor–mentee relationship, the mentor enhances the quality of the relationship by sharing both experiences that have been successful and those that have failed. Like preceptors, mentors must possess expert knowledge and skill in their field because mentees select a mentor from a field in which they too want to learn, develop, and excel (Abbajay, 2019). A mentor recognizes that the relationship takes significant time and commitment and is prepared to dedicate resources and plan for meetings. Mentors are facilitators, sharing resources and networking skills as part of their role (Kowalski, 2019).

Lastly, mentors must be adept in developing and challenging mentees (Abbajay, 2019; Kowalski, 2019). An important aspect of this is creating a safe environment where the mentee can share successes, challenges, concerns, and disappointments (Kowalski, 2019). Mentors need to be willing to address difficult issues, possess the skill of asking open-ended questions that encourage self-reflection, and be able to actively listen (Abbajay, 2019). Mentors provide guidance to the mentee in learning the skill of giving and receiving feedback (Kowalski, 2019). Most importantly, mentors must be willing to be honest in their approach and advice. It is through this type of candor and sincerity that mentees grow and are inspired to reach their goals.

The mentoring relationship is a shared and collaborative relationship, with accountability for its success divided equally between the mentor and mentee. The critical foundation of the relationship is based on mutual trust and respect. Mentees positively influence the outcome of the relationship by being actively involved and asking appropriate questions not only of their mentors but of themselves (Box 16.1). Reflection will help mentees clearly articulate their expectations and desired outcomes. They should possess a vision for what they want in their careers, both professionally and personally. Mentees need to be flexible, open minded, interested in learning, and willing to implement creative ideas in order to enhance their abilities (Abbajay, 2019). Being receptive to feedback is critically important since feedback is used as a stepping stone to further enhance skills and abilities. Most importantly, mentees must demonstrate personal responsibility and accountability (Abbajay, 2019). It is essential for mentees to be fully present and participate in required meetings with their mentors. There may be additional readings or activities recommended and the mentee is responsible for completing these assignments. Meetings with other experts may be suggested by the mentor, and it would be the mentee's responsibility to schedule and attend each session. Since it is a shared relationship, mentors and mentees must be actively involved in all components of the relationship in order for the mentoring relationship to be successful and sustainable.

BOX 16.1 Questions Asked in a Mentoring Relationship

Questions mentees should reflect upon and ask themselves:

What are my nursing career goals?

Where do I see myself in the next few years?

What do I need to accomplish in order to reach my goals?

Where do I see opportunities for growth?

What are my expectations from the mentoring experience?

What traits does this mentor possess that will push me to grow and influence my success?

What skills does the mentor have that I want to learn?

Am I open to all feedback from my mentor?

Am I willing to put in the time, effort, and energy to implement any suggestions provided?

After each meeting with my mentor, am I willing to reflect and assess what was helpful and what needs to change?

Am I able to discuss my thoughts honestly and openly with my mentor?

Questions mentees should ask their mentors:

What is our meeting format? Will we meet in person, virtually, by phone? How often? Length of meetings?

What are the meeting ground rules and expectations?

Do you feel my expectations are realistic?

How can I enhance my skills in order to achieve my goals?

Where do you see my opportunities for growth?

Can you describe what each of us is responsible for accomplishing?

How do I identify key stakeholders who may be instrumental in my learning?

How do I develop relationships with them?

How do I know if my goals are significant for my career and for the organization?

CASE STUDY

A new-to-practice nurse in the third week of nursing orientation in a busy surgical unit is assigned to care for a 65-year-old male who was admitted to the unit after having had total knee replacement surgery. Upon entering the room, the patient is alert and oriented and happy that his procedure has been successful, but while the nurse performs a head-to-toe assessment, the patient becomes diaphoretic with sudden slurred speech. He cannot effectively move his left arm. The new-to-practice nurse realizes something is wrong, and leaves the patient to find the nurse preceptor. The preceptor arrives and immediately calls for the rapid response team. When the team arrives, many questions are being asked quickly, lab tests are being drawn, and the room is filled with controlled chaos. Feeling inadequate, the new-to-practice nurse stays off to the side of the room hoping that no one asks any further questions. The patient is sent for a stat CT scan and then transferred to the neuro ICU. The nurse preceptor seems disappointed in the new-to-practice nurse's care and provides harsh feedback regarding the way the emergency was handled.

1. *Recognizing Benner's levels of proficiency, at what stage of proficiency is the new-to-practice nurse practicing?*
2. *What would have been the professional action for the preceptor to take to prevent feelings of inadequacy for the new-to-practice nurse?*
3. *How can the new-to-practice nurse address concerns regarding the preceptor's approach and delivery of feedback?*
4. *How can the new nurse improve performance?*

REGULATORY AGENCIES AND NATIONAL INITIATIVES FOR QUALITY AND SAFETY

New-to-practice RNs have an expectation of support and guidance as they enter the workforce. Clinical support is often provided from internal venues that include orientation programs, clinical preceptors, and nursing colleagues. Other sources of support are found outside of the clinical setting. Specifically, regulatory agencies develop standards and guidelines for high-quality care delivery that offer national solutions to the complex issues impacting healthcare. The implementation of these standards ensures nursing care delivery is grounded in quality and safety.

The mission of regulatory agencies and quality-focused organizations is to drive national initiatives to continuously improve healthcare and advance improved health outcomes. All play a major role in ensuring high-quality, safe care delivery. Healthcare regulations standardize practices to safeguard the public from adverse events and harm. National agencies have a responsibility to monitor healthcare facilities and providers to ensure compliance and keep them abreast of changes in practice. The Joint Commission (TJC) and the Institute for Healthcare Improvement (IHI) are organizations who share the common goal of continuously evaluating care delivery, developing standards for practice, and promoting enhanced patient outcomes.

THE JOINT COMMISSION

TJC is the oldest and most well-known agency responsible for providing accreditation status to healthcare facilities that meet high-quality standards (TJC, n.d.). TJC is an important driver for quality, safe care, sharing its mission with many other regulatory agencies to reach the goal of zero patient harm. TJC standards serve as foundational tools to objectively evaluate the performance of healthcare organizations. In 2002, TJC became a champion for patient safety by establishing the National Patient Safety Goals program, which continues to this day. Goals are updated regularly and identified for type of healthcare setting to address the inherent dangers and risks of each. The National Patient Safety Goals for Hospitals are unique to the inpatient setting (Box 16.2) and provide a blueprint for delivery of high-quality, safe care.

The National Patient Safety Goals for Hospital Programs help new nurses gain an understanding of essential safety requirements, while also providing strategies for implementing these requirements. Fully comprehending the goals and ways of incorporating them into practice helps to ensure safe care delivery. Nurses are instrumental in integrating the current National Patient Safety Goals into practice settings. The first patient safety goal focuses on correct patient identification and requires the critical use of two patient identifiers, such as name and date of birth, whenever medications and blood or blood products are administered, or treatments and procedures are performed. To fully meet this goal, in addition to using two patient identifiers, nurses must also confirm that all specimens are labeled at the patient's bedside or in the patient's presence (TJC, 2021). New-to-practice nurses can enforce this patient safety goal by developing and consistently following a systematic process of positive patient identification for all patient interventions. It is vitally important that nurses actively ask patients their name and date of birth, then scan their name bands, and finally, confirm the accuracy of this information with what is found in the electronic health record every time with every medication, every intervention, and every treatment. If there is a discrepancy, the nurse must stop and rectify the problem before proceeding.

The second patient safety goal highlights the importance of effective communication among the healthcare team. This goal describes the vital importance of reporting critical results in a timely fashion (TJC, 2021). Hospitals are charged with developing clear and sustainable communication policies and procedures to guarantee that information is delivered promptly. When a significantly abnormal laboratory test or diagnostic test result is reported to the nurse, the provider should be immediately contacted. Prompt reporting of this information can prevent a life-threatening emergency from happening and allow treatment to begin.

BOX 16.2 National Patient Safety Goals 2020 for Hospital Programs

The Joint Commission National Patient Safety Goals

1. Improve the accuracy of patient identification.
2. Improve the effectiveness of communication among caregivers.
3. Improve the safety of using medications.
4. Reduce patient harm associated with clinical alarm systems.
5. Reduce the risk of healthcare-associated infections.
6. Identify patient safety risks.

Source: Data from The Joint Commission. (2021). *National patient safety goals effective January 2021 for the hospital program.* https://www.jointcommission.org/-/media/tjc/documents/standards/national-patient-safety-goals/2021/hap_npsg_jan2021.pdf

The third patient safety goal emphasizes safe medication administration practices, stressing that all medications must be clearly labeled with the drug name, dose, diluent, and expiration information (TJC, 2021). Consistently employing the "rights of medication administration" and labeling all medications, regardless of whether the medication is in a syringe or another type of container, will promote safe practices for the new-to-practice nurse. This goal also includes safety and harm prevention strategies associated with the use of anticoagulant therapy. Anticoagulants are recognized as causing potential patient harm, often due to varied dosing regimens and monitoring requirements. To enhance safety, hospitals must use evidence-based algorithms, protocols, and guidelines when prescribing these medications (TJC, 2021). During the orientation process, new-to-practice nurses are provided with this important information and it is reinforced at the unit level by clinical preceptors.

The fourth patient safety goal centers on enhancing safety with clinical alarm systems. Although initially developed to promote safety, clinical alarm systems, when used incorrectly, result in the potential for harm events especially when the audible alarm is not easy to hear or when the alarm parameters are incorrectly set. Inaccurately set alarm parameters cause continuous nuisance ringing which leads to desensitization of staff. The result is important alarms can be missed or, worse yet, silenced. New-to-practice nurses and other healthcare providers need to know the hospital's policy about alarms and implement safety strategies to prevent patients from becoming compromised (TJC, 2021). Alarm safety is a hospital priority. Criteria regarding alarms are clearly established in policies. Alarm safety education is provided to healthcare personnel during the orientation process. Preceptors should provide information to new nurses about alarm parameters, including information on specific settings, disabling alarms, changing settings, responding to alarms, and procedures for ensuring alarms are working (TJC, 2021).

The fifth patient safety goal impacts millions of patients and focuses on healthcare-associated infections (TJC, 2021). Healthcare providers dedicate themselves to caring for others to provide care without causing harm. The quality of care and the safety of patients are foremost in decision-making and serve as the foundation for healthcare delivery. Unfortunately, despite having goals for quality and safety, the reality is that patients are harmed, often entering hospitals with a genuine fear of becoming sicker or injured. Throughout the nation's hospitals, one out of every 25 patients will develop a hospital-acquired infection, and more than 1,000 hospitalized people will die each day from a preventable adverse event (The Leapfrog Group, 2020). Although there are many components needed to reduce hospital-acquired infections, one of the easiest ways of reducing infections is through hand hygiene. In order to meet this goal, hospitals are expected to have a robust program for educating, monitoring, and assessing compliance with handwashing. As part of professional practice, nurses need to hold each other accountable to consistently perform correct handwashing practices. Feedback should be given to peers who do not adhere to the handwashing policy and if that does not correct the problem, the expectation would be that the nurse would escalate concerns to the department's nurse manager.

The sixth patient safety goal is identifying patient safety risks. It is specifically focused on the prompt identification and management of patients at risk for suicide. According to the Centers for Disease Control and Prevention (CDC), suicide rates have risen in nearly all states, with suicide listed as a leading cause of death in the United States (CDC, n.d.). All healthcare providers are uniquely positioned to screen patients for risk of suicide. TJC expects that professionals are provided with education to enhance their competence with assessing and caring for patients at risk for suicide and that evidence-based screenings are routinely conducted to identify them (TJC, 2021). Additionally, healthcare organizations must have detailed plans to mitigate the risk of suicide for high-risk patients. During the orientation process and then annually thereafter, nurses receive education on correctly utilizing suicide risk assessment scoring systems, communicating concerns with other members of the healthcare team, implementing safety measures, and monitoring through ongoing assessment and hourly rounding. Nursing orientation and residency programs provide new-to-practice nurses with detailed information about how to render the patient's room safe and free of ligature risks, how to identify and remove objects that increase risk of patient self-harm such as silverware on the dietary tray and plastic bags in the trash cans, and requirements for providing one-to-one supervision (TJC, 2021).

Lastly for the hospital-based setting, TJC has developed a universal protocol, applicable to all surgical and invasive procedures that dictates surgery be performed on the correct patient, at the correct site, with the correct procedure (TJC, 2021). This is accomplished by routinely and consistently conducting a preprocedure verification process to confirm that all required documents are complete, and equipment needed to conduct the surgery safely is available as another safety step to ensure that the correct patient is having the correct procedure at the correct site (TJC, 2021). To further enhance patient safety and prevent harm, surgical sites must be marked when there is a possibility of more than one location for the procedure, such as the right eye versus the left eye. Finally, it is a requirement that a time-out be conducted immediately before starting any surgery or invasive procedure. The time-out is performed as a final assessment, confirming that all is correct and the surgery or procedure would only begin when all questions are answered and concerns are rectified (TJC, 2021).

INSTITUTE FOR HEALTHCARE IMPROVEMENT

The IHI is an independent, not-for-profit organization that is a leader in driving quality, safe care and positive outcomes. As a way of fostering the delivery of reliable, safe care, the IHI developed the concept of evidence-based "bundles" (IHI, n.d.-b), which hospitals have adopted as policies. A bundle is composed of approximately three to five evidence-based, standardized practices that, when performed correctly and consistently, have been shown to enhance patient outcomes (IHI, n.d.-a). An important feature to remember is that bundles are considered best practices obtained from robust scientific evidence, but for bundles to improve outcomes, all bundle components must be completed entirely and consistently. If one or more bundle components are not followed, then risks to the patient in terms of infection or injury increase. Specific bundles used in the hospital setting include central line associated bloodstream infection (CLABSI) bundle, ventilator-associated events (VAE) bundle, sepsis bundle, catheter-associated urinary tract infection (CAUTI) bundle, and *Clostridium difficile* (*C-diff*) bundle.

Understanding the components of a bundle, as well as correctly implementing all steps involved, are vitally important to the delivery of quality, safe care. Nursing orientation programs infuse content about these bundles throughout the curricula as hospital policy and newly hired nurses are given opportunities in clinical practice to correctly demonstrate each step included in the various bundles. New-to-practice nurses will also be introduced to the unit-specific data regarding bundles. Many units use this data to identify gaps in care delivery, to develop educational plans to address deficiencies, and to celebrate the length of time their units have been infection-free.

CLABSIs are serious infections where an organism enters the bloodstream from a central line site. These infections have a tremendous human and financial toll, resulting in thousands of deaths annually and significant unreimbursed expenses for hospitals. Most importantly, CLABSIs are preventable with bundle compliance. Bundle components include performing hand hygiene, using full barrier precautions/personal protective equipment during central line insertion, conducting daily evaluations to determine if the central line is still needed, using alcohol-impregnated caps on all IV ports of the central line and scrubbing the hub of all IV ports for 15 seconds before accessing them, applying sterile caps on all tubing, ensuring that chlorohexidine baths are provided to patients, and maintaining integrity of the sterile central line dressing. Nursing orientation programs provide education on each bundle component and require a return demonstration of all skills. As nurses grow in their roles, they can become champions to ensure bundle compliance among colleagues.

Another important bundle used in clinical practice is the CAUTI bundle. Like CLABSIs, CAUTIs can result in increased patient mortality, increased hospital cost, and excessive hospital length of stay. A consistent component of all bundles includes handwashing. Components of the CAUTI bundle include inserting indwelling urinary catheters aseptically and only for defined indications, keeping them in place for the shortest duration possible, and keeping the drainage system closed, with tubing unkinked, and the drainage bag below the level of the bladder but never resting on the floor (CDC, 2019). The catheterized patient requires antibacterial perineal washing daily while the catheter is in place. Lastly the catheter must be secured with a securement device to prevent migration and/or urethral traction (CDC, 2019). The nurse as leader understands that urinary catheters should not be used as the treatment for patients experiencing incontinence and champions for external devices to be considered as alternatives. The daily review for the necessity of the catheter is important and, as a result, many hospitals have developed nurse-driven protocols to allow nurses the autonomy to discontinue catheters when certain criteria are met. The concepts and skills involved in the CAUTI bundle is introduced to new nurses during classroom and clinical orientation. In many organizations, it is included as an annual competency requirement for all nursing personnel thereafter.

National initiatives for quality and safety support scientifically proven, innovative approaches to ensure high-quality safe care. Working in complex, rapidly changing

BOX 16.3 Developing Clinical Judgment

Mrs. Leddy is a 68-year-old female patient admitted to the unit with a diagnosis of unexplained weight loss of 60 pounds over the past 3 months. Mrs. Leddy is quiet and withdrawn and difficult to engage in conversation. As a part of the routine admission assessment process, the nurse asks questions that assess suicide risk. Mrs. Leddy states that she is a widow, lives alone, and has been very sad since losing her 35-year-old son a year ago to lymphoma. He was her only child and lived with her. Mrs. Leddy states that she does not have any other family members or friends that are close to her or that she can count on for support. She tells the nurse that she attempted to kill herself 2 months ago and is upset that her attempt failed—she was hoping to be reunited with her son and husband. After completing the suicide risk assessment, the score indicates that Mrs. Leddy's suicide risk is in the highest category for suicidal ideation.

1. What **CUES (Assessment)** might the nurse identify as risk for suicide?
2. What **HYPOTHESIS (Diagnosis)** will the nurse consider for making a nursing diagnosis?
3. What **ACTION (Plan and Implement)** will be most effective for the nurse to take to assure the patient's safety?
4. How will the nurse evaluate the effectiveness of actions taken and the patient's **OUTCOME (Evaluation)**?

environments, new and seasoned nurses are frequently confronted with issues adversely impacting quality and safety. Nurses need to realize that they are an important line of defense, protecting patients from harm. Nurses can take a leadership role by adhering to the policies that support patient safety, by championing the use of bundles, by monitoring for inconsistencies in care, and by speaking up when they see others not adhering to hospital policy.

CASE STUDY

Mrs. Smith is an 85-year-old female who is admitted with an exacerbation of congestive heart failure. Mrs. Smith has a history of hypertension and diabetes mellitus type 2. In the emergency department (ED), she had difficulty breathing with crackles noted in all lung fields, an oxygen saturation of 91%, and multifocal premature ventricular contractions on her electrocardiogram. The ED physician ordered high doses of furosemide intravenously, an indwelling urinary catheter was placed, and supplemental oxygen via nasal cannula was applied. Within 24 hours, Mrs. Smith diuresed significantly and her physical examination revealed an 8-pound weight loss, crackles only in the bases of her lungs, nonlabored respirations, an oxygen saturation at 94%, and normal sinus rhythm on her electrocardiogram. She was alert and oriented and willing to participate in her care. The new-to-practice nurse is concerned and speaks to a senior nurse about needing to request an order from the physician team to remove Mrs. Smith's indwelling urinary catheter. The senior nurse replies, "I wouldn't do that until her furosemide is stopped. Otherwise, you'll need to be constantly putting her on the bedpan."

1. *How can the new-to-practice nurse best advocate for the patient in this situation?*
2. *What part of the EBP bundle needs to be implemented?*
3. *How can the new-to-practice nurse address concerns like this that are not in the patient's best interest and do not align with best practices? What resources could be used?*

NURSING-SENSITIVE INDICATORS AND THE NURSE'S ROLE

For nurses to ensure excellent care is provided, they must first be able to effectively describe, measure, and evaluate the care they deliver (McIntyre et al., 2020). Measuring ways in which professional nurses contribute to quality care is essential and helps validate the inextricable link between nursing care and patient outcomes (Cantlin & Kronebusch, 2019). The quality of care being delivered is captured by assessing a healthcare organization's structures in place, processes being used, and outcomes being measured. Outcome data drives practice. Organizations use results of this data to benchmark and compare the quality of care being delivered at their own institutions, measured against the quality of care being delivered by other similar organizations through specific indicators that are affected by nursing care.

Nursing-sensitive indicators are measures that clearly demonstrate the structures, processes, and outcomes of nursing care (Table 16.2). These indicators provide a way of measuring and understanding specific aspects of care that are most influenced by the actions of nurses (McIntyre et al., 2020). Two significant outcomes monitored are pressure injuries and patient falls. Most healthcare organizations participate in collecting and reporting

TABLE 16.2 NURSING-SENSITIVE INDICATORS

NURSING-SENSITIVE INDICATOR	MEASURE
• Nursing Hours per Patient Day	STRUCTURE
• Nursing Turnover Rates	STRUCTURE
• Hospital-Acquired Infections Catheter Associated Urinary Tract Infections (CAUTIs) Central Line-Associated Bloodstream Infections (CLABSIs) *Clostridium Difficile* (*C-diff*) Ventilator-Associated Event (VAE)	OUTCOME
• Patient Falls	PROCESS & OUTCOME
• Patient Falls With Injury	PROCESS & OUTCOME
• Pressure Injury Incidence and Prevalence	PROCESS & OUTCOME
• Pediatric Pain Assessment/Intervention Cycle	PROCESS
• Pediatric Peripheral IV Infiltration	OUTCOME
• Psychiatric Physical/Sexual Assault	OUTCOME
• RN Degrees and Certifications	STRUCTURE
• RN Survey	PROCESS & OUTCOME
• Restraint Prevalence	OUTCOME
• Staff Mix (RN, LPN/LVN, UAP, Percent Agency Staff)	STRUCTURE

this data to measure practice outcomes. Nursing-sensitive indicators are reliable and valid ways to identify gaps in care and support, evaluate, and measure improvement for nursing care performance.

Each nursing-sensitive indicator focuses on a serious health risk to patients that not only negatively impacts recovery, but also impacts the financial health of the institution. Consider the extent of pressure injuries as a nursing-sensitive indicator. The development of pressure injuries is a significant problem afflicting over one in ten adult patients and is considered a type of patient harm (Li et al., 2020). Li et al. (2020) studied the prevalence and incidence of pressure injuries in adult patients and found that 62% of all pressure injuries were hospital-acquired, with the sacrum, heels, and hips being the most frequently affected body locations. More than 2.5 million patients develop a hospital-acquired pressure injury (HAPI) each year, and of those, approximately 60,000 will die or be left to experience chronic pain, permanent disfigurement, and/or disability (Agency for Healthcare Research and Quality [AHRQ], 2011; Padula & Delarmente, 2018). Some argue that in severely debilitated patients, pressure injuries are unavoidable, while the vast majority of experts view it as not only preventable, but reflective of the quality of care delivered (AHRQ, 2011; TJC, 2016). The physical and psychological cost to the patient is substantial; however, the cost to healthcare organizations is staggering. Padula and Delarmente (2018) estimate HAPIs cost the U.S. healthcare system over $26.8 billion annually. Prevention of HAPIs requires the nurse to be vigilant and adhere to policies in place aimed at prevention, which is why pressure injuries are a nursing-sensitive indicator; they are an indicator of the nursing care rendered to the patient.

Another nursing-sensitive indicator is patient falls, a significant healthcare issue which can result in serious patient injury (TJC, 2019). Research supports that there are hundreds of thousands of falls each year with over half of the falls resulting in varying degrees of injury, ranging from minor lacerations to major fractures (TJC, 2019). Research also supports that most falls are preventable, with older adult patients accounting for the majority of the falls population (TJC, 2019). Prevention of falls requires prompt identification of patients at risk and action to mitigate those risks. The responsibility of nurses to take interventions to mitigate fall risk is what makes it a nursing-sensitive indicator of care.

New-to-practice nurses receive extensive education regarding nursing-sensitive indicators throughout their nurse residency, which then continue as life-long learning and annual competency assessments. Many facilities have developed a "Nurse Champion" model, which is a quality and safety model whereby nurses self-select to be a part of the safety culture team in their organizations and assume a leadership role regarding a nursing-sensitive indicator they feel passionate about. These Nurse Champions are provided additional education and support from mentors to become unit-based experts. New-to-practice nurses can also play an active role in the auditing process required for each nursing-sensitive indicator by participating in monthly data collection and analysis. Nurse Champions review unit-specific data and assist in identifying issues and developing plans for correction. New-to-practice nurses are encouraged to become Nurse Champions and play a leadership role in improving patient outcomes by enhancing safety and preventing harm.

All nurses, especially Nurse Champions, can prevent falls or the development of HAPIs by assuming a leadership role and becoming the unit expert. Prevention is key and requires the expertise of interprofessional teams to foster the best outcomes. Nurses play a significant role in identifying those at risk, communicating concerns, and implementing appropriate evidence-based interventions that manage care by following hospital protocol to prevent harm or injury. Nurse Champions and new-to-practice nurses can conduct safety huddles on their units every shift to highlight those patients who are at increased risk of falling or developing a pressure injury so that all members of the team can have a heightened awareness. These actions not only keep patients safe from harm but protect the financial well-being of the organization.

The AHRQ identify nursing bedside shift report (NBSR) as a national best practice for patient safety as it provides an opportunity for nurses to address concerns, communicate interventions, and discuss prevention. NBSR is an evidence-based process that involves a face-to-face conversation shared between the offgoing and oncoming nurses at the patient's bedside, ensuring the smooth transfer of care and accountability between nurses. Because it is conducted at the patient's bedside, it works to include the patient as a partner in the plan of care (Becker et al., 2020). The goals of NBSR are to improve communication between caregivers, enhance patient safety, improve patient satisfaction, provide patient-centered care, and promote quality outcomes (Becker et al., 2020; Sun et al., 2020). When NBSR is standardized and consistently utilized, the quality of care is enhanced, while errors and adverse events, such as falls, decrease (Becker et al., 2020; Sun et al., 2020). NBSR provides benefits that include an opportunity for a thorough assessment and to identify patient-specific concerns. Additionally, it invites patients to add and clarify information and voice questions. Despite the benefits of NBSR, there have been barriers to it being fully implemented. Some nurses fear breaching confidentiality of information that the patient does not know. Other nurses claim that this method of report takes more time to conduct, while others have an overall resistance and general dislike of the process and do not want to change from their long-time method of shift report (Becker et al., 2020).

Unfortunately, the opposition to conduct NBSR may manifest as nursing incivility and disrespect when one nurse wants to comply with implementation and the other nurse does not. Respect for one another is key in promoting a healthy work environment. If incivility or disrespect occur, the nurses should have a peer conversation where the benefits of NBSR are discussed, the reasons for noncompliance identified, and explanations for disrespectful behaviors provided. If the peer conversation does not result in a positive change, then it should be escalated to a trusted mentor and the nurse leader. Healthcare organizations have strict zero tolerance policies prohibiting incivility and disrespect in the workplace as well as policies requiring the delivery of EBP, such as NBSR. The nurse leader would be instrumental in enforcing the policies which prohibit these kinds of behaviors.

As vital members of the healthcare team and effective patient advocates, nurses can influence outcomes for patients in a positive way. New-to-practice nurses are encouraged to actively participate in unit activities and become unit-based Nurse Champions and data collectors. By being proactive members of the team and fostering a safety culture, new-to-practice nurses can effectively identify gaps in practice and work to find solutions to address them. Providing nurses, especially new-to-practice nurses, with education about nursing-sensitive indicators, framed in the knowledge, skills, and attitudes of quality and safety, is a significant component of Transition to Practice Programs.

QUALITY AND SAFETY-FRAMED NURSING ORIENTATION PROGRAMS

Many nursing orientation and Nurse Residency Programs are framed in the QSEN competencies. The pioneering work of QSEN occurred primarily in academia, with the integration of QSEN competencies in the practice domain being sporadic and sparse. Regrettably, the benefits of learning about quality and safety in prelicensure nursing programs may be fleeting if newly graduated RNs work in an environment where quality and safety competencies are not integrated into nursing practice (Olds & Dolansky, 2017). With numbers reaching over three million, RNs are considered the largest division of the health profession's work force (U.S. Bureau of Labor Statistics, 2020). Of that total number, 60% of RNs are employed in hospital settings (U.S. Bureau of Labor Statistics, 2020), with those educated prior to 2005 having little information about quality and safety competencies (James et al., 2017). Incorporating content on the QSEN competencies into nursing orientation programs further enhances nursing knowledge and promotes individual and organizational success in achieving positive healthcare outcomes.

BOX 16.4 Developing Clinical Judgment

Mr. Luigi, an 85-year-old patient, is ready to be discharged after having colon resection surgery 4 days ago. Mr. Luigi still has a Jackson Pratt drain in place, a Stage III hospital-acquired pressure injury on his sacrum, and a peripherally inserted central catheter (PICC). The unit is very busy with four discharges and eight new admissions, and everyone seems short-tempered and stressed. The oncoming nurse overhears that there were two staff members who called out sick, leaving the unit short-staffed. The oncoming nurse receiving report on this patient has never worked with Mr. Luigi before and requests that bedside shift report take place so that she can assess Mr. Luigi's incision, wound, drain, and PICC line. The offgoing nurse feels that bedside shift report takes too much time and refuses to leave the nurse's station. The offgoing nurse tells the oncoming nurse, "Bedside shift report isn't worth the trouble, so I'm giving you report at the desk."

1. What **CUES (Assessment)** can the oncoming nurse identify that might explain the offgoing nurse's behavior?
2. What **HYPOTHESIS (diagnosis)** can the oncoming nurse make in thinking about how to address the offgoing nurse's concerns?
3. What **ACTION (Plan and implement)** can the oncoming nurse take to help address the situation?
4. What **OUTCOME (Evaluation)** would support that the offgoing nurse is reflecting on the feedback from the oncoming nurse?

ONE HOSPITAL'S STORY OF A QUALITY AND SAFETY EDUCATION FOR NURSES-FRAMED NURSING ORIENTATION PROGRAM

A tertiary-care academic medical center redesigned its orientation program to be framed in the QSEN competencies and studied its feasibility and effects on new-to-practice nurses (Hopkins-Pepe, 2019). During a 4-day program, all newly hired nurses engaged in content focused on the six quality and safety competencies and specific practice-focused objectives that were infused throughout the curriculum with presentations and interactive learning activities. The goal of this QSEN-framed orientation program was to shift from a task-oriented focus to one with an increased emphasis on quality and safety competence.

The newly hired RNs participating in this study were predominantly female, white, and BSN-prepared, with ages ranging from 21 years to 50 years (Hopkins-Pepe, 2019). Forty-five percent of the new nurses recently graduated from nursing school and the mean years of employment as an RN was 2.26 years (*SD* = 3.75; Hopkins-Pepe, 2019). After attending the orientation program, newly hired nurses were invited to attend a focus group session where they evaluated the program. Four themes emerged (Box 16.5). The identified themes exemplified what newly hired RN participants believed about the acceptability, satisfaction, and sufficiency of having a QSEN-framed orientation (Box 16.5).

The newly hired RN participants voiced that after attending the QSEN-framed nursing orientation, they viewed quality and safety through a different lens, ultimately beginning to shift their nursing focus from learning specific tasks to putting quality and safety at the forefront of their care delivery. They described how their appreciation for all that was taught during the 4-day nursing orientation was not fully realized until they began working in their clinical units. Many acknowledged the value of learning about the various infection control care "bundles" in an interactive learning environment. The participants explained how these standardized EBP fostered their critical thinking skills, while also enhancing their understanding of the quality and safety measures needed to improve the reliability of care delivery and the added enhancement of positive patient outcomes.

Newly hired RN participants in this study identified the critical importance of communication strategies and their influence in promoting safe care delivery. They described how safety was enhanced through use of NBSR and they described the value in seeking clarity when communicating with healthcare teams. Participants described how the tactic, CUS ("I'm Concerned, I'm Uncomfortable, this is a Safety issue"), an acronym used to improve communication and teamwork, provided them with the professional language to disagree. Newly hired RN participants recounted clinical instances, with medication orders and

BOX 16.5 Themes Related to Newly Hired RNs' Perceptions of a Quality and Safety Education for Nurses-Framed Nurse Orientation Program

Recognizing the Meaning of Quality, Safe Nursing Care
- Developing New Ways of Thinking to Foster Quality, Safe Nursing Care
- Deepening Understanding of the Influence of Quality and Safety Strategies on Care Delivery
- Applying Quality and Safety Knowledge to Impact Nursing Care

Source: From Hopkins-Pepe, L. (2019). *The feasibility and effects of an orientation program framed by QSEN competencies for registered nurses.* (Publication No. 13865408) [Doctoral dissertation, Widener University]. ProQuest Dissertations Publishing. Reprinted with permission.

obtaining patient-informed consent, when use of the CUS strategy enabled them to advocate for their patients while expressing concerns to the physicians.

Newly hired RNs in this study recognized that understanding quality and safety strategies, along with developing new ways of thinking, were influential in promoting optimal patient care (see Box 16.6). They voiced that safety is a priority and can be enhanced through the provision of person-centered care. Teamwork and collaboration were viewed as critical strategies necessary to ensure safety. Various communication tactics and psychomotor skills were identified as impactful in enhancing patient outcomes. Learning and utilizing strategies, such as NBSR, and hourly rounding were described as effective tools which fostered a safe clinical environment. Participants expressed how these strategies provided the structure needed when challenging conversations were necessary. EBP knowledge, in conjunction with utilizing EBP bundles and protocols, was highlighted as an essential foundation for delivering the highest quality care, while also improving outcomes.

This study provided valuable information about the benefits of a QSEN-framed nursing orientation program. Quality and safety competencies infused into the program enabled

BOX 16.6 Newly Hired Registered Nurses Interview Responses After Attending a Quality and Safety Education for Nurses-Framed Nursing Orientation Program

"I think orientation gave me a different lens in that when I come to work, I'm working with safety and quality always on my mind. . . . I can better bring that all together in having safety and quality as a leading force in what I do."

"I feel like going from the beginning of the orientation until now as I mentioned before I'm not just task oriented. I take my time. I think through everything. I think what is best for this patient, what can we do, collaborate with everybody. And I feel like yes, that is reflecting quality and safety and I'm understanding more about it rather than just like having read it in nursing school. So, I am getting the meaning of it now."

"I really liked the CUS thing, because if you have any apprehensive feelings to talk to like residents or doctors, it gives you a way to say it professionally. I'm concerned this is a safety issue. So, I really like that I have it written on my binder, so if I have that come up, I can say it that way, even though it might not be something – like maybe I should say like an emergency situation, but I can still say, well, hey, I'm still concerned. This could become a safety issue. It gives you that phrase to say if you have concern about your patient."

"Lessons we learned about evidence-based practice encouraged us to always ask why. Why are we doing this? Why is this a best practice? And to answer that 'why' question, you need the best evidence you can get out there."

"I think just one specific example was that activity we did when we split into groups and we came up with the bundles for CAUTIs and CLABSIs. And I think it just pushed us to do our little mini research and critically think about what is important for the patient in reducing those infection rates."

"I think the orientation encouraged that just culture where it's the no blame and it's more about how to make the patient safe and encourage those PSN [Patient Safety Network-incident reporting system] that we fill out. It's for the patient. It's not to penalize anybody. It's to make sure that this doesn't happen again. And I think that orientation really encouraged us to really use that as a resource and a tool to improve care."

Source: From Hopkins-Pepe, L. (2019). *The feasibility and effects of an orientation program framed by QSEN competencies for registered nurses.* (Publication No. 13865408) [Doctoral dissertation, Widener University]. ProQuest Dissertations Publishing. Reprinted with permission.

new nurses to view safety as a priority, identifying that without safety, other interventions become less important. The orientation program highlighted the inextricable link between quality and safety and communication strategies. These newly hired RNs recognized how essential communication was in preventing errors and ensuring safety. Integrating education and simulation about the evidence-based care bundles into the program reinforced how influential these strategies are in fostering safe patient care and by implementing and applying the bundles, newly hired nurses described feelings of legitimacy behind their care delivery (Hopkins-Pepe, 2019). The QSEN-framed nursing orientation helped define and enhance the meaning of quality, safe nursing care and provided these newly hired RNs with the preparation needed for heightened awareness of their role in enhancing quality care and preventing harm.

STRATEGIES TO FOSTER NURSING PROFESSIONAL DEVELOPMENT

Safety and quality are critical elements in the provision of patient care, requiring professional nurses to engage in life-long learning to stay current with EBP. Working in fast-paced, high acuity environments requires a competent nursing workforce with the knowledge and capabilities to address complex issues. Professional nurses are the healthcare leaders who assume responsibility for implementing national initiatives, addressing unsafe practices, and championing the safety culture of their organizations. As new-to-practice nurses become acclimated to their direct care roles, they will begin to expand their nursing portfolio, focusing on their personal and professional development to prepare them to assume leadership roles in the continually changing healthcare landscape.

Nurses should begin their professional development journey with a strategy. A **professional development plan** is a detailed plan which includes clear expectations, a sensible timeline, available and needed resources, and identified measures of success as proposed outcomes (Hill, 2020). This plan begins by reflecting on the individual's vision of their nursing future and then developing goals and strategic ways of accomplishing those goals. Goals that are developed must be SMART goals—Specific, Measurable, Attainable, Relevant, and Timely (Hill, 2020). A professional development plan needs to be detailed, yet flexible, and include clear expectations, a sensible timeline, and needs to identify available and needed resources. Measures of success and proposed outcomes should be included in professional development plans because they serve as guides for advancement in nursing so that new opportunities can be recognized while also serving as milestones in fulfilling one's future career goals.

Professional development plans can be challenging to create if the nurse is unsure of how to begin or where to seek support. Successful plans need to be thoughtful and a good place to start might be with reflection to recognize one's specific learning needs and knowledge gaps. Valuable information can be obtained from peer review conversations, a process by which honest, thoughtful feedback is provided between nursing colleagues as a vehicle for professional growth and development. Through honest feedback, learning needs can be identified and prioritized. Prioritization should focus on the areas which most greatly impact quality and safety of care. With the assistance of a nurse educator, clinical nurse specialist, nurse manager, or a senior colleague, these prioritized learning needs can be formed into goals, assigned measurable objectives, and connected to specific activities for achieving success.

Professional development goals can be identified and nurtured through participation in organizational activities and hospital committees. Joining unit-based and hospital-wide committees creates an opportunity to share nursing's perspective on important issues. Committees focused on nursing research and EBP create opportunities for nurses to learn the processes involved in nursing research and EBP. Experienced committee members provide support for novice nurses to develop their own projects with the goal of presenting them to colleagues locally and nationally. Many hospitals have a shared governance structure whereby nurses, as committee members, are actively involved in decisions that further enhance nursing care delivery and promote positive patient outcomes.

Professional development is further enhanced when nurses become part of a professional network or join a national nursing organization for nurses engaged in similar types of healthcare work. Professional organizations exist for almost every healthcare specialty. In addition to promoting life-long learning, these professional networks are a forum where EBP are discussed, and quality care is encouraged (Sherman & Cohn, 2018). Benefits of participating as a member of a network include enhanced collaboration among professionals, breaking down silos between disciplines for interprofessional collaboration, sharing best-practices, and identifying opportunities for career advancement (Sherman & Cohn, 2018). The networking process begins with active involvement in committee work. Joining national professional nursing organizations creates a pathway for widening networking opportunities through conversations and meetings that occur with nurses from other healthcare organizations.

National and specialty professional nursing organizations afford nurses opportunities for enhancing knowledge and promoting professional development. Many professional organizations have continuing education offerings which provide tools to achieve the advanced knowledge and skills nurses need for specialty certification. Certification in one's specialty further validates that the professional nurse has attained advanced specialty training and possesses a higher level of knowledge and competence. Certification of nurses has been recognized as a significant strategy to enhance the quality and safety of healthcare (Coelho, 2019). In fact, nursing certification was found to positively influence nursing-sensitive indicator outcomes such as decreasing patient falls and reducing rates of hospital-acquired infections (Coelho, 2019). The American Nurses Credentialing Center (ANCC) fosters excellence in nursing by offering numerous certification preparation resources and programs, providing nurses with the knowledge needed to be successful when taking their certification examination.

The safety and quality of care delivered to patients can be greatly enhanced by professional nurses. Nurses need to engage in life-long learning and actively participate in research and implementation of EBP, both of which are crucial for enhancing care and promoting the best outcomes. By being an active member of committees, nurses can be the voice of both the patient and the nurse. Becoming a member of local and national professional nursing organizations connects nurses to a larger network where best practices are shared, and further collegial support is provided. Finally, nurses need to achieve specialty certification, appreciating that nurses holding advanced certifications promote better patient outcomes and deliver quality care.

PATHWAYS FOR TRANSITIONING TO LEADERSHIP ROLES AFTER ORIENTATION

Orientation and residency programs provide new-to-practice nurses with support and education while marking the beginning of the nurse's professional journey. The next phase of professional development includes progressing to various leadership roles within the nurse's assigned unit and beyond through participation in committees, attendance at continuing education courses, developing EBP projects, or conducting research. Being an active member of hospital-based committees enables nurses to be well-informed, participate in decision-making, and enhance clinical practice. Information about committee participation is easily obtained from the unit nurse manager and the nursing leadership team. Many hospitals have a Nurse Residency Advisory Board, which is a committee that welcomes nurses who have recently completed the Nurse Residency Program to share their perspective about the nurse residency experience through meaningful conversations that often lead to improvements to the program.

After nurses become organized in their bedside care and comfortable in reacting appropriately to changing patient conditions, there are opportunities to assume greater leadership responsibilities for care of the patients and smooth operations of the nursing unit. Transitioning to a leadership role can begin by functioning in the roles of preceptor and charge nurse. Although healthcare facilities may differ, most nurses are eligible to become a preceptor or charge nurse after 1 to 2 years of nursing experience. Interested nurses schedule meetings with their managers to have further discussions and enroll in courses that support those roles. Specifically, a Preceptor Workshop Program is offered to nurses who are interested in working with newly hired nurses. The most effective preceptors are those who have been afforded the opportunity to attend courses focused on the nuances of the role. Preceptor education programs include topics such as effective communication techniques, giving and receiving constructive feedback, adult learning principles, conflict management, emotional intelligence, coaching techniques, and teaching strategies.

The role of charge nurse is an opportunity for unit leadership. Successful transition into this role is enhanced by attending a specialized program which provides advanced knowledge and skills related to management of not only the unit, but of the people working in it. A charge nurse needs to be a nurse leader who is accountable, responsive to the team, trustworthy, and flexible. Charge nurses are often viewed as clinical experts who possess effective communication and conflict resolution skills. These nurses promote cooperation of team members by having a fair and consistent approach to problem-solving. Most hospitals provide programs for charge nurses that include topics such as team-building, communication styles, delegation, supervision, legal considerations, and conflict and resource management.

Conducting nursing research or EBP projects is another facet of nurse leadership. Nursing research and EBP are the underpinnings essential for making informed decisions and delivering quality patient care. New-to-practice nurses can enroll in courses at local universities to further advance their knowledge in these areas. Additionally, facilities which have research departments are an excellent resource for novice nurse researchers. Often these departments can guide and mentor new nurses starting this type of work. Involvement in these projects often fosters interprofessional collaboration, since many projects require involvement from multiple disciplines, in addition to nursing.

Lastly, an important pathway into nursing leadership is through attainment of an advanced practice graduate degree, such as a master's or doctoral degree. Advanced practice nursing degrees can be obtained in one of four roles, specifically clinical nurse specialist (CNS), certified nurse midwife (CNM), certified registered nurse anesthetist (CRNA), or a certified registered nurse practitioner (CRNP). To assist in clarifying future goals, a nurse can request to shadow an advanced practice RN to better understand all facets of the role before selecting a program of advanced study. Additionally, hospitals promote the achievement of advanced degrees by providing tuition support and scholarship funding. Specialty organizations are instrumental in assisting with the completion of advanced nursing degrees by offering additional scholarship funds through their organizations. The professional development, expert knowledge, and highly developed skills that nurses with advanced degrees possess significantly benefit the nursing profession and the organizations in which they are employed.

END-OF-CHAPTER RESOURCES

KEY CONCEPTS

1. Nursing orientation is a formal program offered to all newly hired RNs and is influential in the successful transition of new RNs to the practice setting.
2. Orientation is composed of different components, specifically the initial classroom-based orientation program followed by a unit-based clinical orientation. Although the classroom component is usually 4 to 7 days, the unit-based component varies between 12 weeks to 12 months, depending on nursing specialty.
3. Transition to Practice Programs, also known as Nurse Residency Programs, are considered the "gold standard" for supporting transition of new-to-practice nurses into the clinical setting.
4. Nurse Residency Programs share the universal goal of bridging new-to-practice nurses from academia to the practice arena. They also support delivery of quality and safe care, optimize patient outcomes, and foster job satisfaction.
5. Nurse Residency Programs include strategies to enhance critical thinking, clinical decision-making, and interprofessional teamwork abilities of new nurses.
6. Nurse Residency Programs include both technical and nontechnical skills, such as resiliency education and stress management seminars. These programs also help fortify new nurses with the tools to better understand and complete an EBP project.
7. Preceptorship involves the selection of a preceptor who is willing to work with a new nurse, also known as an orientee. It is ideal for a new orientee to have two preceptors so that the new orientee can be exposed to various teaching styles, clinical skill sets, and different approaches to nursing work.
8. Clinical preceptors assume a teaching role in the successful transition of new nurses into practice. Preceptors must be good role models who possess competency in various skills.
9. RNs interested in fulfilling the preceptor role should attend a preceptor course. This course provides the tools necessary for assessing competency, understanding diverse learning styles, providing constructive feedback, promoting effective communication, and managing conflict.
10. Preceptors need to understand the experience level of the new nurse orientee. Most new-to-practice nurses or nurses new to a specialty are at the advanced beginner stage of proficiency.
11. Novice nurses find themselves overwhelmed by most clinical circumstances and are preoccupied with missing something of importance. Advanced beginners may be better able to recognize components of situations; however, they lack sufficient in-depth experiences from which to draw upon.
12. Novices and advanced beginners thrive in a learning environment which allows them opportunities to make mistakes without fear of harming a patient, which is why simulation sessions, skills labs, and observational experiences can facilitate their learning.
13. Mentoring is a relationship built on trust and formed between a novice and an experienced professional with the goal of providing support and strategies for personal and professional growth.

14. Although there are certain similarities between a preceptor and mentor, there are also distinct important differences in the roles.
15. A mentoring relationship is a shared relationship where the mentor and mentee work collaboratively and openly share successes, challenges, concerns, and disappointments.
16. In 2002, TJC addressed patient safety by establishing the National Patient Safety Goals program. This program continues today and was developed to help various healthcare organizations address safety concerns.
17. Care "bundles" are grouped evidence-based interventions that, when consistently employed, significantly reduce risk of harm and enhance positive patient outcomes.
18. Through working in interdisciplinary teams, nursing-sensitive indicators such as hospital-acquired infections, pressure injuries, and falls can be significantly reduced or prevented.
19. Professional development ensures that contemporary nurses keep pace with the continually changing healthcare landscape.
20. Professional development plans are guides for advancement in nursing, creating opportunities to fulfill future career goals.
21. A professional development plan needs to be detailed, yet flexible, and include clear expectations, a sensible timeline, and available and needed resources with measures of success and proposed outcomes identified.
22. Professional development includes progressing to leadership roles through participation in hospital-based committees, attendance at continuing education courses, developing EBP projects, or conducting research.

CRITICAL DISCUSSION POINTS

1. During the nursing student's clinical experiences, the student nurse was assigned to work with different primary nurses. Select one of those nurses and describe what characteristics the primary nurse possessed that would make them a good preceptor.
2. Nurses and other members of the interprofessional team need to fully implement all elements of a bundle. What tools or resources can nurses utilize to enhance their understanding of bundle components?

KEY TERMS

- Clinical preceptors
- Mentor
- Nursing orientation
- Nursing-sensitive indicators
- Preceptorship
- Professional development plan
- Transition to Practice Programs/Nurse Residency Programs

REVIEW QUESTIONS

Answers to Review Questions appear in the Instructor's Manual. Qualified instructors should request the Instructor's Manual from textbook@springerpub.com.

1. The clinical preceptor is teaching the new nurse about the alarm system on the intravenous infusion pump. Which information should the clinical preceptor reinforce during the demonstration? *Select all that apply.*
   A. When alarms are used improperly, healthcare providers become desensitized and miss warnings.
   B. All healthcare providers require appropriate education before using equipment with alarms.
   C. Policies must address who has the authority to set, change, and turn off alarm parameters.
   D. Alarm volumes can be lowered to decrease noise and promote patient rest.
   E. Alarms cannot be trusted to work properly with certain medications.
2. The nurse is preparing to administer medications. Upon entering the patient's room, the nurse must perform patient identification. The patient is confused and is unable to state his name. Which action should the nurse take next?
   A. Tell the patient, "Try again and tell me your name and date of birth."
   B. Check the patient's identification band for name and date of birth and compare that information to the medication administration record (MAR).
   C. Hold the medication and document "not given" in the MAR.
   D. Notify the provider.
3. A clinical preceptor is observing a new nurse preparing medications and sees the new nurse crushing an extended-release medication. The preceptor questions the new nurse and the new nurse appears to not understand the type of medication being administered, the reason for the medication, or the specific nursing interventions. As a nurse leader, the preceptor should do which of the following? *Select all that apply.*
   A. Instruct the new nurse to find clinical resources and get information on the medication.
   B. Call the pharmacy to obtain another dose of the medication.
   C. Ask questions of the new nurse, probing for a deeper understanding and evaluating the critical thinking that led to the decision.
   D. Stop the new nurse and have the preceptor administer the medication.
   E. Report the incident immediately to the nurse manager for discipline.
4. Following an increase in CLABSI rates on the nursing unit, the nurse manager asks staff nurses to audit all patients who have a central venous access device. The staff nurse notices that many of the nurses are disregarding components of the CLABSI bundle. Which actions would be most effective in changing unit culture?
   A. Perform the audits and provide the nurse manager with the results.
   B. Perform audits, then provide "real time" education to the nurses focusing on opportunities for improvement.
   C. Discuss with peers their reasons for not following the bundle.
   D. Let someone else address it because it may promote negative feelings and cause an uncomfortable work environment.

5. The nurse receives morning report and is told that Mr. Maxwell has an indwelling urinary catheter and needs to be transported to the radiology department for an x-ray. How would the nurse demonstrate an understanding of the CAUTI prevention bundle? *Select all that apply.*
   A. The indwelling urinary catheter tubing is free of kinks.
   B. The indwelling urinary catheter bag is placed on the patient's bed.
   C. The nurse reviews the nurse-driven protocol to see if the indwelling urinary catheter can be removed.
   D. The catheter is secured with an external securement device.
   E. The nurse irrigates the urinary catheter with normal saline to clear sediment.
6. A new-to-practice nurse is caring for a debilitated patient who is at risk for developing pressure injuries. This nurse notices that the patient has had a 40-pound weight loss over the last 3 months and does not have an appetite. Additionally, the patient is frequently incontinent of urine. What is the new-to-practice nurse's highest priority that would be most effective in preventing the development of pressure injuries for this patient?
   A. Discuss use of incontinence products, such as adult briefs.
   B. Participate in interprofessional team rounds to discuss concerns.
   C. Enter routine times for massaging bony prominences into patient's plan of care.
   D. Develop schedule for every 2-hour repositioning.
7. Mrs. Vesci recently suffered a stroke and is scheduled to be discharged to home tomorrow. Although Mrs. Vesci is still able to walk and complete her activities of daily living, her stroke has caused residual weakness in her right leg. She lives with her son; however, he works full-time outside of the house. As the new-to-practice nurse caring for this patient, what should be included in the discharge plan for this patient? *Select all that apply.*
   A. Instruction about environmental falls risks, such as removal of throw rugs
   B. Discussion about safety monitoring systems that can be implemented
   C. Appropriate use of furniture to assist with balance
   D. Encouragement to hire a daily companion
   E. Daily visits from a home health nurse to check status of the patient
8. Nurses are instrumental in ensuring quality patient care. A nurse can best exhibit this through which of the following ways? *Select all that apply.*
   A. Consistently implement most of the process measures found in a bundle.
   B. Complete falls risk assessments each shift.
   C. Read nursing journals to stay current with best practices.
   D. Keep a patient's indwelling urinary catheter in place to prevent incontinence.
   E. Participate in bedside nursing shift report.
9. A nurse is interested in developing a professional development plan but is unsure where to begin. As the nurse's mentor, what strategies would be the most helpful in assisting this nurse in developing an individualized plan? *Select all that apply.*
   A. Reflect on nursing practice and identify areas of uncertainty.
   B. Schedule meetings with several peers and ask for feedback about opportunities for growth.
   C. Consult the nurse manager or nursing educator.
   D. Become a member of hospital committees.
   E. Offer to work overtime to help meet unit staffing needs.

10. An emergency department nurse is interested in achieving specialty certification. The nurse obtained a study guide and other resources to sufficiently prepare for the certification examination. What is the most significant result of obtaining specialty certification?

   A. Certified nurses receive an annual bonus for obtaining certification.

   B. Certified nurses have better patient outcomes with falls and healthcare-associated infections.

   C. Certified nurses attend more continuing education offerings.

   D. Certified nurses are promoted more quickly into different positions.

REVIEW ACTIVITIES

1. Data for this quarter's nursing-sensitive indicators has been sent to the nursing leadership team. After reviewing the information, the charge nurse identifies that there are more CAUTIs in the department as compared to the national average. What strategies might the charge nurse use to champion a positive change in the department?

2. The nurse has successfully completed 2 years in critical care nursing and is interested in growing as a professional nurse. She has discussed her ideas with her peers and her nurse manager. Everyone encouraged this nurse to begin the process of obtaining certification in critical care nursing. Give examples of goals that could be included in the nurse's professional development plan. What strategies could be implemented to assist in successfully meeting those goals?

3. A new-to-practice nurse successfully completed her clinical orientation and is now taking assignments independently. This nurse began experiencing anxiety on certain days as she was nearing the end of the shift while preparing to give NBSR. A nursing peer approaches the new-to-practice nurse to discuss the observations. The new-to-practice nurse confides in her peer and describes how a seasoned nurse openly ridicules and humiliates her during report. The seasoned nurse chooses to do this at the nurses' station where many of the staff are watching. What steps can be implemented to prevent this behavior from continuing to happen?

EXPLORING THE WEB

1. Locate "Chasing Zero: Winning the War on Healthcare Harm" at the QSEN website, https://qsen.org/publications/videos/chasing-zero-winning-the-war-on-healthcare-harm. This 53-minute video is narrated by Dennis Quaid and includes discussions about healthcare harm and preventable medical errors. It contains a series of short stories from the perspective of families and discusses how healthcare providers addressed the challenges and overcame them.

2. Explore the Joint Commission website at www.jointcommission.org/standards/national-patient-safety-goals. Review the National Patient Safety Goals for hospitals. Which of the National Patient Safety Goals are the most frequently seen in action in a hospital setting?

3. Search the ANCC certification programs website at www.nursingworld.org/our-certifications. Scroll down and select "Medical-Surgical Nursing Certification," then scroll down and select "Certification General Testing and Renewal Handbook." then Discuss the requirements for initial certification and include steps for preparing for the examination.

A robust set of instructor resources designed to supplement this text is located at **http://connect.springerpub.com/content/book/978-0-8261-6145-1.** Qualifying instructors may request access by emailing **textbook@springerpub.com.**

REFERENCES

Abbajay, M. (2019). *Mentoring matters: Three essential elements of success.* https://www.forbes.com/sites/maryabbajay/2019/01/20/mentoring-matters-three-essential-element-of-success/?sh=1aa8a7045a9f

Agency for Healthcare Research and Quality. (2011). Preventing pressure ulcers in hospitals. https://www.ahrq.gov/patient-safety/settings/hospital/resource/pressureulcer/tool/pu1.html

Becker, S., Hagle, M., Amrhein, A., Bispo, J., Hopkins, S., Kogelmann, M., Porras, E., & Smith, M. (2020). Implementing and sustaining bedside shift report for quality patient-centered care. *Journal of Nursing Care Quality, 36*, 125–131. https://doi.org/10.1097/NCQ.0000000000000509

Benner, P. (1984). *From novice to expert: Excellence and power in clinical nursing practice.* Addison-Wesley.

Cantlin, D., & Kronebusch, B. (2019). In pursuit of meaningful nurse-sensitive indicators. *ViewPoint, 41,* 8–19.

Centers for Disease Control and Prevention. (n.d.). *Vital signs: Suicide rising across the US.* https://www.cdc.gov/vitalsigns/suicide/index.html

Centers for Disease Control and Prevention. (2019, June 6). *Catheter-associated urinary tract infections (CAUTI).* https://www.cdc.gov/infectioncontrol/guidelines/cauti/index.html

Chesak, S. S., Morin, K. H., Cutshall, S., Carlson, M., Joswiak, M. E., Ridgeway, J. L., Vickers, K. S., & Sood, A. (2019). Stress management and resiliency training in a nurse residency program. *Journal for Nurses in Professional Development, 35*, 337–343. https://doi.org/10.1097/NND.0000000000000589

Coelho, P. (2019). Relationship between nurse certification and clinical patient outcomes. *Journal of Nursing Care Quality, 35*, E1–E5. https://doi.org/10.1097/NCQ.0000000000000397

Dimino, K., Louie, K., Banks, J., & Mahon, E. (2020). Exploring the impact of a dedicated education unit on new graduate nurses' transition to practice. *Journal for Nurses in Professional Development, 36,* 121–128. https://doi.org/10.1097/NND.0000000000000622

Hill, T. (2020). *Professional development plan template with completed examples.* https://www.seoptimer.com/blog/professional-development-plan-template

Hopkins-Pepe, L. (2019). *The feasibility and effects of an orientation program framed by QSEN competencies for registered nurses.* (Publication No. 13865408) [Doctoral dissertation, Widener University]. ProQuest Dissertations Publishing.

Huston, C. L., Phillips, B., Jeffries, P., Todero, C., Rich, J., Knecht, P., Sommer, S., & Lewis, M. P. (2018). The academic-practice gap: Strategies for an enduring problem. *Nursing Forum, 53*, 27–34. https://doi.org/10.1111/nuf.12216

Institute for Healthcare Improvement. (n.d.-a). *Evidence-based care bundles.* Author. http://www.ihi.org/Topics/Bundles/Pages/default.aspx

Institute for Healthcare Improvement. (n.d.-b). *What is a bundle?* Author. http://www.ihi.org/resources/Pages/ImprovementStories/WhatIsaBundle.aspx

Institute of Medicine. (2011). *The future of nursing: Leading change, advancing health.* National Academies Press. https://doi.org/10.17226/12956

James, D., Patrician, P., & Miltner, R. (2017). Testing for Quality and Safety Education for Nurses (QSEN). *Journal for Nurses in Professional Development, 33*, 180–184. https://doi.org/10.1097/NND.0000000000000365

Kowalski, K. (2019). Differentiating mentoring from coaching and precepting. *The Journal of Continuing Education in Nursing, 50*, 493–494. https://doi.org/10.3928/00220124-20191015-04

The Joint Commission. (n.d.). *Joint Commission FAQs*. https://www.jointcommission.org/about-us/facts-about-the-joint-commission/joint-commission-faqs/

The Joint Commission. (2016). *Quick safety: Preventing pressure injuries*. https://www.jointcommission.org/-/media/tjc/documents/quick-safety-issue-25-july-2016-final3-w-addendumrev2.pdf

The Joint Commission. (2019). *The Joint Commission launches educational campaign on preventing falls*. https://jointcommission.new-media-release.com/2019_speak_up_falls/downloads/printfriendly.pdf

The Joint Commission. (2021). *National Patient Safety Goals® effective January 2021 for the hospital program*. https://www.jointcommission.org/-/media/tjc/documents/standards/national-patient-safety-goals/2021/npsg_chapter_hap_jan2021.pdf

The Leapfrog Group. (2020, April 30). Leapfrog hospital safety grade: Errors, injuries, accidents, infections. https://www.hospitalsafetygrade.org/what-is-patient-safety/errors-injuries-accidents-infections

Li, Z., Lin, F., Thalib, L., & Chaboyer, W. (2020). Global prevalence and incidence of pressure injuries in hospitalized adult patients: A systematic review and meta-analysis. *International Journal of Nursing Studies, 105*, 1–13. https://doi.org/10.1016/j.ijnurstu.2020.103546

Mathen, G. C., & Hoke, L. M. (2020). An innovative action-learning plan designed for the struggling orientee. *Journal for Nurses in Professional Development, 36*, 146–155. https://doi.org/10.1097/NND.0000000000000623

McIntyre, D., Coyer, F., & Bonner, A. (2020). Identifying nurse sensitive indicators specific to haemodialysis nursing: A Delphi approach. *Collegian, 27*, 75–91. https://doi.org/10.1016/j.colegn.2019.06.003

National Council of State Boards of Nursing. (2008, August). *Regulatory model for transition to practice report*. https://www.ncsbn.org/Final_08_reg_model.pdf

National Council of State Boards of Nursing. (2017). *Transition to practice*. https://www.ncsbn.org/transition-to-practice.htm

Nursing Solutions, Inc. (2020). National health care retention & RN staffing report. https://www.nsinursingsolutions.com/Documents/Library/NSINational_HealthCare_Retention_Report.pdf

Olds, D., & Dolansky, M. (2017). Quality and safety research: Recommendations from the quality and safety education for nursing (QSEN) institute. *Applied Nursing Research, 35*, 126–127. https://doi.org/10.1016/j/apnr.2017.04.001

Padula, W. V., & Delarmente, B. A. (2018). The national cost of hospital-acquired pressure injuries in the United States. *International Wound Journal, 26*, 634–640. https://doi.org/10.1111/iwj.13071

Quek, G. J. H., & Shorey, S. (2018). Perceptions, experiences, and needs of nursing preceptors and their preceptees on preceptorship: An integrative review. *Journal of Professional Nursing, 34*, 417–428. https://doi.org/10.1016/j.profnurs.2018.05.003

Sherman, R. O., & Cohn, T. M. (2018). Why your nursing networks matter: Networks help you advance your career, provide high-quality care, and support your colleagues. *American Nurse Today, 13*, 1-9. https://link.gale.com/apps/doc/A534879705/AONE? u=drexel_main&sid=AONE&xid =7a804310

Slate, K. A., Stavarski, D. H., Romig, B. J., & Thacker, K. S. (2018). Longitudinal study transformed onboarding nurse graduates. *Journal for Nurses in Professional Development, 34*, 92–98. https://doi.org/10.1097/NND.0000000000000432

Sun, C., Fu, C., O'Brien, J., Cato, K., Stoerger, L., & Levin, A. (2020). Exploring practices of bedside shift report and hourly rounding. Is there an impact on patient falls? *Journal of Nursing Administration, 50*, 355–362. https://doi.org/10.1097/NNA.0000000000000897

U.S. Bureau of Labor Statistics. (2020). *Occupational outlook handbook—registered nurses, September 2020*. https://www.bls.gov/ooh/healthcare/registered-nurses.htm

Van Patten, R. R., & Bartone, S. S. (2019). The impact of mentorship, preceptors, and debriefing on the quality of program experiences. *Nurse Education in Practice, 35*, 63–68. https://doi.org/10.1016/j.nepr.2019.01.007

SUGGESTED READINGS

Boyer, S., Mann-Salinas, E., Valdez-Delgado, K., & VanFosson, C. (2019). Using the Delphi technique to determine core components of a nurse competency program. *Journal for Nurses in Professional Development, 35,* 261–267. https://doi.org/10.1097/NND.0000000000000569

Chan, H. Y., So, W. K., Aboo, G., Sham, A., Fung. G., Law, W., Wong, H., Chau, C. L. T., Tsang, L. F., Wong, C., & Chair, S. Y. (2019). Understanding the needs of nurse preceptors in acute hospital care setting: A mixed-method study. *Nurse Education in Practice, 38*, 112–119. https://doi.org/10.1016/j.nepr.2019.06.013

Kennedy, J. A., Jenkins, S. H., Novotny, N. L., Astroth, K. M., & Woith, W. M. (2020). Lessons learned in implementation of an expert nurse mentor program. *Journal for Nurses in Professional Development, 36,* 141–145. https://doi.org/10.1097/NND.0000000000000624

Keys, Y. (2020). Mitigating the adverse effects of 12-hour shifts: Nursing leaders' perspectives. *Journal of Nursing Administration, 50*, 539–545. https://doi.org/10.1097/NNA.0000000000000931

Lovegrove, J., Fulbrook, P., & Miles, S. (2020). International consensus on pressure injury preventative interventions by risk level for critically ill patients: A modified Delphi study. *International Wound Journal, 17,* 1112–1127. https://doi.org/10.1111/iwj.13461

McGarity, T., Reed, C., Monahan, L., & Zhao, M. (2020). Innovative frontline nurse leader professional development program. *Journal for Nurses in Professional Development, 5*, 277–282. https://doi.org/10.1097/NND.0000000000000628

Monforto, K., Perkel, M., Rust, D., Wildes, R., King, K., & Lebet, R. (2020). Outcome-focused critical care orientation program: From unit based to centralized. *Critical Care Nurse, 40*, 54–65. https://doi.org/10.4037/ccn2020585

Sezgunsay, E., & Basak, T. (2020). Is moulage effective in improving clinical skills of nursing students for the assessment of pressure injury? *Nurse Education Today, 94*, 104572. https://doi.org/10.1016/j.nedt.2020.104572

Willman, A., Bjuresater, K., & Nilsson, J. (2020). Newly graduated nurses' clinical competencies and need for further training in acute care hospitals. *Journal of Clinical Nursing, 29*, 2209–2220. https://doi.org/10.1111/jocn.15207

Appendix

PRELICENSURE Knowledge, Skills, and Attitudes (KSA) Targets
http://qsen.org/competencies/pre-licensure-ksas

Listed in the text that follows are the Prelicensure Quality and Safety Education for Nurses (QSEN) Competencies and Targets. The chapter with information related to the competency is identified.

<table>
<tr><th colspan="3">PATIENT-CENTERED CARE (PCC)</th></tr>
<tr><td colspan="3">Definition: Recognize the patient or designee as the source of control and full partner in providing compassionate and coordinated care based on respect for the patient's preferences, values, and needs.</td></tr>
<tr><th>KNOWLEDGE</th><th>SKILLS</th><th>ATTITUDES</th></tr>
<tr>
<td>Integrate understanding of multiple dimensions of patient-centered care:
• patient/family/community preferences, values
• coordination and integration of care
• information, communication, and education
• physical comfort and emotional support
• involvement of family and friends
• transition and continuity

• Chapter 6

Describe how diverse cultural, ethnic, and social backgrounds function as sources of patient, family, and community values.

• Chapter 6</td>
<td>Elicit patient values, preferences, and expressed needs as part of clinical interview, implementation of care plan, and evaluation of care.

• Chapter 6

Communicate patient values, preferences, and expressed needs to other members of healthcare team.

• Chapter 5
• Chapter 6

Provide patient-centered care with sensitivity and respect for the diversity of the human experience.

• Chapter 6</td>
<td>Value seeing healthcare situations "through patients' eyes."

• Chapter 6
• Chapter 9

Respect and encourage individual expression of patient values, preferences, and expressed needs.

• Chapter 6
• Chapter 9

Value the patient's expertise with own health and symptoms.

• Chapter 6
• Chapter 9

Seek learning opportunities with patients who represent all aspects of human diversity.

• Chapter 6

Recognize personally held attitudes about working with patients from different ethnic, cultural, and social backgrounds.

• Chapter 6

Willingly support patient-centered care for individuals and groups whose values differ from own.

• Chapter 6</td>
</tr>
</table>

(continued)

PATIENT-CENTERED CARE (PCC) (***CONTINUED***)		
KNOWLEDGE	**SKILLS**	**ATTITUDES**
Demonstrate comprehensive understanding of the concepts of pain and suffering, including physiological models of pain and comfort. • Chapter 6	Assess presence and extent of pain and suffering. • Chapter 6 Assess levels of physical and emotional comfort. • Chapter 6 Elicit expectations of patient and family for relief of pain, discomfort, or suffering. • Chapter 6 Initiate effective treatments to relieve pain and suffering in light of patient values, preferences, and expressed needs. • Chapter 6	Recognize personally held values and beliefs about the management of pain or suffering. • Chapter 6 Appreciate the role of the nurse in relief of all types and sources of pain or suffering. • Chapter 6 Recognize that patient expectations influence outcomes in management of pain or suffering. • Chapter 6
Examine how the safety, quality, and cost effectiveness of healthcare can be improved through the active involvement of patients and families. • Chapter 6 Examine common barriers to active involvement of patients in their own healthcare processes. • Chapter 6 Describe strategies to empower patients or families in all aspects of the healthcare process. • Chapter 6	Remove barriers to the presence of families and other designated surrogates based on patient preferences. • Chapter 6 Assess level of patient's decisional conflict and provide access to resources. Engage patients or designated surrogates in active partnerships that promote health, safety and well-being, and self-care management. • Chapter 6	Value active partnership with patients or designated surrogates in planning, implementation, and evaluation of care. • Chapter 6 • Chapter 9 Respect patient preferences for degree of active engagement in care process. • Chapter 6 Respect patient's right to access to personal health records. • Chapter 6 • Chapter 8
Explore ethical and legal implications of patient-centered care. • Chapter 6 Describe the limits and boundaries of therapeutic patient-centered care.	Recognize the boundaries of therapeutic relationships. • Chapter 6 Facilitate informed patient consent for care. • Chapter 6	Acknowledge the tension that may exist between patient rights and the organizational responsibility for professional, ethical care. • Chapter 6 Appreciate shared decision-making with empowered patients and families, even when conflicts occur. • Chapter 6

(continued)

PATIENT-CENTERED CARE (PCC) (***CONTINUED***)		
KNOWLEDGE	**SKILLS**	**ATTITUDES**
Discuss principles of effective communication. • Chapter 6 • Chapter 7 Describe basic principles of consensus building and conflict resolution. • Chapter 6 • Chapter 7 Examine nursing roles in assuring coordination, integration, and continuity of care. • Chapter 6	Assess own level of communication skill in encounters with patients and families. • Chapter 6 Participate in building consensus or resolving conflict in the context of patient care. • Chapter 6 • Chapter 7 Communicate care provided and needed at each transition in care. • Chapter 6	Value continuous improvement of own communication and conflict resolution skills. • Chapter 6 • Chapter 7

TEAMWORK AND COLLABORATION		
Definition: Function effectively within nursing and interprofessional teams, fostering open communication, mutual respect, and shared decision-making to achieve quality patient care.		
KNOWLEDGE	**SKILLS**	**ATTITUDES**
Describe own strengths, limitations, and values in functioning as a member of a team. • Chapter 7	Demonstrate awareness of own strengths and limitations as a team member. • Chapter 7 Initiate plan for self-development as a team member. • Chapter 7 Act with integrity, consistency, and respect for differing views. • Chapter 7	Acknowledge own potential to contribute to effective team functioning. • Chapter 7 Appreciate importance of intra- and interprofessional collaboration. • Chapter 7

(continued)

TEAMWORK AND COLLABORATION (***CONTINUED***)		
KNOWLEDGE	**SKILLS**	**ATTITUDES**
Describe scopes of practice and roles of healthcare team members. • Chapter 7 Describe strategies for identifying and managing overlaps in team member roles and accountabilities. • Chapter 7 Recognize contributions of other individuals and groups in helping patient/family achieve health goals. • Chapter 7	Function competently within own scope of practice as a member of the healthcare team. • Chapter 7 Assume role of team member or leader based on the situation. • Chapter 2 • Chapter 7 Initiate requests for help when appropriate to the situation. • Chapter 7 Clarify roles and accountabilities under conditions of potential overlap in team member functioning. • Chapter 7 Integrate the contributions of others who play a role in helping patient/family achieve health goals. • Chapter 7	Value the perspectives and expertise of all health team members. • Chapter 7 Respect the centrality of the patient/family as core members of any healthcare team. • Chapter 7 Respect the unique attributes that members bring to a team, including variations in professional orientations and accountabilities. • Chapter 7
Analyze differences in communication style preferences among patients and families, nurses, and other members of the health team. • Chapter 7 Describe impact of own communication style on others. • Chapter 7 Discuss effective strategies for communicating and resolving conflict. • Chapter 7	Communicate with team members, adapting own style of communicating to needs of the team and situation. • Chapter 7 Demonstrate commitment to team goals. • Chapter 7 Solicit input from other team members to improve individual, as well as team, performance. • Chapter 7 Initiate actions to resolve conflict. • Chapter 7	Value teamwork and the relationships upon which it is based. • Chapter 7 Value different styles of communication used by patients, families, and healthcare providers. • Chapter 7 Contribute to resolution of conflict and disagreement. • Chapter 7

(continued)

TEAMWORK AND COLLABORATION (***CONTINUED***)		
KNOWLEDGE	**SKILLS**	**ATTITUDES**
Describe examples of the impact of team functioning on safety and quality of care. • Chapter 7 • Chapter 11 Explain how authority gradients influence teamwork and patient safety. • Chapter 7	Follow communication practices that minimize risks associated with handoffs among providers and across transitions in care. • Chapter 7 Assert own position/ perspective in discussions about patient care. • Chapter 7 Choose communication styles that diminish the risks associated with authority gradients among team members. • Chapter 7	Appreciate the risks associated with handoffs among providers and across transitions in care. • Chapter 7
Identify system barriers and facilitators of effective team functioning. • Chapter 7 Examine strategies for improving systems to support team functioning. • Chapter 7	Participate in designing systems that support effective teamwork. • Chapter 7	Value the influence of system solutions in achieving effective team functioning. • Chapter 7

EVIDENCE-BASED PRACTICE (EBP)		
Definition: Integrate best current evidence with clinical expertise and patient/family preferences and values for delivery of optimal healthcare.		
KNOWLEDGE	**SKILLS**	**ATTITUDES**
Demonstrate knowledge of basic scientific methods and processes. • Chapter 9 • Chapter 11 • Chapter 12 Describe evidence-based practice (EBP) to include the components of research evidence, clinical expertise, and patient/family values. • Chapter 9	Participate effectively in appropriate data collection and other research activities. • Chapter 9 • Chapter 12 Adhere to Institutional Review Board (IRB) guidelines. Base individualized care plan on patient values, clinical expertise, and evidence. • Chapter 9	Appreciate strengths and weaknesses of scientific bases for practice. • Chapter 9 Value the need for ethical conduct of research and quality improvement. • Chapter 9 Value the concept of EBP as integral to determining best clinical practice, • Chapter 9 • Chapter 11

(continued)

EVIDENCE-BASED PRACTICE (EBP) (***CONTINUED***)		
KNOWLEDGE	**SKILLS**	**ATTITUDES**
Differentiate clinical opinion from research and evidence summaries. • Chapter 9 Describe reliable sources for locating evidence reports and clinical practice guidelines. • Chapter 9	Read original research and evidence reports related to area of practice. • Chapter 9 Locate evidence reports related to clinical practice topics and guidelines. • Chapter 9	Appreciate the importance of regularly reading relevant professional journals. • Chapter 9
Explain the role of evidence in determining best clinical practice. • Chapter 9 Describe how the strength and relevance of available evidence influences the choice of interventions in provision of patient-centered care. • Chapter 9	Participate in structuring the work environment to facilitate integration of new evidence into standards of practice. • Chapter 9 • Chapter 11 Question rationale for routine approaches to care that result in less-than-desired outcomes or adverse events. • Chapter 9 • Chapter 11	Value the need for continuous improvement in clinical practice based on new knowledge. • Chapter 9 • Chapter 11 • Chapter 12
Discriminate between valid and invalid reasons for modifying evidence-based clinical practice based on clinical expertise or patient/family preferences. • Chapter 9	Consult with clinical experts before deciding to deviate from evidence-based protocols. • Chapter 9	Acknowledge own limitations in knowledge and clinical expertise before determining when to deviate from evidence-based best practices. • Chapter 9

<table>
<tr><th colspan="3">QUALITY IMPROVEMENT (QI)</th></tr>
<tr><td colspan="3">Definition: Use data to monitor the outcomes of care processes and use improvement methods to design and test changes to continuously improve the quality and safety of healthcare systems.</td></tr>
<tr><th>KNOWLEDGE</th><th>SKILLS</th><th>ATTITUDES</th></tr>
<tr><td>Describe strategies for learning about the outcomes of care in the setting in which one is engaged in clinical practice.
• Chapter 1
• Chapter 2
• Chapter 3
• Chapter 5
• Chapter 8
• Chapter 9
• Chapter 10
• Chapter 11
• Chapter 12</td><td>Seek information about outcomes of care for populations served in care setting.
• Chapter 9
• Chapter 11
• Chapter 12
• Chapter 15

Seek information about quality improvement projects in the care setting.
• Chapter 11</td><td>Appreciate that continuous quality improvement (QI) is an essential part of the daily work of all health professionals.
• Chapter 1
• Chapter 2
• Chapter 3
• Chapter 4
• Chapter 7
• Chapter 8
• Chapter 9
• Chapter 11
• Chapter 12
• Chapter 14
• Chapter 15
• Chapter 16</td></tr>
<tr><td>Recognize that nursing and other health professions students are parts of systems of care and care processes that affect outcomes for patients and families.
• Chapter 11
• Chapter 12

Give examples of the tension between professional autonomy and system functioning.
• Chapter 3
• Chapter 11</td><td>Use tools (such as flow-charts, cause-effect diagrams) to make processes of care explicit.
• Chapter 12

Participate in a root cause analysis of a sentinel event.
• Chapter 12</td><td>Value own and others' contributions to outcomes of care in local care settings.
• Chapter 3
• Chapter 7
• Chapter 11
• Chapter 12</td></tr>
<tr><td>Explain the importance of variation and measurement in assessing quality of care.
• Chapter 12</td><td>Use quality measures to understand performance.
• Chapter 11
• Chapter 12

Use tools (such as control charts and run charts) that are helpful for understanding variation.
• Chapter 12

Identify gaps between local and best practice.
• Chapter 9
• Chapter 11
• Chapter 12</td><td>Appreciate how unwanted variation affects care.
• Chapter 12

Value measurement and its role in good patient care.
• Chapter 12</td></tr>
</table>

(continued)

QUALITY IMPROVEMENT (QI) (***CONTINUED***)		
KNOWLEDGE	**SKILLS**	**ATTITUDES**
Describe approaches for changing processes of care. • Chapter 3 • Chapter 9 • Chapter 11 • Chapter 12	Design a small test of change in daily work (using an experiential learning method such as Plan-Do-Study-Act). • Chapter 11 • Chapter 12 Practice aligning the aims, measures, and changes involved in improving care. • Chapter 11 • Chapter 12 Use measures to evaluate the effect of change. • Chapter 12	Value local change (in individual practice or team practice on a unit) and its role in creating joy in work. • Chapter 9 • Chapter 11 Appreciate the value of what individuals and teams can do to improve care. • Chapter 7 • Chapter 11 • Chapter 12

SAFETY		
Definition: Minimizes risk of harm to patients and providers through both system effectiveness and individual performance.		
KNOWLEDGE	**SKILLS**	**ATTITUDES**
Examine human factors and other basic safety design principles as well as commonly used unsafe practices (such as work-arounds and dangerous abbreviations). • Chapter 3 • Chapter 10 • Chapter 11 Describe the benefits and limitations of selected safety-enhancing technologies (such as Computer Provider Order Entry, barcodes, medication pumps, and automatic alerts/alarms). • Chapter 10 Discuss effective strategies to reduce reliance on memory. • Chapter 10	Demonstrate effective use of technology and standardized practices that support safety and quality. • Chapter 8 • Chapter 10 • Chapter 11 Demonstrate effective use of strategies to reduce risk of harm to self or others. • Chapter 10 Use appropriate strategies to reduce reliance on memory (such as forcing functions, checklists). • Chapter 10 • Chapter 11	Value the contributions of standardization/reliability to safety. • Chapter 3 • Chapter 10 • Chapter 11 Appreciate the cognitive and physical limits of human performance. • Chapter 10

(continued)

SAFETY (***CONTINUED***)		
KNOWLEDGE	**SKILLS**	**ATTITUDES**
Delineate general categories of errors and hazards in care. • Chapter 10 Describe factors that create a culture of safety (such as open communication strategies and organizational error reporting systems). • Chapter 3 • Chapter 10 • Chapter 11	Communicate observations or concerns related to hazards and errors to patients, families, and the healthcare team. • Chapter 7 • Chapter 10 Use organizational error reporting systems for near miss and error reporting. • Chapter 10 • Chapter 11	Value own role in preventing errors. • Chapter 3 • Chapter 10 • Chapter 11
Describe processes used in understanding causes of error and allocation of responsibility and accountability (such as Root Cause Analysis and Failure Mode and Effect Analysis). • Chapter 3 • Chapter 10 • Chapter 11	Participate appropriately in analyzing errors and designing system improvements. • Chapter 10 • Chapter 11 Engage in root cause analysis rather than blaming when errors or near misses occur. • Chapter 10 • Chapter 11	Value vigilance and monitoring (even of own performance of care activities) by patients, families, and other members of the healthcare team. • Chapter 3 • Chapter 10
Discuss potential and actual impact of national patient safety resources, initiatives, and regulations. • Chapter 3 • Chapter 10 • Chapter 11	Use national patient safety resources for own professional development and to focus attention on safety in care settings. • Chapter 1 • Chapter 10 • Chapter 11	Value relationship between national safety campaigns and implementation in local practices and practice settings. • Chapter 3 • Chapter 10

INFORMATICS		
Definition: Use information and technology to communicate, manage knowledge, mitigate error, and support decision-making.		
KNOWLEDGE	**SKILLS**	**ATTITUDES**
Explain why information and technology skills are essential for safe patient care. • Chapter 8 • Chapter 10	Seek education about how information is managed in care settings before providing care. • Chapter 8 Apply technology and information management tools to support safe processes of care. • Chapter 3 • Chapter 8 • Chapter 11	Appreciate the necessity for all health professionals to seek life-long, continuous learning of information technology skills. • Chapter 8 • Chapter 16
Identify essential information that must be available in a common database to support patient care. • Chapter 8 Contrast benefits and limitations of different communication technologies and their impact on safety and quality. • Chapter 8	Navigate the electronic health record. • Chapter 8 Document and plan patient care in an electronic health record. • Chapter 8 Employ communication technologies to coordinate care for patients. • Chapter 8	Value technologies that support clinical decision-making, error prevention, and care coordination. • Chapter 3 • Chapter 8 • Chapter 10 • Chapter 11 Protect confidentiality of protected health information in electronic health records. • Chapter 8
Describe examples of how technology and information management are related to the quality and safety of patient care. • Chapter 3 • Chapter 8 • Chapter 11 Recognize the time, effort, and skill required for computers, databases, and other technologies to become reliable and effective tools for patient care. • Chapter 8	Respond appropriately to clinical decision-making supports and alerts. • Chapter 8 Use information management tools to monitor outcomes of care processes. • Chapter 8 Use high-quality electronic sources of healthcare information. • Chapter 8 • Chapter 9	Value nurses' involvement in design, selection, implementation, and evaluation of information technologies to support patient care. • Chapter 8

Source: Reprinted from Cronenwett, L., Sherwood, G., Barnsteiner, J., Disch, J., Johnson, J., Mitchell, P., Sullivan, D. T., & Warren, J. (2007). Quality and Safety Education for Nurses. *Nursing Outlook*, *55*(3), 122–131. https://doi.org/10.1016/j.outlook.2007.02.006

Glossary

A **delegated responsibility** is the transfer of a nursing activity, task, or procedure from a nurse to another member of the healthcare team (NCSBN, 2019).

Accountability is to be answerable to self and others, based on the agreed upon standards of professional nursing ethics (NCSBN, 2019).

Adverse event is an incident that occurs during healthcare delivery when the patient suffers injury resulting in prolonged hospitalization, disability, or death.

Adverse Event Any injury caused to a patient by the care received (AHRQ Glossary, nd)

Advocacy refers to any activity that helps a person achieve and maintain good health as well as receive the "best" healthcare needed depending on the person's needs and wishes.

Aggregate data is the summary of data collected. It is grouped together based on the process under measurement. It may be aggregated by minute, hour, day, week, month, year, or multiple years depending on the variable. Aggregated data is commonly presented in a table format.

Assignment involves the transfer of routine RN or LPN/LVN care activities and/or part of the routine to another healthcare member (NCSBN, 2019).

Attitude a mental position with regard to a fact or state (Merriam-Webster, 2021, Merriam-webster.com).

Audit is a documented, systematic process to obtain objective evidence of conformity or nonconformity to established procedures or requirements (ISO, 2015b).

Authority is the right to act or to command the action of others. Authority comes with the job and is required for a nurse to take action (NCSBN, 2019).

Bar-code medication administration a system that receives orders from the CPOE (computerized physician order entry) system, which prints bar-coded labels that contain the patient's identification number (usually the patient's healthcare record number) that is scanned and compared against a patient's wristband when administering medications.

Barrier a structure structure, process, belief system, cultural aspect, or behavior that inhibits or limits progress towards successful innovation, improvement, or implementation. https://cfirguide.org/

Baseline data are the before, or pre-intervention measurements that indicated the need for improvement. Without baseline data, there is no ability to assess if an improvement intervention succeeded or failed.

Baseline Data is data generated from processes that is used to determine if the process is meeting expectation. If not, it may stimulate a QI intervention to improve where the process currently is. Once QI is conducted and studied, the outcome or postintervention data is used to compare to the baseline data to determine the effect of the intervention on the process.

Bedside nurses nurses that provide direct patient care; the designation is often used interchangeably with staff nurse or frontline nurse. Maryville University (2021). Bedside nursing and beyond: The other side of nursing. https://online.maryville.edu/blog/bedside-nursing

Best available evidence implies that someone must conduct a thorough search of the literature and then judge the quality of the evidence to determine if it truly is the "best available."

Bibliographic databases a basic record, or citation, for an article that often includes an abstract or brief summary of the article but may not include a full text of the article.

Boolean operators terms such as "AND," "OR," or "NOT" that are used to expand or limit literature search results.

Breach in Duty occurs when a nurse or other healthcare professional has a duty of care toward another person but fails to live up to the accepted standard of care.

Budget an estimate of revenues and expenses for a set amount of time, often annualized. Johnson, J. E. (2017). Financial terms 101. *American Nurse Today, 12*(4), 16.

Causal Loop Diagram stories about a problem or issue created through the linking of loops which represent variables within the system and the links between them. In Lannon, C. (2018). *Causal loop construction: The basics.* https://thesystemsthinker.com/causal-loop-construction-the-basics

Chief Nursing Officer (CNO) oversees a department of nursing to maintain standards of care. Gaines, K. (2021). Chief nursing officer. nurse.org. https://nurse.org/resources/chief-nursing-officer/

CINAHL Cumulative index to Nursing and Allied Health Literature a bibliographic database which indexes thousands of journals in the fields of nursing, biomedicine, alternative/complementary medicine, consumer health and numerous allied health fields.

Citation chasing using a citation or reference from one literature source to locate the full-text for another relevant piece of literature.

Clinical decision support system an integrated database of clinical and scientific information to aid healthcare professionals by examining a set of data (such as assessment data) and then leading the user through a decision-making process for interventions based on evidence.

Clinical expertise develops as the nurse tests and refines both theoretical and practical knowledge in actual clinical situations (Benner, 1984).

Clinical practice guidelines (CPG) are summaries of information developed by practitioners, professional organizations, expert groups and others who critically analyze and synthesize information about a clinical topic, procedure or scenario and make recommendations for clinical practice. Rosenfeld, R. M., & Shiffman, R. N. (2009). Clinical practice guideline development manual: a quality-driven approach for translating evidence into action. *Otolaryngology--head and neck surgery : official journal of American Academy of Otolaryngology-Head and Neck Surgery, 140*(6 Suppl 1), S1–S43. https://doi.org/10.1016/j.otohns.2009.04.015

Clinical Preceptors Skilled nurses who are responsible for assessing, supporting, and evaluating the learning and skill acquisition of newly hired RNs. The preceptor is assigned by a nurse manager or clinical nurse specialist/nurse educator. *Mathen, & Hoke, 2020*

Closed System A system that does not interact with the environment. In Cordon, C. (2013). System theories: An overview of various system theories and its application in healthcare. *American Journal of Systems Science,* 2(1), 13–22 https://doi.org/10.5923/j.ajss.20130201.03

Collaboration Healthcare professionals working cooperatively together, sharing responsibilities for problem solving and carrying out the plan of care. Professional communication and team collaboration. In *Patient safety and quality: An evidence-based handbook for nurses.* https://www.ncbi.nlm.nih.gov/books/NBK2637

Common cause variation is the variability seen in a process that is inherent or expected to that process. When common cause variability exists within a process, that process is stable or "in control."

Common Law is the body of law that has been created through the application of prior court decisions.

Complex System a system that consists of many parts or smaller systems that interact with each or the environment. In Cordon, C. (2013). System theories: An overview of various system theories and its application in healthcare. *American Journal of Systems Science, 2*(1), 13–22. https://doi.org/10.5923/j.ajss.20130201.03

Computerized physician (provider) order entry (CPOE) a computerized physician (provider) order entry is considered any system that allows the physician to directly transmit an order electronically to a recipient (AHRQ PSNet (2019)).

Concept map visual representation of information often used in nursing coursework to help students organize and represent knowledge of a subject. In *The University of North Texas Health Science Center.* (n.d). https://www.unthsc.edu/center-for-innovative-learning/concept-mapping/

Consolidated Framework for Implementation Research (CFIR) A commonly used implementation science research framework which emphasizes the study of how to optimize a successful implementation. The CFIR includes a focus on barriers and facilitators to implementation and includes the study of four key aspects: (1) inner environment; (2) outer setting; (3) intervention; and (4) processes. https://cfirguide.org/

Control chart is a graphical display of data in a time-series design using the mean as the centerline. In addition, the control chart includes an upper (3 standard deviations above the mean) and lower (3 standard deviations below the mean) control limit line. Using interpretation rules, common cause and special cause variation in a data set can be identified.

Corrective Action is action taken to eliminate the cause(s) of an error with the goal to prevent recurrence (ISO. 2015a).

Crisis standards of care describes the significant change in operations or ability to provide the established level of care because of a catastrophic or emergency event such as a pandemic or earthquake. Watkins, S. (2020). What are crisis standards of care? *Washington State Nurses Association.* https://www.wsna.org/news/2020/what-are-crisis-standards-of-care

Cross-monitoring The process of monitoring the actions of other team members for the purpose of sharing the workload and reducing or avoiding errors. *Agency for Healthcare Research and Quality* Team*STEPPS.* (n.d.) https://www.ahrq.gov/teamstepps/instructor/fundamentals/index.html

C-Suite refers to the executive managers of the team. Most common C-suite members include the Chief Executive Officer (CEO), Chief Operating Officer (COO), Chief Financial Officer (CFO), and Chief Nursing Officer (CNO). Workable Technology. (2021). What is a C-level executive? Workable Technology. https://resources.workable.com/hr-terms/c-level-executive

Cultural competence "the ability of systems to provide care to patients with diverse values, beliefs and behaviors, including the tailoring of healthcare delivery to meet patients' social, cultural, and linguistic needs" (AHA, 2019, para 1).

Culture of safety a culture that generates trust related to transparency of processes, including reporting, and learning from unsafe conditions to pursue safety. AHRQ. (2019, September). *Patient safety primer. Culture of safety.* Patient Safety Network. Agency for Healthcare Research and Quality. https://psnet.ahrq.gov/primer/culture-safety

Culture proficiency is the ability to effectively deliver healthcare services that meet the social, cultural, and linguistic needs of a patient.

Data are the raw numbers or results collected to monitor a variety of processes within the organization or those provided to the organization from an outside source. Data are used to determine if performance meets the expected goal.

Data display refers to the visual picture or graphing of data that best illustrates the story you want that data to exhibit. It is important to display data in ways staff, patients, and families can understand it. Both graphs and tables are acceptable methods of displaying data.

Debriefing Recounting key events and analyzing why they occurred; include what worked, what didn't work, leading to a discussion of lessons learned and how they will alter the plan next time. *Agency for Healthcare Research and Quality* Team*STEPPS.* (n.d.) https://www.psnet.ahrq.gov/primer/debriefing-clinical-learning

De-escalation Strategies In healthcare, actions that decrease aggressive behaviors during challenging communications which include refocusing attention on the patient. Altmiller, 2011

De-implementation The process or practice of removing a process, intervention, technology or other element previously implemented into a healthcare process or system. van Bodegom-Vos, L., Davidoff, F., Marang-van de Mheen, P.J. Implementation and de-implementation: two sides of the same coin?*BMJ Quality & Safety* 2017;**26**:495–501.

Delegation is allowing a delegatee to perform a specific nursing activity, task, or procedure that is beyond the delegatee's traditional role and not routinely performed (NCSBN, 2019).

Descriptive statistics are useful when evaluating aggregate data sets. Several basic descriptive statistics commonly calculated when doing quality improvement activities include mean, median, mode, range, and standard deviation (SD) of a set of data.

Duty of Care is the legal obligation of professionals to deliver a certain standard of care when performing acts which could directly or indirectly harm others.

Dynamic Sustainability Framework (DSF) An implementation science research framework which focuses on the study of sustaining an implementation over time. The DSF includes four major components: (1) intervention; (2) practice setting; (3) ecological system; and (4) PDSA improvement cycles. Chambers D. A., Glasgow R. E., & Stange, K.C. (2013). The dynamic sustainability framework: Addressing the paradox of sustainment amid ongoing change. *Implementation Science, 8*, 117. doi.org/10.1186/1748-5908-8-117.

Ecological system A term used in the Dynamic Sustainability Framework (DSF) referring to the context of an implementation effort and its surrounding and influencing environment. Chambers D.A., Glasgow R.E., & Stange, K.C. (2013). The dynamic sustainability framework: Addressing the paradox of sustainment amid ongoing change. *Implementation Science, 8*, 117. doi.org/10.1186/1748-5908-8-117.

Electronic health record a legal record of what happened to a patient during one care encounter at a healthcare organization.

Electronic medical record a longitudinal electronic record of patient health information generated by one or more encounters in any care delivery setting.

Emotional intelligence is the process of reflection and analysis of emotion within self and others, as well as the ability to self-regulate emotions (Marquis & Huston, 2021).

Empathetic communication the act of communicating with someone else from the vantage point of their feelings, values, perspective, and it is at the foundation of establishing relationships that are consistent with PCC.

E-patient informed healthcare consumers who are equipped, enabled, empowered, and engaged in their health and healthcare decisions.

Error An act of commission where someone does something wrong or an act of omission where someone fails to do what is required, with either type of event leading to an undesirable outcome or injury (AHRQ Glossary, n.d.).

Evidence-based practice is the delivery of optimal healthcare through the integration of best current evidence, clinical expertise and patient/family values (QSEN, 2012).

Executive Branch of the Federal Government consists of the office of the President of the United States.

External data are those data provided to the organization from those outside the organization.

Facilitator A structure, process, belief system, cultural aspect, or behavior that enables, empowers, accelerates, or maximizes progress towards successful innovation, improvement, or implementation. https://cfirguide.org

Failure to rescue is when clinicians fail to notice patient symptoms, or they fail to respond adequately or quickly enough to clinical signs that may indicate that a patient is dying of preventable complications in a hospital.

Federal Anti-Kickback Statute is a law that prohibits the payment or receipt of any gift or remuneration in exchange for the referrals of a patient for designated healthcare services reimbursed by Medicare.

Feedback is one of four major elements of a system. Feedback is the information produced that can be used to evaluate the system. Von Bertalanffy, L. (1968). *General system theory.* George Braziller.

Fee-for-service model provides payment for each service that is rendered. Examples are diagnostic tests such as laboratory samples, x-rays, or office visits. AHA. (2020). Current and emerging payment models. *American Hospital Association.* https://www.aha.org/advocacy/current-and-emerging-payment-models

Flow map sometimes referred to as a process map, allows the team to visualize, or diagram the actual flow or sequence of a process from the beginning to the end of that process.

Followership is demonstrated through critical thinking, assertive but respectful communication, and by raising concerns to supervisors.

Frontline nurse a designation used to describe nurses that provide direct patient care; often used interchangeably with bedside nurse or clinical staff nurse. SMARP. (2020, December 1). Who are frontline workers and how to set them up for success. https://blog.smarp.com/who-are-frontline-workers-and-how-to-enable-their-success

Gantt chart is a graph depicting the phases of a project as they are planned over the projects time frame and are periodically reviewed by the team in determining if the team is staying on schedule.

Hand searching the process of electronically or physically browsing a relevant journal cover-to-cover to locate relevant literature.

Hand-off The process of one healthcare professional updating another on the status of one or more patients for the purpose of taking over their care. *Agency for Healthcare Research and Quality Glossary of Terms.* (n.d.). https://psnet.ahrq.gov/glossary?glossary%5B0%5D=term%3AH

Healthcare Failure Mode and Effect Analysis (HFEMA™) is a proactive approach to mitigate harm that involves a comprehensive risk assessment of a select high-risk process that the organization has identified. The goal of the team is to improve the high-risk processes before an adverse event occurs.

Healthcare Failure Mode and Effect Analysis (HFEMA™) is a proactive step-by-step process that examines activities having a high possibility of a negative outcome.

Healthcare quality How well healthcare services for individuals and populations achieve desired health outcomes that are consistent with current professional knowledge and standards (IOM, 2001).

Healthcare Systems Science The application of systems thinking to the healthcare setting to improve quality, outcomes, and costs for patients and populations. In Dolansky, M. A., Moore, S. M., Palmieri, P. A., & Singh, M. K. (2020). Development and validation of the systems thinking scale. *Journal of General Internal Medicine, 35*(8), 2314–2320. http://doi.org/10.1007/s11606-020-05830-1

Health information exchanges The coordination of the access and exchange of patient information occurs through the establishment of health information exchanges (HIEs), where a patient's vital health data is shared electronically on both a regional and national level (HealthIT, 2020).

Health Insurance Portability and Accountability Act (HIPAA) are national standards for the protection of patient information.

Health literacy the degree to which individuals can obtain, process, and understand basic health information and services they need to make appropriate health decisions.

Hierarchies of evidence (also known as levels of evidence) provide a visual representation of evidence from the least reliable (at the bottom) to the most reliable (at the top) (Ingham-Broomfield, 2016).

High Reliability Organization a learning health system dedicated to the goal of zero error or in the context of healthcare, zero harm. In *Agency for Healthcare Research and Quality Glossary of Terms.* (n.d.). https://psnet.ahrq.gov/glossary?glossary%5B0%5D=term%3AH

High Reliability Organizations are organizations that have a preoccupation with failure, reluctance to simplify, sensitivity to operations, commitment to resilience, and deference to expertise.

High-quality care Care that is Safe, Timely, Effective, Efficient, Equitable, and Patient-centered (also referred to as STEEEP) with no disparities between racial or ethnic groups (IOM, 2001).

High-reliability organization an organization that experiences fewer than anticipated harmful events despite working in highly complex environments such as healthcare. AHRQ. (2019, September). *Patient safety primer. High reliability.* Patient Safety Network. Agency for Healthcare Research and Quality. https://psnet.ahrq.gov/primer/high-reliability

HIPAA (Health Insurance Portability and Accountability Act) a federal law requiring healthcare providers to protect an individual's identifiable health information by using several privacy protections for patients and their records.

Histogram is a bar graph that displays the frequency distribution of a process or event. Data displayed using a histogram allows for easier visualization of large, aggregate data sets.

HITECH a federal law that provides money to healthcare providers, institutions, and organizations to encourage the meaningful use of certified EHRs (electronic health records).

Home healthcare is the provision of limited health care services by a nurse or other healthcare professional in the home of the patient.

Hospital Value-Based Purchasing (HVBP) Program incentive payments system that rewards providers on the quality care outcomes delivered. The program also adjusts reimbursement to hospitals based on quality care outcomes achieved, Payment is made by CMS to hospitals who either demonstrate improvement in performance of quality measures from a baseline period, or by how well benchmarks are achieved (Centers for Medicaid and Medicare Services, 2020).

Hospital-acquired infection (HAI) is an infection that a patient did not have at the time of admission but is acquired after being admitted to the hospital.

Hybrid research designs are research designs that focus on the implementation of an evidence-based intervention and its effectiveness and/or utility. The three major hybrid research designs are effectiveness, feasibility, and a combination of effectiveness and feasibility. *Medical Care*, *50*(3): 217–226. doi.org/10.1097/MLR.0b013e3182408812.

Iceberg Model Challenge a method for viewing a problem holistically rather than focusing on a single individual problem by considering what lies beneath the actual problem that is visible. Waters Center for System Thinkers. (2021). *Tools course #4: The iceberg* [MOOC] Thinking Tools Studio. https://thinkingtoolsstudio.org/courses/04-iceberg

Impairing conditions are substance use disorders, psychiatric conditions, and physical conditions that can impact a nurse's ability to practice safely.

Implementation framework Conceptual models developed to help implementation science researchers to: (1) learn how to conduct successful implementation efforts; (2) determine what elements are essential to and resultant from a successful implementation; and (3) discover how to sustain implementation efforts over time. Adapted and synthesized by the authors based on definitions in the following: (1) Damschroeder, L., Aron, D., Keith, R. et al. (2009). Fostering implementation of health services research findings into practice: a consolidated framework for advancing implementation science. *Implementation Science*; 4, 50. https://doi.org/10.1186/1748-5908-4-50; (2) https://cfirguide.org/; (3) https://www.re-aim.org; and (3) Birken, S. A., Powell, B. J., Shea, C. M. et al. (2017). Criteria for selecting implementation science theories and frameworks: results from an international survey. *Implementation Science, 12*, 124. https://doi.org/10.1186/s13012-017-0656-y

Implementation Science refers to the study of adopting, installing, or integrating evidence-based interventions into an existing practice or healthcare to beneficially affect outcomes. Adapted and synthesized by the authors based on definitions in the following: (1) Damschroeder, L., Aron, D., Keith, R. et al. (2009). Fostering implementation of health services research findings into practice: a consolidated framework for advancing implementation science. *Implementation Science, 4*, 50. https://doi.org/10.1186/1748-5908-4-50; (2) https://cfirguide.org

Implementation strategies methods to enhance the adoption, implementation, sustainment, and scale-up of an innovation. Adapted and synthesized by the authors based on the following sources: (1) https://cfirguide.org/; (2) https://www.re-aim.org/; (3) https://www.ahrq.gov/patient-safety/settings/long-term-care/resource/ontime/pruhealing/impmenu.html; and (4) Boehm, L. M., Stolldorf, D. P., & Jeffery, A. D. (2019). Implementation Science Training and Resources for Nurses and Nurse Scientists. *J Nurs Scholarsh, 52*(1), 47–54. doi:10.1111/jnu.12510

Improvement activities which iteratively refine, optimize, or standardize an existing process, product, method, or approach to improve performance and outcomes. Adapted by the authors from the AHRQ definition "Quality improvement (QI) consists of systematic and continuous actions that lead to measurable improvement in healthcare services and the health status of targeted patient groups." https://www.hrsa.gov/sites/default/files/quality/toolbox/508pdfs/qualityimprovement.pdf

Improvement Sustainability is the goal of all QI that meets the goal. Once the goal is accomplished, maintaining that goal is the most difficult aspect of QI.

Incidence data are the actual counts of every event that occurred. For example, falls incidence data includes the actual number of falls that occurred over a specific timeframe.

Individuals refers to the population of interest.

Infant Mortality Rate (IMR) is the number of infant deaths for every 1,000 live births, and it is a measurable outcome

Information is collected and analyzed data, such as trends in blood pressure that is used to act.

Information privacy is the patient's right to limit the amount of personal health care information accessible to and known by others (HIPAA, 1996).

Inner Setting a term used in the Consolidated Framework for Implementation Research (CFIR) referring to the context and lived experience of the "front line," e.g. a clinical unit and the professionals who work in it. https://cfirguide.org

Innovation the creation of a novel idea (concept, service, process, or product) not previously used in a particular setting, with the goal of helping to solve an identified problem. Adapted by the authors, from Rogers, E. M. (1995). *Diffusion of innovations* (Fourth). Free Press.

Input is one of four major elements of a system. It is the material or energy that goes into the system. In Von Bertalanffy, L. (1968). *General system theory.* George Braziller.

Internal data are those data generated by staff within the organization.
Interoperability is an agreed-upon standard of communication between hardware and software companies that allows for the effective exchange of patient information between various health information systems (HIMSS, 2013).
Interprofessional Collaborative Practice (IPCI) is when multiple health workers from different professional backgrounds provide comprehensive services by working with patients, their families, [caregivers], and communities to deliver the highest quality of care across settings
Interprofessional Education Two or more professions that learn with, from, and about each other simultaneously in the same environment to improve collaboration and the quality of care.
Inter-rater-reliability is a process used that provides evidence that those collecting the data are doing so following the same procedures. When Inter-rater-reliability exists, the data are considered more reliable because data are collected in a consistent manner.
Intervention a term often used in implementation science applications describing a process, practice, technology, change, or other exposure applied to a system context and population. https://cfirguide.org/
Judicial Branch of the federal government has the responsibility of interpreting federal laws and assuring that the laws are in compliance with the U.S. Constitution.
Just culture of safety is an environment where the high-risk nature of the organization's activities is acknowledged, where there is a determination to achieve consistently safe operations in a blame-free environment or just culture, where individuals can report errors or near misses without fear of reprimand or in punishment, where there is encouragement of collaboration across healthcare positions and disciplines to seek solutions to patient safety problems, and where there is an organizational commitment of resources to address safety concerns.
Keyword is a search term that uses natural language terminology to search the literature.
Knowledge the fact or condition of having information and being learned (Merriam-Webster, 2021, Merriam-webster.com).
Leadership the ability to motivate a person or persons to achieve common goals. Gustafsson, L., & Stenberg, M. (2017). Crucial contextual attributes of nursing leadership towards a care ethics. *Nursing Ethics, 24*(4), 419–429.
Lean thinking, originating from the Toyota Motor Corporation, strives to eliminate forms of waste within a process to increase efficiency while enhancing effectiveness. There are eight identified sources of waste in organizations that include unused human potential, waiting, transportation, defects, inventory, motion, overproduction, and processing.
Learning Health System one in which all members of the healthcare team are acting as change agents; engaging in consistent, holistic evaluation of the organization. Agency for Healthcare Research and Quality. (2019, May). *About learning health systems.* https://www.ahrq.gov/learning-health-systems/about.html
Learning system a system that learns from adverse event reporting to optimize performance to deliver greater value through focusing on continual improvement, innovation, quality, and safety. Cross, S.R.H. (2018). The systems approach at the sharp end. *Future Healthcare Journal, 3*, 176–180.
Left hand column technique is a way to analyze difficult conversations by visualizing spoken words in relation to personal perceptions, opinions, or thoughts that were occurring at the same time. Senge, P. (2006). *The fifth discipline.* Doubleday.
Legislative Branch of the federal government has the responsibility under the U.S. Constitution to make laws.
Levels of evidence provide a visual representation of evidence from the least reliable (at the bottom) to the most reliable (at the top) (Ingham-Broomfield, 2016).

Lower control limit is the line three standard deviations below the mean on a control chart. If a data point falls below this line, special cause variability is occurring in the process under study.

Macrosystem includes the mesosystem, community members and agencies, regional culture and values, and regulatory and governmental agencies

Magnet Status granted by the American Nurses Credentialing Center (ANCC) to hospitals who have exemplary nursing care based on criteria to ensure excellent patient outcomes and high job satisfaction. ANCC. (n.d.) ANCC magnet recognition program. American Nurses Credentialing Program. https://www.nursingworld.org/organizational-programs/magnet/

Malpractice is one form of negligence and is defined as improper, illegal, or negligent professional activity or treatment by a healthcare practitioner, lawyer, or other professional.

Management in business, refers to the structure that maintains an environment so that members of the organization can work to achieve the mission and vision of the organization. Business Jargons. (2021). Management. *Business Jargons*. https://businessjargons.com/management.html

Mean is a descriptive statistic that is the average of a set of data points. To calculate the mean, add the data points together and divide by the number of data points in the data set.

Meaningful Use was an initiative designed to encourage the use of EHRs by using data collected in the clinical setting such as hospitals, clinics or physician offices, to improve patient care outcomes (HealthIT.gov, 2019).

Median is a descriptive statistic that represents the data point exactly in the middle of a set of data. To calculate the median, the data is sorted from lowest to highest values, thus dividing the data into two groups.

MEDLINE the U.S. National Library of Medicine's (NLM's) bibliographic database, indexing thousands of journals in the fields of medicine, nursing, dentistry, veterinary medicine, healthcare systems and the preclinical sciences.

Mentor An experienced, trusted, respected professional that possesses expert knowledge and skill in his or her field and provides personal, professional, and career support to another, often referred to as the mentee. *Van Patten & Bartone, 2018*

MeSH (medical subject headings) are the current controlled vocabulary thesaurus of biomedical terms used to describe the subject(s) of each piece of literature in MEDLINE; contains approximately 28,000 subject heading descriptors; it is updated regularly to reflect changes in medical terminology.

Mesosystem community members and agencies, regional culture and values, and regulatory and governmental agencies.

Microsystem is the team that includes the patient and their caregivers, a medical provider, RN, and administrative support person. May also include a number of other health care staff (e.g. LPN, Medical Assistant, social worker, behavioral health specialists, and clinical pharmacist) who are involved in the patient's care.

Mindfulness Staying focused with the ability to see the significance of early and weak signals and to take strong and decisive action to prevent harm. Weick & Sutcliff, 2001

Misuse of healthcare services is when incorrect diagnoses, medical errors, and avoidable healthcare complications occur.

Mode is a descriptive statistic that is the value repeated most frequently in a set of data, the "typical" value observed.

Near miss An event or situation that did not produce a patient injury but only because of chance; considered a *close call. Agency for Healthcare Research and Quality Glossary of Terms.* (n.d.). https://psnet.ahrq.gov/glossary?glossary%5B0%5D=term%3AN

Negligence is the failure to exercise the care that a reasonably prudent person would exercise in like circumstances.

Nurse Care Coordinator a nurse who deliberately organizes patient care activities between participants involved in a patient's care to facilitate the appropriate delivery of healthcare services.

Nurse Managers nurses that are responsible for controlling part, such as one or more patient care units, of a healthcare organization. Nurse.Org. (2021). Nurse manager. Nurse.Org. https://nurse.org/resources/nurse-manager/

Nurse practice acts (NPAs) are laws that have been enacted by state governments to protect the public's health, safety, and welfare by overseeing and ensuring the safe practice of nursing.

Nursing informatics is "the specialty that integrates nursing science with multiple information and analytical sciences to identify, define, manage, and communicate data, information, knowledge, and wisdom in nursing practice" (American Nurses Association [ANA], 2016).

Nursing Orientation A formal program offered to all newly hired RNs which is influential in the success, retention, and transition of new RNs. Orientation is comprised of different components, specifically the initial classroom-based orientation program followed by a unit-based clinical orientation. Although the classroom component is usually four to seven days, the unit-based component varies between 12 weeks to 12 months, depending on nursing specialty. *Mathen & Hoke, 2020*

Nursing surveillance the process to identify threats to safety and quality care such as physiologic deterioration and adverse events, including unintended injury, complications, or harm in the hospital healthcare setting. Boamah, 2018

Nursing-Sensitive Indicators measures that clearly demonstrate the structure, processes, and outcomes of nursing care. They measure aspects of care that are most influenced by the actions of the nurse. Nursing-sensitive indicators are reliable and valid ways to identify gaps in care and support, evaluate, and improve nursing care performance. Two examples of nursing-sensitive indicators include pressure injuries and falls. *McIntyre, Coyer, & Bonner, 2020*

Objective data is what the healthcare worker can see or measure, such as the patient's blood pressure or glucose results, and is collected and analyzed to make conclusions about whether the patient is getting better, worse, or if the data requires physician notification.

Open System a system that interacts with its environment. Cordon, C. (2013). System theories: An overview of various system theories and its application in healthcare. *American Journal of Systems Science,* 2(1), 13–22. https://doi.org/10.5923/j.ajss.20130201.03

Operational definition is a clear, unambiguous definition that specifies measurement methods and the conditions in which that variable is measured or not.

Outcome Data is the data generated from healthcare delivery processes. Outcomes are inherent to care delivery and healthcare systems.

Outcomes refer to the "changes (desirable or undesirable) in individuals and populations that can be attributed to healthcare" such as patient satisfaction results or outcomes of care (Donabedian, 2003, p.46).

Outer Setting a term used in the Consolidated Framework for Implementation Research (CFIR) referring to the external environment surrounding and influencing the context and the intervention under study in an implementation effort. https://cfirguide.org/

Outliers are data point(s) that are observed abnormally away from other data points in a random sample.

Output is one of four major elements of a system. The output is what results from the process. Von Bertalanffy, L. (1968). *General system theory.* George Braziller.

Overuse of healthcare services is when a healthcare service is provided even though it is not justified by the patient's healthcare needs.

Panel a group of patients assigned to each care team in the practice. The average panel size for a care team is between 1,500-2,000 patients.

Panel Management a population nurse role, in a primary care setting, where there is a shared responsibility for a panel, or a group of patients.

Pareto chart is another type of bar graph and similar to the histogram because it depicts a frequency distribution. The Pareto chart orders findings in a descending order with the most frequent issue contributing to the results furthest to the left of the X-axis. Visualizing results from high to low allows for prioritizing as to what data is most impacting the variable in question.

Patient acuity is the degree of healthcare service complexity needed by a patient related to his or her physical or mental status.

Patient-centered care "recognizes the patient or designee as the source of control and full partner in providing compassionate and coordinated care based on respect for patient's preferences, values, and needs" (Cronenwett et al., 2007, p. 123).

Patient decision aids are defined by the International Patient Decision Aid Standards [IPDAS] Collaboration as "tools designed to help people participate in decision-making about healthcare options" (IPDAS, 2019, para. 1). http://ipdas.ohri.ca/what.html

Patient navigator a clinical nursing staff member who is paired with a patient at the time of admission to support, educate, and facilitate the patient's interactions throughout their hospitalization, experience of care, treatment, and discharge from the hospital.

Patient portals allow patients timely access to health data and education (CMS, 2020).

Patient preferences refer to the involvement of the patient and family with a consideration of their values and beliefs in clinical shared decisions (Hopp & Rittenmeyer, 2012).

Patient-Centered Medical Home Model (PCMH) a model of care in which patients are engaged in a direct relationship with a chosen healthcare provider who coordinates a cooperative team of healthcare professionals, takes collective responsibility for the comprehensive integrated care provided to the patient, and advocates and arranges appropriate care with other qualified providers and community resources as needed.

Person approach to safety is when blame is assigned to the person at the end of a long chain of errors for making an error that caused an adverse event from overuse, underuse, or misuse of healthcare services.

Personal Representative is a person that is legally authorized to make healthcare decisions on an individual's behalf or to act for a deceased individual or an estate (such as acting under a power of attorney or as a guardian.

Person-centered care care that focuses "on the individual within multiple complicated contexts, including family and/or important others," and that is "holistic, just, respectful, compassionate, coordinated, evidence-based and developmentally appropriate" (p. 11).

Phrase searching a search for a specific phrase that is enclosed within quotes in the literature search box.

PICO an effective way to generate a searchable question and systematically identify and retrieve relevant nursing and healthcare published papers, where "P" represents the patient or population of interest, "I" represents the intervention of interest, "C" represents the comparison of interest, "O" represents the desired outcome of interest.

Plan-Do-Study-Act (PDSA) incorporates knowledge of engineering, operations, and management with the goal of improving accuracy, reducing costs, increasing efficiency and safety, and is composed of four parts: (1) appreciation for a system, (2) understanding process variation, (3) applying theory of knowledge, and (4) using psychology.

Pluralistic approach considers all the literature when searching for evidence (Pearson, Wiechula, Court & Lockwood, 2007).

Point-of-care databases contain evidence summaries, literature reviews, and enhanced content such as pictures, videos, and patient education materials that are readily accessible during care delivery at the bedside.

Population Health defined by the Centers for Disease Control (CDC, 2020) as an interdisciplinary, tailored approach that connects health departments, healthcare institutions, and policy to achieve positive health outcomes locally.

Population Health Nursing Model Practice Nursing interventions targeted at three levels, i.e., "1) serving and coordinating care for individuals and families in the context of their environment; 2) identifying determinants of health and gaps in resources (trends) and advocating for remedies[solutions]; and 3) designing and implementing population-level interventions[to improve health]."

Postintervention Data is collected after an intervention is applied to confirm the success or failure of the intervention.

Postintervention Data is the measure obtained when studying the impact an improvement intervention has toward the QI goal. It is used to decide if the goal is met or if additional PDSA cycles are warranted.

Practice guidelines summaries of information developed by practitioners, professional organizations, expert groups, and others who critically analyze and synthesize information about a clinical topic, procedure, or scenario and make recommendations for clinical practice.

Practice setting a term used in the Dynamic Sustainability Framework (DSF) referring to the context in which an intervention or implementation is being conducted or studied. Chambers D.A., Glasgow R.E., & Stange, K.C. (2013). The dynamic sustainability framework: Addressing the paradox of sustainment amid ongoing change. *Implementation Sci*; 8:117. doi.org/10.1186/1748-5908-8-117.

Preceptorship a widely used clinical learning method for practice-based professions, such as nursing that involves the selection of a clinical preceptor who is willing to teach and work with a new nurse orientee. *Quek & Shorey, 2018*

Prevalence data are measures of the collection of data taken on one single day.

Process is one of four major elements of a system. The process is the actions that happen within the system to create an output. Von Bertalanffy, L. (1968). *General system theory.* George Braziller.

Process refers to "the activities that constitute health care," such as healthcare policies and standards of care (Donabedian, 2003, p.46).

Processes actions conducted by people (patients and/or professionals) and/or health systems which utilize resources to generate services and or products that influence health outcomes. https://cfirguide.org

Professional Development Plan a detailed plan which includes clear expectations, a sensible timeline, available and needed resources, and identified measures of success as proposed outcomes. *Hill, 2020*

Project a temporary task undertaken to create a unique product, service, or result

Project management the application of knowledge, skills, tools, and techniques to project activities to meet the project requirements

Psychological safety is an aspect of teamwork when a person can speak up or ask questions without being afraid of being criticized, ostracized, or punished.

Public health what, "we as a society do collectively to assure the conditions in which people can be healthy."

PubMed provides free Internet access to MEDLINE citations and abstracts for those who do not have subscription access to electronic databases through their college, university, hospital, or organization, although not full text articles.

Qualitative data is non-numeric data often gathered during an interview.

Quality improvement (QI) is defined by the Quality and Safety Education for Nurses (QSEN) as to "use data to monitor the outcomes of care processes and use improvement methods to design and test changes to continuously improve the quality and safety of healthcare systems" (2020).

Quality improvement a framework for utilizing data to track process outcomes, then implementing improvement methods to continuously improve quality and safety

Quality Improvement the use of data to monitor outcomes and apply tests of change to continuously improve healthcare outcomes, taking into consideration the system in which care is delivered.

Quality improvement Use of data to monitor the outcomes of care processes and use improvement methods to design and test changes to continuously improve the quality and safety of healthcare systems.

Quality is the degree to which health services for individuals and populations increases the likelihood of desired health outcomes and is consistent with current professional knowledge (IOM, 2011).

Quantitative data are numeric data commonly collected during QI activities.

RACI Matrix: a project management tool used to understand the relationships between roles and decision-making. The RACI acronym stands for Responsible, Accountable, Consulted, and Informed. ASQ. (2016). RACI matrix. American Society for Quality. https://asqservicequality.org/glossary/rasic-or-raci-matrix/

Radio frequency identification a technology that uses radio waves to transfer data from an electronic tag to an object for the purpose of identifying and tracking the object.

Range is a descriptive statistic that represents the lowest and highest values within the data points.

Rapid Response Team A team of providers summoned to a bedside when a patient demonstrates signs of imminent deterioration to assess and treat the patient with the goal of preventing adverse clinical outcomes. *Agency for Healthcare Research and Quality Glossary of Terms.* (n.d.). Retrieved from: https://psnet.ahrq.gov/glossary?glossary%5B0%5D=term%3AR

Reach, Effectiveness, Adoption, Implementation, Maintenance (RE-AIM) A commonly utilized implementation science research framework which emphasizes the study of the critical elements required for successful implementation and what aspects of implementation must be evaluated to assess for successful implementation. RE-AIM has five core components: (1) reach (scope); (2) effectiveness (impact); (3) adoption (spread); (4) implementation (fidelity); and (5) maintenance (sustainability). https://www.re-aim.org/

Responsibility is the acceptance and maintenance of overall accountability for the patient, even when tasks are delegated; although the delegatee shares responsibility for the completed delegated activity, task, or procedure (NCSBN, 2019).

Risk adjustment is a statistical process that identifies and adjusts for variation in patient outcome data due to differences in patient characteristics (or risk factors) across healthcare organizations.

Risk is an effect of uncertainty, a deviation from what is expected. Risk may be quantified by likelihood of occurrence (ISO, 2015a).

Risk Management is a program that protects the assets of the organization by identifying potential threats or actual harm and seeking to prevent and reduce injury to the organization, patients, and employees.

Risk-Based-Thinking is the proactive assessment of identifying risks and taking action to mitigate them before error occurs.

Root Cause Analysis (RCA) is an investigative approach of what caused a problem and why the problem occurred. A root cause is a system or process finding that has redesign capability to reduce the risk of a repeat error. The Joint Commission requires that a RCA take place whenever a sentinel event occurs (The Joint Commission, 2020).

Root cause analysis Initially developed to analyze industrial accidents but is now widely deployed as an error analysis tool in health care to identify underlying problems that increase the likelihood of errors while avoiding the trap of focusing on mistakes by individuals. In *Agency for Healthcare Research and Quality Glossary of Terms.* (n.d.). https://psnet.ahrq.gov/glossary?glossary%5B0%5D=term%3AR

Root Cause Analysis An error analysis tool in healthcare whose central tenet is to identify the underlying problems that increase the likelihood of errors while avoiding the trap of focusing on mistakes of individuals. *Agency for Healthcare Research and Quality Glossary of Terms.* (n.d.). https://psnet.ahrq.gov/glossary?glossary%5B0%5D=term%3AR

Run chart is a graphical display of data over time using a median as the centerline. Using interpretation rules, common cause variation and special cause variation in a data set can be identified. Run charts are often used in QI because they can visually show effectiveness of a QI change.

Safety initiatives are programs that use standardized clinical practice tools and strategies and focus on reducing healthcare errors and improving patient safety in selected areas of health care.

Safety is the process of minimizing risk of harm to patients and providers through both system effectiveness and individual performance.

Safety science knowledge about safety related issues, and the development of concepts, theories, principles and methods to understand, assess, communicate and manage safety (Terge, 2014)

Scatter plot diagrams display relationships between two variables. Scatter plots provide a visual means to test the strength of the relationship between the two variables.

Scope the essential work to accomplish the project

Search limits a method to help refine search results, for example date range, type of publication, or language can be used.

Security is the set of protections placed on a computer system to prohibit unauthorized access and to prevent any loss or distortion of the data (HIPAA, 1996).

Self-concept the conception an individual holds about his or her own particular traits, aptitudes, and unique characteristics; it typically includes physical, social, and personal components (Shpigelman & HaGani, 2019).

Sentinel Event: referred to as never events, any unanticipated event in a healthcare setting that reaches a patient and results in the patient's death, permanent harm, or severe temporary harm requiring intervention to sustain life (The Joint Commission [TJC], 2017a).

Separation of Powers puts in place strategic checks and balances designed to prevent one branch of government from overpowering other branches of government.

Shared decision-making a collaborative process in which both the patient and interprofessional team members work together to agree on healthcare decisions that are aligned with the patient's health and life preferences (Kamal et al., 2018).

Shared decision-making a collaborative interprofessional approach to patient-and family centered care. AHRQ. (2020, September). *The SHARE approach – essential steps of shared decision making: Quick reference guide.* Agency for Healthcare Research and Quality. https://www.ahrq.gov/health-literacy/professional-training/shared-decision/tools/resource-1.html

Shared governance a practice model designed to integrate core values of nursing as a means to achieve quality care (Anthony, 2004).

Sharp end refers to the point in a healthcare system where any healthcare provider works and gives care to patients; it is where errors may occur.

Simple System a system that has a single path to only one answer. In Cordon, C. (2013). System theories: An overview of various system theories and its application in healthcare. *American Journal of Systems Science, 2*(1), 13–22. https://doi.org/10.5923/j.ajss.20130201.03

Simplification of work processes is the act of reducing a work process to its basic components and, in so doing, making it easier to complete the work and to understand it.

Situational awareness is when a nurse knows what is happening in the work environment and is ready to help quickly as the nurse is aware of situations that threaten safety.

Situational Awareness The degree to which one's perception of a situation matches reality; i.e., fatigue and stress of team members, environmental factors that threaten safety, deteriorating status of the patient. *Agency for Healthcare Research and Quality Glossary of Terms.* (n.d.). https://psnet.ahrq.gov/glossary?glossary%5B0%5D=term%3AS

Six Sigma methodologies, adopted by healthcare organizations from the business sector, encompass interventions with the goal to reduce variation in existing processes. Six Sigma incorporates several problem-solving steps to reduce variation in the process referred to as DMAIC (Define, Measure, Analyze, Improve, and Control).

Skill the ability to use one's knowledge effectively and readily in execution or performance (Merriam-Webster, 2021, Merriam-webster.com).

Social Determinant of Health (SDOH) The U.S. Department of Health and Human Services (2020a) defines Social Determinant of Health as "the conditions in the environment where people are born, live, learn, work, play, worship, and age, that affect a wide range of health, functioning, and quality-of-life outcomes and risks."

Special cause variation may occur when a change in a process occurs. It is unexpected variation within a process. Special cause variability signals that something happened, that the process changed for the better or worse, or that the process is "out-of-control."

Stakeholders persons, groups, or organizations who have an interest in, are affected by, or can affect a practice change

Standard deviation is a common statistical method used to describe variation of a data set. It is sometimes referred to as sigma and may be represented by the Greek letter for sigma: σ. Standard deviation represents the square root of the variance. Variance is defined as the average of the squared difference from the mean.

Standardization of simplified work processes is use of a single set of standardized terms, definitions, practices, and/or clinical tools to reduce variation in patient care delivery.

Stark Law prohibits a physician from making a Medicare or Medicaid referral to a healthcare provider or organization with whom the physician or his family member has a financial relationship.

Statistical process control is a type of statistic that when applied demonstrates a statistical approach to quality improvement decision-making. Statistical process control is used to monitor a process over time (time-series design) but adds the ability to scientifically identify variation within that process by plotting data points within a run or control chart.

Statutory Laws are written laws that derive from a legislative body such as those written statutes from the U.S. Congress, a state legislative body, or a municipal board of trustees of a city or town.

Stratification is the process of breaking the data down into sub-sets to better interpret what is happening. It can help focus improvement efforts on specific areas where problems are found.

Structure refers to "the conditions under which care is provided" such as, nursing staff ratios, supplies available to provide patient care, etc. (Donabedian, 2003, p. 46).

Subject heading a search term or phrase that is standardized for consistency in results.

Subjective data may include the patient's description of how they feel. For example, the patient may state they feel dizzy, hot, or lightheaded.

Supervision is the active process of directing, guiding, and influencing the outcome of an individual's performance of a task (Duffy & Fields, 2014, p. 23). Supervision includes guidance or direction, oversight, evaluation, and follow-up by the RN for the accomplishment of a delegated nursing task by assistive personnel; the delegatee is responsible for communicating patient information to the RN during the delegation situation (NCSBN, 2019).

Survey Readiness is the organization's ability to determine survey readiness, or ensuring all staff know and follow regulatory requirements and that the processes to meet requirements are followed.

Sympathy defined as a reactive emotional concern or distress for another, and it does not involve imagining their perspective or being in their situation.

System a group of interconnected parts that when combined form a whole that works or moves as a unit. Merriam-Webster. (n.d.). System. In *Merriam-Webster.com dictionary*. https://www.merriam-webster.com/dictionary/system

System approach to safety looks at the total context in which the adverse event took place and considers how to prevent future occurrences through improvement in the total health care system.

Systems Science an interdisciplinary field that studies the nature of systems and applies systems concepts to improve outcomes. In Mobus, G.E. & Kalton, M.C. (2015). *Principles of systems science.* Springer

Systems Thinking a mental model to solving problems within a complex system that considers structures, patterns, and cycles. In Cordon, C. (2013). System theories: An overview of various system theories and its application in healthcare. *American Journal of Systems Science* 2(1), 13-22 https://doi.org/10.5923/j.ajss.20130201.03

Systems thinking Understanding and synthesizing the interactions and interdependencies within the healthcare system and how they influence care of the individual patient (Dolansky & Moore, 2013)

Telehealth the use of electronic information and communications technologies to support and facilitate clinical and population-based healthcare, patient health education, and health administration from long distances.

Tracer Methodology is a process used by the Joint Commission when conducting an onsite survey. The surveyor will use information from the organization to trace an individual patient or a system to determine if staff is following their defined policies and procedures while providing care and services. The surveyor will speak with the intraprofessional teams the patient encountered across all settings starting with the current team. The patient's care and services are traced back until the surveyor concludes the tracer after speaking with the team where the patient accessed the organization. (The Joint Commission, 2020).

Transition to Practice Programs/Nurse Residency Programs structured programs of active learning for newly licensed nurses, designed to support the transition from education to practice. *Van Patten & Bartone, 2018*

Triple Aim improving the patient experience of care (including quality and satisfaction); improving the health of populations; and reducing the per capita cost of healthcare."

Truncation a literature search using symbols to look for variations of the same word.

Underuse of healthcare services is when a healthcare service is not provided even though it would have benefited the patient.

Upper control limit is defined as the line three standard deviations above the mean on a control chart. If a data point falls above this line, special cause variability is occurring in the process under study.

Upstream Factors Social Determinants of Health that encompass government, societal, economic, and environmental factors that impact health outcomes.

Utilization management is a process of hospitalized patient case management using evidence-based and standardized criteria to evaluate a patient's level of care from hospital admission to discharge.

Value-based purchasing (VBP) an incentive program that rewards quality of services provided including patient outcomes. VBP is an alternative payment model to fee-for-service. AHA. (2020). Current and emerging payment models. *American Hospital Association.* https://www.aha.org/advocacy/current-and-emerging-payment-models

Variability of data refers to the spread of the data. Determining the high and low values within a data set (range) is one way to assess for variability. There are more sophisticated statistical process control methods in assessing for variation in data points.

Voltage drop the gradual degradation of the implementation over time, a loss of its fidelity and/or effectiveness. Chambers D.A., Glasgow R.E., & Stange, K.C. (2013). The dynamic sustainability framework: Addressing the paradox of sustainment amid ongoing change. *Implementation Sci*; 8:117. doi.org/10.1186/1748-5908-8-117.

Whistleblower claim is a formal complaint that exposes or describes certain types of misconduct from a hospital or healthcare facility. Another word for qui tam.

Wildcards a literature search using symbols to replace different letters for words that may be spelled differently, a letter is replaced with a ? to capture spellings that use the letter "s" instead of "z."

Work-arounds are when one does not follow the rules and/or works around the rules or correct actions of a patient care process or a work process to save time or solve a problem

Workforce bullying is unwelcome negative behavior in the workplace meant to harm someone who feels powerless to respond.

Index

accessible care, 207
accountability, 147–148
accountability data, 372
adverse event, 6, 319
advocacy, 186
Agency for Healthcare Research and Quality (AHRQ), 5, 90
aggregate data, 406
AHRQ. *See* Agency for Healthcare Research and Quality
alarm fatigue, 277
alarm safety, 341
AMA. *See* American Medical Association
American Association of Colleges of Nursing (AACN) Essentials Domains, 30–31
American Association of Retired Persons (AARP), 63
American Medical Association (AMA), 366
American Nurses Association (ANA) Code of Ethics, 131
American Nurses Credentialing Center (ANCC) Magnet Recognition Program, 28
American Organization for Nursing Leadership, 65
Appraisal of Guidelines for Research and Evaluation (AGREE) II instrument, 302
assistive personnel, 52
audit, 389
authentic leadership, 48
authority, 148
autonomy, 133

Baldrige Health Care Criteria for Performance Excellence, 17
bar-code medication administration (BCMA), 275
barrier, 446
baseline data, 372, 405
basic literature search strategies, 290
BCMA. *See* bar-code medication administration
bedside nurse, 43, 49
  COVID-19 unit, 67
  direct-care, 4
  direct responsibility and accountability, 53
  patient- and family-centered approach, 54
  positions of power, 56
  SHARE approach, 53
  supportive environment, 44
Behavioral Emergency Support Team (BEST) code response, 58
beneficence, 131
Benner's professional development model, 534–535
best available evidence, 290–294
BEST code response. *See* Behavioral Emergency Support Team code response
bibliographic databases, 291
Boolean operators, 296
business skills, 490

callout, 235
case-control study, 303
CASP. *See* Critical Appraisal Skills Program
catheter-associated urinary tract infection (CAUTI), 94, 547
  dynamic sustainability framework analysis, 457
  hybrid research designs, 458
causal loop diagrams, 97, 99
cause-effect diagram, 384
CDSS. *See* clinical decision support system
Center for Care Innovation and Transformation, 65
Centers for Medicare and Medicaid Services (CMS), 5
central line associated bloodstream infections (CLABSI), 91, 546–547
certified executive nursing practice (CENP), 52
certified medication assistants (CMA), 147
certified nurse manager and leader (CNML), 52
CFIR. *See* Consolidated Framework for Implementation Research
chain of command, 153–154
Chaos Theory, 45
chief nursing officer, 51
chief nursing officer (CNO), 49, 55–56
CHNA. *See* Community Health Needs Assessment
CINAHL. *See* Cumulative Index to Nursing and Allied Health Literature
citation chasing, 297–298

civil law, 117–118
Civil Monetary Penalties Law, 129
classroom-based hospital-wide nursing orientation program, 535
Cleveland Clinic, 90–91
clinical alarm systems, 545
clinical decision support system (CDSS), 272
clinical expertise, 304–306
clinical informatics, 264
clinical judgment, 95, 96
  interprofessional teamwork and collaboration, 233
  person-centered care, 186, 191
Clinical Judgment Model, 239
clinical nurse leader, 51
clinical practice guidelines (CPG), 294, 303
clinical preceptors, 535
Clinical Process Guides, 264
closed system, 81
Cochrane Library, 292
code, 115
cognitive rehearsal, 245
cognitive science, 259
cognitive skills, 490
cohort study, 303
collaboration, 180, 228
common cause variation, 416
common law, 118
communication
  empathetic, 188–189
  person-centered care (PCC), 187–191
  technologies, 274–275
communication science, 259
communication strategies
  barriers, 240–241
  cognitive rehearsal, 245
  destructive events, 242
  difficult situations, 242
  documentation, 242
  horizontal violence, 243–244
  hospital and nursing leadership, 245–247
  interprofessional teamwork and collaboration, 234–237
  negative/difficult communication, 242–243
  patient's partnership, 240
  preceptors, 244–245
Community Health Needs Assessment (CHNA), 504
comparative negligence, 122
compensatory damages, 122–123
complex system, 81, 82
compliance process, 60
comprehensive care, 207
Comprehensive Unit-Based Safety Program (CUSP), 341
computerized physician (provider) order entry, 275
computer science, 259
concept map, 97
concept mapping
  concept map, 97
  iceberg model challenge, 101, 102
  left-hand column technique, 100–101
concerned, uncomfortable, and safety (CUS), 235–236
Consolidated Framework for Implementation Research (CFIR), 449–452
constructive feedback
  clinical judgment models, 239
  debriefing, 238
  reflection, 238–239
contributory negligence, 122
control chart, 386
coordinated care, 207
Core Measures, 8
corrective action, 382
COVID-19 pandemics
  anecdotal support, 68
  bedside nurse, 67
  crisis standards of care, 68
  disinformation campaign, 66
  ICU and the progressive care unit (PCU), 67
  leadership and management skills, 66–68
  safety leadership, 350–351
  telehealth/telemedicine, 277–279
  transparent communication, 67
  unit-based nurse managers, 68
  U.S. response, 66
CPG. *See* clinical practice guidelines
crew resource management (CRM), 233
criminal law, 117–118
crisis standards of care, 68
Criteria for Performance Excellence, 17
critical appraisal of evidence, 302
Critical Appraisal Skills Program (CASP), 302–303
cross-monitoring process, 235
C-suite, 49
culture of safety, 62
culture proficiency, 344
Cumulative Index to Nursing and Allied Health Literature (CINAHL), 291–292
CUS. *See* concerned, uncomfortable, and safety
customs and beliefs, 184, 185

damages, 122–123
data, 404–405
data capture, 271–272
data display
  format, 410
  histogram, 412
  Pareto chart, 413–415
  scatter plot diagrams, 413, 414

data, information, knowledge, and wisdom model, 259
de-escalation strategies, 244
Define, Measure, Analyze, Improve, And Control (DMAIC), 381, 386, 488–490
de-implementation, 461
delegated responsibility, 146–147
delegation
  accountability, 147–148
  American Nurses Association (ANA), 154–156
  assignment, 147
  authority, 148
  chain of command, 153–154
  communication factors, 158–159
  community settings, 159–160
  definition, 145
  interprofessional teamwork and collaboration, 233
  national guidelines, 149
  NCSBN Five Rights, 150–152
  NCSBN National Guidelines, 154–156
  patient assignment sheet, 160–164
  responsibility, 146–147
  right supervision and evaluation, 165
  right task and right circumstances, 165
  right tasks assigned, 165
  Scope of Nursing Practice Decision-Making Framework, 156–157
  State Nurse Practice Acts, 145–146
  supervision, 148–149
deliberate practice, 536
Deming's Theory of Management, 45
deontology, 134
Department of Health and Human Services (DHHS), 127, 262, 264
descriptive statistics, 409–410
designated project leader, 474
DHHS. *See* Department of Health and Human Services
dietary customs, 185
Diffusion of Innovations, 445
dignity, 180
Director of Nursing, 51
discharge planning, 178, 200–202
disruptive behavior, 341
DMAIC. *See* Define, Measure, Analyze, Improve, And Control
Donabedian's model
  outcomes, 374
  Plan-Do-Study-Act (PDSA) model, 375–378
  process, 374
  structure, 374
Dreyfus Model of Skill Acquisition, 534
duty of care, 120–121
DynaMed, 293
Dynamic Sustainability Framework (DSF), 449, 450, 455–456

EBP. *See* evidence-based practice
ecological system, 456
economic issues, interprofessional collaboration, 228
Effective Followership Algorithm, 332
EHR. *See* electronic health record
electronic health record (EHR), 61
  accurate and reliable data, 265
  easy to use, 265
  enhanced workflow, 266
  health information exchanges (HIEs), 266–267
  historical basis, 262–263
  inefficiencies, 266
  intuitive data displays, 265
  Meaningful Use, 269
  native data, 265
  navigation, 265–266
  point of care evidence, 266
  Safety Assurance Factors for EHR Resilience, 264
  timely data, 265
electronic medical record (EMR), 262
Electronic Quality Metrics (EQM), 520
Embase, 292
Emergency Care Research Unit (ECRI), 319
emergency department patient flow map, 428
emotional intelligence, 144
empathetic communication, 188–189
empathy, 188
Employee Health Department services, 414
environmental safety, 348
environment, healthcare delivery, 89
e-patient, 205
e-Prescribing, 273–274
ethical codes, 130–134
ethical decision-making process, 135
ethnic customs, 185
evidence appraisal, 301–302
evidence-based Nurse Residency Programs, 538
evidence-based nursing practice model, 289
evidence-based practice (EBP), 24, 569–570
  best available evidence, 290–294
  clinical expertise, 304–306
  clinical practice guidelines (CPG), 294
  definition, 288–290
  electronic databases, 291–292
  full-text databases, 291
  literature search, 294–304
  literature search strategies, 290
  nurse's role, 307–308
  patient preferences, 306–307
  PICO/PICOT question, 290–291

evidence-based practice (EBP) (*cont.*)
point-of-care databases, 293
quality improvement (QI), 371–374
search engines, 292
evidence types, 300–301
executive branch, U.S. federal government, 115
external auditor, 390
external data, 405

facilitator, 446
failure to rescue, 346
falls, operational definition, 407–408
Federal Anti-Kickback Statute, 128–129
feedback, 81, 238–239
fee-for service model, 60
feminism, 133
fidelity, 133
financial consequences and safety, 320–321
fishbone diagram, 384
fishbone technique, 97
Florence Nightingale's work, 42
flow map, 426, 428–429
followership, 332
forest ecosystem, 80
forming stage, team development, 232
Foundational Guides, 264
four-level nested system, healthcare delivery, 88–89
fragmented patient care, 200
frontline nurse, 43
full-text databases, 291

Gantt chart, 426, 427, 483
gender issues, interprofessional collaboration, 228
general systems theory (GST), 81
Good Samaritan laws, 120–121
GST. *See* general systems theory

hand hygiene, 346–347
handoff reports, 163–164
handoffs, 231
hand searching, 297–298
hashtag, 294–295
health beliefs, 185
healthcare delivery, four-level nested system, 88–89
healthcare excellence, 17
Healthcare Failure Mode and Effect Analysis (HFMEA), 381, 384–386
Healthcare Failure Mode and Effect Assessment (HFMEA), 337
Healthcare Financial Management Association (HFMA), 9
Health Care Information Management and Systems Society (HIMSS), 262
Healthcare Information Technology Standards Panel (HITSP), 270
healthcare quality, 5
healthcare staff safety
nurse leadership, 351
nurses' safety risks, 349, 350
safe patient handling, 349–351
serious safety threats, 348–349
healthcare systems science, 88
health customs, 185
health information exchanges (HIEs), 266–267
Health Information Technology for Economic and Clinical Health (HITECH) Act, 269
Health Insurance Portability and Accountability Act (HIPAA), 60, 114
authorized disclosure, patient information, 128
goal of, 127
penalties, 128
permitted usage, patient information, 127
health literacy, 192–193
Health on the Net Foundation (HON), 270–271
health-related websites, 270–271
Healthy People 2030 Initiative, 193, 199
Heath Insurance Portability and Accountability Act (HIPAA), 267
information privacy, 267–268
security, 268
Hersey and Blanchard Situational Leadership, 47
HFMEA. *See* Healthcare Failure Mode and Effect Analysis; Healthcare Failure Mode and Effect Assessment
HHS. *See* U.S. Department of Health and Human Services
hierarchical organizational structures, 60
hierarchies of evidence, 300
HIEs. *See* health information exchanges
high-alert medications, 340
high-quality care, 5
high-quality healthcare environment, 320
high-reliability organizations (HROs), 62, 90–91, 322, 324
HIPAA. *See* Health Insurance Portability and Accountability Act
histogram, 412
HITECH Act. *See* Health Information Technology for Economic and Clinical Health Act
HITSP. *See* Healthcare Information Technology Standards Panel
Home healthcare, 128
homelessness, 83
horizontal violence, 243–244
hospital-acquired infection (HAI), 126–127

hospital-acquired infections, 94
hospital-acquired pressure injury (HAPI), 405, 549
Hospital Consumer Assessment of Health Care Providers and Systems [HCAHPS] Survey, 211–212
Hospital Value-Based Purchasing (HVBP) Program, 367
HROs. *See* high-reliability organizations
hybrid research designs, 456, 458–459

iceberg model challenge, 101, 102
impairing conditions, 346
implantable cardioverter defibrillator (ICD), 276
implementation science, 447
  bedside nurses, 464
  Consolidated Framework for Implementation Research, 450–452
  Dynamic Sustainability Framework, 455–457
  evidence-based practice barriers, 460–461
  frameworks, 449–450
  hybrid research designs, 456, 458–459
  in nursing practice, 462, 464
  quality and safety education, 459
  RE-AIM, 452–454
  theoretical frameworks, 461–462
incidence data, 405
infant mortality rate (IMR), 503
informatics, 26, 574. *See also* nursing informatics
information, 405
information privacy, 267–268
information sharing, 180
Infrastructure Guides, 264
innovation, 445
innovation, improvement, and implementation science approaches
  barrier, 446
  characteristics, 445
  facilitator, 446
  implementation strategies, 446–449
  improvement, 446–447
  innovation, 445
  models and methods, 445
Inpatient Quality Indicators, 8
input, 81
Institute for Healthcare Improvement (IHI), 9, 230, 504, 546–548
Institute for Safe Medication Practice (ISMP), 7, 322
Institute of Medicine (IOM), 5
  recommendations, 28–30
integrative review, 303
internal audit, 390
internal data, 405
International Council of Nurses (ICN) Code of Ethics, 130–131
interoperability, 269–270
interpersonal customs, 185
interprofessional collaborative practice (IPCP), 511
interprofessional education (IPE), 229, 240
Interprofessional Education Collaborative (IPEC) Core Competencies
  interprofessional teamwork and collaboration, 227–228
interprofessional skills, 490
interprofessional team, 88–89
  nurse's role as, 476
interprofessional teamwork and collaboration
  clinical judgment, 242
  cognitive rehearsal, 245
  communication barriers, 240–241
  communication strategies, 234–237
  constructive feedback, 238–240
  crew resource management (CRM), 233
  delegation, 233
  destructive events, 242
  difficult situations, 242
  horizontal violence, 243–244
  hospital and nursing leadership, 245–247
  informatics, 237–238
  interprofessional team, 227
  near miss event, 230
  negative/difficult communication, 242–243
  nursing's evolving role, 228–230
  preceptors, 244–245
  rapid response team (RRT), 230
  role and core competencies, 227–228
  root cause analysis (RCA), 230
  team coordinated care, 230–231
  team development, 232
  Team*STEPPS*, 226, 234–237
interrater reliability (IRR), 408
intuitive data displays, 265
IPCP. *See* interprofessional collaborative practice

Joanna Briggs Institute (JBI) EBP Database, 292
judicial branch, U.S. federal government, 115–116
just culture of safety
  behaviors, 322–324
  in healthcare, 323
  high reliability, 330
  key features, 321
  leadership, 324–326
  measurement, 325–327
  medication safety, 322

just culture of safety (*cont.*)
risk identification and reduction, 327–330
similar medication vials, 321, 322
teamwork, 331–333
utilization management (UM), 323–335
justice, 132

key driver diagram (KDD), 430
keyword, 294
keyword searching, 294
knowledge, skills, and attitudes (KSAs), 179, 364
knowledge utilization process, 266

lateral violence, 243–244
leadership, 43
just culture of safety, 324–326
quality improvement (QI), 390–391
systems thinking, 101–103
leadership and management skills
bedside nurse, 43
crisis management, 66–68
leadership theory, 46–48
learning system, 65–66
management theory, 44–45
membership benefits, 64–65
nurse roles and education, 49–57
organization's culture, 62
organization's structure, 58–61
professional development and education, 64
quality improvement, 57–58
leadership theory, 46–48
lean healthcare, 82
Lean methodologies, 486
sources of organization waste, 378–379
5S process, 380
work-around, 379–380
Leapfrog Group, 9
learning system, 65–66, 90
left-hand column technique, 100–101
legal and ethical aspects
civil law, 117–118
common law, 118
criminal law, 117–118
ethical codes, 130–134
ethical decision-making process, 135
Health Insurance Portability and Accountability Act, 127–128
Medicare Certification requirement, 128–130
negligence, 119–123
nurse practice act, 118–119
nurse's responsibilities, 123–127
statutory law, 118
whistleblower claims, 130
legislative branch, U.S. federal government, 115
levels of evidence, 300
Lewin's Leadership Styles, 47
library science, 259
licensed practical nurse/licensed vocational nurse (LPN/LVN), 147
literature search
AGREE II, 302
citation chasing and hand searching, 297–298
critical appraisal of evidence, 302
Critical Appraisal Skills Program (CASP), 302–303
evidence appraisal, 301–302
evidence types, 300–301
keyword searching, 294
lifelong learning resources, 304
search limits, 296–297
search structure, 298–299
search techniques, 296
subject headings/MeSH subject headings, 294–295
truncation and wildcards, 297, 298
lower control limit (LCL), 421

MACRA. *See* Medicare Access and CHIP Reauthorization Act
macrosystem, 89, 512–515
Magnet Recognition Program, 28
Magnet status, 63
malpractice. *See also* negligence/malpractice
common causes, 124
definition, 119
elements, 120
management, 43
management theory, 44–45
mean, 409
Meaningful Use, 269
median, 409
Medicaid Health Homes Model, 208
medical assistants (MA), 147
Medical Error Recognition and Revision Strategies program, 8
medical errors, 13–14
medical subject headings (MeSH), 294–295
Medicare Access and CHIP Reauthorization Act (MACRA), 269
Medicare home healthcare certification
Civil Monetary Penalties Law, 129
exclusions, 129–130
Federal Anti-Kickback Statute, 128–129
requirements, 128
medication administration, systems thinking, 93
medication safety, 322
MEDLINE, 291–292
Medscape, 304

mentee, 542
mentors, 541–542
MeSH. *See* medical subject headings
mesosystem, 89, 512–515
meta-analysis, 303
Mhealth app characteristics, 271
microsystem, 89, 512–515
mindfulness, 239
misuse of healthcare services, 335
mobile app characteristics, 271

National Academy of Medicine (NAM), 5, 8–9
National Center for Biotechnology Information (NCBI), 304
National Council of State Boards of Nursing (NCSBN), 145, 537–538
National Database of Nursing Quality Indicators (NDNQI), 370, 371
National Health Information Network (NHIN), 262
National League for Nursing (NLN), 230
National Nanotechnology Initiative, 276
National Patient Safety Goals (NPSG), 341, 544
  clinical alarm systems, 545
  effective communication, 544
  healthcare-associated infections, 545
  hospital-based setting, 546
  patient identification, 544
  patient safety risk assessment, 545–546
  safe medication administration practices, 545
National Quality Forum (NQF), 7, 9, 371
National Student Nurse Association (NSNA), 65
NBSR. *See* nursing bedside shift report
NCBI. *See* National Center for Biotechnology Information
NDNQI. *See* National Database of Nursing Quality Indicators
near miss event, 230
negative/difficult communication, 242–243
negligence/malpractice
  breach in duty of care, 121
  damages, 122–123
  duty of care, 120–121
  proximate cause of injury, 121–122
Neuman's System Model, 82
new-to-practice nurses, 536, 537
nonempathetic communication behaviors, 189
non-experimental research, 303
nonmaleficence, 132
nonvalue added (NVA), 489
norming stage, team development, 232
novice nurses, 537

NPA. *See* nurse practice act
NPSG. *See* National Patient Safety Goals
nurse care coordinator, 517
nurse champion, 50, 550
nurse educator, 50
nurse managers, 48
Nurse Practice Act (NPA), 118–119, 146
nurse preceptor, 50
nurse residencies, 537–538
Nurse Residency Program, 537–539
Nurses on Boards Coalition (NOBC), 63
nurse's responsibilities, hospital-acquired infection prevention, 126–127
nurse-to-nurse aggression, 243–244
nursing bedside shift report (NBSR), 550
Nursing Brain, 163
Nursing Excellence, 28
nursing informatics, 517
  clinical judgment, 261
  definition, 258
  electronic health record, 262–267
  electronic medical record, 262
  health-related websites, 270–271
  information and analytical sciences, 258–259
  legislation needed, 267–270
  metastructure, 259–260
  technologies and information systems, 274–277
  technology initiatives, 271–274
  telehealth, 277–279
nursing knowledge, 228–229
nursing orientation, 535–536
nursing professional development (NPD) specialist, 52
nursing responsibilities, 149–150
nursing-sensitive indicators, 548–551
nursing student, 52
nursing surveillance, 43

objective data, 405–407
occupational hazards, 350
OCR. *See* Office for Civil Rights
Office for Civil Rights (OCR), 278
Office of the National Coordinator for Health Information Technology (ONC), 264
online e-patient communities, 205
open system, 81
operational definition, 406–408
  falls, 407–408
  hand hygiene guidelines, 407
organizational chain of command, 153–154
organizational leaders, quality improvement (QI), 390–391
organization, healthcare delivery, 89

organizations structure, hospital healthcare settings
community hospitals, 58
compliance process, 60
fee-for service model, 60
hierarchical organizational structures, 60
hospital organizational chart, 59
risk management, 61
strategic planning, 60
technological advances, 61
value-based purchasing (VBP), 60
orientation programs, 535–536
outcome data, 372
outcomes, 374
outcomes research, 303
outliers, 418
output, 81
overuse of healthcare services, 335

panel, 517
panel management, 517
Pareto chart, 413–415
participation, 180
paternalism, 133
paternalistic healthcare decisions, 179
patient acuity, 344
patient assignment sheet, 160–164
patient-centered care communication
culture and language influence, 189–190
empathetic communication, 188–189
interprofessional communication, 190–191
verbal and nonverbal communication, 187–188
Patient-Centered Medical Home (PCMH), 206–208
patient-centered medical home (PCMH) model, 517
Patient-Centered Primary Care Collaborative (PCPCC), 206
patient decision aids
implementation, 198
IPDAS collaboration, 197–198
knowledge to action framework, 198
websites, 199
patient-driven research (PDR), 203–204
patient information
authorized disclosure, 128
permitted usage, 127
patient journals, 203
patient navigator, 202–203
patient portals, 274
patient preferences, 306–307
Patient Protection and Affordable Care Act (PPACA), 178, 206, 504
patient safety
care delivery variation reduction, 337–339
disparity, safety outcomes, 344
and high-quality outcomes, 319–321
just culture of safety. *see* just culture of safety
national and international organizations, 340
person approach, 335–337
safety initiatives, 340–348
system approach, 335–337
utilization management (UM), 318
Patient Safety Indicators, 8
patient safety movement
adverse event, 14
culture, 14–15
financial penalties, 15
healthcare costs, 16–17
healthcare excellence, 17
improvement process, 14
medical errors, 13–14
PDR. *See* patient-driven research
PDSA. *See* Plan-Do-Study-Act
Pediatric Quality Indicators, 8
people-centered health services, 181
performing stage, team development, 232
personal representative, HIPAA, 128
person approach to safety, 335–337
person-centered care (PCC), 22, 565–567
advocacy, 186
barriers and resistance, 180
characteristics, 180–181
communication, 187–191
core concepts, 180
cultural competence, 185
customs and beliefs, 184, 185
definition, 178
discharge planning, 200–202
health literacy barriers, 192–193
history, 178–180
innovations to support, 203
legislative efforts, 205–206
Medicaid Health Homes Model, 208
nursing practice implications, 194
online e-patient communities, 205
organizational structures, 181–184
Patient-Centered Medical Home, 206–208
Patient-Centered Primary Care Collaborative, 206
patient decision aids, 197–199
patient-driven research, 203–204
patient journals, 203
patient navigator, 202–203
Patient Protection and Affordable Care Act, 206
patient satisfaction, 210, 211
Picker's principles, 182–183
QSEN competency, 179

quality improvement (QI), 209
resources, 210
shared decision-making, 195–197
social determinants of health, 199–201
strategies to support, 192
World Health Organization framework, 181
phrase searching, 294
physical therapist (PT), 152
Plan-Do-Study-Act (PDSA)
cycle, 456
model, 375–378
Planetree international's person-centered care hospital certification program elements, 211
planning phase, project management
budget, 484
communication, 484
risk management, 484
time schedule, 482–484
work breakdown structure (WBS), 482–484
pluralistic approach, 300
PM. *See* project management
point-of-care databases, 293
population-focused nursing competencies, 509–510
population health
definition, 500
emerging nursing roles, 511–517
evolution, 501–504
interprofessional team, 511
nursing model, 505
nursing practice, 504–506
patient-centered medical home (PCMH) model, 517
population-focused nursing competencies, 509–510
public health, 506–507
quality improvement (QI), 519–520
registered nurse roles, 512–516
Population Health Nursing Model, 505, 506
postintervention data, 372, 405
PPACA. *See* Patient Protection and Affordable Care Act
practice guidelines, 293
practice setting, 456
pre-appraised evidence, 301
preceptors, 540–541
preceptorship, 540
Preceptor Workshop Progra, 556
preference-sensitive care, 337
preintervention process mapping, 386
Press Ganey survey, 212, 213
prevalence data, 406
prevention levels, 506–507
Prevention Quality Indicators, 8
primary prevention, 507
process, 81, 374
process maps, 386
professional development plan, 554
professional role development
Benner's professional development model, 534–535
certification, 555
Institute For Healthcare Improvement, 546–548
The Joint Commission, 543–546
mentors, 541–542
national initiatives, 543
networking process, 555
nursing-sensitive indicators, 548–551
preceptors, 540–541
professional development plan, 554
quality and safety-framed nursing orientation programs, 551–554
regulatory agencies, 543
project management (PM)
benefits and limitations, 491
closing phase, 488
definition, 475
executing phase, 485–486
five-step methodology (5S), 486
initiating phase, 478–480
leadership and management skill, 490–491
Lean method, 486
monitoring and controlling, 487
planning phase, 480–484
Six Sigma, 486
systematic phases, 476, 478
systematic steps, 488–490
projects, 475
Promoting Action on Research Implementation in Health Services (PARIHS) framework, 305
prospective study, 303
psychological safety, 331
public health, 506–507
PubMed, 292
punitive damages, 122–123

qualitative data, 405
qualitative research, 303
quality and safety
adverse event, 6
cost of achieving, 16–17
drivers, 6–7
errors, 6
global advances, 11–12
initiatives, 5
levels, 5–6
national organizations, 7–9
nurse education, 18
nurse leaders, 28–30

quality and safety (*cont.*)
nurses' role in, 27–30
patient safety movement, 13–17
QSEN competencies, 18–26
sentinel event, 6
sharp end, 6
STEEEP, 5
Quality and Safety Education for nurse (QSEN) competencies
accreditation and evaluation, 30–31
evidence-based practice, 24
faculty development and sustainability, 19
informatics, 26
Knowledge, Skills, and Attitudes (KSA), 19–20
patient-centered care, 22
purpose, 18
quality improvement, 25
safety competency, 25, 26
teamwork and collaboration, 23
quality and safety-framed nursing orientation programs
newly hired RN participants, 552–554
QSEN competencies, 551
quality errors, 6
quality improvement (QI), 25, 404, 571–572
academic barriers, 391–392
auditing, 389–390
care delivery aims, 363
clinical judgment, 364
data, 404–405
data collection, 408–409
data display, 410–414
definition, 362, 475
descriptive statistics, 409–410
Donabedian's model, 374–378
evidence-based practice, 371–374
flow map, 426, 428–429
formal projects, 363
Gantt chart, 426
history and evolution, 366–370
internal auditing, 391
knowledge, skills, and attitudes (KSAs), 364
leadership support, 390–391
Lean methodologies, 378–380
nurse QI attitude survey, 391
nurse role, 388–389
in nursing, 370–371
objective data, 405–407
organizations with healthcare quality, 363
performance measurement, 372–373
population health, 519–520
QSEN competencies, 392
retroactive approach, 382–387
risks and failures, 378
shared governance, 391
Six Sigma, 380–381
standards, 363
statistical process control, 414–424
triggers, 363
Quality Indicators, 8
quantitative data, 405
quantitative research, 303

RACI Matrix, 53
radio frequency identification (RFID), 275–276
randomized controlled trial (RCT), 303
range, 410
rapid response team (RRT), 230
RCA. *See* root cause analysis
Reach, Effectiveness, Adoption, Implementation, and Maintenance (RE-AIM) framework, 449, 450, 452–454
regional health information organizations (RHIOs), 267
registered nurse (RN)
clinical preceptors, 535
population health, 512–516
regulatory agencies, 543
relativism, 133
religious beliefs, 185
research terminology, 303
respect, 180
RFID. *See* radio frequency identification
RHIOs. *See* regional health information organizations
risk adjustment, 325
risk-based-thinking, 384
risk management, 337, 484
root cause analysis (RCA), 97, 230
causal statements and recommended changes, 384, 385
cause-effect diagram, 384
corrective action, 382
flowchart creation, 383, 384
Healthcare Failure Mode and Effect Analysis, 384–386
medication administration error, 336
risk-based-thinking, 384
stages, 382
Roy's Adaptation Model, 82
run chart
advantage, 420
benefits, 418
clinical judgment, 420
pain reassessment compliance, 416, 417
prioritization, 419
QI intervention, 419
time-series format, 416

safe patient handling, 349–351
SAFER. *See* Safety Assurance Factors for EHR Resilience

Safe, Timely, Efficient, Equitable, Effective, Patient-centered (STEEEP), 5
safety, 319, 572–573
Safety Assurance Factors for EHR Resilience (SAFER), 264
safety huddles, 236
safety initiatives, 318
  avoidance of workplace violence, 341–342
  environmental safety, 348
  hand hygiene, 346–347
  healthcare ranking and information sources, 343–344
  high-alert medications, 340
  nurses with impairing conditions, 346
  safe nurse staffing, 344–346
  sampling, 340, 341
  suicide prevention, 347–348
Safety Management System, 82–83
safety science, 18
scatter plot diagrams, 413, 414
Scope of Nursing Practice Decision-Making Framework, 156–157
SDOH. *See* Social Determinants of Health
secondary prevention, 507
security, 268
self-concept, 192
sentinel event, 6
separation of powers, 115
servant leadership, 48
SHARE approach, 53, 54
shared decision-making, 44, 195–197, 306–307
  activities, 197
  collaborative process, 195
  nursing practice, 197
  three-talk model, 195, 196
shared governance, 63, 391
sharp end, 6
Shewhart control chart
  control limits, 421
  data display formats, 421
  medication errors, 422
  PDSA cycle, 422–423
  software, 421
Sigma Theta Tau International, 65
simple system, 81
simplification of work processes, 338
situational awareness, 233, 320
Situation, Background, Assessment, and Recommendation (SBAR), 234, 235
Six Sigma, 380–381, 486
smart healthcare devices, 276
Social Determinants of Health (SDOH), 199–200, 501–503
  definition, 199
  resources, 201
  team-based approach, 200
socially distanced nurse leaders and managers, 66
social science, 259
Social Security Act, 367
SPC. *See* statistical process control
special cause variation, 416
SQUIRE Guidelines. *See* Standards for Quality Improvement Reporting Excellence Guidelines
stakeholder engagement, 485
stakeholders, 478
standard deviation (SD), 410
standardization of simplified work processes, 338, 339
Standards for Quality Improvement Reporting Excellence (SQUIRE) Guidelines, 388–389
Stark Law, 129
State Nurse Practice Acts, 145–146
statistical process control (SPC), 404
  common cause variation, 416
  Pareto chart, 414–415
  PDSA cycle, 422–423
  run chart, 416–420
  Shewhart control chart, 421–423
  special cause variation, 416
  stratification, 423–424
  tardiness, 415
statute, 115
statutory law, 118
storming stage, team development, 232
strategic skills, 490
stratification, 423–424
Strengths, Weaknesses, Opportunities, and Threats (SWOT) analysis, 484
structure, 374
STS. *See* Systems Thinking Scale
subject heading, 294
subjective data, 405
suicide prevention, 347–348
supervision, 148–149
Survey Analysis for Evaluating Risk (SAFER) Matrix, 369
survey readiness, 389
sympathy, 188
system, 80–82
system approach to safety, 335–337
systematic review (SR), 303
Systems Addressing Frail Elders (SAFE) Care Model, 511
systems science, 82
Systems Theory, 45, 82–83
systems thinker
  causal loop diagrams, 97, 99
  concept mapping, 97, 100–102
  habits of mind, 99
  iceberg model challenge, 101, 102
  root cause analysis, 97

systems thinking, 18
clinical judgment, 95
clinical practice, 91
continuum, 86
definition, 80, 83
fostering organizations, 92
four-step model, 86, 87
global perspective, 83
historical development, 89–91
hospital-acquired infections, 94
leadership, 101–103
medication administration, 93
nursing practice, 86–87
origins, 88–89
patient length of stay, 95
pattern recognization, 84
quality and safety processes, 92–95
reflection, 84
self-assessment, 96
system, 80–82
systems theory, 82–83
systems thinker strategies, 97–101
willingness to change, 84–85
Systems Thinking Scale (STS), 96

team-based approach, SDOH, 200
team coordinated care, 230–231
team development, 232
Team*STEPPS*
phases, 234
SBAR, 234, 235
teamwork
and collaboration, 567–569
just culture of safety, 331–333
telehealth, 277–279
Telemedicine IMPACT Plus (TIP) Model, 511
tertiary prevention, 507
The Joint Commission (TJC), 9, 12, 80, 83, 236, 367–368, 543–546
international patient safety goals, 12
The Joint Commission on Accreditation of Healthcare Organizations (JCAHO), 367
Theory X and Theory Y, 44
Three-Talk Model of Shared Decision Making, 195–196
TJC. *See* The Joint Commission
total systems approach, 90
Toyota's production systems, 82
tracer methodology, 368
trait leadership, 46
transactional leadership, 46
transformation, 84
transformational leadership, 46, 48
transition to practice programs
leadership roles, 555–556
nurse residencies, 537–538
nursing orientation, 535–536
Triple Aim, 504
truncation, 297, 298
two-challenge rule, 235

underuse of healthcare services, 335
unit-based nurse manager, 51, 55
unit-based orientation programs, 535–536
unit charge nurse, 50
United States Department of Health and Human Services (USDHHS), 209
United States (U.S.) healthcare system, 4
global perspective, 11–12
surgeries and complications, 16
unlicensed assistive personnel (UAP), 145–147
assignment, 147
competency checklists, 158
responsibilities, 150
upper control limit (UCL), 421
upstream factors, 505
U.S. Department of Health and Human Services (HHS), 116
agencies and functions, 117
U.S. federal government. *See also* legal and ethical aspects
administrative agencies, 116
criminal law and civil law, 117–118
executive branch, 115
judicial branch, 115–116
legislative branch, 115
utilitarianism, 134
utilization management (UM), 318, 323–335

value-based purchasing (VBP), 60
Vancouver 3M Clinical Pathway, 199
variability, 410
VBP. *See* value-based purchasing
verbal and nonverbal communication, 187–188
Voice of the Customer, 387
voltage drop, 455

whistleblower claim, 130
wildcards, 297, 298
work-arounds, 328, 329
work breakdown structure (WBS), 482–484
workforce bullying, 342
workplace violence
avoidance of, 341–342
types, 342
3Ws Method of Communication, 332